BIOMEDICAL ENGINEERING – FROM THEORY TO APPLICATIONS

Edited by **Reza Fazel-Rezai**

INTECHWEB.ORG

Biomedical Engineering – From Theory to Applications
Edited by Reza Fazel-Rezai

Published by InTech
Janeza Trdine 9, 51000 Rijeka, Croatia

Edition 2014

Publishing Process Manager Davor Vidic

Technical Editor Teodora Smiljanic

Cover Designer InTech Design Team

Image Copyright Leigh Prather, 2010. Used under license from Shutterstock.com

Additional hard copies can be obtained from orders@intechopen.com

Biomedical Engineering – From Theory to Applications, Edited by Reza Fazel-Rezai
p. cm.
ISBN 978-953-307-637-9

INTECH

open science | open minds

Contents

Preface

There have been different definitions for Biomedical Engineering. One of them is the application of engineering disciplines, technology, principles, and design concepts to medicine and biology. As this definition implies, biomedical engineering helps closing the gap between"engineering" and "medicine".

There are many different disciplines in engineering field such as aerospace, chemical, civil, computer, electrical, genetic, geological, industrial, mechanical. On the other hand, in the medical field, there are several fields of study such as anesthesiology, cardiology, dermatology, emergency medicine, gastroenterology, orthopedics, neuroscience, pathology, pediatrics, psychiatry, radiology, and surgery. Biomedical engineering can be considered as a bridge connecting field(s) in engineering to field(s) in medicine. Creating such a bridge requires understanding and major cross - disciplinary efforts by engineers, researchers, and physicians at health institutions, research institutes, and industry sectors. Depending on where this connection has happened, different areas of research in biomedical engineering have been shaped.

In all different areas in biomedical engineering, the ultimate objectives in research and education are to improve the quality life, reduce the impact of disease on the everyday life of individuals, and provide an appropriate infrastructure to promote and enhance the interaction of biomedical engineering researchers. In general, biomedical engineering has several disciplines including, but not limited to, bioinstrumentation, biostatistics, and biomaterial, biomechanics, biosignal, biosystem, biotransportation, clinical, tissue, rehabilitation and cellular engineering. Experts in biomedical engineering, a young area for research and education, are working in various industry and government sectors, hospitals, research institutions, and academia. The U.S. Department of Labor estimates that the job market for biomedical engineering will increase by 72%, faster than the average of all occupations in engineering. Therefore, there is a need to extend the research in this area and train biomedical engineers of tomorrow.

This book is prepared in two volumes to introduce a recent advances in different areas of biomedical engineering such as biomaterials, cellular engineering, biomedical devices, nanotechnology, and biomechanics. Different chapters in both volumes are stand-alone and readers can start from any chapter that they are interested in. It is hoped that this book brings more awareness about the biomedical engineering field and helps in completing or establishing new research areas in biomedical engineering.

As the editor, I would like to thank all the authors of different chapters. Without your contributions, it would not be possible to have a quality book and help in the growth of biomedical engineering.

Dr. Reza Fazel-Rezai
University of North Dakota
Grand Forks, ND,
USA

1

Biomedical Web, Collections and Meta-Analysis Literature Applications

Layla Michán, Israel Muñoz-Velasco,
Eduardo Alvarez and Lyssania Macías
Universidad Nacional Autónoma de México, Facultad de Ciencias
México

1. Introduction

Cause and effect of the digital revolution is the production of a lot and different kinds of web tools, applications and resources that permit optimization the retrieve, management and analysis of biomedical bibliography. The information revolution is a cause and effect of scientific and technological progress of the twentieth century, amount of information that is now produced on different scientific topics is huge plus: It can be electronic or printed, there is text, images and sounds is systematized in databases data, catalogs or lists, your query can be free or restricted, is on life or their parts, phenomena and explanations, cover publications, researchers, projects, groups and research lines, agreements, grants, scientific, institutions research and teaching, biological collections, educational institutions and societies science, to name a few. Refer to information in the twenty-first century involves the mention of terms, methods, novel and innovative theories as knowledge society, information society, globalization, info diversity, access to information, e-science, e-research, grid, collaboratories, repositories, knowledge based on literature, text mining, semantic web, impact index, cocitation, web 2.0 and 3.0, social networking, plagiarism, and free access. Those changes have been dramatically impacted the contemporary world view, scientific practice and scientific relations, social, economic, political and cultural (Russell, 2001).

Scientific society generates and receives information, it is exposed to it as a representation of thought and knowledge in all cases creates a conscious or unconscious interest transmits individually or collectively. The scientific communities recognize the value of the information, required it as a condition to perform fundamental research. Published information on biology and medicine is not exception, the quantity, diversity and complexity of digital information are so many and so different, some electronic resources through which you can access it are not simple, which has made it necessary to be informed and update on the continuing emergence and modification of these tools, while it has become a problem to solve: continuously published magazines in a large number of items. Recover strategies and analysis of information on the specific area of interest of researchers and design programs and websites constantly to achieve this (Larson, 2010a).

Electronic resources with biomedical literature can be consulted electronically Internet allows instant access to digital data collections updated with information generated by the specialists (Faciola, 2009). The power of the new electronic technologies has increased exponential, we have designed a lot of applications that allow you to group, sort and display documents which have reduced power, cost and time required to analyze literature specialized (Hey & Trefethen, 2005). Not only that, in less than ten years has changed the practice of science, is no longer explores the reality only through experiments and models *in vivo* and / or *in vitro* but made *in silico* tools and computational methods (Atkins *et al.*, 2003). This phenomenon has affected both the way we produce scientific knowledge that have developed new fields of knowledge practiced by specialists, such as bioinformatics, medical informatics, biological informatics, neuroinformatics, and literature-based discovery, among others. The change has been important even in the way recovered and analyzed the literature so much that you have proposed new ways to access the information to put aside the reductionist approach and adopt a system according to the progress of own biological discipline.

The search, access, analysis and updating of the literature in databases has become a daily task. It is usually necessary to consult several indexes to have more complete representation of the literature on the topic of interest (Zhou *et al.*, 2006). But such is the quantity and diversity of papers on biomedicine, there are so many, so different and complex electronic resources (especially bibliographic databases) through which you can access that information, not just that, but change, progress and constantly updated, it is difficult to keep track of them all and identify which and how many can and should use.

2. Biomedical web

The Biomedical Science is one of the most innovative and cutting-edge in science, excellence and is recognized today. The literature in this field is applied in several biomedical practice areas, ranging from the production of new biological knowledge to resource management, assessment, management and science policy (Labarga, 2009). For these reasons essential to include an innovative course in art, sort and classify all electronic resources for the recovery and analysis of specialized information effectively and efficiently, in a review of the types and characteristics of digital information, explaining definitions basic, to explore its importance and implications, are synthesized and explain the electronic resources online more relevant and practical, especially databases and specialized software, are presented source's compendiums from which information can be extracted and understanding (Rizkallah & Sin, 2010; Weeber *et al.*, 2005; Henderson, 2005) like scientometrics studies (Cokol & Rodriguez-Esteban, 2008; Uthman, 2008; Li *et al.*, 2009; Boyack, 2004).

Also allow stakeholders to introduce the necessary tools to make reports to information and documents indexed journals, impact, collaboration and citation of own production commonly requested by the evaluation committees of National Foundations and councils.

This chapter presents the application of an interdisciplinary and integrative approach to use biomedical literature to extract, analyze and manage specialized literature efficient, prompt, timely, comprehensive and organized.

Contrary to common understanding now exist a lot of friendly electronic tools for non informatics specialist's that permit literature Biomedicine management, designed from informatics specialist's to all others. Previous knowledge it's not needed to use this web tools and services (Hull, *et al.*, 2008; Renear, & Palmer, 2009). Most of them are open access resources. Some of their advantages are:

1. Explain in detail the cyberinfrastructure (resources, tools and services) available for the management of literature specializes in biomedicine, keeping with the needs and challenges of our time and explains the characteristics of each, Biomedicine.
2. Present the stages of document retrieval electronics and how to handle this is done in an efficient, effective and updated.
3. State the main bibliometric indicators are frequently used to evaluate literature.
4. Apply new techniques to analyze the references, the contents of scientific papers and large quantities of documents simultaneously, including network analysis and discovery based on the literature.

In this chapter we will classify, systematize and describe the most useful web-based applications for innovative retrieval and processing of biomedical literature; all of them are friendly and can be used by any scholar or biomedical specialist. We will present all resources in three categories: 1) general web applications, 2) literature collections and 3) meta-analysis tools in logic retrieval and processing literature order (Fig. 1).

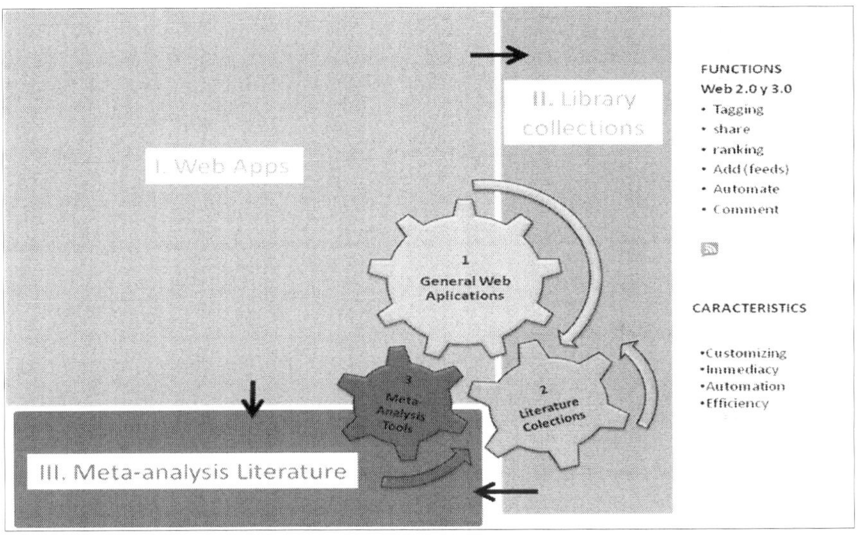

Fig. 1. The resource's classification for retrieval biomedical information.

2.1 Web literature retrieval

Digital information retrieval from the Web, in a modern sense is a personalized, automatic, multitask, integrated and immediacy process (Larson, 2010b) the stages of document retrieval electronics and how to handle this is done in an efficient, effective and updated form with specific apps. The process consists of: search (browser, search engines and collections), bookmark (Bookmarks), manage (reference management) share and analyze (Meta-analysis apps).

Every day a lot of innovative web apps appeared with Biomedical scholar interest like web pages, wikis, blogs and search engines (web 2.0 and web 3.0), social networks, feeds, reference management software and mobile resources, the most relevant for biomedicine.

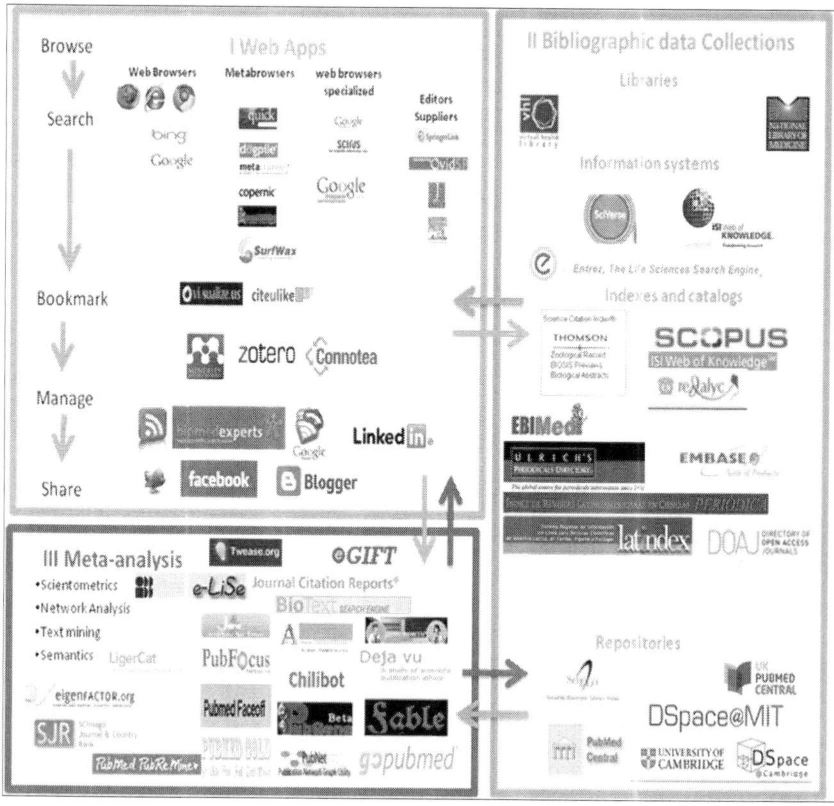

Fig. 2. Process for retrieval information.

The process for retrieve literature on the web begins with the web browser, the Merriam-Webster's dictionary (2011) defines a web browser as a computer program used for accessing sites or information on a network (as the World Wide Web). This is a simple, yet accurate description. Web browsers come in many different styles, each with their own nuances. However, the main reason a person utilizes a web browser is to view web pages on the Internet, similar to the way you are viewing this book right now. Today there are the two main open source web browsers with add-on options (something as an accessory or added feature that enhances the thing it is added to) that the search experience, Firefox from Mozilla (http://www.mozilla.com/en-US/firefox/) and Chrome from Google (http://www.google.com/Chrome) (Fig. 3), right now our favorite is the second one, because is easy and speed, but right now the first one has the most bigger gallery of complement options.

There are a lot of resources, tools and services available for the management of literature Biology specializes in keeping with the needs and challenges of our time, the most efficient could be installed in the browser for better and faster use.

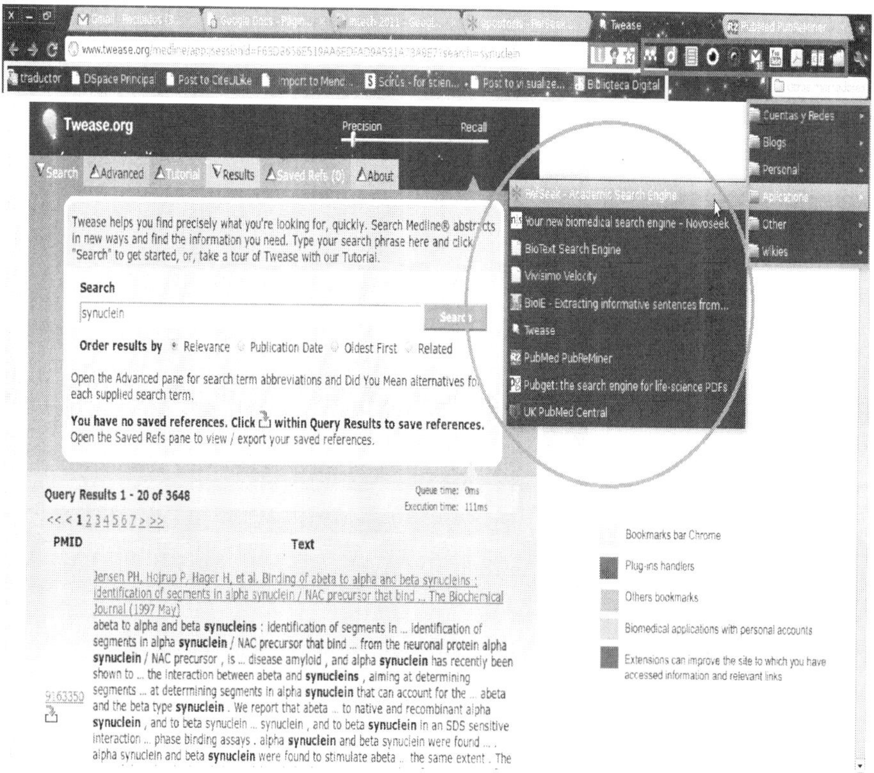

Fig. 3. Chrome personalized browser for biomedical literature retrieval.

2.1.1 Search engines and meta-searchers

There are thousands of search engines in the Internet, a program that searches documents for specified keywords and returns a list of the documents where the keywords were found. They create a web pages database that use any algorithm to classify the web pages (wikis, blogs, sites, …), the most biggest and also the most used for general research are Google, Bing, Yahoo, Altavista, Lycos, and Ask. But there are some scholar biomedical search engines that filter and index specialized and certified web pages like Scirus, Scientific WebPlus, Orefil, Nextbio or Quertle (Table 1).

Biomedical search engine	Total records	URL
Scientific WebPlus	Is an open Web search engine created by Thomson Reuters that harnesses the power of our editorial expertise, controlled vocabularies, and proprietary relevancy algorithms. It is designed to complement your search results, bringing the most relevant Web resources to the forefront for the professional researcher. WebPlus allows you to search the Web by Topic, Person/Author, Source, Institution, Organism, Drug, and Gene. Displays the 250 most important results, was help of windows live search.	http://scientific.thomsonwebplus.com/BasicSearch.aspx
Scirus	Covers over 410 million science-related Web pages.	http://www.scirus.com/
Orefil	OReFiL uses DBCLS's (Database Center for Life Science). Whatever the query, which displays the maximum score is 1,000 to 10,000 results.	http://orefil.dbcls.jp/
Nextbio	NextBio indexes over 19 million abstracts from PubMed and over 130,000 full-text publications from PubMed Central. For its literature search, NextBio uses a number of heuristics, including: 1. Extensive ontology with relationships between terms, synonyms, as well as a term hierarchy 2. A customized domain-specific stop word list and analyzer that emphasizes ontology terms 3. The authority of the journal where the paper was published 4. Publication date	http://www.nextbio.com/b/nextbio.nb
Quertle	Creating its own database of about 250 million of relationships.	http://www.quertle.info/v2/

Table 1. The Most popular scientific search engines. General search, retrieval from 16 February 2011, *Papers published in journals

2.2 Biomedical collections

Computing tool of choice for systematizing the documents and metadata are the databases, a computerized bibliographic records stored in tables with an established order that allows you to save, sort, retrieve and generate information. We will divide the main biomedical literature collections in five kinds: 1) Libraries, 2) Information systems, 3) Index and catalogs, 4) Bookstores or editorials (press) and 5) Repositories. We classified a sample of each one.

Literature Collection	Example	URL
e-Library	MedLine	http://www.nlm.nih.gov/databases /databases_medline.html
Information system	Entrez	http://www.ncbi.nlm.nih.gov/sites/gquery
Paper index o catalog, Journal index o catalog	PubMed Journals NCBI	http://www.ncbi.nlm.nih.gov/nlmcatalog/journals
Press	Biomed Central	http://www.biomedcentral.com/
Repository	PubMed central	http://www.ncbi.nlm.nih.gov/pmc/

Table 2. Kinds of biomedical collections

A digital library (e-Library) comprises digital collections, services and infrastructure to support lifelong learning, research, scholarly communication and preservation and conservation of our knowledge recorded and democratization, has a clear goal and are formed with a selection of content organized through a descriptive metadata (cataloging) and also associated with some facilities for search and use of services (Borgman, 1999), makes use of telecommunications and particularly the Internet to facilitate access to its contents remotely or locally through various connected systems that provide control and preservation of resources, while providing added services around the needs of users and information collected managed and preserved.

If a Web application allows you to consult more than one library collection simultaneously, we have named the information system (Villanova-Oliver *et al.*, 2003). We define all information collection systematized into a digital database with immediate access, designed with the intention of making them available for those interested in his consultation with academic and made available through the Web.

We define also a library collections or literature as all those documents that record information about scientific research product is the result of a process of planning and balanced acquisition of library materials in various formats, mainly primary literature consists of books, magazines and conference proceedings, online resources, and other media, bibliographies, references, stored, structured and inter-linked for retrieval using a computer system.

Press is the process of production and dissemination of literature or information, the activity of making information available for public view. In some cases, authors may be their own publishers, meaning: originators and developers of content also provide media to deliver and display the content. Traditionally, the term refers to the distribution of printed works such as books (the "book trade") and newspapers. With the advent of digital information systems and the Internet, the scope of publishing has expanded to include electronic resources, such as the electronic versions of books and periodicals, as well as micropublishing, websites, blogs and video games.

There is necessary for a better information retrieval to know the main characteristics of the datasets for search like temporal coverage, geographic coverage, topic coverage, size coverage and typological coverage. For better understand we present a key card with the dissection of PubMed the most used bibliographic biomedical database (Table 3).

CHARACTERISTICS	DESCRIPTION
Name	PubMed
Editor/Producer	National Center for Biotechnology Information, U.S. National Library of Medicine.
Access	Free
Language	English
Typological coverage	Scientific articles, online books, case reports, clinical conferences, clinical trials, comparative studies, conferences, commentaries, dictionaries, directories, editorials, evaluation studies, government publications, historical articles, interactive tutorials, interviews, letters, newspaper articles, revisions, retractions of publications, technical reports, twin studies, web-cast. Is accompanied by other resources contained in other databases under the responsibility of NCBI as sequences of genes and proteins, and analysis.
Subject coverage	Biomedical and life sciences. As well as dentistry, nursing, veterinary, pharmaceutical, and other related.
Temporal coverage	1951
Start date	1997
Geographical coverage	"World" (70 countries)
Language of documents	Usually in English. Also French, German, Italian, Japanese, Russian, Spanish, Albanian, Catalan, Korean, Polish, Portuguese, Romanian, Serbian, Slovenian, Turkish, and Vietnamese among others.
Thesaurus	Yes, through MeSH.
Total records	Journals: 23,000. Records: 20 million.
Update	Every 2 days
Number of records displayed per page	5, 10, 20, 50, 100 y 200
Access full text	Yes, when the document is freely available, is in PubMed Central, or have the relevant subscription to the journal.
Search fields	Title, abstract, author, book, corporate author, creation date, number EC / RN, editor, filter, first author, author's full name, full name of investigator, ISBN, issue, volume, journal, language , last author, ID, location, name of substances.
Save the query	If you have a My NCBI account.
Advanced search	Affiliation [AD] Article Identifier [AID] All Fields [ALL]

	Author [AU] Book [book] Comment Corrections Corporate Author [CN] Create Date [CRDT] EC/RN Number [RN] Editor [ED] Entrez Date [EDAT] Filter [FILTER] First Author Name [1AU] Full Author Name [FAU] Full Investigator Name [FIR] Grant Number [GR] Investigator [IR] ISBN [ISBN] Issue [IP] Journal Title [TA] Language [LA] Last Author [LASTAU] Location ID [LID] MeSH Date [MHDA] MeSH Major Topic [MAJR] MeSH Subheadings [SH] MeSH Terms [MH] NLM Unique ID [JID] Other Term [OT] Owner Pagination [PG] Personal Name as Subject [PS] Pharmacological Action MeSH Terms [PA] Place of Publication [PL] PMCID & MID Publication Date [DP] Publication Type [PT] Secondary Source ID [SI] Subset [SB] Substance Name [NM] Text Words [TW] Title [TI] Title/Abstract [TIAB] Transliterated Title [TT] UID [PMID] Volume [VI]
Export records	Yes, via e-mail and bibliography managers EndNote, Reference Manager, and ProCite.
Citation analysis	No.
List of journal indexed	Yes, by downloading a file.

Displayed documents references	No
Links to full text electronic document	Yes
Search by keyword	No
Abstract	Yes
Interface language	English
URL	http://www.ncbi.nlm.nih.gov/pubmed
Related document	Yes
Web 2.0 apps	RSS, bookmarks, alerts, saved search results by e-mail.
Document selection criteria	Is based on the magazine Coverage: Articles mainly on basic biomedical research. Quality: validity, relevance, originality and contribution to the field coverage of content. Editorial quality, objectivity, credibility and quality of its contents, peer review, ethical quality, timely correction of errors. Production Quality: Design, printing, graphics and illustrations (but not pre-requisite) Audience: health professions: researchers, practitioners, educators, administrators and students. Content type: Reports of original research, original clinical observations accompanied by analysis and discussion, analysis of philosophical, ethical, social or health professions or biomedical sciences, critical commentaries, statistical compilations, descriptions of evaluation methods or procedures, case reports with discussions. Language: At least title and abstract in English. Geographic coverage: Generally not be selected for indexing if the contents are subjects already well represented in MEDLINE or published to a local audience.
Records meta-analysis*	No
Tools	My NCBI. Save searches, results, bibliography, and has an automatic update option. My NCBI preferences. Storage, highlight search terms, abstract screen, additional data. Furthermore, filtering of search results, view recent activity and the establishment of Link Out, document delivery service.
Advantages	Database more important, most used, most popular in biomedical information. Very short time to upgrade. It is complemented with other resources and information bases by the NCBI. Using multiple and varied fields of search.
Disadvantages	Few or no options for meta-analysis. Ambiguity in the identification of authors and documents.

Table 3. Characteristics of PubMed database. *Meta-analysis details are explained below.

Index and catalog. Although the biomedical community uses mainly PubMed database for literature retrieval, there are a lot of restricted/open, regional/global and monothematic/multithematic collections that are important to obtain an exhaustive review of the publisher papers. There are more useful catalogs: with documents and journals (Table 4).

Collection	Temporal coverage	Geographic coverage	Topic coverage	Total records
Web of Science http://apps.isiknowledge.com/WOS_GeneralSearch_input.do?highlighted_tab=WOS&product=WOS&last_prod=WOS&search_mode=GeneralSearch&SID=1CpkLf29P65GF7GiHI9	1899	Global	Scholarly literature in the sciences, social sciences, arts, and humanities; examined proceedings of international conferences, symposia, seminars, colloquia, workshops, and convention. Original research articles, reviews, editorials, chronologies, abstracts, and more.	Over 40 million records
Scopus http://www.scopus.com/home.url	20.5 millions of records previous 1996 which go back as far as 1823.	Global	Scopus covers the following subject areas: Life Sciences, Health Sciences, Social Sciences and Physical Sciences. Through international publishers, conference proceedings, trade publications, book series and patents.	More than 42.5 million records
Biological Abstracts http://apps.isiknowledge.com/BIOABS_GeneralSearch_input.do?highlighted_tab=BIOABS&product=BIOABS&last_prod=BIOABS&SID=1CpkLf29P65GF7GiHI9&search_mode=GeneralSearch	1926	Global	Citations, meetings, conferences, references to review articles, patents, reviews and references for books, CD-ROMs and other life sciences media. */RRM® (Reports, Reviews, Meetings)*	More than 11.3 million records.
PubMed http://www.ncbi.nlm.nih.gov/pubmed/	1950	Global emphasis on research in the U.S.	Books, electronic journals, scientific articles, brochures and web pages	20,603,313

Bireme http://regional.bvsalud.org/php/index.php?lang=en	1967	Latin America and Caribbean, Portugal and Spain	Systematic Reviews, Clinical Trials, Evidence Summaries, Economic Evaluations in Health, Health Technology Assessments, Clinical Practice Guidelines	19,643,741 of records 1,749,767 full text
Embase http://www.embase.com/info/	1988	Global	Agriculture & Food Sciences, Bioengineering & Biotechnology, Clinical Medicine, Computer Science & Technology, Dentistry, Earth & Environmental Sciences, Enginery, Evidence-Based Medicine, Geology, Life Sciences, Neurology & Neurosciences, Nursing & Allied Health, Pharmacy & Pharmacology Philosophy & Religion, Physics, Psychology & Psychiatry, Social Sciences & the Humanities, Technical Sciences, Veterinary Medicine, Zoology	Over 100 bibliographic and full-text databases

Table 4. The most popular databases for biomedical literature (Date of access: March 2011).

The Merriam Webster dictionary (2011) defines a repository as one that contains or stores something nonmaterial<considered the book a *repository* of knowledge>. Repositories of literature are understood as large files that store digital texts composed of a group of services designed to capture, store, manage, preserve and redistribute the documentation to a certain audience or a specific user community (Pappalardo and Fitzegerald, 2007). Emerged from the so-called e-print community, concerned to maximize the spread and impact of scientific works deposited in them (Melero, 2005). An e-print (e-paper) is the digital version of a research paper (usually a journal article, but could be a thesis, papers, book chapters, or book) is available online because it has been deposited in a digital repository (Swan and Brown, 2005), which comprises five components essential to its operation: interactivity, design, integration, aggregation and mobility. Digital versions of research papers called e-prints include both pre-prints (articles before they are evaluated by peers) and post-prints (version result of peer review).

Repositories whose main function the storage of files and their creation is linked with the movement of information from open access (open access), a term that describes the online public access without restriction to scientific articles (Suber et al., 2010), has two forms: free and open. Repositories are dynamic tools, consisting of the infrastructure, programs, personal information and keeping it and consultation. They constantly recorded and scholars put their scientific production, as are the basic units of construction of the global scholarly communication, and therefore of scientific collaboration (Table 5).

Repository	Kind	Total Records
PubMed Central http://www.ncbi.nlm.nih.gov/pmc/	National	2 million articles
PubMed UK http://ukpmc.ac.uk/	National	1.8 million full text, peer reviewed published journal articles covering all fields of biomedical and health research (the UK PubMed Central repository) 24 million PubMed and PubMed Central abstracts
Dspace MIT http://dspace.mit.edu/	Institutional	47,133 titles 2,500 scholar articles 25,000 theses completed

Table 5. The biggest repositories

2.3 Automatic meta-analysis apps

We will present in meta-analysis topic around five dozens of web applications that process thousands of bibliographic records simultaneously, automatic and instantaneous for patterns identification, visualization or better retrieval goals. Apply new techniques of analysis of the references and the contents of scientific papers to analyze large quantities of documents simultaneously, including bibliometrics, text mining, semantic or networks analysis (Table 6).

Method	Description
Bibliometrics	Bibliometrics involves the quantitative assessment of certain events in the literature and therefore scientific literatures, main bibliometric indicators (publication counts, impact factors and received citations, for example) are frequently used to retrieve and evaluate literature (Koskinen *et al.*, 2008). In this way the bibliometric analysis is a good tool to assess the impact of an investigation in the context of others scientific investigations and it's possible compares the relative contributions of research groups or institutions, infer patterns and trends (Rosas *et al.*, 2011).
Text mining	Text mining involves the processes of information retrieval, automated information extraction and data mining from electronically published sources. It is used to generate new knowledge interesting, plausible, and intelligible (Ananiadou *et al.*, 2006). Linking two or more literature concepts that have so far not been linked (i.e., disjoint) through the use of software and algorithms designed for this purpose (Rodriguez-Esteban, 2009).

	To perform text mining, it must be structured (pre-processing) to analyze texts or discovering interesting patterns that generate new knowledge (Krallinger *et al.*, 2008). Depending on the methods used in the pre-processing is the type of representation of the contents of the texts constructed, and according to this representation, is the kind of patterns discovered (Harmston *et al.*, 2010).
Semantic	Based on the ontologies, that formulate a conceptual scheme (a map of concepts and their relationships) in a given domain, the semantic expresses the meaning of data, the properties of objects and the complex relationships between them by a series of formal rules (Robu *et al.*, 2006).
Networks analysis	Networks are open structures that can expand without limit of integration of new nodes based on the communication possibilities that exist in your environment and share communications code compatible. It is done through the study of theories of structural behavior, the dynamics, and influence within the biomedical issues, to establish a likely explanation for the growth and evolution of real networks in any advanced biomedical subject.

Table 6. Most frequent literature automatic meta-analysis methods.

Right now exist dozens of scholar free web programs that process literature with one or more bibliographic meta-analysis methods. Most of those resources are based on PubMed literature because it is open access records, normalized and robustness information. For this chapter we choose some of them for details, a list with most of them is in Append.

2.3.1 Bibliometric analysis

HubMed

HubMed: pubmed rewired

HubMed (http://www.hubmed.org/) retrieval information from the PubMed´s database and produces one interface focused basically on browsing, organizing and gathering information from the biomedical literature. Shows the results arranged by relevance, you can perform grouping and graphic representation of related articles, can export metadata in different formats for further analysis.

Twease

Twease.org

Twease is a web-based tool to search in the abstracts for Medline. Index the words of Medline and provides features to expand a query and thereby find what you are looking for. Finally, Twease can automatically discover common abbreviations for search phrases.

(http://twease.org/medline/app;jsessionid=2ACC96312364DDB1E50519CE8EC316BB?component=clearSettingsDirectLink&page=Home&service=direct&session=T)

2.3.2 Text-mining

PubReMiner

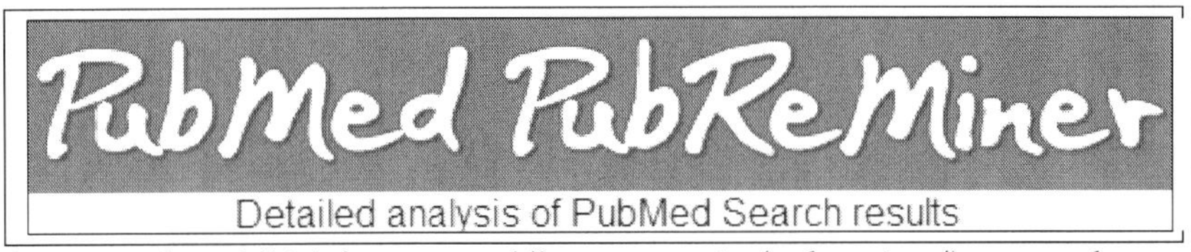
PubMed PubReMiner
Detailed analysis of PubMed Search results

PubReMiner (http://bioinfo.amc.uva.nl/human-genetics/pubreminer/) process the results of a query based in PubMed´s database and display its results in frequency tables, get all abstracts and generate metric statistics that include journals, authors and most productive countries, analyze your query words in the title, abstract, keywords and name of substances, allows extract metadata for further metric analysis.

LitMiner

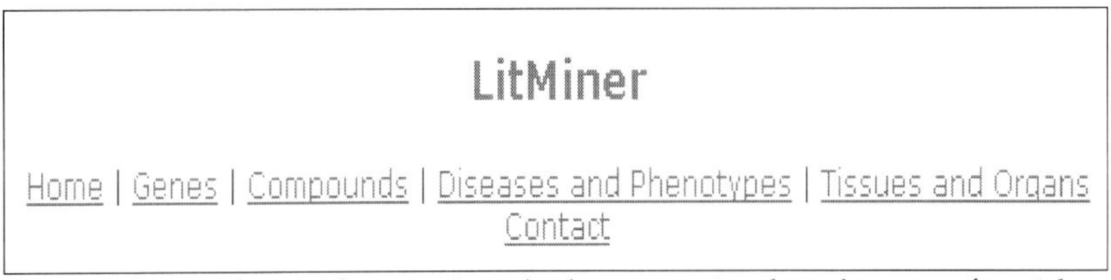

Application that is known for scoring the key terms in the abstracts of articles and predict the relationships between key terms from biomedical literature into four categories: genes, chemicals, diseases and organs.
Also performs statistical analysis of co-citation of annotated key terms to infer relationships (http://andromeda.gsf.de/litminer).

2.3.3 Ontology-based literature search (semantic)

Go PubMed

gopubmed
Searching is now sorted!

Search PubMed for biomedical research articles (http://www.gopubmed.org/web/gopubmed/1?WEB10O00h00100090000). Your keywords are submitted to PubMed and the resulting abstracts are classified using Gene Ontology and Medical Subject Headings (MeSH).

MeSH is a hierarchical vocabulary covering biomedical and health-related topics.
GeneOntology is a hierarchical vocabulary for molecular biology covering cellular components, biological processes and molecular functions.

PIKB: Pathways and Interaction Knowledge Base

PIKB (http://linkedlifedata.com/) allows you to execute arbitrary queries in the semantic network. For example: "Select pathways controlled by the expression of genes located in a specific chromosome". You can also use sets of declarative rules to customize the criteria for identifying redundant information. For example: "All molecular interactions composed by a related Uniprot accession number, a Uniprot cross-reference identifier or an Entrez-Gene identifier and coming from different data sources are equivalent".

2.3.4 Networks analysis

Ali Baba PubMed

Shows the connection of separate record of terms such as cells, drugs, tissues, diseases, reactions, enzymes and compounds of the KEGG (Kyoto encyclopedia of genes and genomes), nutrients, proteins and genes, UniProt and NCBI Taxonomy species. Once the sample has identified links of the articles found as protein-protein interactions, localization of proteins, nutrients and genes (http://alibaba.informatik.hu-berlin.de/).

PubGene

Find the proteins and genes related documents. It shows the quantity of items for each node and its relationships (http://www.pubgene.org/tools/Network/Subset.cgi).

3. Conclusion

The use of web apps investigated in this work makes it possible to extract, analyze and manage an automated literature, efficient, prompt, timely, comprehensive and organized to facilitate handling of large amounts of documentary records simultaneously, choose from the vast amount of the most relevant information available, handle the selected records and learn the ways of analysis of latest digital literature, from which it can and must extract information according to the needs and challenges of our time. Because the constantly actualization and the release of new and innovative internet tools, we have a blog with news about Biomedical Web, Collections and Meta-Analysis Literature Applications: http://biiiogeek.blogspot.com/

4. Acknowledgements

Roberto Calderón for retrieval information and discussions, Claudia Itzel Pedraza for some data about retrieval information, Jack Guillén, Teresita Amezcua and Francisco Castillo for revisions and corrections to the text.
Founds DGAPA, UNAM Project PAPIME PE 201509 and CONACYT 13276.

5. Append

Web apps that process literature with one or more bibliographic meta-analysis methods
Batch Citation Matcher
http://www.ncbi.nlm.nih.gov/entrez/citmatch_help.html#JournalLists
PubMed Retractions
http://pmretract.heroku.com/journals
e-LiSe - text mining tool for Medline data - run
http://miron.ibb.waw.pl/elise/run.html
eGIFT - extracting Gene Information From Text
http://biotm.cis.udel.edu/eGIFT/index.php
Biomedical Informatics Group : PubDNA Finder
http://servet.dia.fi.upm.es:8080/pubdnafinder
BOND Web Portal
http://bond.unleashedinformatics.com/Action?
eGIFT - extracting Gene Information From Text
http://biotm.cis.udel.edu/eGIFT
MEDSUM - THE MEDLINE/PubMed SUMMARY TOOL: research PubMed and Medline data
http://webtools.mf.uni-lj.si/public/medsum.html
Meva - MedLine Postprocessor
http://www.med-ai.com/meva/index.html
Twease
http://twease.org/medline/app?component=clearSettingsDirectLink&page=Home&service=direct&session=T
BioText: Project Homepage
http://biotext.berkeley.edu/
BITOLA - Biomedical Discovery Support System
http://ibmi.mf.uni-lj.si/bitola/?oe=bitola

EBIMed
http://www.ebi.ac.uk/Rebholz-srv/ebimed
FABLE - Fast Automated Biomedical Literature Extraction
http://fable.chop.edu/?hgsid=null&submitbutton=View+browser&submithit=true
LitMiner
http://www.litminer.com
MEDIE - Semantic retrieval engine for MEDLINE
http://www-tsujii.is.s.u-tokyo.ac.jp/medie
MedKit
http://metnetdb.gdcb.iastate.edu/medkit
MedMiner - MetaBase
http://biodatabase.org/index.php/MedMiner
PubMed-EX
http://bws.iis.sinica.edu.tw/PubMed-EX
XplorMed: eXploring Medline abstracts
http://www.ogic.ca/projects/xplormed
eTBLAST 3.0
http://etest.vbi.vt.edu/etblast3
Skill Kit: Searching Full Author Names in PubMed. NLM Technical Bulletin. 2009 Mar–Apr
http://www.nlm.nih.gov/pubs/techbull/ma09/ma09_skill_kit_full_author_names.html
NCBI ESpell Utility
http://eutils.ncbi.nlm.nih.gov/corehtml/query/static/espell_help.html
PubFocus
http://pubfocus.com/pubfocus/images/p...
PubMed Tools
http://www.google.com.mx/gwt/x?source=m&u=http%3A%2F%2Feblas.kisti.re.kr/eblas/index.php%3Foption%3Dcom_weblinks%26view%3Dcategory%26id%3D19%26Itemid%3D98&wsi=5c68445d6e82ae59&ei=8bkXTOTRIqearAOJ2ZT-CA&wsc=pr&ct=pg1&whp=30
Home - PubMed Alternatives - Research Guides at Virginia Commonwealth University
http://guides.library.vcu.edu/content.php?pid=111410&sid=839044
PubMed On Tap
http://www.referencesontap.com
Unbound MEDLINE | Free MEDLINE/PubMed Journal Article Search
http://www.unboundmedicine.com/medline/ebm
LigerCat
http://ligercat.ubio.org/articles
EGQuery Entrez Utility
http://eutils.ncbi.nlm.nih.gov/corehtml/query/static/egquery_help.html
Pubget: the search engine for life-science PDFs
http://pubget.com
Taxonomy Home
http://www.ncbi.nlm.nih.gov/sites/entrez?db=taxonomy
medical Subject Headings (MeSH)
http://www.campusvirtual-hgm.net/alfin/contenido/3-3.html
PubSearch Fast, efficient PubMed® searching on your Mac and your iPhone / iPod Touch
http://www.deathraypizza.com/deathraypizza/PubSearch_Home.html
Deja vu

http://dejavu.vbi.vt.edu/dejavu/duplicate

ConceptLink
http://project.cis.drexel.edu/conceptlink

ARMiner Info Index
http://www.cs.umb.edu/%7Elaur/ARMiner

PubGene. Browse literature or sequence neighbours.
http://www.pubgene.org/tools/Network/Subset.cgi

Kleio @ NaCTeM
http://www.nactem.ac.uk/software/kleio

Acromine dictionary
http://www.nactem.ac.uk/software/acromine

XTractor
http://www.xtractor.in

PolySearch
http://wishart.biology.ualberta.ca/polysearch

PubMatrix
http://pubmatrix.grc.nia.nih.gov

NLM Mobile
http://www.nlm.nih.gov/mobile/

Pubget Mobile
http://pubget.com/mobile

MD on Tap
http://palmdoc.net/?p=417

Bionlp search page
http://www.ccs.neu.edu/home/futrelle/bionlp/search.html

University of Geneva - EAGL System
http://129.194.97.165/EAGL

LitLinker - Home
http://litlinker.ischool.washington.edu

Telemakus Home
http://www.telemakus.net

SLIM v.2 - BETA
https://pmi.nlm.nih.gov/slim

Anne O'Tate
http://arrowsmith.psych.uic.edu/cgi-bin/arrowsmith_uic/AnneOTate.cgi

GoPubMed®
http://www.gopubmed.com/web/gopubmed/1?WEB10O00h01000900001

PubMed Gold
http://www.neurotransmitter.net/ftsearch.html

< *MEDLINE/PubMed Multilanguage Search*
http://babelmesh.nlm.nih.gov

PubMed global biomedical research community - BioWizard
http://www.biowizard.com

BITOLA - Biomedical Discovery Support System
http://ibmi.mf.uni-lj.si/bitola

PubCrawler Web Service
http://pubcrawler.gen.tcd.ie

askMEDLINE
http://askmedline.nlm.nih.gov/ask/ask.php
iHOP - Information Hyperlinked over Proteins
http://www.ihop-net.org/UniPub/iHOP
NCBO BioPortal: Welcome to the NCBO BioPortal
http://bioportal.bioontology.org
Gene-L'EXPO
http://www.genelexpo.jp/genelexpo
Home - BioMedLib™ search engine
http://www.relemed.com
BioIE - Extracting informative sentences from the biomedical literature
http://www.bioinf.manchester.ac.uk/dbbrowser/bioie
PubMed Assistant
http://metnet.vrac.iastate.edu/browser
e-LiSe - text mining tool for Medline data
http://miron.ibb.waw.pl/elise/index.html
FACTA - Finding Associated Concepts with Text Analysis
http://text0.mib.man.ac.uk/software/facta/main.html
FABLE - Fast Automated Biomedical Literature Extraction
http://fable.chop.edu
Journal / Author Name Estimator
http://biosemantics.org/jane
Ali Baba – PubMed as a graph
http://alibaba.informatik.hu-berlin.de
PubNet: Publication Network Graph Utility
http://pubnet.gersteinlab.org
Pubget: the search engine for life-science PDFs
http://pubget.com/search
PolySearch: a web-based text mining system for...
http://www.ncbi.nlm.nih.gov/pubmed/18487273?dopt=AbstractPlus
Deja vu > Browse
http://spore.swmed.edu/dejavu/duplicate
Non-Bibliographic LinkOut Providers
http://www.ncbi.nlm.nih.gov/projects/linkout/journals/htmllists.cgi?type_id=9
Bio Saga: 18 Ways to improve your PubMed searches
http://lukeskywaran.blogspot.com/2008/07/18-ways-to-improve-your-pubmed-searches.html
PathBinder
http://metnet.vrac.iastate.edu/MetNet_PathBinder.htm
www.scitrends.net
http://www.scitrends.net
Manjal - Mining MEDLINE for New Ideas
http://sulu.info-science.uiowa.edu/cgi-bin/ManjalMain.cgi
MScanner
http://mscanner.stanford.edu
PubMed search: A free individualized PubMed software search
http://www.pubmedreader.com
Anne O'Tate
http://128.248.65.210/cgi-bin/arrowsmith_uic/AnneOTate.cgi

6. References

Atkins, D. E., Droegemeier, K. K., Feldman, S. I., Garcia-molina, H., Klein, M. L., Messina, P., Messerschmitt, D. G., Ostriker, J. P. and Wright, M. H. (2003). Revolutionizing Science and Engineering Through Cyberinfrastructure: Report of the National Science Foundation Blue-Ribbon Advisory Panel on. *Science*.

Ananiadou, S., Kell, D. B., & Tsujii, J.-i. (2006). Text mining and its potential applications in systems biology. Trends in biotechnology, 24(12), 571–579. URL http://dx.doi.org/10.1016/j.tibtech.2006.10.002

Borgman, C. L . (1999). What are Digital Libraries, Who is Building Them, and Why? In Aparac, T. (Ed.), *Digital libraries: Interdisciplinary concepts, challenges and opportunities* (pp. 29-42). Zagreb : Benja.

Boyack, K. W. (2004). Mapping knowledge domains: Characterizing PNAS. *Proceedings of the National Academy of Sciences of the United States of America, 101* (Suppl 1), 5192-5199.

Cokol, M., & Rodriguez-Esteban, R. (2008). Visualizing evolution and impact of biomedical fields. *Journal of Biomedical Informatics, 41*(6), 1050-1052.

Elsevier. (2011). Scopus. In: *Sciverse*. Frebuary 2011. Available from: <http://www.info.sciverse.com/scopus/scopus-training/faqs>

European Bioinformaticas Institute. (2011). CiteExplore Statistics. In:*CiteExplore*, March 2011, Available from: <http://www.ebi.ac.uk/citexplore/showStatistics.do>

Falciola, L. (2009). Searching biotechnology information: A case study. *World Patent Information, 31(1)*, 36-47.

Harmston, N., Filsell, W., & Stumpf, M. P. H. (2010). What the papers say: Text mining for genomics and systems biology. *Human Genomics*, 5(1), 17–29.

Henderson, J. (2005). Google scholar: A source for clinicians? *CMAJ, 172*(12), 1549-1550.

Hey, T., & Trefethen, A. E. (2005). Cyberinfrastructure for e-Science. *Science, 308(5723)*, 817-821.

Hull, D., Pettifer, S. R., & Kell, D. B. (2008). Defrosting the digital library: Bibliographic tools for the next generation web. *PLoS Computational Biology, 4*(10), e1000204+.

Koskinen, J., Isohanni, M., Paajala, H., Jääskeläinen, E., Nieminen, P., Koponen, H., Tienari, P., & Miettunen, J. (2008). How to use bibliometric methods in evaluation of scientific research? an example from finnish schizophrenia research. *Nordic Journal of Psychiatry, 62(2)*, 136–143. URL http://dx.doi.org/10.1080/08039480801961667

Krallinger, M., Valencia, A., & Hirschman, L. (2008). Linking genes to literature: text mining, information extraction, and retrieval applications for biology. *Genome Biology*, 9 Suppl 2(Suppl 2), S8. URL http://dx.doi.org/10.1186/gb-2008-9-s2-s8

Labarga, A. (2009). Comunicación y uso de la literatura científica en biomedicina. In *II Seminario EC3 sobre evaluación y comunicación de la ciencia*. Retrieved from http://ec3.ugr.es/seminario2009/

Larson, R. R. (2010a). Information retrieval: Searching in the 21st century; human information retrieval. *Journal of the American Society for Information Science and Technology, 61*(11), 2370-2372.

Larson, R. R. (2010b). Introduction to information retrieval. *Journal of the American Society for Information Science and Technology, 61*(4), 852-853.

Li, L.-L., Ding, G., Feng, N., Wang, M.-H., & Ho, Y.-S. (2009). Global stem cell research trend: Bibliometric analysis as a tool for mapping of trends from 1991 to 2006. *Scientometrics, 80*(1), 39-58.

Melero, R. (2005). Acceso abierto a las publicaciones científicas: definición, recursos, copyright e impacto. *El profesional de la información*, vol. 14, n. 4 (jul.-ago.), p. 255-266.

Merriam-Webster. (2011). Dictionary on-line. Merriam-Webster, Incorporated. http://www.merriam-webster.com/

Michán-Aguirre, L., Calderón-Rojas, R., Nitxin-Castañeda-Sortibrán, A., & Rodríguez-Arnáiz, R. (2010). Aplicaciones web para recuperación y análisis de bibliografía de *PubMed. El Profesional de la Informacion, 19*(3), 285-291. doi: 10.3145/epi.2010.may.09.

Pappalardo,K. and Fitzgerald, A. (2007). *A Guide to Developing Open Access Through Your Digital Repository*. QUT Printing Services.

Renear, A. H., & Palmer, C. L. (2009). Strategic reading, ontologies, and the future of scientific publishing. *Science (New York, N.Y.), 325(5942)*, 828-832.

Rizkallah, J., & Sin, D. D. (2010). Integrative approach to quality assessment of medical journals using impact factor, eigenfactor, and article influence scores. *PloS one*, *5*(4), e10204+.

Robu, I., Robu, V., & Thirion, B. (2006). An introduction to the semantic web for health sciences librarians. Journal of the Medical Library Association : JMLA, 94(2), 198–205.

Rodriguez-Esteban, R. (2009). Biomedical text mining and its applications. *PLoS Computational Biology*, *5*(12), e1000597+.

Romary, L., & Armbruster, C. (2009). Beyond institutional repositories. Social Science. Research Network Working Paper Series.

Rosas, S. R., Kagan, J. M., Schouten, J. T., Slack, P. A., & Trochim, W. M. K. (2011). Evaluating research and impact: A bibliometric analysis of research by the NIH/NIAID HIV/AIDS clinical trials networks. PLoS ONE, 6(3), e17428.

Russell, J. M. (2001). Scientific communication at the beginning of the 21st century. *International Social Science Journal*, 168, 271-282.

Suber, P. (2010). Open Access Overview. Last revised November 6, 2010 Available from: <http://www.earlham.edu/~peters/fos/overview.htm>

Swan, A. & Brown, S. (2005) Open Access self archiving: an author study. Truro, UK: *Key Perspectivas*. Date of access: February 25, 2011, Available from: <http://eprints.ecs.soton.ac.uk/10999/>.

Thomson Reuters. (2011). Products A-Z. In: *Web of Knowlegde*, February 2011, Available from:<http://wokinfo.com/products_tools/products/>

Uthman, O. (2008). HIV/AIDS in nigeria: a bibliometric analysis. *BMC Infectious Diseases*, *8*(1), 19+.

Villanova-Oliver, M., Gensel, J., & Martin, H. (2003). Models and guidelines for the design of progressive access in web-based information systems. *Lecture Notes in Computer Science*, *2817*, 238-249+.

Weeber, M., Kors, J. A., & Mons, B. (2005). Online tools to support literature-based discovery in the life sciences. *Briefings in Bioinformatics*, *6*(3), 277-286.

Zhou, X., Hu, X., Li, G., Lin, X., & Zhang, X. (2006). Relation-Based document retrieval for biomedical IR. In C. Priami, X. Hu, Y. Pan, & T. Lin (Eds.) *Transactions on Computational Systems Biology V*, vol. 4070 of *Lecture Notes in Computer Science*, chap. 9, (pp. 112-128). Berlin, Heidelberg: Springer Berlin / Heidelberg.

2

Biomedical HIV Prevention

Gita Ramjee and Claire Whitaker
HIV Prevention Research Unit, South African Medical Research Council
South Africa

1. Introduction

In 2009, an estimated 33.3 million adults and children worldwide were living with HIV, while 2.6 million were newly infected that year (UNAIDS, 2010). The epidemic most severely affects sub-Saharan Africa, where 22.5 million people live with the virus, and 1.8 million were newly infected in 2009 (UNAIDS, 2010). The predominant mode of HIV transmission in this hardest hit area is heterosexual intercourse, with young women particularly vulnerable to acquisition of the virus (Laga et al., 2001), a result of intersecting biological, social and cultural vulnerabilities (Coovadia et al., 2009; Hladik & Hope, 2009).

Although initially considered a fatal diagnosis, HIV is fast becoming a chronic disease, manageable through the use of antiretroviral (ARV) medications. Under good health-care conditions, people living with HIV may now enjoy a life-span that is not significantly different from that of an uninfected person, even without ARV treatment (van Sighem et al., 2010).

Over the past 25 years since the identification of the causative agent of HIV, researchers have investigated many methods for the prevention of acquisition of the virus. It has become increasingly clear that a combination HIV prevention approach to combating the epidemic will be necessary, since no single intervention has yet been shown to have more than approximately 60% effectiveness in preventing infection (Klausner et al., 2008; Vermund et al., 2009). Biomedical prevention encompasses the use of medical treatments such as ARVs for prevention or post-exposure prophylaxis, barrier methods such as male and female condoms, procedures such as medical male circumcision or other methods to reduce the chance of transmission of HIV (Padian et al., 2008). Rather than dichotimising the response to the epidemic into separate biomedical and behavioural interventions, the most effective intervention is likely to incorporate both behavioural change and widespread provision of one or more biomedical prevention options for both men and women.

2. Biomedical HIV prevention technologies

2.1 Vaccines

Although vaccines may appear to be a ubiquitous facet of modern medical care, their development has required prolonged experimentation in several cases. The earliest and most famous vaccination experiment is perhaps Edward Jenner's deliberate infection in 1796 of a young boy with cowpox which conferred protection against the related, but much more deleterious smallpox (Dunn, 1996). Later in 1885, Louis Pasteur developed a post-exposure rabies anti-toxin which he also called a vaccine (Hoenig, 1986), thus broadening the definition of the term to include any applied substance which induced an immune response and conferred protection against subsequent infection (Atkinson et al., 2002). Vaccine development and production continued apace from that point onwards, although some diseases have proved more amenable to development of a vaccine than others. For example, although the causative agent of poliomyelitis was identified in 1908, an effective vaccine was not developed until 1955, an elapsed time of 47 years; it took 105 years to develop a vaccine against typhoid subsequent to identification of the causative organism, while the elapsed times to vaccine for *Haemophilus influenza* and pertussis were 92 years and 89 years respectively (Markel, 2005). Comparatively quicker has been the 16 year developmental pathway to a vaccine against hepatitis B (Markel, 2005).

Vaccines are generally formulated in the following ways:

- attenuated (live organisms which have lowered or disabled virulence)
- conjugate (combination of antigenic substances)
- killed (heat or chemically destroyed whole organism)
- inactivated toxoid (organismal products which would normally produce illness)
- subunit (specific fragments of the organism of interest)

Successful vaccines have been developed against viruses which follow a particular course of infection: a certain degree of initial replication and dissemination after infection is followed by migration to the target organ and the development of illness (Johnston & Fauci, 2007). Should previous exposure to viral antigens have occurred, an endogenous immune reaction can occur, preventing the development of illness (Johnston & Fauci, 2007). This response has two broad components: humoral and cellular. The humoral response involves the production of antibodies which neutralise the virus and prevent new infection of cells, while the cellular response recruits specific CD8+ cytotoxic T lymphocytes to destroy virally infected cells (Markel, 2005). The classic approach to vaccine design has been to elicit the production of high levels of neutralising antibodies which prevent the establishment of infection in target cells or organs (Johnston & Fauci, 2007).

The search for an effective HIV vaccine has been hampered by the high genetic plasticity of HIV and its ability to escape the effects of neutralising antibodies through conformational shielding of vulnerable antigenic sites on the HIV envelope protein (Richman et al., 2003; Burton et al., 2004). HIV is able to establish a pool of latently infected cells in the early stages of infection (Chun et al., 1998), a feature of the infectious process which complicates the development of an effective vaccine, since infection in latent cells provides a reservoir of infection which cannot be cleared by the neutralising antibody response. In HIV infection, the natural production of neutralising antibodies only occurs weeks to years after the initial infecting event (Wyatt & Sodroski, 1998; Johnston & Fauci, 2007), and even then, the constant mutation of the virus renders the antibodies ineffective (Johnston & Fauci, 2008). The approach in the context of HIV vaccines may have to be modified towards the elicitation of T-cell responses rather than neutralising antibodies. This may not provide protection against infection, but will rather reduce the viral load set point and early viral load should the vaccine recipient become infected, with associated positive effects on progression to AIDS or length of time to initiation of ARV therapy (Amara et al., 2001; Letvin et al., 2006; Padian et al., 2008). Reduction of viral load set point and early viral load could also have important implications for transmission, since most transmission events are hypothesised to occur during acute infection of the transmitting partner, due to high viral load levels (Pilcher et al., 2004).

HIV vaccines strategies have included live attenuated vaccines, inactivated vaccines, virus-like particles, subunit vaccines, naked DNA and live recombinant vaccines (Girard et al., 2006). Of these, only subunit vaccines (gp120 protein) and live recombinant vaccines (MRKAd5 HIV-1 gag/pol/nef and ALVAC) have advanced to late stage human clinical testing, the results of which will be summarised below.

Five candidate vaccines have advanced to late stage safety and/or efficacy testing (see table 1). Two, the STEP and Phambili trials, were of the MRKAd5 HIV-1 gag/pol/nef vaccine (Buchbinder et al., 2008; Gray et al., 2008); these vaccines utilised a mixture of three adenovirus vectors expressing the *gag, pol* and *nef* genes of HIV. *Gag, pol* and *nef* were selected for inclusion in the vaccine as they are commonly recognised during natural HIV infection, and are conserved across HIV clades (thus potentially providing protection against more than one HIV sub-type) (Buchbinder et al., 2008). Two trials were of rgp120 vaccines (Flynn et al., 2005; Pitisuttithum et al., 2006); rgp120 is a purified recombinant form of an HIV outer envelope protein, which, it was hoped, would elicit an effective immune response in vaccine recipients. A combination prime (ALVAC-HIV) + boost (AIDSVAX B/E) strategy was also investigated in a large trial in Thailand (known as RV 144) (Rerks-Ngarm et al., 2009). The ALVAC component comprised a recombinant canarypox vector genetically engineered to express subtype B HIV-1 Gag and Pro proteins and gp120 from subtype CRF01_AE linked to the transmembrane anchoring portion of gp41. AIDSVAX consisted of a combination of gp120 proteins from subtype B and E viruses. The hope of the prime + boost technique was that both T-cell and antibody responses could be generated by the vaccine, as opposed to antibody responses alone (Hu et al., 1991), the effectiveness of which is compromised by the innate behaviour of HIV (described in the preceding paragraph).

Vaccine	Study location	Approximate sample size	Result
B/B rgp120 (Flynn et al., 2005)	North America; The Netherlands	5000+	No significant effect on HIV acquisition
MRKAd5 HIV-1 gag/pol/nef (B) (Buchbinder et al., 2008)	North America; South America; Caribbean, Australia	3000	No significant effect on HIV acquisition, possible harm
MRKAd5 HIV-1 gag/pol/nef (B) (Gray et al., 2008)	South Africa	801	Trial stopped early
AIDSVAX B/E rgp120	Thailand	2500	No significant effect on HIV acquisition
ALVAC-HIV (vCPI521) HIV-1 gag/pro (B) & rgp120/gp41 (E) prime + AIDSVAX B/E (rgp 120) boost (Rerks-Ngarm et al., 2009)	Thailand	16000+	Modest protective effect against acquisition of HIV

* "B" and "E" in Vaccine column refer to HIV clades that vaccine products were derived from.

Table 1. Advanced stage safety and efficacy trials of HIV vaccines

Of these trials, the STEP, Phambili and rgp120 trials, produced "flat" results, indicating neither benefit nor harm of the interventions in terms of HIV prevention. Both the STEP and Phambili trials were prematurely terminated due to concerns over safety, while both of the rgp120 trials were completed. However, the recent RV 144 trial provided tantalising evidence of a significant positive effect for preventing the acquisition of HIV (Rerks-Ngarm et al., 2009). The effect was modest, however, and further research will be necessary to expand on several questions raised by the study results: vaccine efficacy was found to decrease over the first year after vaccination, and may have been greater in persons at lower risk (Rerks-Ngarm et al., 2009). Overall, the results of these advanced stage trials tend to indicate that more pre-clinical studies should be undertaken to gain improved understanding of immune response to the virus before products are tested in large-scale human clinical trials. A significant limitation of the vaccine trials conducted to date has been that the vaccines are derived from less prevalent HIV subtypes: as shown in table 1, most contained derivatives of subtype B or E virus, while subtype C is most prevalent in Africa, the region with the worst HIV epidemic (UNAIDS, 2010).

As with most biomedical technologies, vaccines are unlikely to be 100% effective. Even if we reduce self-reported adherence challenges by using vaccines, consumer and epidemiological models suggest that individual perception of protection by the vaccine is likely to increase risk behaviour by 25% to 50% (Newman et al., 2004; Crosby & Holtgrave, 2006). Behavioural changes will be necessary to demonstrate effectiveness of the vaccine.

2.2 Medical male circumcision

Medical male circumcision has been regarded as one of the success stories in the battle against HIV over the past decade. Based on ecological and observational evidence (Weiss et al., 2000) it was hypothesised that male circumcision had a significant effect on the prevalence of HIV. There are several possible causes for this effect: circumcision removes the foreskin, thus resulting in keratinisation of the underlying epithelium. The non-keratinized inner epithelium is more susceptible to infection by HIV than the keratinised outer epithelium of the foreskin (Patterson et al., 2002), which could provide a point of entry for the virus. However, some evidence contradicting this hypothesis has recently been presented: Dinh et al (Dinh et al., 2010) found no significant difference between the degree of keratinisation of the inner and outer foreskin in 16 donor tissue samples; those authors and others (Kigozi et al., 2009) suggest that the surface area of the foreskin may play a more important role in susceptibility to HIV - the larger the foreskin, the higher the risk of acquiring the virus. The proliferation of HIV target cells (such as Langerhans cells) in the foreskin may also explain the reduction in vulnerability to HIV following its removal (McCoombe & Short, 2006). Circumcision also reduces the risk of men acquiring certain other sexually transmitted infections such as chancroid, syphilis (Weiss et al., 2006), human papillomavirus (HPV) and herpes simplex virus type 2 (HSV2) (Tobian et al., 2009) which may themselves increase the risk of infection with HIV (Fleming & Wasserheit, 1999).

An earlier meta-analysis of studies conducted in sub-Saharan Africa which included circumcision as a potential risk factor found that the evidence for an effect was compelling, but also noted significant heterogeneity between the studies, which the authors concluded indicated that effects might vary between populations (Weiss et al., 2000). Despite this, three large-scale clinical trials monitoring the incidence of female-to-male transmission of HIV following circumcision showed strong evidence for a reduction in risk of acquisition of HIV ranging from 48% to 61% (Auvert et al., 2005; Bailey et al., 2007; Gray et al., 2007). This level of protection was projected to potentially be capable of preventing 2 million new HIV infections and 0,3 million deaths in the ten years after 2006 (Williams et al., 2006), and has even been described as "as good as the HIV vaccine we've been waiting for" (Klausner et al., 2008). Despite the positive benefits for men, male circumcision does not appear to protect women from acquiring HIV from an already infected man (Wawer et al., 2009). This may be due to resumption of sexual activity prior to complete wound healing, or risk compensation (an increase in risky behaviour owing to perceptions of the protective effect of the intervention) (Wawer et al., 2009). Medical male circumcision has, however, been found to reduce the prevalence and incidence of HPV infections in female partners (Wawer et al., 2011). Safer sex counselling and condom provision are recommended as companions to circumcision services.

Despite clear evidence for efficacy of this intervention in preventing female-to-male HIV transmission, evidence for effectiveness in preventing male-to-male transmission is less certain - although some evidence suggests that circumcision may protect against HIV acquisition in men who prefer the insertive role, overall, circumcision has not been found to protect against HIV infection in men who have sex with men (MSM) (Millett et al., 2008; Templeton et al., 2009). Further research on the potential role of circumcision in HIV prevention for MSM is warranted.

Scaling up of this intervention has been challenging due to lack of health infrastructure capacity in countries most in need of this intervention, which impacts on both safety and cost-effectiveness. In addition, cultural beliefs may hinder the uptake of this intervention in many societies worldwide.

2.3 Barrier methods for HIV prevention

Condoms provide an effective physical barrier to HIV infection, the evidence for which is consistent and compelling (Carey et al., 1992; Lytle et al., 1997; Pinkerton & Abramson, 1997; Weller & Davis-Beaty, 2002). In addition, condoms also reduce the transmission of many other sexually transmitted infections such as *Chlamydia trachomatis*, syphilis, HSV2 and *Neisseria gonorrhoeae* (Holmes et al., 2004), infection with which may in turn increase susceptibility to HIV infection (Wasserheit, 1992). *In vitro* testing of the male latex condom has shown that in a worst case scenario, use of a condom is 10^4 times better at preventing semen transfer than not using a condom at all (Carey et al., 1992).

Male condoms have been pivotal in HIV prevention programs since HIV was first identified. When correctly and consistently used, condoms are estimated to reduce the per contact probability of male-to-female infection by as much as 95% (Pinkerton & Abramson, 1997). Among the general population in Rakai, Uganda, consistent condom use was associated with reduced HIV incidence (Ahmed et al., 2001), while meta-analysis of condom use among sero-discordant couples has shown that consistent use results in an incidence rate for male-to-female transmission of 0.9 per 100 person years compared with 6.8 per 100 person years in persons who never used condoms (Davis & Weller, 1999). Davis and Weller also found in their review that breakage rates varied between 0.5% and 6.7%, while rates of slippage ranged from 0.1% to 16.6% (Davis & Weller, 1999). Despite widespread condom promotion, their use is often incorrect and inconsistent (Foss et al., 2004), which reduces their effectiveness. Usage has been found to vary by partner type, with condoms more frequently used with casual or short-term partners, but not with marital or long-term partners (Maharaj & Cleland, 2004; Chimbiri, 2007; Hargreaves et al., 2009). In contexts in which multiple concurrent partnering may be normalised, this pattern of behaviour puts the partners at risk of both contracting and rapidly transmitting HIV (Halperin & Epstein, 2007; Epstein, 2008).

Uganda has served as an example of the possible success of an aggressive "ABC" approach - abstinence, behavioral change and condom use campaigns can be successful in curbing HIV infections (Stoneburner & Low-Beer, 2004). This has also been demonstrated by the "100% condom program" in Thailand (Rojanapithayakorn & Hanenberg, 1996; Park et al., 2010), which sought to encourage condom use at every commercial sexual encounter and was also accompanied by an extensive advertising campaign. However, in many countries gender relations, social inequality and economic dependence do not allow young women to negotiate safe sex (with condoms) with their partners (Laga et al., 2001; Hunter, 2007; Ramjee et al., 2008). Hence, other woman-initiated prevention options are urgently needed (Stein, 1990).

The efficacy of the female condom in preventing transmission of STIs has provided support for its hypothetical efficacy in preventing HIV, although no clinical trials specifically to test this have been conducted (Vijayakumar et al., 2006). Early testing showed that the female condom was impermeable to both HIV and cytomegalovirus (Drew et al., 1990). Measures of semen exposure during female condom use have been found to vary between 5 and 19% when no problems were reported, but this rose to between 17 and 30% if a problem *was* reported during use (Macaluso et al., 2003). Complete protection from semen exposure occurred in 79-93% of sex acts. In that study, 83% of women who used one or more female condoms reported experiencing a problem with the condom, indicating that mechanical and acceptability challenges may seriously limit the uptake of the female condom. However, the incidence of problems did decline over time, suggesting that greater experience reduced problems with usage (Macaluso et al., 2003). Incidence of semen exposure has also been found to vary with both couple- and intercourse-specific features, indicating that achieving consistent results across a population may prove difficult unless intensive counselling and education accompany distribution of the female condom (Lawson et al., 2003). The female condom is relatively more expensive than male condoms as it is made of polyurethane rather than latex, but could in turn prove highly cost effective when implemented in a strategic public health programme targeting users at high risk of contracting HIV (Warren & Philpott, 2003). Despite evidence of demand for the female condom, production levels remain low, and the price accordingly high (Peters et al., 2010), an untenable situation for such a promising prevention method. It may be possible to circumvent the problems of cost and availability by re-using female condoms - washing, drying and re-lubricating them between *in vivo* uses has been shown not to affect the burst and seam strength up to eight washes, while the breakage rate associated with multiple washing and re-use was slightly lower than that found in the case of single use followed by washing. While it is preferable to use a new female condom for each instance of intercourse, re-use may be possible where a new female condom cannot be obtained (Beksinska et al., 2001).

The urgent need to develop woman-initiated methods which can be used covertly led to testing of the HIV prevention potential of cervical barriers. Observational data suggested that covering the cervix with a diaphragm may reduce the risk of HIV (Padian et al., 2007). The epithelium of the cervix is composed of a comparatively thinner and more delicate unilayer of columnar epithelium, in contrast to the stratified squamous epithelium of the vagina, which may be more robust in resisting infection (Hladik & Hope, 2009). The cervix is also rich in HIV target cells - particularly in the transformation zone, which is richly supplied with macrophages and CD4+ T cells (Pudney et al., 2005). However, a randomized controlled trial (RCT) testing the hypothesis that covering the cervix may protect against HIV infection failed to show effectiveness (Padian et al., 2007) - the HIV seroconversion rates were similar in diaphragm users and control participants. Some challenges experienced during implementation of the trial included low adherence and risk compensation among diaphragm users. It is proposed that diaphragms could be an additional tool in the "HIV prevention tool-box" and used as a delivery device for products such as microbicides (see below) (Padian et al., 2007). Despite the lack of evidence for efficacy in preventing HIV infection, the diaphragm has shown efficacy in prevention of gonococcal infections (Ramjee et al., 2008).

2.4 Microbicides

Microbicides are intravaginal products designed to be used discreetly by women to prevent HIV; the products are formulated in a variety of ways, including gels, films, tablets and as intravaginal rings (IVR) (Ndesendo et al., 2008; Buckheit Jr et al., 2010). Although a variety of dosage forms have been developed, the gel and IVR have lately come to dominate the development pipeline. The development of microbicides was prompted by Zena Stein's call for a woman-initiated means of preventing HIV infection, in recognition of the fact that men had ultimate control of the (then) only biomedical means of preventing HIV infection - the male condom (Stein, 1990).

The first generation of microbicides to be tested in large-scale clinical trials were surfactant in nature - nonoxynol-9 (N9) was one of the first compounds to be tested. Surfactant products act by non-specifically disrupting biological membranes resulting in organism lysis. This spermicide was found to have *in vitro* anti-HIV activity (Polsky et al., 1988; Jennings & Clegg, 1993) and prevented infection of cats by feline immunodeficiency virus (Moench et al., 1993) and macaques with simian immunodeficiency virus (SIV)(Miller et al., 1992), but failed to prevent HIV infection in women (van Damme et al., 2002). N9 was found to disrupt the epithelium of the vagina in women who made frequent use of the product, thus *enhancing* rather than protecting against HIV infection. This result encouraged the adoption of more rigorous and extensive pre-clinical studies in an attempt to prevent the advancement into human stage testing of potentially harmful products. N9 was succeeded by another surfactant gel product called SAVVY, which although safe, was not conclusively found to be of utility in preventing HIV infection (Peterson et al., 2007; Feldblum et al., 2008).

Alongside the surfactants, the following polyanionic compounds were also tested as microbicidal agents: cellulose sulphate, Carraguard and PRO 2000. Polyanions interfere with the attachment of HIV to target cells - PRO 2000, for example, binds to the viral coat protein gp120, and also to host cellular receptors such as CD4 and CXCR4 (Huskens et al., 2009). However, all three polyanions (as well as the surfactants) were non-specific to HIV, a characteristic which is now thought to have had a profound impact on the utility of the compounds for the prevention of infection. Although Carraguard and PRO 2000 were both found to be safe to use, they had no discernable effect on HIV infection (Skoler-Karpoff et al., 2008; Abdool Karim et al., 2011), while cellulose sulphate may have increased the risk of infection in a similar manner to that of N9 - by disrupting tight junctions between cells and increasing viral replication (Mesquita et al., 2009). However, Carraguard has been found to have utility in preventing infection with HPV (Marais et al., 2010) - the causative agent of cervical cancer (Ho et al., 1995; Nobbenhuis et al., 1999), and further investigations for this application are underway. Gels which are found to be safe may also be used as carriers for other compounds - the combination of Carraguard and the ARV MIV-150 has shown some efficacy in preventing SHIV-RT infection in macaques (Aravantinou et al., 2010).

Recently, there has been a major leap forward in the microbicide field, with the use of ARV-based agents for HIV prevention. The Centre for the AIDS Programme of Research In South Africa (CAPRISA) 004 safety and effectiveness study compared 1% tenofovir gel with a placebo, and found that the active gel reduced HIV infections by 39% overall, and by 54% in highly adherent trial participants (Abdool Karim et al., 2010). This result is at the forefront of a major sea change in the microbicide field away from non-specific compounds and towards the use of specific ARV drugs for application prior to exposure to HIV. Trials are currently planned to confirm the effect of 1% tenofovir gel, and several trials are ongoing to test the safety and/or efficacy of other ARVs such as dapivirine and UC781 (see table 2 below).

Study /Phase	Location	Population	Candidate substance
VOICE (MTN 003) Phase IIb, safety and effectiveness	Malawi, South Africa, Uganda, Zimbabwe	5,000 heterosexual women	Tenofovir gel; oral TDF; oral TDF/FTC
IPM 014A Phase I/II, safety	Kenya, Malawi, Rwanda, South Africa	320 women	Dapivirine vaginal gel
IPM 014B Phase I/II, safety	South Africa	320 women	Dapivirine vaginal gel
IPM 020 Phase I/II, safety	United States	180 women	Dapivirine vaginal gel
IPM 015 Phase I/II, safety	South Africa (ongoing), Kenya, Malawi, Rwanda, Tanzania, Zambia (planned)	280 women	Dapivirine vaginal ring
IPM 013 Phase I, P/K	Belgium	48 women	Dapivirine vaginal ring
Pilot Study Phase I	United States	15 women	UC-781 gel

Table adapted from Alliance for AIDS Vaccine Advocacy Coalition website at www.avac.org accessed March 29, 2011 FTC - emtricitabine; TDF - tenofovir disoproxil fumarate

Table 2. Ongoing ARV-based microbicide trials

The ARV-based microbicides in Table 2 are all reverse transcriptase inhibitors (RTIs), although of two different classes. Tenofovir is a nucleoside reverse transcriptase inhibitor or "chain terminator" which interferes with the synthesis of the viral DNA by interpolation into the growing strand. Both dapivirine and UC-781 are non-nucleoside reverse transcriptase inhibitors (NNRTIs) which bind to a non-active site on reverse transcriptase, inducing a conformational change which prevents further activity of the enzyme (D'Cruz & Uckun, 2006). Other prospective ARV-based microbicides may include maraviroc (a cell entry inhibitor) (Fletcher et al., 2010; Herrera et al., 2010), protease inhibitors (Evans et al., 2010) and other NNRTIs such as MIV-150 (Kenney et al., 2011).

Recent innovations in microbicide delivery have included the development of intravaginal rings (IVRs). These rings are similar to those currently marketed for contraceptive use, but have instead as their active ingredient an antiretroviral agent. The rings have been formulated in two ways - as matrix or reservoir types. In the matrix type, the active ingredient is homogenously distributed throughout the ring material, while in the reservoir type, a central core containing the ARV is surrounded by an unmedicated outer layer (Malcolm et al., 2010). Matrix type IVRs may have a less favourable drug release profile than the reservoir type, since the release of the drug is less controlled, resulting in an early spike in concentration. The addition of rate controlling layers may assist in minimising this characteristic (Malcolm et al., 2010). Most IVRs are made of silicone elastomer (eg. polydimethylsiloxane) or thermoplastic elastomer (eg. poly[ethylene vinyl acetate] and segmented polyurethane) (Malcolm et al., 2010). Formulation of IVRs both with and without contraceptives will provide women with the option of preventing acquisition/transmission of HIV without affecting fertility - a feature which is particularly important in contexts where fertility is highly valued.

Although microbicides were initially proposed for vaginal use, there has recently been an increase in research on microbicides for rectal application, since it is recognised that this is a significant route of exposure to HIV infection for both women and men who have sex with men (Ramjee et al., 2010). The development of microbicides for application to the rectum has resulted in research comparing the effect of microbicides on the vaginal and rectal mucosa which has shown that the rectal mucosa may be relatively more delicate (Patton et al., 2009). Vaginal microbicides should not be assumed to be safe for rectal use. Future work on rectal microbicides will require specific *in vitro* and animal models to assess the impact of the products on the target tissue type.

Challenges in the clinical trials of microbicides have included lack of appropriate animal models to assess safety prior to human trials, high pregnancy rates (women are taken off the product when pregnant), products with low HIV specificity, and achieving high adherence to the product by trial participants (Ramjee et al., 2010). The promising effectiveness demonstrated by an ARV-based microbicide has re-invigorated the field (Abdool Karim et al., 2010). However, these products remain unlikely to be 100% effective, hence correct and consistent use of additional prevention options may be required.

2.5 Oral antiretroviral therapy for prevention

Development and use of ARV agents has had a significant impact on improving lifespan and quality of life of people living with HIV. These agents have also played a ground-breaking role in prevention of mother to child transmission (MTCT) (Connor et al., 1994) with MTCT in the developed world almost eradicated owing to this success. The use of ARVs for prevention of MTCT has been shown to be both feasible and cost effective (Chigwedere et al., 2008) - but treatment may not be available to women living in less developed countries.

The success of prevention of MTCT suggests that antiretroviral therapy (ART) could be used as a chemoprophylactic method to prevent sexual HIV transmission due to its ability to suppress viral load and viral replication both prior to and post exposure to HIV. There is evidence that post-exposure prophylaxis (PEP) can reduce the risk of acquisition of HIV (Mackie & Coker, 2000). Research into ART for pre-exposure prophylaxis (PrEP) has gained momentum recently with several trials in various population groups under way in many countries. All these trials (see Table 3) have used the drug tenofovir disoproxil fumarate (TDF) or tenofovir disoproxil fumarate/emtricitabine (TDF/FTC) due to its good safety profile and infrequent side effects (Paxton et al., 2007). Tenofovir disoproxil fumarate is the prodrug form of tenofovir, a nucleotide reverse transcriptase inhibitor which prevents elongation of the transcribed HIV DNA by interpolation into the growing chain in place of adenosine 5′-monophosphate (Gilead, 2010). Emtricitabine functions in a similar manner and is the (-) enantiomer of a thio analog of cytidine (Gilead, 2008).

Trial	Products	Population	Countries
Phase IIb and III			
Parallel comparison of Tenofovir and Emtricitabine/Tenofovir PrEP to prevent HIV-1 acquisition within HIV-1 discordant couples (Partners PrEP)	TDF/FTC: Oral, TDF: Oral	4700 discordant heterosexual couples	Kenya, Uganda
Safety and efficacy of daily tenofovir to prevent HIV infection (Bangkok Tenofovir Study	TDF: Oral	2400 IV drug users	Thailand
Safety and effectiveness study of tenofovir 1% gel, tenofovir disoproxil fumarate tablet and emtricitabine/tenofovir disoproxil fumarate tablet for the prevention of HIV infection in women (VOICE/MTN 003)	TDF/FTC:Oral TDF: Oral TDF: Gel	5000 women	South Africa, Uganda, Zimbabwe
Phase I and II			
Extended safety trial (PrEP in young MSM)	TDF: Oral	99 young MSM	United States
Safety and efficacy of daily and oral antiretroviral use for the prevention of HIV infection in heterosexually active young adults (TDF2)	TDF/FTC: Oral	1200 heterosexual men and women	Botswana
IAVI E001 & E002 Phase I/II	TDF/FTC: Oral daily and coitally dependent	150 serodiscordant couples	Kenya, Uganda

Table adapted from Alliance for AIDS Vaccine Advocacy Coalition website at www.avac.org accessed 22 February 2011.
TDF/FTC: tenofovir disoproxil fumarate/emtricitabine; TDF: tenofovir disoproxil fumarate

Table 3. Oral pre-exposure prevention candidates in clinical trials

The results of the iPrEx trial of oral TDF/FTC showed that oral PrEP may be able to reduce HIV incidence among men who have sex with men (Grant et al., 2010). However, the effectiveness of the treatment is likely to be heavily influenced by the adherence of the persons taking the medication - low adherence among participants in the iPrEx trial may have affected the level of protection afforded by the study drugs (Grant et al., 2010). If consensus emerges that PrEP is safe and effective, there will be several challenges for wide-spread roll-out of the method to the population that needs it, including identifying the appropriate target population, monitoring of adherence and side-effects, and development of potential drug resistance. PrEP is unlikely to be 100% effective, so monitoring of adherence and risk compensation will be critical and will require behavioural intervention.

2.6 Treatment of Sexually Transmitted Infections

Many observational studies have suggested that sexually transmitted infections (STIs), including HSV2, enhance HIV acquisition (Wasserheit, 1992; del Mar Pujades Rodríguez et al., 2002; Freeman et al., 2006). The mechanism by which infection is thought to be facilitated varies depending on the particular STI. Rebbapragada and Kaul (Rebbapragada & Kaul, 2007) summarise five mechanisms by which STIs might enhance susceptibility to HIV: macro or micro-scale breach of the genital epithelium; alteration of the levels of innate immune proteins and/or mucosal environment; enhancing susceptibility to other genital infections; attraction of activated HIV target cells to the site of HIV exposure; and by increasing inflammation which in turn enhances HIV replication. Ulcerative STIs such as HSV2 and syphilis may facilitate HIV infection directly through discontinuities in the genital epithelium (Wasserheit, 1992), but may also have mechanisms in common with other non-ulcerative STIs such as gonorrhoea and *Chlamydia trachomatis* which are thought to facilitate infection both through micro-ulcerations and by increasing inflammation within the genital tract with subsequent proliferation of HIV target cells (Rebbapragada & Kaul, 2007).

Treatment of STIs for prevention of HIV can include antibiotic or viral suppressive medications, or a combination of both.

Randomised controlled trials of STI treatment have found a significant reduction in HIV in only one instance - for a community randomised trial of syndromic treatment of bacterial infections in Mwanza, Tanzania (Grosskurth et al., 1995). Monthly provision of 1g of azithromycin to female commercial sex workers in a RCT in Nairobi, Kenya did not result in a reduction in subsequent acquisition of HIV, although significant reductions in gonorrhoea, *Chlamydia* and *Trichomonas vaginalis* infections were noted (Kaul et al., 2004). A large scale community intervention with three arms (including an STI treatment arm) carried out near Masaka, Uganda, found that although the trial activities may have positively influenced sexual behaviour and incidence of certain STIs, no detectable influence on HIV was noted (Kamali et al., 2003). In a trial comparing the effects of intensive versus standard STI care and treatment, a lower but not significantly different HIV seroconversion rate was noted in participants randomized to the intensive care regimen (Ghys et al., 2001). Two recent large-scale trials showed no evidence for an effect of HSV2 suppressive therapy on HIV acquisition (Celum et al., 2008; Watson-Jones et al., 2008). HSV2 suppressive therapy was also unable to prevent transmission of HIV from infected to uninfected partners, despite a reduction in their HIV viral load (Celum et al., 2010).

It has been proposed that STI treatment may only be effective in concentrated epidemics, and that the effectiveness of such interventions decreases with increasing generalization of the epidemic (Grosskurth et al., 2000). Despite overwhelming biological evidence for STI treatment as a potential HIV prevention option, efficacy has not been demonstrated in trials due to limitations in treatment approach, adherence and acceptability (Grosskurth et al., 2000; Lagakos & Gable, 2008). This should not preclude the inclusion of effective STI treatment in HIV prevention plans, as this approach is important for preventing other significant causes of morbidity, and may also have the effect of normalising the need for safe sexual behaviour.

2.7 Harm reduction for intravenous drug users

Although the primary mode of HIV transmission in the world is heterosexual sex, there remain concentrated HIV epidemics among intravenous drug users (IDUs) in parts of Asia and South America, while the epidemic among IDUs in Europe and North America is declining (UNAIDS, 2010).

HIV may remain viable in blood residue in used needles and syringes for several weeks (Abdala et al., 1999), providing an efficient mechanism for transmitting virus between multiple individuals who re-use such equipment. Mechanisms introduced to reduce the incidence of HIV infection in this population include behavioral risk reduction (Copenhaver et al., 2006), clean needle and syringe exchange programs, and opioid substitution (Vlahov et al., 2010).

Although it is possible to clean needles with bleach for re-use (Shapshak et al., 1994; Abdala et al., 2001), greater success in lowering HIV risk has been achieved through needle exchange programs (NEPs). Such programs provide IDUs with sterile needles and syringes and promote other interventions such as referral to treatment programs. Although there is a lack of experimental data (Wodak & Cooney, 2005), it is apparent that such programs impact on risky injection behavior and thus transmission of HIV and other infections (Holtzman et al., 2009). Ecological studies have shown that a reduction in HIV infections followed the introduction of combined opioid substitution therapy and needle and syringe exchange programs in the European Union and five middle and higher income countries (Wiessing et al., 2009); similarly, cities worldwide that have needle exchange programs have experienced a drop in HIV prevalence (Hurley et al., 1997; MacDonald et al., 2003).

Opioid substitution therapy is largely based on the provision of methadone or a buprenorphine/naloxone combination (Vlahov et al., 2010). Methadone is a synthetic compound, which, although differing in structure from morphine, also has significant analgesic effects (Toombs & Kral, 2005). The drug may be administered by a variety of routes, but is most commonly applied orally or intravenously (Toombs & Kral, 2005), with oral administration favored for use in opioid substitution therapy (Doweiko, 2009). Methadone has two primary properties which make it useful in treatment of opioid addiction: first, it ameliorates the discomfort associated with withdrawal from the illicit drugs, and second, oral doses block the craving for opioids (Doweiko, 2009). The use of methadone provides the opportunity for the IDU to resume a more normal life, but must be accompanied by other supportive interventions to promote behavior change and integration into mainstream society. Combination of methadone treatment with needle exchange programs may be the most effective intervention for lowering incidence of HIV and other infections among IDUs (Van Den Berg et al., 2007).

Buprenorphine in combination with naloxone is also used in the treatment of IDUs; buprenorphine is a long-acting derivative of the morphine alkaloid thebaine which blocks the effects of morphine with infrequent induction of physical dependence (Jasinski et al., 1978; Ruiz et al., 2007). Although buprenorphine has poor oral bioavailability, it was thought important that it not be intravenously administered to former IDUs due to their previous abuse of injection equipment; the drug is therefore formulated as an oral tablet, either alone or in combination with naloxone (Ruiz et al., 2007). The addition of naloxone is intended to reduce the potential for abuse of buprenorphine (known as treatment "diversion"), since intravenously administered naloxone precipitates unpleasant withdrawal symptoms (Mendelson et al., 1996); naloxone has poor oral bioavailability and few effects when taken via this route (Walsh & Eissenberg, 2003).

Opioid substitution therapy has been shown to have significant positive effects in reducing HIV acquisition through reductions in both drug use and risky behaviors associated with injection drug use (Metzger et al., 1993; Metzger & Navaline, 2003). Refinements to treatment regimens are on-going, including the investigation of the possibility of treatment in physician's offices (Gunderson & Fiellin, 2008) (as opposed to in-program treatment) and contingent provision of treatment to be taken at home (Gerra et al., 2011).

3. Conclusion

Of the many trials of biomedical interventions to prevent sexual HIV acquisition completed, six to date have shown a statistically significant reduction in HIV incidence (three on male circumcision, one on STI control, one microbicide trial and one oral PrEP trial). Challenges encountered while testing these interventions included lack of appropriate animal models to measure safety and efficacy in pre-clinical testing (Dhawan & Mayer, 2006; Buckheit Jr et al., 2010), lack of appropriate measures of adherence to product use by participants (non-vaccine trials) (Tolley et al., 2009), the confounding effect of heterosexual anal sex (Mâsse et al., 2009), high pregnancy rates (Mâsse et al., 2009), and generally falling HIV incidence rates in countries where these efficacy trials are conducted (Ramjee et al., 2008). It is now widely accepted that a single biomedical intervention is unlikely to be 100% effective in preventing HIV acquisition, and all will have the potential to be confounded by risk compensation, poor adherence, and acceptability issues. The potential effectiveness of many biomedical prevention interventions tested to date is undermined by risk compensation - unintended changes in behaviour which arise from a change in the perception of risk. As Richens et al. describe it, introduction of a safety device could lead to a lowered perception of risk; the rewards of risk-taking are subsequently heightened and an increase in risky behaviour may result (Richens et al., 2000). This is a prime concern as we develop new biomedical HIV prevention tools.

There is currently a move towards the development, assessment and implementation of combination approaches to HIV prevention which will provide a combination of the effective interventions outlined in this chapter. Future research will focus on determining the most appropriate and effective elements for inclusion in combination packages targeted at different vulnerable population groups and risk profiles (i.e. single women, single men, couples, and young people). The combination approach may also require revision of traditional mechanisms for delivery of primary health care, particularly in resource-limited settings, since this will likely be the most feasible venue in which to introduce such integrated care options.

Despite recent successes in the HIV prevention field (microbicides and oral PrEP), there are numerous implementation challenges ahead. Confirmation of the positive results will be necessary before these new prevention modalities can be widely rolled out, whether that be alone or in combination with other interventions. However, there is now renewed hope that biomedical intervention coupled with behaviour change may turn the tide against new HIV infections worldwide.

4. References

Abdala, N., Gleghorn, A.A., Carney, J.M. & Heimer, R. (2001). Can HIV-1-contaminated syringes be disinfected?: Implications for transmission among injection drug users. *Journal of Acquired Immune Deficiency Syndromes* 28, 5: 487-494.

Abdala, N., Stephens, P.C., Griffith, B.P. & Heimer, R. (1999). Survival of HIV-1 in syringes. *Journal of Acquired Immune Deficiency Syndromes* 20, 1: 73-80.

Abdool Karim, Q., Abdool Karim, S.S., Frohlich, J.A., Grobler, A.C., Baxter, C., Mansoor, L.E., Kharsany, A.B.M., Sibeko, S., Mlisana, K.P., Omar, Z., Gengiah, T.N., Maarschalk, S., Arulappan, N., Mlotshwa, M., Morris, L., Taylor, D. & on behalf of the CAPRISA 004 Trial Group (2010). Effectiveness and safety of tenofovir gel, an antiretroviral microbicide, for the prevention of HIV infection in women. *Science* 329, 5996: 1168-1174

Abdool Karim, S.S., Richardson, B.A., Ramjee, G., Hoffman, I.F., Chirenje, Z.M., Taha, T., Kapina, M., Maslankowski, L., Coletti, A., Profy, A., Moench, T.R., Piwowar-Manning, E., Mâsse, B., Hillier, S.L., Soto-Torres, L. & on behalf of the HIV Prevention Trials Network 035 Study Team (2011). Safety and effectiveness of BufferGel and 0.5% PRO2000 gel for the prevention of HIV infection in women. *AIDS* ePublished Ahead of Print: 10.1097/QAD.1090b1013e32834541d32834549.

Ahmed, S., Lutalo, T., Wawer, M., Serwadda, D., Sewankambo, N.K., Nalugoda, F., Makumbi, F., Wabwire-Mangen, F., Kiwanuka, N., Kigozi, G., Kiddugavu, M. & Gray, R. (2001). HIV incidence and sexually transmitted disease prevalence associated with condom use: a population study in Rakai, Uganda. *AIDS* 15, 16: 2171-2179.

Amara, R.R., Villinger, F., Altman, J.D., Lydy, S.L., O'Neil, S.P., Staprans, S.I., Montefiori, D.C., Xu, Y., Herndon, J.G., Wyatt, L.S., Candido, M.A., Kozyr, N.L., Earl, P.L., Smith, J.M., Ma, H.-L., Grimm, B.D., Hulsey, M.L., Miller, J., McClure, H.M., McNicholl, J.M., Moss, B. & Robinson, H.L. (2001). Control of a mucosal challenge and prevention of AIDS by a multiprotein DNA/MVA vaccine. *Science* 292, 5514: 69-74.

Aravantinou, M., Kenney, J., Singer, R., Gettie, A., Lifson, J., Piatak Jr, M., Fernandez-Romero, J., Zydowsky, T., Blanchard, J. & Robbiani, M. (2010). Temporal association of protection by Carraguard-based gels containing MIV-150 after single versus repeated vaginal application in macaques [Abstract no. 38]. *Microbicides 2010*, Pittsburgh, Pennsylvania, USA, 22-25 May 2010.

Atkinson, W.L., Pickering, L.K., Schwartz, B., Weniger, B.G., Iskander, J.K. & Watson, J.C. (2002). General recommendations on immunization. *Morbidity and Mortality Weekly Report* 51, RR02: 1-36.

Auvert, B., Taljaard, D., Lagarde, E., Sobngwi-Tambekou, J., Sitta, R. & Puren, A. (2005). Randomized, controlled intervention trial of male circumcision for reduction of HIV infection risk: The ANRS 1265 trial. *PLoS Medicine* 2, 11: e298.

Bailey, R., Moses, S., Parker, C., Agot, K., Maclean, I., Krieger, J., Williams, C., Campbell, R. & Ndinya-Achola, J. (2007). Male circumcision for HIV prevention in young men in Kisumu, Kenya: A randomised controlled trial. *The Lancet* 369, 9562: 643-656.

Beksinska, M.E., Rees, H.V., Dickson-Tetteh, K.E., Mqoqi, N., Kleinschmidt, I. & McIntyre, J.A. (2001). Structural integrity of the female condom after multiple uses, washing, drying, and re-lubrication. *Contraception* 63, 1: 33-36.

Buchbinder, S., Mehrotra, D., Duerr, A., Fitzgerald, D., Mogg, R., Li, D., Gilbert, P., Lama, J., Marmor, M. & Delrio, C. (2008). Efficacy assessment of a cell-mediated immunity HIV-1 vaccine (the Step Study): A double-blind, randomised, placebo-controlled, test-of-concept trial. *The Lancet* 372, 9653: 1881-1893.

Buckheit Jr, R.W., Watson, K.M., Morrow, K.M. & Ham, A.S. (2010). Development of topical microbicides to prevent the sexual transmission of HIV. *Antiviral Research* 85, 1: 142-158.

Burton, D.R., Desrosiers, R.C., Doms, R.W., Koff, W.C., Kwong, P.D., Moore, J.P., Nabel, G.J., Sodroski, J., Wilson, I.A. & Wyatt, R.T. (2004). HIV vaccine design and the neutralizing antibody problem. *Nature Immunology* 5, 3: 233-236.

Carey, R.F., Herman, W.A., Retta, S.M., Rinaldi, J.E., Herman, B.A. & Athey, T.W. (1992). Effectiveness of latex condoms as a barrier to human immunodeficiency virus-sized particles under conditions of simulated use. *Sexually Transmitted Diseases* 19, 4: 230-234.

Celum, C., Wald, A., Hughes, J., Sanchez, J., Reid, S., Delany-Moretlwe, S., Cowan, F., Casapia, M., Ortiz, A. & Fuchs, J. (2008). Effect of aciclovir on HIV-1 acquisition in herpes simplex virus 2 seropositive women and men who have sex with men: A randomised, double-blind, placebo-controlled trial. *The Lancet* 371, 9630: 2109-2119.

Celum, C., Wald, A., Lingappa, J.R., Magaret, A.S., Wang, R.S., Mugo, N., Mujugira, A., Baeten, J.M., Mullins, J.I., Hughes, J.P., Bukusi, E.A., Cohen, C.R., Katabira, E., Ronald, A., Kiarie, J., Farquhar, C., Stewart, G.J., Makhema, J., Essex, M., Were, E., Fife, K.H., de Bruyn, G., Gray, G.E., McIntyre, J.A., Manongi, R., Kapiga, S., Coetzee, D., Allen, S., Inambao, M., Kayitenkore, K., Karita, E., Kanweka, W., Delany, S., Rees, H., Vwalika, B., Stevens, W., Campbell, M.S., Thomas, K.K., Coombs, R.W., Morrow, R., Whittington, W.L.H., McElrath, M.J., Barnes, L., Ridzon, R., Corey, L. & the Partners in Prevention HSV/HIV Transmission Study Team (2010). Acyclovir and transmission of HIV-1 from persons infected with HIV-1 and HSV-2. *New England Journal of Medicine* 362, 5: 427-439.

Chigwedere, P., Seage, G.R., Lee, T.-H. & Essex, M. (2008). Efficacy of antiretroviral drugs in reducing mother-to-child transmission of HIV in Africa: A meta-analysis of published clinical trials. *AIDS Research and Human Retroviruses* 24, 6: 827-837.

Chimbiri, A.M. (2007). The condom is an 'intruder' in marriage: Evidence from rural Malawi. *Social Science and Medicine* 64, 5: 1102-1115.

Chun, T.-W., Engel, D., Berrey, M.M., Shea, T., Corey, L. & Fauci, A.S. (1998). Early establishment of a pool of latently infected, resting CD4+ T cells during primary HIV-1 infection. *Proceedings of the National Academy of Sciences of the United States of America* 95, 15: 8869-8873.

Connor, E.M., Sperling, R.S., Gelber, R., Kiselev, P., Scott, G., O'Sullivan, M.J., VanDyke, R., Bey, M., Shearer, W., Jacobson, R.L., Jimenez, E., O'Neill, E., Bazin, B., Delfraissy, J.-F., Culnane, M., Coombs, R., Elkins, M., Moye, J., Stratton, P., Balsley, J. & The Pediatric AIDS Clinical Trials Group Protocol 076 Study Group (1994). Reduction of maternal-infant transmission of human immunodeficiency virus type 1 with zidovudine treatment. *New England Journal of Medicine* 331, 18: 1173-1180.

Coovadia, H., Jewkes, R., Barron, P., Sanders, D. & McIntyre, D. (2009). The health and health system of South Africa: Historical roots of current public health challenges. *The Lancet* 374, 9692: 817-834.

Copenhaver, M.M., Johnson, B.T., Lee, I.C., Harman, J.J. & Carey, M.P. (2006). Behavioral HIV risk reduction among people who inject drugs: Meta-analytic evidence of efficacy. *Journal of Substance Abuse Treatment* 31, 2: 163-171.

Crosby, R.A. & Holtgrave, D.R. (2006). Will sexual risk behaviour increase after being vaccinated for AIDS? *International Journal of STD & AIDS* 17, 3: 180-184.

D'Cruz, O.J. & Uckun, F.M. (2006). Dawn of non-nucleoside inhibitor-based anti-HIV microbicides. *Journal of Antimicrobial Chemotherapy* 57, 3: 411-423.

Davis, K.R. & Weller, S.C. (1999). The effectiveness of condoms in reducing heterosexual transmission of HIV. *Family Planning Perspectives* 31, 6: 272-279.

del Mar Pujades Rodríguez, M., Obasi, A., Mosha, F., Todd, J., Brown, D., Changalucha, J., Mabey, D., Ross, D., Grosskurth, H. & Hayes, R. (2002). Herpes simplex virus type 2 infection increases HIV incidence: A prospective study in rural Tanzania. *AIDS* 16, 3: 451-462.

Dhawan, D. & Mayer, K.H. (2006). Microbicides to prevent HIV transmission: Overcoming obstacles to chemical barrier protection. *The Journal of Infectious Diseases* 193, 1: 36-44.

Dinh, M.H., McRaven, M.D., Kelley, Z., Penugonda, S. & Hope, T.J. (2010). Keratinization of the adult male foreskin and implications for male circumcision. *AIDS* 24, 6: 899-906

Doweiko, H.E. (2009). *Concepts of Chemical Dependancy* (Seventh edition), Brooks/Cole Cengage Learning, Belmont.

Drew, W.L., Blair, M., Miner, R.C. & Conant, M. (1990). Evaluation of the virus permeability of a new condom for women. *Sexually Transmitted Diseases* 17, 2: 110-112.

Dunn, P.M. (1996). Dr Edward Jenner (1749-1823) of Berkeley, and vaccination against smallpox. *Archives of Disease in Childhood - Fetal and Neonatal Edition* 74, 1: F77-F78.

Epstein, H. (2008). AIDS and the irrational. *BMJ* 337: a2638.

Evans, A., Fletcher, P., Herrera, C. & Shattock, R. (2010). Protease inhibitors darunavir, lopinavir and ritonavir as potential microbicides [Abstract no. 24]. *Microbicides 2010*, Pittsburgh, Pennsylvania, USA, 22-25 May 2010.

Feldblum, P., Adeiga, A., Bakare, R., Wevill, S., Lendvay, A., Obadaki, F., Olayemi, M., Wang, L., Nanda, K. & Rountree, W. (2008). SAVVY vaginal gel (C31G) for prevention of HIV infection: A randomized controlled trial in Nigeria. *PLoS One* 3, 1: e1471.

Fleming, D.T. & Wasserheit, J.N. (1999). From epidemiological synergy to public health policy and practice: The contribution of other sexually transmitted diseases to sexual transmission of HIV infection. *Sexually Transmitted Infections* 75, 1: 3-17.

Fletcher, P., Herrera, C., Armanasco, N., Nuttall, J., Romano, J. & Shattock, R. (2010). Anti-HIV activity of the candidate microbicide maraviroc, a CCR5 receptor antagonist [Abstract no. 21]. *Microbicides 2010*, Pittsburgh, Pennsylvania, USA, 22-25 May 2010.

Flynn, N.M., Forthal, D.N., Harro, C.D., Judson, F.N., Mayer, K.H., Para, M.F. & rgp, H.I.V.V.S.G. (2005). Placebo-controlled phase 3 trial of a recombinant glycoprotein 120 vaccine to prevent HIV-1 infection. *The Journal of Infectious Diseases* 191, 5: 654-665.

Foss, A.M., Watts, C.H., Vickerman, P. & Heise, L. (2004). Condoms and prevention of HIV. *BMJ* 329, 7459: 185-186.

Freeman, E., Weiss, H., Glynn, J., Cross, P., Whitworth, J. & Hayes, R. (2006). Herpes simplex virus 2 infection increases HIV acquisition in men and women: Systematic review and meta-analysis of longitudinal studies. *AIDS* 20, 1: 73-83.

Gerra, G., Saenz, E., Busse, A., Maremmani, I., Ciccocioppo, R., Zaimovic, A., Gerra, M.L., Amore, M., Manfredini, M., Donnini, C. & Somaini, L. (2011). Supervised daily consumption, contingent take-home incentive and non-contingent take-home in methadone maintenance. *Progress in Neuro-Psychopharmacology and Biological Psychiatry* 35, 2: 483-489.

Ghys, P.D., Diallo, M.O., Ettiègne-Traoré, V., Satten, G.A., Anoma, C.K., Maurice, C., Kadjo, J.-C., Coulibaly, I.-M., Wiktor, S.Z., Greenberg, A.E. & Laga, M. (2001). Effect of interventions to control sexually transmitted disease on the incidence of HIV infection in female sex workers. *AIDS* 15, 11: 1421-1431.

Gilead (2008). *Emtriva package insert.*

Gilead (2010). *Viread package insert.*

Girard, M.P., Osmanov, S.K. & Kieny, M.P. (2006). A review of vaccine research and development: The human immunodeficiency virus (HIV). *Vaccine* 24, 19: 4062-4081.

Grant, R.M., Lama, J.R., Anderson, P.L., McMahan, V., Liu, A.Y., Vargas, L., Goicochea, P., Casapía, M., Guanira-Carranza, J.V., Ramirez-Cardich, M.E., Montoya-Herrera, O., Fernández, T., Veloso, V.G., Buchbinder, S.P., Chariyalertsak, S., Schechter, M., Bekker, L.-G., Mayer, K.H., Kallás, E.G., Amico, K.R., Mulligan, K., Bushman, L.R., Hance, R.J., Ganoza, C., Defechereux, P., Postle, B., Wang, F., McConnell, J.J., Zheng, J.-H., Lee, J., Rooney, J.F., Jaffe, H.S., Martinez, A.I., Burns, D.N. & Glidden, D.V. (2010). Preexposure chemoprophylaxis for HIV prevention in men who have sex with men. *New England Journal of Medicine* 363, 27: 2587-2599.

Gray, G., Allen, M., Bekker, L., Churchyard, G., Mlisana, K., Nchabeleng, M., Moodie, F., Metch, B. & Cassis-Ghavami, F. (2008). Results from the Phambili (HVTN 503) study: A multicenter double-blind placebo-controlled Phase IIB test-of-concept study to evaluate the safety and efficacy of the MRKad5 HIV-1 gag/pol/nef vaccine in HIV-1 uninfected South Africans. *AIDS Vaccine*, Cape Town, South Africa, 13-16 Ocober 2008.

Gray, R., Kigozi, G., Serwadda, D., Makumbi, F., Watya, S., Nalugoda, F., Kiwanuka, N., Moulton, L., Chaudhary, M. & Chen, M. (2007). Male circumcision for HIV prevention in men in Rakai, Uganda: A randomised trial. *The Lancet* 369, 9562: 657-666.

Grosskurth, H., Gray, R., Hayes, R., Mabey, D. & Wawer, M. (2000). Control of sexually transmitted diseases for HIV-1 prevention: Understanding the implications of the Mwanza and Rakai trials. *The Lancet* 355, 9219: 1981-1987.

Grosskurth, H., Todd, J., Mwijarubi, E., Mayaud, P., Nicoll, A., ka-Gina, G., Newell, J., Mabey, D., Hayes, R., Mosha, F., Senkoro, K., Changalucha, J., Klokke, A. & Mugeye, K. (1995). Impact of improved treatment of sexually transmitted diseases on HIV infection in rural Tanzania: Randomised controlled trial. *The Lancet* 346, 8974: 530-536.

Gunderson, E.W. & Fiellin, D.A. (2008). Office-based maintenance treatment of opioid dependence: How does it compare with traditional approaches? *CNS Drugs* 22: 99-111.

Halperin, D. & Epstein, H. (2007). Why is HIV prevalence so severe in southern Africa? The role of multiple concurrent partnerships and lack of male circumcision: Implications for AIDS prevention. *The Southern African Journal of HIV Medicine* 8: 19-25.

Hargreaves, J.R., Morison, L.A., Kim, J.C., Busza, J., Phetla, G., Porter, J.D., Watts, C. & Pronyk, P.M. (2009). Characteristics of sexual partnerships, not just of individuals, are associated with condom use and recent HIV infection in rural South Africa. *AIDS Care* 21, 8: 1058-1070.

Herrera, C., Armanasco, N., Fletcher, P., Nuttall, J., Romano, J. & Shattock, R. (2010). Combinations of maraviroc and reverse transcriptase inhibitors as potential microbicides [Abstract no. 22]. *Microbicides 2010*, Pittsburgh, Pennsylvania, USA, 22-25 May 2010.

Hladik, F. & Hope, T. (2009). HIV infection of the genital mucosa in women. *Current HIV/AIDS Reports* 6, 1: 20-28.

Ho, G.Y.F., Burk, R.D., Klein, S., Kadish, A.S., Chang, C.J., Palan, P., Basu, J., Tachezy, R., Lewis, R. & Romney, S. (1995). Persistent genital Human Papillomavirus infection as a risk factor for persistent cervical dysplasia. *Journal of the National Cancer Institute* 87, 18: 1365-1371.

Hoenig, L.J. (1986). Triumph and controversy: Pasteur's preventive treatment of rabies as reported in JAMA. *Archives of Neurology* 43, 4: 397-399.

Holmes, K., Levine, R. & Weaver, M. (2004). Effectiveness of condoms in preventing sexually transmitted infections. *Bulletin of the World Health Organization* 82: 454-461.

Holtzman, D., Barry, V., Ouellet, L.J., Jarlais, D.C.D., Vlahov, D., Golub, E.T., Hudson, S.M. & Garfein, R.S. (2009). The influence of needle exchange programs on injection risk behaviors and infection with hepatitis C virus among young injection drug users in select cities in the United States, 1994-2004. *Preventive Medicine* 49, 1: 68-73.

Hu, S.-L., Klaniecki, J., Dykers, T., Sridhar, P. & Travis, B.M. (1991). Neutralizing antibodies against HIV-1 BRU and SF2 isolates generated in mice immunized with recombinant vaccinia virus expressing HIV-1 (BRU) envelope glycoproteins and boosted with homologous gp160. *AIDS Research and Human Retroviruses* 7, 7: 615-620.

Hunter, M. (2007). The changing political economy of sex in South Africa: The significance of unemployment and inequalities to the scale of the AIDS pandemic. *Social Science and Medicine* 64, 3: 689-700.

Hurley, S.F., Jolley, D.J. & Kaldor, J.M. (1997). Effectiveness of needle-exchange programmes for prevention of HIV infection. *The Lancet* 349, 9068: 1797-1800.

Huskens, D., Vermeire, K., Profy, A.T. & Schols, D. (2009). The candidate sulfonated microbicide, PRO 2000, has potential multiple mechanisms of action against HIV-1. *Antiviral Research* 84, 1: 38-47.

Jasinski, D.R., Pevnick, J.S. & Griffith, J.D. (1978). Human pharmacology and abuse potential of the analgesic buprenorphine: A potential agent for treating narcotic addiction. *Archives of General Psychiatry* 35, 4: 501-516.

Jennings, R. & Clegg, A. (1993). The inhibitory effect of spermicidal agents on replication of HSV-2 and HIV-1 *in-vitro*. *Journal of Antimicrobial Chemotherapy* 32, 1: 71-82.

Johnston, M. & Fauci, A. (2007). An HIV vaccine--evolving concepts. *New England Journal of Medicine* 356, 20: 2073-2081.

Johnston, M.I. & Fauci, A.S. (2008). An HIV vaccine—challenges and prospects. *New England Journal of Medicine* 359, 9: 888-890.

Kamali, A., Quigley, M., Nakiyingi, J., Kinsman, J., Kengeya-Kayondo, J., Gopal, R., Ojwiya, A., Hughes, P., Carpenter, L. & Whitworth, J. (2003). Syndromic management of sexually-transmitted infections and behaviour change interventions on transmission of HIV-1 in rural Uganda: A community randomised trial. *The Lancet* 361, 9358: 645-652.

Kaul, R., Kimani, J., Nagelkerke, N.J., Fonck, K., Ngugi, E.N., Keli, F., MacDonald, K.S., Maclean, I.W., Bwayo, J.J., Temmerman, M., Ronald, A.R. & Moses, S. (2004). Monthly antibiotic chemoprophylaxis and incidence of sexually transmitted infections and HIV-1 infection in Kenyan sex workers: A randomized controlled trial. *JAMA* 291, 21: 2555-2562.

Kenney, J., Aravantinou, M., Singer, R., Hsu, M., Rodriguez, A., Kizima, L., Abraham, C.J., Menon, R., Seidor, S., Chudolij, A., Gettie, A., Blanchard, J., Lifson, J.D., Piatak, M., Jr., Fernández-Romero, J.A., Zydowsky, T.M. & Robbiani, M. (2011). An antiretroviral/zinc combination gel provides 24 hours of complete protection against vaginal SHIV infection in macaques. *PLoS One* 6, 1: e15835.

Kigozi, G., Wawer, M., Ssettuba, A., Kagaayi, J., Nalugoda, F., Watya, S., Mangen, F.W., Kiwanuka, N., Bacon, M.C., Lutalo, T., Serwadda, D. & Gray, R.H. (2009). Foreskin surface area and HIV acquisition in Rakai, Uganda (size matters). *AIDS* 23, 16: 2209-2213

Klausner, J.D., Wamai, R.G., Bowa, K., Agot, K., Kagimba, J. & Halperin, D.T. (2008). Is male circumcision as good as the HIV vaccine we've been waiting for? *Future HIV Therapy* 2, 1: 1-7.

Laga, M., Schwärtlander, B., Pisani, E., Sow, P.S. & Caraël, M. (2001). To stem HIV in Africa, prevent transmission to young women. *AIDS* 15: 931-934.

Lagakos, S.W. & Gable, A.R. (2008). Challenges to HIV prevention -- seeking effective measures in the absence of a vaccine. *New England Journal of Medicine* 358, 15: 1543-1545.

Lawson, M.L., Macaluso, M., Duerr, A., Hortin, G., Hammond, K.R., Blackwell, R., Artz, L. & Bloom, A. (2003). Partner characteristics, intensity of the intercourse, and semen exposure during use of the female condom. *American Journal of Epidemiology* 157, 4: 282-288.

Letvin, N.L., Mascola, J.R., Sun, Y., Gorgone, D.A., Buzby, A.P., Xu, L., Yang, Z.-y., Chakrabarti, B., Rao, S.S., Schmitz, J.E., Montefiori, D.C., Barker, B.R., Bookstein, F.L. & Nabel, G.J. (2006). Preserved CD4+ central memory T cells and survival in vaccinated SIV-challenged monkeys. *Science* 312, 5779: 1530-1533.

Lytle, D.C., Routson, L.B., Seaborn, G.B., Dixon, L.G., Bushar, H.F. & Cyr, H.W. (1997). An *in vitro* evaluation of condoms as barriers to a small virus. *Sexually Transmitted Diseases* 24, 3: 161-164.

Macaluso, M., Lawson, M.L., Hortin, G., Duerr, A., Hammond, K.R., Blackwell, R. & Bloom, A. (2003). Efficacy of the female condom as a barrier to semen during intercourse. *American Journal of Epidemiology* 157, 4: 289-297.

MacDonald, M., Law, M., Kaldor, J., Hales, J. & J. Dore, G. (2003). Effectiveness of needle and syringe programmes for preventing HIV transmission. *International Journal of Drug Policy* 14, 5-6: 353-357.

Mackie, N. & Coker, R. (2000). Post-exposure prophylaxis following non-occupational exposure to HIV: Risks, uncertainties, and ethics. *International Journal of STD & AIDS* 11, 7: 424-427.

Maharaj, P. & Cleland, J. (2004). Condom use within marital and cohabiting partnerships in KwaZulu-Natal, South Africa. *Studies in Family Planning* 35, 2: 116-124.

Malcolm, R.K., Edwards, K.-L., Kiser, P., Romano, J. & Smith, T.J. (2010). Advances in microbicide vaginal rings. *Antiviral Research* 88, Supplement 1: S30-S39.

Marais, D., Gawarecki, D., Rutenberg, N., Allan, B., Ahmed, K., Altini, L., Cassim, N., Gopolang, F., Hoffman, M. & Williamson, A.-L. (2010). Carraguard, a vaginal microbicide, protects women against HPV infection. *26th International Papillomavirus Conference & Clinical and Public Health Workshops*, Montréal, Canada, 3-8 July 2010.

Markel, H. (2005). The search for effective HIV vaccines. *New England Journal of Medicine* 353, 8: 753-757.

Mâsse, B., Boily, M.-C., Dimitrov, D. & Desai, K. (2009). Efficacy dilution in randomized placebo-controlled vaginal microbicide trials. *Emerging Themes in Epidemiology* 6, 1: 5.

McCoombe, S.G. & Short, R.V. (2006). Potential HIV-1 target cells in the human penis. *AIDS* 20, 11: 1491-1495

Mendelson, J., Jones, R.T., Fernandez, I., Welm, S., Melby, A.K. & Baggott, M.J. (1996). Buprenorphine and naloxone interactions in opiate-dependent volunteers. *Clinical Pharmacology and Therapeutics* 60, 1: 105-114.

Mesquita, P.M.M., Cheshenko, N., Wilson, S.S., Mhatre, M., Guzman, E., Fakioglu, E., Keller, M.J. & Herold, B.C. (2009). Disruption of tight junctions by cellulose sulfate facilitates HIV infection: Model of microbicide safety. *The Journal of Infectious Diseases* 200, 4: 599-608.

Metzger, D.S. & Navaline, H. (2003). Human immunodeficiency virus prevention and the potential of drug abuse treatment. *Clinical Infectious Diseases* 37, Supplement 5: S451-S456.

Metzger, D.S., Woody, G.E., McLellan, A.T., O'Brien, C.P., Druley, P., Navaline, H., DePhilippis, D., Stolley, P. & Abrutyn, E. (1993). Human immunodeficiency virus seroconversion among intravenous drug users in- and out-of-treatment: An 18-month prospective follow-up. *Journal of Acquired Immune Deficiency Syndromes* 6, 9: 1049-1056.

Miller, C., Alexander, N., Gettie, A., Hendrickx, A. & Marx, P. (1992). The effect of contraceptives containing nonoxynol-9 on the genital transmission of simian immunodeficiency virus in rhesus macaques. *Fertility and Sterility* 57, 5: 1126-1128.

Millett, G.A., Flores, S.A., Marks, G., Reed, J.B. & Herbst, J.H. (2008). Circumcision status and risk of HIV and sexually transmitted infections among men who have sex with men. *JAMA* 300, 14: 1674-1684.

Moench, T.R., Whaley, K.J., Mandrell, T.D., Bishop, B.D., Witt, C.J. & Cone, R.A. (1993). The cat/feline immunodeficiency virus model for transmucosal transmission of AIDS: Nonoxynol-9 contraceptive jelly blocks transmission by an infected cell inoculum. *AIDS* 7, 6: 797-802.

Ndesendo, V., Pillay, V., Choonara, Y., Buchmann, E., Bayever, D. & Meyer, L. (2008). A review of current intravaginal drug delivery approaches employed for the prophylaxis of HIV/AIDS and prevention of sexually transmitted infections. *AAPS PharmSciTech* 9, 2: 505-520.

Newman, P.A., Duan, N., Rudy, E.T. & Johnston-Roberts, K. (2004). HIV risk and prevention in a post-vaccine context. *Vaccine* 22, 15-16: 1954-1963.

Nobbenhuis, M.A.E., Walboomers, J.M.M., Helmerhorst, T.J.M., Rozendaal, L., Remmink, A.J., Risse, E.K.J., van der Linden, H.C., Voorhorst, F.J., Kenemans, P. & Meijer, C.J.L.M. (1999). Relation of human papilloma virus status to cervical lesions and consequences for cervical-cancer screening: A prospective study. *The Lancet* 354, 9172: 20-25.

Padian, N., van der Straten, A., Ramjee, G., Chipato, T., de Bruyn, G., Blanchard, K., Shiboski, S., Montgomery, E., Fancher, H. & Cheng, H. (2007). Diaphragm and lubricant gel for prevention of HIV acquisition in southern African women: A randomised controlled trial. *The Lancet* 370, 9583: 251-261.

Padian, N.S., Buvé, A., Balkus, J., Serwadda, D. & Cates Jr, W. (2008). Biomedical interventions to prevent HIV infection: Evidence, challenges, and way forward. *The Lancet* 372, 9638: 585-599.

Park, L.S., Siraprapasiri, T., Peerapatanapokin, W., Manne, J., Niccolai, L. & Kunanusont, C. (2010). HIV transmission rates in Thailand: Evidence of HIV prevention and transmission decline. *Journal of Acquired Immune Deficiency Syndromes* 54, 4: 430-436

Patterson, B.K., Landay, A., Siegel, J.N., Flener, Z., Pessis, D., Chaviano, A. & Bailey, R.C. (2002). Susceptibility to human immunodeficiency virus-1 infection of human foreskin and cervical tissue grown in explant culture. *American Journal of Pathology* 161, 3: 867-873.

Patton, D.L., Sweeney, Y.T. & Paul, K.J. (2009). A summary of preclinical topical microbicide rectal safety and efficacy evaluations in a pigtailed macaque model. *Sexually Transmitted Diseases* 36, 6: 350-356.

Paxton, L., Hope, T. & Jaffe, H. (2007). Pre-exposure prophylaxis for HIV infection: What if it works? *The Lancet* 370, 9581: 89-93.

Peters, A., Jansen, W. & van Driel, F. (2010). The female condom: The international denial of a strong potential. *Reproductive Health Matters* 18, 35: 119-128.

Peterson, L., Nanda, K., Opoku, B.K., Ampofo, W.K., Owusu-Amoako, M., Boakye, A.Y., Rountree, W., Troxler, A., Dominik, R., Roddy, R. & Dorflinger, L. (2007). SAVVY® (C31G) gel for prevention of HIV infection in women: A phase 3, double-blind, randomized, placebo-controlled trial in Ghana. *PLoS One* 2, 12: e1312.

Pilcher, C.D., Tien, H.C., Eron Jr, J.J., Vernazza, P.L., Leu, S.Y., Stewart, P.W., Goh, L.E. & Cohen, M.S. (2004). Brief but efficient: Acute HIV infection and the sexual transmission of HIV. *The Journal of Infectious Diseases* 189, 10: 1785-1792.

Pinkerton, S. & Abramson, P.R. (1997). Effectiveness of condoms in preventing HIV transmission. *Social Science and Medicine* 44, 9: 1303-1312.

Pitisuttithum, P., Gilbert, P., Gurwith, M., Heyward, W., Martin, M., van Griensven, F., Hu, D., Tappero, J. & Choopanya, K. (2006). Randomized, double-blind, placebo-controlled efficacy trial of a bivalent recombinant glycoprotein 120 HIV-1 vaccine among injection drug users in Bangkok, Thailand. *The Journal of Infectious Diseases* 194, 12: 1661-1671.

Polsky, B., Baron, P., Gold, J.M., Smith, J., Jensen, R. & Armstrong, D. (1988). *In vitro* inactivation of HIV-1 by contraceptive sponge containing nonoxynol-9. *The Lancet* 331, 8600: 1456-1456.

Pudney, J., Quayle, A.J. & Anderson, D.J. (2005). Immunological microenvironments in the human vagina and cervix: Mediators of cellular immunity are concentrated in the cervical transformation zone. *Biology of Reproduction* 73, 6: 1253-1263.

Ramjee, G., Kamali, A. & McCormack, S. (2010). The last decade of microbicide clinical trials in Africa: From hypothesis to facts. *AIDS* 24, Suppl 4: S40-S49.

Ramjee, G., Kapiga, S., Weiss, S., Peterson, L., Leburg, C., Kelly, C., Mâsse, B. & HPTN Study Team (2008). The value of site preparedness studies for future implementation of phase 2/IIb/III HIV prevention trials - Experience from the HPTN 055 study. *Journal of Acquired Immune Deficiency Syndromes* 47, 1: 93-100.

Ramjee, G., van der Straten, A., Chipato, T., de Bruyn, G., Blanchard, K., Shiboski, S., Cheng, H., Montgomery, E., Padian, N. & for the, M.t. (2008). The diaphragm and lubricant gel for prevention of cervical sexually transmitted infections: Results of a randomized controlled trial. *PLoS One* 3, 10: e3488.

Rebbapragada, A. & Kaul, R. (2007). More than their sum in your parts: The mechanisms that underpin the mutually advantageous relationship between HIV and sexually transmitted infections. *Drug Discovery Today: Disease Mechanisms* 4, 4: 237-246.

Rerks-Ngarm, S., Pitisuttithum, P., Nitayaphan, S., Kaewkungwal, J., Chiu, J., Paris, R., Premsri, N., Namwat, C., de Souza, M., Adams, E., Benenson, M., Gurunathan, S., Tartaglia, J., McNeil, J.G., Francis, D.P., Stablein, D., Birx, D.L., Chunsuttiwat, S., Khamboonruang, C., Thongcharoen, P., Robb, M.L., Michael, N.L., Kunasol, P., Kim, J.H. & the MOPH-TAVEG Investigators (2009). Vaccination with ALVAC and AIDSVAX to prevent HIV-1 infection in Thailand. *New England Journal of Medicine* 361, 23: 2209-2220.

Richens, R., Imrie, J. & Copas, A. (2000). Condoms and seat belts: The parallels and the lessons. *The Lancet* 355, 9201: 400-403.

Richman, D.D., Wrin, T., Little, S.J. & Petropoulos, C.J. (2003). Rapid evolution of the neutralizing antibody response to HIV type 1 infection. *Proceedings of the National Academy of Sciences of the United States of America* 100, 7: 4144-4149.

Rojanapithayakorn, W. & Hanenberg, R. (1996). The 100% condom program in Thailand. *AIDS* 10, 1: 1-8.

Ruiz, P., Strain, E.C. & Langrod, J. (2007). *The Substance Abuse Handbook* Lippincott Williams & Wilkins, Philadelphia.

Shapshak, P., McCoy, C.B., Shah, S.M., Page, J.B., Rivers, J.E., Weatherby, N.L., Chitwood, D.D. & Mash, D.C. (1994). Preliminary laboratory studies of inactivation of HIV-1 in needles and syringes containing infected blood using undiluted household bleach. *Journal of Acquired Immune Deficiency Syndromes* 7, 7: 754-759.

Skoler-Karpoff, S., Ramjee, G., Ahmed, K., Altini, L., Plagianos, M., Friedland, B., Govender, S., Dekock, A., Cassim, N. & Palanee, T. (2008). Efficacy of Carraguard for prevention of HIV infection in women in South Africa: A randomised, double-blind, placebo-controlled trial. *The Lancet* 372, 9654: 1977-1987.

Stein, Z.A. (1990). HIV prevention: The need for methods women can use. *American Journal of Public Health* 80, 4: 460-462.

Stoneburner, R. & Low-Beer, D. (2004). Population-level HIV declines and behavioral risk avoidance in Uganda. *Science* 304, 5671: 714-718.

Templeton, D.J., Jin, F., Mao, L., Prestage, G.P., Donovan, B., Imrie, J., Kippax, S., Kaldor, J.M. & Grulich, A.E. (2009). Circumcision and risk of HIV infection in Australian homosexual men. *AIDS* 23, 17: 2347-2351

Tobian, A.A.R., Serwadda, D., Quinn, T.C., Kigozi, G., Gravitt, P.E., Laeyendecker, O., Charvat, B., Ssempijja, V., Riedesel, M. & Oliver, A.E. (2009). Male circumcision for the prevention of HSV-2 and HPV infections and syphilis. *New England Journal of Medicine* 360, 13: 1298-1309.

Tolley, E.E., Harrison, P.F., Goetghebeur, E., Morrow, K., Pool, R., Taylor, D., Tillman, S.N. & van der Straten, A. (2009). Adherence and its measurement in phase 2/3 microbicide trials. *AIDS and Behavior* 14, 5: 1124-1136.

Toombs, J.D. & Kral, L.A. (2005). Methadone treatment for pain states. *American Family Physician* 71, 7: 1353-1358.

UNAIDS (2010). *Report on the global AIDS epidemic 2010* Joint United Nations Programme on HIV/AIDS, Geneva.

van Damme, L., Ramjee, G., Alary, M., Vuylsteke, B., Chandeying, V., Rees, H., Sirivongrangson, P., Tshibaka, L., Ettiegnetraore, V. & Uaheowitchai, C. (2002). Effectiveness of COL-1492, a nonoxynol-9 vaginal gel, on HIV-1 transmission in female sex workers: A randomised controlled trial. *The Lancet* 360, 9338: 971-977.

Van Den Berg, C., Smit, C., Van Brussel, G., Coutinho, R. & Prins, M. (2007). Full participation in harm reduction programmes is associated with decreased risk for human immunodeficiency virus and hepatitis C virus: Evidence from the Amsterdam Cohort Studies among drug users. *Addiction* 102, 9: 1454-1462.

van Sighem, A., Gras, L., Reiss, P., Brinkman, K., de Wolf, F. & on behalf of the ATHENA national observational cohort study (2010). Life expectancy of recently diagnosed asymptomatic HIV-infected patients approaches that of uninfected individuals. *AIDS* 24, 10: 1527-1535

Vermund, S.H., Allen, K.L. & Karim, Q.A. (2009). HIV-prevention science at a crossroads: Advances in reducing sexual risk. *Current Opinion in HIV and AIDS* 4, 4: 266-273.

Vijayakumar, G., Mabude, Z., Smit, J., Beksinska, M. & Lurie, M. (2006). A review of female-condom effectiveness: Patterns of use and impact on protected sex acts and STI incidence. *International Journal of STD & AIDS* 17, 10: 652-659.

Vlahov, D., Robertson, Angela M. & Strathdee, Steffanie A. (2010). Prevention of HIV infection among injection drug users in resource-limited settings. *Clinical Infectious Diseases* 50, S3: S114-S121.

Walsh, S.L. & Eissenberg, T. (2003). The clinical pharmacology of buprenorphine: Extrapolating from the laboratory to the clinic. *Drug and Alcohol Dependence* 70, 2, Supplement 1: S13-S27.

Warren, M. & Philpott, A. (2003). Expanding safer sex options: Introducing the female condom into national programmes. *Reproductive Health Matters* 11, 21: 130-139.

Wasserheit, J.N. (1992). Epidemiological synergy: Interrelationships between human immunodeficiency virus infection and other sexually transmitted diseases. *Sexually Transmitted Diseases* 19, 2: 61-77.

Watson-Jones, D., Weiss, H.A., Rusizoka, M., Changalucha, J., Baisley, K., Mugeye, K., Tanton, C., Ross, D., Everett, D., Clayton, T., Balira, R., Knight, L., Hambleton, I., Le Goff, J., Belec, L. & Hayes, R. (2008). Effect of herpes simplex suppression on incidence of HIV among women in Tanzania. *New England Journal of Medicine* 358, 15: 1560-1571.

Wawer, M., Makumbi, F., Kigozi, G., Serwadda, D., Watya, S., Nalugoda, F., Buwembo, D., Ssempijja, V., Kiwanuka, N. & Moulton, L. (2009). Circumcision in HIV-infected men and its effect on HIV transmission to female partners in Rakai, Uganda: A randomised controlled trial. *The Lancet* 374, 9685: 229-237.

Wawer, M.J., Tobian, A.A.R., Kigozi, G., Kong, X., Gravitt, P.E., Serwadda, D., Nalugoda, F., Makumbi, F., Ssempiija, V., Sewankambo, N., Watya, S., Eaton, K.P., Oliver, A.E., Chen, M.Z., Reynolds, S.J., Quinn, T.C. & Gray, R.H. (2011). Effect of circumcision of HIV-negative men on transmission of human papillomavirus to HIV-negative women: A randomised trial in Rakai, Uganda. *The Lancet* 377, 9761: 209-218.

Weiss, H., Quigley, M. & Hayes, R. (2000). Male circumcision and risk of HIV infection in sub-Saharan Africa: A systematic review and meta-analysis. *AIDS* 14, 15: 2361.

Weiss, H.A., Thomas, S.L., Munabi, S.K. & Hayes, R.J. (2006). Male circumcision and risk of syphilis, chancroid, and genital herpes: A systematic review and meta-analysis. *Sexually Transmitted Infections* 82, 2: 101-110.

Weller, S. & Davis-Beaty, K. (2002). Condom effectiveness in reducing heterosexual HIV transmission. *Cochrane Database of Systematic Reviews*, 1.

Wiessing, L., Likatavicius, G., Klempova, D., Hedrich, D., Nardone, A. & Griffiths, P. (2009). Associations between availability and coverage of HIV-prevention measures and subsequent incidence of diagnosed HIV infection among injection drug users. *American Journal of Public Health* 99, 6: 1049-1052.

Williams, B.G., Lloyd-Smith, J.O., Gouws, E., Hankins, C., Getz, W.M., Hargrove, J., de Zoysa, I., Dye, C. & Auvert, B. (2006). The potential impact of male circumcision on HIV in sub-Saharan Africa. *PLoS Medicine* 3, 7: e262.

Wodak, A. & Cooney, A. (2005). Effectiveness of sterile needle and syringe programmes. *The International journal on drug policy* 16: 31-44.

Wyatt, R. & Sodroski, J. (1998). The HIV-1 envelope glycoproteins: Fusogens, antigens, and immunogens. *Science* 280, 5371: 1884-1888.

3

Physiological Cybernetics: An Old-Novel Approach for Students in Biomedical Systems

Alberto Landi, Marco Laurino and Paolo Piaggi
University of Pisa, Italy

1. Introduction

Wiener in a seminal book (Wiener, 1948) associated the ancient Greek word 'κυβερνητικος' to the control of physiological systems. "Thus, as far back as four years ago, the group of scientists about Dr. Rosenblueth and myself had already become aware of the essential unity of the set of problems centering about communication, control and statistical mechanics, whether in the machine or in the living tissue. [...] We have decided to call the entire field [...] by the name Cybernetics, which we form from the Greek κυβερνητης or steersman. In choosing this term, we wish to recognize that the first significant paper on feed-back mechanisms is an article on governors, which was published by Clerk Maxwell in 1868 and that governor is derived from a Latin corruption of κυβερνητης. We also wish to refer to the fact that the steering engines of a ship are indeed one of the earliest and best developed forms of feed-back mechanisms."

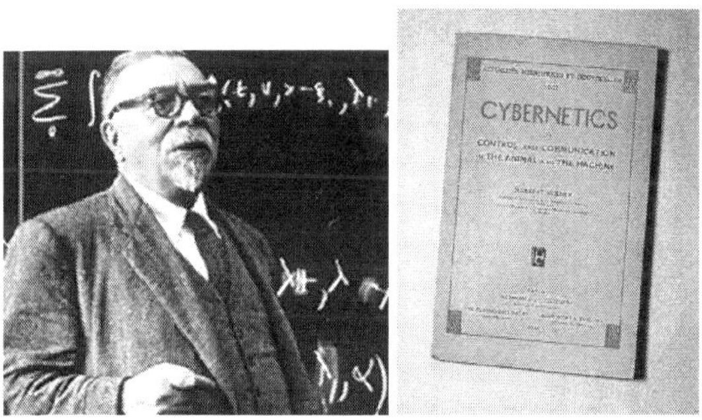

Fig. 1. Norbert Wiener (1894-1964) and his book on cybernetics

The increasing knowledge in each sector of science led to a huge diversification of scientific research, especially in a borderline sector like cybernetics applied to physiological systems. A first problem to solve was the following: let's suppose that two groups, one with a control engineering experience and the other one with a medical background (e.g., physicians), decide to cooperate, because they strongly believe that a joined research could be useful for developing mathematical and statistical models. Usually physicians do not have enough time to study and apply advanced modelling.

Wiener approached the communication between scientists belonging to different disciplines: "If a physiologist, who knows no mathematics, works together with a mathematician, who knows no physiology, the one will be unable to state his problem in terms that the other can manipulate, and the second will be unable to put the answers in any form that the first can understand. [...] The mathematician need not have the skill to conduct a physiological experiment, but he must have the skill to understand one, to criticize one, and to suggest one. The physiologist need not be able to prove a certain mathematical theorem, but he must be able to grasp its physiological significance and to tell the mathematician for what he should look."

A correct interaction in terms of a clear communication and reciprocal comprehension of the objectives of the research activity between groups with different competences is a crucial aspect in any interdisciplinary research.

In 2003 at the University of Pisa it was decided to introduce a new course for undergraduate students in biomedical engineering, based on the Wiener 'utopia', in order to teach a novel discipline useful for helping biomedical students to communicate and cooperate effectively with physicians. We named this new course as Physiological Cybernetics, remembering the old Wiener definition.

The organization of this course was a difficult task, and it required to gain experience in order to integrate so different disciplines and to produce a common language between students in biomedical engineer and physicians. At a first glance this attempt seemed to be too ambitious, because the different approaches of biomedical engineers with respect to physicians seemed incompatible and even the languages of the two groups were so different to remember the Babel tower…

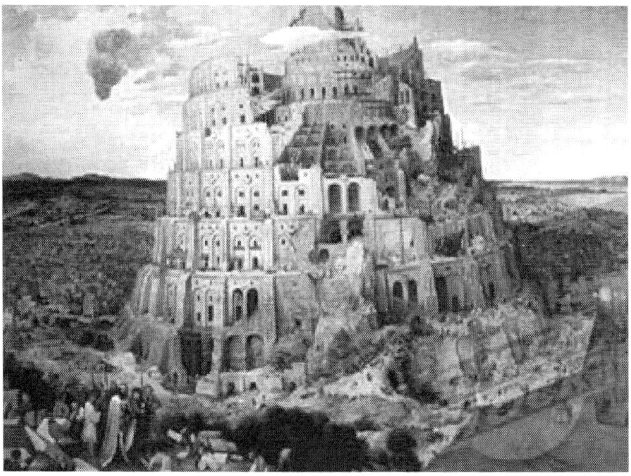

Fig. 2. Tower of Babel (1563) Pieter Bruegel the Elder, Oil on Wood Panel - Kunsthistorisches Museum, Vienna, Austria.

A great deal of effort and attention was required to produce appealing and stimulating lectures, but after many years we can affirm that this challenge is successful, especially for the enthusiastic answers of the students: their number was increasing year after year (about seventy students per year are now attending the course).

A strict and trusted cooperation between different groups of physicians is growing up and several groups of physicians belonging to different medical fields are going to join us for new interactions.

The aim of this chapter is to describe how the approach to physiological cybernetics has led to integrate academic lessons with research activities. To be more specific, the basic idea of Physiological Cybernetics was to search for models able to emulate physiological systems based on the feedback theory and/or the system theory.

In fact, recently, the widespread use of friendly software packages for modelling, along with the development of powerful identification and control techniques has led to a renewed interest in control (Khoo, 2011; Hoppensteadt & Peskin, 2002; Cobelli & Carson, 2008) and identification (Westwick & Kearney, 2003) of physiological systems. Unfortunately physiological systems are intrinsically time variant and highly non linear. Moreover, an effective balance of the model complexity is a difficult task: low order models are usually too simple to be useful, on the other hand high order models are too complex for simulation purposes and they have too many unknown parameters to be identified.

Each model selected for investigation was studied by a group of biomedical students supervised by physicians. Each model required several iterations and reformulations, due to the continuous adjustment of the research objectives, changing their final horizon, because of the gap between experimental data and theoretical models, so that the answers to the doubts and questions were continuously moving with the obtained partial results.

A final goal of the research was to apply a mathematical framework for helping medical diagnostic techniques and for testing new therapeutic protocols.

The procedure of model extraction followed two main pathways: the first one (pathway A) led to a formulation of a mathematical model usually based on differential equations and on an as deep as possible insight into physiological mechanisms (Marmarelis, 2004; Ottesen et al., 2004; Edelstein-Keshet, 2005; Jones et al., 2009) via a physical description of the system.

The second one (pathway B) was founded on a model description based on a black-box and data-driven identification (Westwick & Kearney, 2003; Cobelli & Carson, 2008), usually leaving to stochastic models with a parametric or non-parametric structure (Ljung, 1987), depending on the a-priori knowledge of constitutive laws governing the observed system.

In this paper we will describe two examples of research activity based on the Physiological Cybernetics, both of them addressed to produce a biomedical framework for predicting the effects of therapeutic actions, but following the two different pathways. The first example follows a statistical non parametric approach, the second one a mathematical model based on differential equations

2. Therapies in obese patients: A statistical approach

In 2004, some lessons of the Physiological Cybernetics course were addressed to describe metabolic dynamics of thyroid hormones T_3 and T_4.

It was an emblematical example regarding physiological feedback theory, intrinsically embedded inside human body.

We decided to focus some lessons on the model presented by Di Stefano et al. (1975), in an interesting paper, showing how this hormonal regulatory system could be described in terms of differential equations. This item was so intriguing for students, to require the support of physicians belonging to the Department of Endocrinology and Metabolism of the University of Pisa, in order to gain a better understanding of the physiology related to the

feedback regulation of thyroid hormones. It was a representative example of pathway A, typical of classic physiological feedback, with a controller -the thyroid gland- embedded in the human body.
One of the physicians proposed a different challenging test to students: how to model another pathology with growing interest in endocrinology, i.e. the obesity?
This challenge was very complex and unsolved from a mathematical viewpoint. It was a classical example of Babel tower, because what physicians expected from us was impossible to be fulfilled in a deterministic framework, similar to the approach leading to the thyroid model.
First, we tried to consider differential equations for modelling dynamics of hormones, like leptin and ghrelin, playing an important role in controlling our weight, but the results obtained were too qualitative, simple and poor to mimic the multi-factorial aspects of obesity. It seemed to be a failed attempt, because it produced a useless model.
Hence we decided to change our approach to the challenge: if a deterministic model was inadequate, a data-driven black box model could be an alternative solution and we decided to follow pathway B. We came to the conclusion that the first and reachable step for coping with obesity was to build an interactive, user-friendly and graphically oriented toolbox for classifying obese patients. Therefore a SW tool, named Obefix, was developed for helping physicians in the classification of obese patients from physiological and psychological data.
Obefix program (Landi et al., 2007) was designed in order to produce an easy-to-use software tool for capturing all essential information on the patients using a reduced data set, solving the problem related to the high data dimensionality.

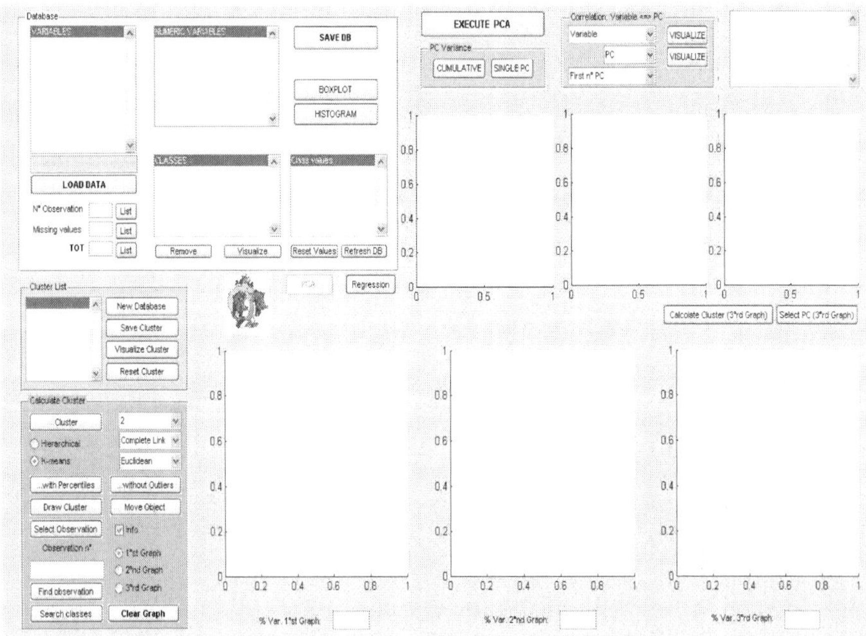

Fig. 3. Obefix window for a classification of obese patients: the interface

An interesting outcome was that this software tool was able to classify patients in a limited and user-selected number of clusters.
Consider to analyze a numerous group of patients. First Obefix's user may use the toolbox for searching a blind unsupervised partition of the treated data in different clusters, using a reduced set of variables, valuable for a correct classification of the patients.
After this first step, a supervised action is possible: physicians, after an evaluation of the unsupervised classification, can ask Obefix to repeat the analysis on a restricted subset of the initial individuals, in order to eventually exclude out-of-range patients (the outliers).
In this framework, physicians can easily load data, select variables of interest, run a fast analysis and visualize results. Clusters are represented in planes, the principal planes, and single patients can be followed, automatically classified as belonging to a cluster, and grouped in Excel spreadsheets.
Obefix employs PCA (Principal Component Analysis) (Jolliffe, 2002) as an engineering statistical tool for reducing data dimensionality: users can then select either hierarchical or k-means clustering methods, for classification of patients on selected principal planes.
A clinical example of Obefix application was presented in Landi et al., (2007) the case study was the *a-posteriori* analysis of a dataset of severe obese women, submitted to adjustable gastric banding surgery. Obese individuals were initially candidate for gastric bariatric surgery; a presurgical preparation included also psychological evaluation.
At first, Obefix toolbox was applied for a multiple regression analysis (Mardia et al., 1979) with delta BMI (variation of the Body Mass Index expressed in %) six months after the gastric banding surgery as a dependent variable, associated with changes in pre-operative psychological data tests as independent variables.
The administrated questionnaire included 567 statements and subjects had to answer "true" or "false" according to what was predominantly true or false for them. It must be remarked that these results have been obtained using only psychological data and that in the literature the quantitative extraction of effective similarities in groups of patients in the case of a so complex and multi-factorial pathology is considered a critical and unsolved problem.
Three main homogeneous clusters were identified, representing subgroups of patients with working problems, with antisocial personality disorder and with obsessive-compulsive disorder. A strict correlation was statistically verified between the variations of BMI six months after surgery with the patients belonging to each subgroup.
All conclusions regarding the similarities between individuals belonging to different clusters were in a good accordance with medical experience and with clinical literature.
Since Obefix development was considered a winning experience, we proceeded toward a following step, more interesting for the aims of the physiological cybernetics, i.e., produce and use a model able not only to classify the patients, but also to predict individual therapeutic outcome in terms of Excess Weight Loss (EWL, another common index for evaluating the loss of weight) after two years from surgery, using a set of pre-surgical data.
To be clearer, the more interesting aspect of this research was to set up a software tool able to predict the effects of a therapy and to address clinical researchers in choosing the patients that will maximally benefit from surgery.
A success in this task could represent the demonstration that the novel vision of Wiener was not a utopia, but a first example of dream coming true.
The research was again addressed to the study of the loss of weight for patients submitted to adjustable gastric banding surgery, because it was intriguing to consider a case study characterized by a high level of uncertainty in the prediction of long term effects.

Nowadays, in the medical literature it is still debated which categories of patients are better suited to this type of bariatric procedure and the selection of candidates for gastric banding surgery doesn't follows standardized guidelines.

In order to create a predictive model, the use of Artificial Neural Networks (ANNs) (Bishop, 1995; Rojas, 1996) appeared to be the best solution for predicting the weight loss after bariatric surgery, with respect to more traditional and used mathematical tools, e.g., the multiple linear regression. Therefore, a particular ANN was developed (see Figure 4) to improve the predictability of the linear model using a multi-layer Perceptron (MLP) with non linear activation functions (Rumelhart et al., 1986).

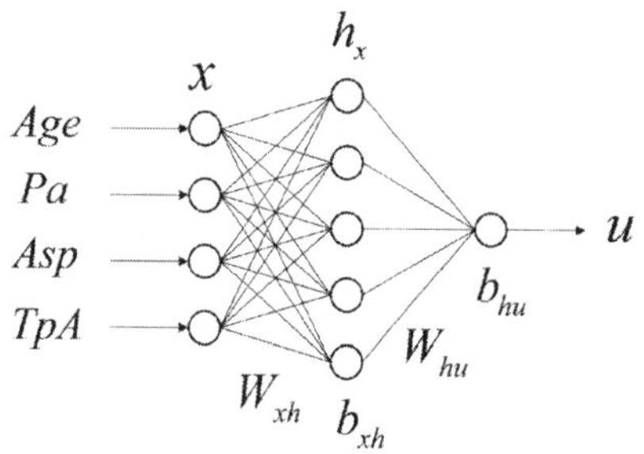

Fig. 4. Architecture of the MLP model for calculating non linear WL predictive score u

A preliminary study on the feasibility of the statistical approach for obese patients was presented in Landi et al., (2010) while, a paper considering the application of ANNs in the outcome prediction of adjustable gastric banding in obese women was published in Piaggi et al., (2010).

In the following, an outline on the engineering approach to this predictive tool is briefly sketched.

The first step was to select the most significant predictors of long term weight loss (the dependent variable) among the psychological scales, age and pre-surgical BMI (independent variables) (Van Hout et al., 2005).

In order to choose the most predictive inputs of a ANN with a limited data set and several potential predictors, a best-subset algorithm based on multiple linear regression (Neter, 1975) was employed. Namely, all combinations of the independent variables (subsets including from one to four variables, in order to avoid over-fitted solutions due to a large number of parameters, with respect to observations) were separately considered as models for computing the best linear fit of the dependent variable.

The best predictive subset was selected from all these models as that with the highest adjusted R^2 and a p-value less than 0.05.

The result was that age and the three psychological scales Paranoia - Pa, Antisocial practices - Asp and type-A behaviour - TpA constituted the best subset, and a predicted weight loss (WL) score was estimated through the formula

$$WL = -0.15 \cdot Age - 0.24 \cdot Pa - 0.26 \cdot Asp + 0.18 \cdot TpA \tag{1}$$

based on the linear combination of their regression coefficients, i.e., regression coefficients of (1) were a measure of the linear relationship between each independent variable and WL.

A non linear model was then built upon the same variables: the aim was to increase the goodness of prediction, taking advantage of ANNs data fitting capability.
For doing this, the four selected variables were used as inputs of a standard MLP for obtaining a non linear predictive score named u (see Figure 5).

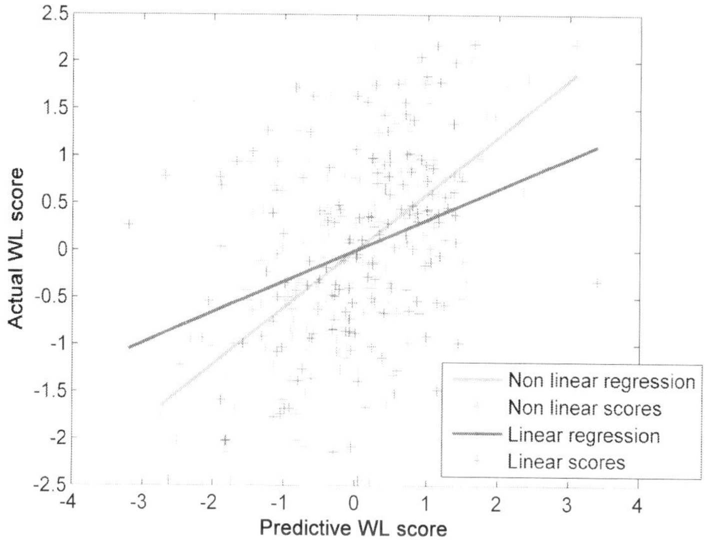

Fig. 5. Figure shows predicted WL on x-axis versus actual WL on y-axis. A comparison between the non linear (green solid line) and linear (red solid line) regressions show the better fit in the non linear case

A non linear activation function (i.e., the hyperbolic tangent function) was employed at the hidden layer units of the MLP to obtain a non linear combination of the inputs, as following:

$$h_x = tanh\left(W_{xh} \cdot x + b_{xh}\right) \tag{2}$$

This ANN architecture extended the regression performance of the previous linear model, which can be still obtained by replacing the nonlinear activation functions with the identity functions in the MLP, removing the nonlinear capability of the model.
The u score was then obtained as:

$$u = W_{hu} \cdot h_x + b_{hu} \tag{3}$$

The global cost function - minimized by the ANN training process - was based on the correlation between u and WL scores, including their standardization terms, as following:

$$J_m = -corr(u, WL) + \langle u \rangle + \langle WL \rangle + \sqrt{\langle u^2 \rangle - 1} + \sqrt{\langle WL^2 \rangle - 1} \tag{4}$$

In this way, the ANN found the optimal values of weights (W_{xh} and W_{hu}) and bias (b_{xh} and b_{hu}), which accounted the maximum correlation between the two scores.

The non linear solution accounted for 36% of WL variance, significantly higher than 10% of the linear model using the same independent variables: this indicated a better fit for the non linear model.
Furthermore, subjects were assigned to different groups according to actual WL quartiles in order to evaluate the classification (ROC curves) and prediction (cross-validation) capabilities of the estimated models. In Figure 6, the sensitivity and specificity of both models in relation to WL outcome are plotted for each possible cut-off in the so-called ROC curves and the Area Under each ROC Curve (AUC) is estimated. AUC measures the discriminating accuracy of the model, i.e., the ability of the model to correctly classify patients in their actual quartile of WL.
As a result, the non linear model achieved better results in terms of accuracy and mis-classification rates (70% and 30% vs. 66% and 34%, respectively) than the linear model.

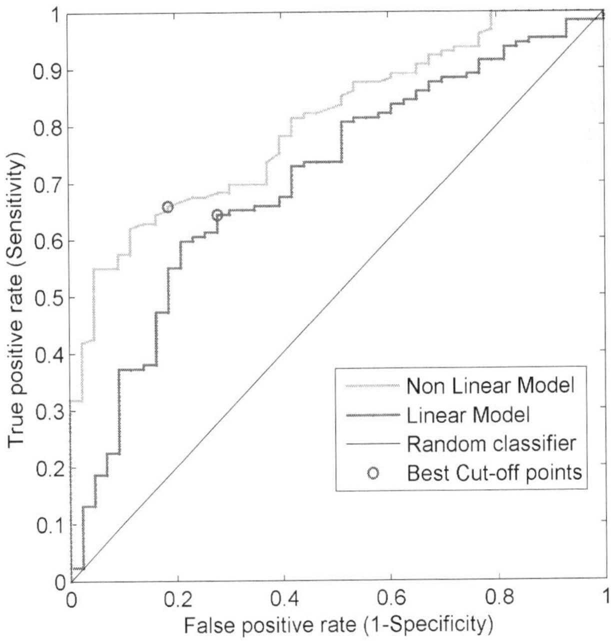

Fig. 6. ROC curves for nonlinear and linear models

So far, both linear and nonlinear predictive models were built by considering all patients of the data set, i.e., each model was estimated from a database with known input and output data.
After this model-building step, the linear and nonlinear models were applied to new patients, with unknown output values, in order to have a quantitative check on the effectiveness of the proposed method on the correct selection of the therapeutic effects.
Two additional statistic tools were introduced: the cross-validation method and the confusion matrix.

Both in case of linear and nonlinear model, patients were randomly subdivided in two groups, used for building and testing the models. A training data set was considered for calculating linear regression coefficients in the case of linear model and for selecting the optimal weights and bias in the case of the MLP. A test data set was used to make a prediction of the WL two years after the bariatric surgery.

Confusion matrix was the tool used for the validation of the prediction. The cross-validation method was repeated 100 times, changing the subsets of patients for training and test sets. It was surprising to verify that after this blind test on the whole dataset, it was possible to establish with over 70% of reliability if the patients will either maximally or minimally benefit from the intervention after two years, in the case of the nonlinear model. Conversely, the reliability was reduced of about 30% in the case of the linear model (Piaggi et al., 2010). Considering that the analysis was restricted to psychological presurgical tests and to age, this result seems to be a surprising success of a research derived from the physiological cybernetics course.

3. Therapies in HIV disease: A predictive control approach

The second example shows the application of model predictive control (MPC) for an optimization of the therapy in HIV disease. It applies the subject of a group of lessons held during the physiological cybernetics course, in which the predictive control theory was presented to students as an effective tool for helping (and emulating) physicians in the selection of an optimal therapy, based on the patients' responses.

The origin of this activity was born when some students asked to study a mathematical model for HIV.

It was easy to find HIV models existing in literature: many of them are well known and accepted from mathematical and from biomedical engineers as gold standards for studies in viral models.

In the literature, (Wodarz & Nowak, 1999) the simplest model presented for mathematical modelling of HIV considers only three state variables and it is mathematically described by:

$$\begin{cases} \dot{x} = \lambda - dx - \beta xv \\ \dot{y} = \beta xv - ay \\ \dot{v} = ky - uv \end{cases} \tag{5}$$

System (5) consists of three differential equations. The state variables are: x, the concentration of healthy $CD4^+$ T-cells; y, the concentration of HIV-infected $CD4^+$ cells; v, the concentration of free HIV copies.

Healthy cells have a production constant rate λ and a death rate d. Infected cells have a death rate a, free virions are produced by the infected cells at a rate k and u is their death rate. In the case of active HIV infection the concentration of healthy cells decreases proportionally to the product xv, with a constant rate β representing a coefficient that depends on various factors, including the velocity of penetration of virus into cells and the frequency of encounters between uninfected cells and free virus.

A five-state model was developed in Wodarz & Nowak (1999). This model offers important theoretical insights into immune control of the virus based on treatment strategies, which can be viewed as a fast subsystem of the dynamics of HIV infection. It is mathematically described by:

$$\begin{cases} \dot{x} = \lambda - dx - \beta xv \\ \dot{y} = \beta xv - ay - pyz \\ \dot{v} = ky - uv \\ \dot{w} = cxyw - cqyw - bw \\ \dot{z} = cqyw - hz \end{cases} \tag{6}$$

Two states are added to (5) to describe the dynamics of w, the concentration of precursor cytotoxic T-lymphocytes (CTLp) responsible for the development of immune memory and z, the concentration of effector cytotoxic T-lymphocytes (CTLe) responsible for killing virus-infected cells cytotoxic T-lymphocyte precursors CTLp.

In the fourth and fifth differential equations c, q, b and h are relative production rate, conversion rate to effector CTLs, death rate of precursor CTLs, and of effector CTLs, respectively.

This model can discriminate the trend of infection as a function of the rate of viral replication: if the rate is high a successful immune memory cannot establish; conversely, if the replication rate is slow, the CTL-mediated immune memory helps the patient to successfully fight the infection.

In Landi & al. (2008) model (6) was modified as:

$$\begin{cases} \dot{x} = \lambda - dx - rxv \\ \dot{y} = rxv - ay - pyz \\ \dot{v} = k\left(1 - \mu_P f_P\right) y - uv \\ \dot{w} = cxyw - cqyw - bw \\ \dot{z} = cqyw - hz \\ \dot{r} = r_0 - \mu_T f_T \end{cases} \tag{7}$$

Model (7) differs from previous W-N in the new state variable r, an index of the aggressiveness of the virus, which substitutes the constant β.

An arbitrary assumption is that r increases linearly with time in untreated HIV-infected individuals, with a growth rate that depends on the constant r_0 (a higher r_0 value indicates a higher virulence growth rate). This hypothesis was verified consistent with the simulation results obtained in the case of infected people who do not show significant disease progression for many years without treatment (long-term non Progressors - LTNP).

Different typologies of patients may require to change the law describing the aggressiveness dynamics. We evaluated the possibility to adapt the model (7) to patients with different clinical progressions, changing the values of some parameters. In particular, we supposed to vary the coefficients b and h, which represent the death rate of immune defensive cells (effector CTLs and precursor CTLs). We considered the two extreme cases for HIV progression (see Figure 7): the lower values correspond to the model dynamics of LTNP patients; the higher values model the dynamics of fast progressor patients (FP).

The coefficients μ_T and μ_P represent the drug effectiveness weights for specific external inputs f_T and f_P, which represent the drug uptakes in case of Highly Active Antiretroviral Therapy (HAART).

HAART is a combination therapy that includes:

- Reverse Transcriptase Inhibitors (RTI), to prevent cell-to-cell transmission, inhibiting reverse transcriptase activity.
- Protease Inhibitors (PI), to prevent the production of virions by infected cells, inhibiting the production of viral protein precursors.

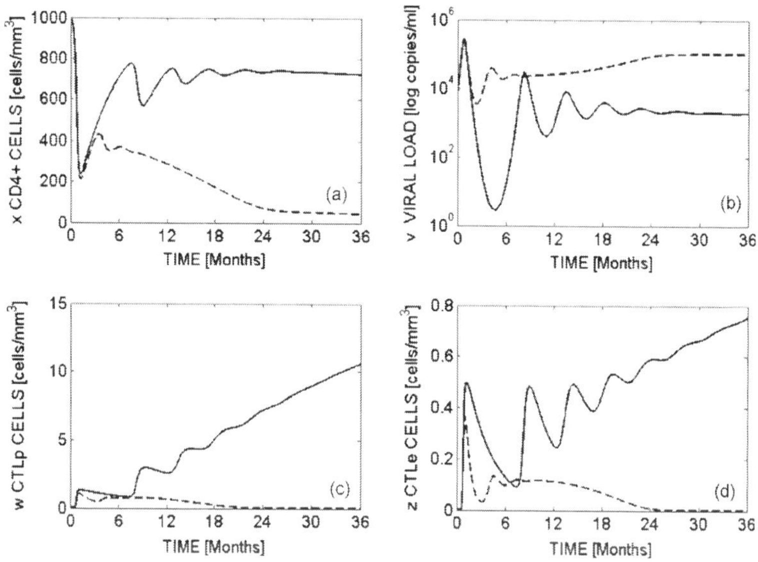

Fig. 7. Dynamic behaviour of the state variables x, v, w and z vs. time in the case of untreated LTNP (solid line) and FP (dashed line) patients.

In different models presented in literature, the effects of RTI and PI drugs have been aggregated, nevertheless we decided to mimic the effects of PI drugs reducing the rate of virus production, i.e., modifying the rate coefficient k of production of new infected cells in the dynamical equation. Instead the effect of RTI drugs is simulated by reducing the infection rate of $CD4^+$ cells by free virus. So, in model (7) the RTI drugs act in virulence equation, because their main role is halting cellular infection.

Another important feature differentiating the proposed model from standard literature is that it does not admit stable steady states, since the model parameters are such that, i.e., the aggressiveness never becomes a constant, since a slow increase of r describes well a real progression of the HIV infection. This hypothesis originates from the observation that the possibility of eradicating completely the virus has not been demonstrated and the HIV disease cannot be long-term controlled.

The inclusion of aggressiveness as a new state variable represented the main outcome of the study: this simple extension to Wodarz & Nowak models allowed us to mirror the natural history of HIV infection and to introduce a new state equation useful for introducing in the model the effects of pharmacologic control.

In Fig. 8 are shown the time courses of CD4 cells and virions obtained in simulation with model (7); for a qualitative validation of the model, compare the results with the plotted experimental data shown in Fig. 9 (Abbas et al., 2000).

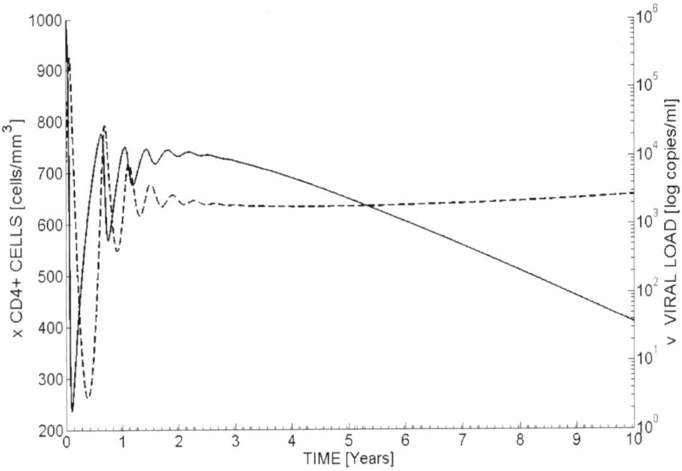

Fig. 8. Simulated behaviour of untreated LTNP HIV-infected patients for ten years with model described in (4). The graph shows viral load (dashed line) and CD4$^+$ cells (solid line)

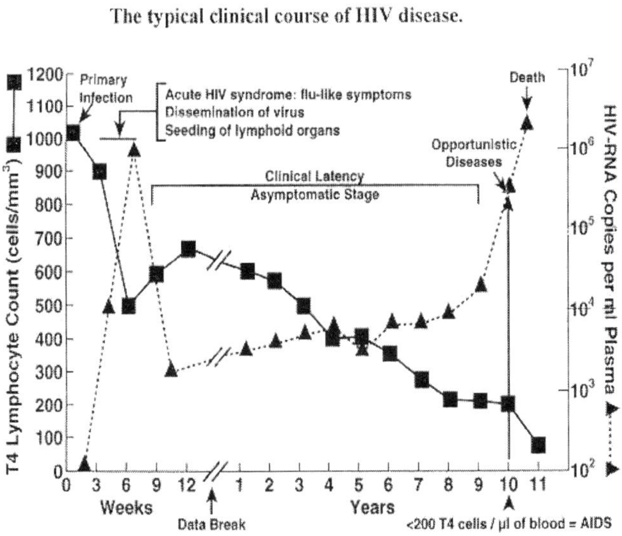

Fig. 9. Typical clinical behaviour of HIV infection for about ten years. Figure shows HIV copies (triangles) and CD4$^+$ cells (squares), in case of untreated HIV-infected human

A straightforward application of the control theory to model (7) was proposed in Pannocchia et al., (2010), with the application of a MPC strategy in anti-HIV therapy.

MPC algorithms (Mayne et al., 2000) utilize a mathematical model of the system to be controlled, to generate the predicted values of the future response. Predicted values are then used to compute a control sequence over a finite prediction horizon, in order to optimize the future behaviour of the controlled system. The control sequence is chosen minimizing a suitable cost function, including a measure of the deviation of the future state variables from reference target values and a measure of the control effort, while respecting state and control constraints. In plain words, the core of the control algorithm is an optimization algorithm, keeping the controlled variables close to their targets and within suitable constraints. The first output in the optimal sequence of control actions is then injected into the system, and the computation is repeated at subsequent control intervals.

The problem was how to adapt MPC to determine the optimal drug scheduling in anti-HIV therapy.

Some examples of MPC applied to biomedical applications like control of the glucose-insulin system in diabetics (Parker et al., 1999), anaesthesia (Ionescu et al., 2008), and HIV (Zurakowski & Teel., 2006) have been presented in literature, but all applications were considered for models admitting a steady-state stable equilibrium. On the other hand, MPC emerged as the more suitable solution for solving the drug optimal administration problem in anti-HIV therapy, even if the model was unstable. MPC algorithm pursued the following logic:

a. future outputs of the control algorithm are generated by the HIV model; measurements on individual patient are considered and compared with the predictions of the model.
b. the cost function to be minimized keeps the controlled variables – e.g., $CD4^+$ cells and free virions concentration – close to the targets and respecting suitable soft constraints on the manipulated variables.
c. the cost function of the future control movements is minimized using a sequence of future PI and RTI drugs over the chosen control horizon, but only the first element of the suggested control sequence is applied to the system.
d. at the successive decision time, the algorithm is solved again if measurements of $CD4^+$ cells and free virions concentration are available and the drug sequence is updated, repeating step c)

Some practical issues were considered (see Pannocchia et al., (2010) for a detailed study), because MPC was applied considering the two different cases of continuous applications of drugs, or of a structured interruption of therapy (STI) for patients. STI is a treatment strategy in HIV-infected patients, involves interrupting HAART in controlled clinical settings, for a specified duration of time. The possible explanation of the effectiveness of this clinical protocol was an induced autovaccination in the patients. The use of STI is currently debated between clinical researchers and most studies agree that STI may be successful if therapy is initiated early in HIV infection, but unsuccessful for people who started therapy later.

Furthermore, a discrete dosage approach required to modify the control algorithm using a non linear MPC: this was due to the clinical request to maintain a maximum dosage of drugs, as in standard HAART protocol, in order to reduce the risks of virus mutations.

Some comments are mandatory to stress the results of this model based on a differential equation deterministic approach. From the viewpoint of a model builder, two different situations have to be usually considered: basal and pathological conditions. In the case of infections, like HIV, the mathematical model have to mirror the natural evolution of HIV infection, and the pathological model must be more accurate, because today it is the only one that can be validated by experimental data, since patients are all maintained under therapy. The impact of therapy into HIV models must be introduced in a way as simple as possible, if we have to satisfy the task to formulate a model suitable for use in feedback control.

Simulation results were coherent with the medical findings: the comments of clinical researchers expert in HIV therapies were essential in testing the model and for evaluating the effectiveness of the proposed control methods.

Obtaining reliable models is relevant from a diagnostic and prognostic point of view, because it allows the physician to prove the therapeutic action using the model for testing the treatment in terms of optimal dosage and administration of drugs.

In 2008, the FDA approved an *in silico* model of diabetes as a pre-clinical testing tool for closed loop research at the seven JDRF Artificial Pancreas Consortium sites. The overall goal of the Artificial Pancreas project was to accelerate the development, regulatory approval, health insurance coverage, and clinical acceptance of continuous glucose monitoring and artificial pancreas technology (Juvenile Diabetes Research Foundation, 2008).

We strongly believe that also a simple but reliable *in silico* model of HIV can lead to an acceleration of the experimental tests for a clinical acceptance of new drugs in HIV disease.

Future activity will be devoted to develop models of HIV infection, able to include the issues of drug resistance and viral mutation, key issues for the HIV studies, and the interest of many clinical researchers in our work is encouraging in the upcoming research.

4. Conclusion

The Physiological Cybernetics course represents an example of integration between different disciplines, in order to produce a common language between students in biomedical engineer and physicians. It offers students an opportunity to verify in practice how to move theoretical lectures, based on the development of mathematical models, to a practical interaction with physicians. This fact seems obvious from an educational viewpoint, but it isn't so usual in practice, because it requires a preliminary long period for preparing a common language between researchers in different fields. Judging from the students' excellent results, if compared to students attending under-graduated courses in previous years, the example proposed was very successful.

In this chapter we presented two examples of research applications, derived from this educational experience, demonstrating that the old-novel vision of Wiener was not a utopia, and that a synergic cooperation between biomedical engineers and physicians can lead to interesting results.

5. Acknowledgment

The authors wish to thank all people cooperating with the activities of the Physiological Cybernetics course over many years, the physicians for their support and clinical supervision and the undergraduate active students for their enthusiasm.

6. References

Abbas, A.K, Lichtman, A.H. & Pober, J.S. (2000). *Cellular and Molecular Immunology,* IV ed., WB Saunders Company, ISBN 07216823323, Philadelphia, US

Bishop, C.M. (1995). *Neural Networks for Pattern Recognition,* Clarendon Press, ISBN 0198538642, Oxford, UK

Cobelli, C. & Carson, E. (2008). *Introduction to Modelling in Physiology and Medicine*, Elsevier/Academic Press, ISBN 978-0-12-160240-62008, New York

Di Stefano III, J.J., Wilson, K.C, Jang, M. & Mak, P.H. (1975). Identification of the Dynamics of Thyroid Hormone Metabolism. *Automatica*, Vol. 11, No. 2, (March 1975) 149-159, ISSN 0005-1098

Edelstein-Keshet, L. (2005). *Mathematival Models in Biology*, SIAM, Classics in Applied Mathematics, ISBN 13-978-0898715-54-5, Philadelphia, PA

Hoppensteadt, F.C. & Peskin, C.S. (2002). *Modeling and Simulation in Medicine and the Life Sciences*, Springer Science series, II edition, ISBN 0-387-95072-9, New York

Ionescu, C. M., Keyser, R. D., Torrico, B. C., De Smet, T., Struys, M. M. & Normey-Rico, J. E. (2008). Robust Predictive Control Strategy Applied for Propofol Dosing Using Bis as a Controlled Variable During Anesthesia. *IEEE Transactions on Biomedical Engineering*, Vol. 55, No. 9, (September 2008), pp. 2161–2170, ISSN 0018-929

Jolliffe, I.T. (2002). *Principal Component Analysis*, Springer Verlag, II edition, ISBN 978-0-387-95442-4, New York.

Jones, D.S., Planck, M.J. & Sleeman, B.D. (2008). *Differential Equations and Mathematical Biology*, CRC Press, Taylor & Francis Group, II edition, ISBN 978-1-4200-8357-6, London, UK

Juvenile Diabetes Research Foundation (2008). Emerging Technologies in Diabetes Research JDRF *Emerging Technologies E-Newsletter*, No. 7, May 2008.

Khoo, M.C.K. (2001). *Physiological Control Systems*, Prentice Hall of India Pvt. Ltd., ISBN 81-203-18-447, New Delhi.

Kutner, M., Neter, J., Nachtsheim, C., & Wasserman, W (2005). *Applied Linear Statistical Models*, V edition, McGraw-Hill/Irwin, ISBN 0071122214, Boston, MA. *Models*, McGraw Hill, Boston, MA. 1985

Landi, A., Pacini, L., Piaggi, P., Lippi, C., Santini, F. & Pinchera, A. (2007). Obefix: a Friendly Toolbox for Obesity Classification, *Proceedings of 2007 International Conference on Cybernetics and Information Technologies, Systems and Applications*, pp.1-6, ISBN 1-934272-07-8, Orlando, Florida, 12-15 July 2007

Landi, A., Mazzoldi, A., Andreoni, C., Bianchi, M., Cavallini, A., Laurino M., Ricotti L., Iuliano, R., Matteoli B. & Ceccherini Nelli, L. (2008). Modelling and Control of HIV Dynamics, *Journal Computer Methods and Programs in Biomedicine*, Vol. 89, No. 2, (February 2008), pp. 162–168, ISSN 0169-2607

Landi, A., Piaggi, P., Lippi, C., Santini, F. & Pinchera, A. (2010). Statistical Toolbox in Medicine for Predicting Effects of Therapies in Obesity, *Proceedings of 2010 IEEE Workshop on Health Care Management*, pp.1-6, ISBN 978-1-4244-4998-9, Venice, Italy, 18-20 February 2010

Ljung. L. (1987). *System Identification: Theory for the User*, Prentice Hall, Inc., ISBN 0-13-881640-9, Englewood Cliffs, N. J.

Mardia, K.V., Kent, J.T. & Bibby, J.M. (1979) *Multivariate Analysis*, Academic Press, ISBN : 0124712509, London, UK

Marmarelis, V.Z. (2004). *Nonlinear Dynamic Modeling of Physiological Systems*, John Wiley & Sons, Inc, ISBN 0-471-46960-2, Hoboken, NJ

Mayne, D. Q., Rawlings, J. B., Rao, C. V. & Scokaert, P. O. M. (2000). Constrained Model Predictive Control: Stability and Optimality. *Automatica*, Vol. 36, No. 6, (June 2000), pp. 789–814, ISSN 0005-1098

Ottesen, J.T., Olufsen, M.S. & Larsen, J.K. (2004). *Applied Mathematical Models in Human Physiology*, SIAM, Monographs on Mathematical Modeling and Computation, ISBN 0-89871-539-3, Philadelphia, PA

Pannocchia, G., Laurino, M. & Landi A. (2010). A Model Predictive Control Strategy Toward Optimal Structured Treatment Interruptions in Anti-HIV Therapy. *IEEE Transactions on Biomedical Engineering*, Vol. 57, No. 5, (May 2010), pp. 1040-1050, ISSN 0018-929

Parker, R., Doyle, F. J. & Peppas, N. A. (1999). A Model- Based Algorithm for Blood Glucose Control in Type I Diabetic Patients. *IEEE Transactions on Biomedical Engineering*, Vol. 56, No. 2, (February 1999), pp. 148–156, ISSN 0018-929

Piaggi. P, Lippi, C., Fierabracci P., Maffei M., Calderone A., Mauri M., Anselmino M., Cassano, G.,B., Vitti P., Pinchera A., Landi A. & Santini, F. (2010). Artificial Neural Networks in the Outcome Prediction of Adjustable Gastric Banding in Obese Women, *PLoS ONE*, vol 5, October 2010, journal.pone. 0013624, ISSN 1932-6203

Rojas, R. (1996). *Neural Networks - A Systematic Introduction,* Springer-Verlag, ISBN 3-540-60505-3, Berlin.

Rumelhart, D.E., Hinton, G.E. & Williams, R.J. (1986). Learning Internal Representations by Error Propagation. in *Parallel Distributed Processing:Explorations in the Microstructure of Cognition*, ISBN:0-262-68053-X, MIT Press, Cambridge, Massachussets

Van Hout, G.C., Verschure, S.K. & van Heck, G.L. (2005). Psychosocial Predictors of Success Following Bariatric Surgery. *Obesity Surgery,* Vol. 15, No. 4, pp. 552–560, ISSN 0960-8923.

Westwick, D. T. & Kearney, R.E. (2003). *Identification of Nonlinear Physiological Systems*, IEEE Biomedical Engineering Book Series, Metin Akay Ed., IEEE Press/Wiley John Wiley & Sons, ISBN 0-471-27456-9, Piscataway, NJ

Wiener, N. (1948). *Cybernetics: Or Control and Communication in the Animal and the Machine.* MIT Press, ISBN 9780262730099, Paris, (Hermann & Cie) & Cambridge Massachussets

Wodarz D. & Nowak, M. A. (1999). Specific Therapy Regimes Could Lead to Long-Term Immunological Control of HIV, *Proceedings of the National Academy of Sciences*, Vol. 96, No. 25, (December 1999), pp. 14464–14469, ISSN 0027-8424

Zurakowski, R. & Teel, A. R. (2006). A Model Predictive Control-Based Scheduling Method for HIV Therapy. *Journal of Theoretical Biology,* Vol. 238, No. 2, (January 2006), pp. 368–382, ISSN 0022-5193

4

Biomedical Signal Transceivers

Reza Fazel-Rezai, Noah Root, Ahmed Rabbi,
DuckHee Lee and Waqas Ahmad
University Of North Dakota
USA

1. Introduction

With the growing costs of healthcare, the need for mobile health monitoring devices is critical. A wireless transceiver provides a cost effective way to transmit biomedical signals to the various personal electronic devices, such as computers, cellular devices, and other mobile devices. Different kinds of biomedical signals can be processed and transmitted by these devices, including electroencephalograph (EEG), electrocardiograph (ECG), and electromyography (EMG). By utilizing wireless transmission, the user gains freedom to connect with fewer constraints to their personal devices to view and monitor their health condition.

In this chapter, in the first few sections, we will introduce the reader with the basic design of the biomedical transceivers and some of the design issues. In the subsequent sections, we will be presenting design challenges for wireless transceivers, specially using a common wireless protocol Bluetooth. Furthermore, we will share our experience of implementing a biomedical transceiver for ECG signals and processing them. We conclude the discussion with current trends and future work.

The information that is being presented is meant to be applied for all types of biomedical signals. However, some examples are reserved to one type of biomedical signal for simplicity. In this case, the example of an ECG signal and device is used. Even though some sections of the chapter rely heavy on this example, the concepts explored in this chapter can still be extrapolated for other biomedical signals.

1.1 Types of biomedical signal transceivers

Different biomedical signal transceiver device types can be designed. There are several distinctions between the types of the devices and their operation. The distinctions can be based upon how the device is powered and how the device communicates. Despite these design differences, the hardware makeup of a biomedical signal transceiver is very standard.

Before going deeper into the details on the types of biomedical signal transceivers, it is important to understand how the device will operate. Typically, a biomedical signal transceiver device will have two main components, the transmitter and the receiver. The transmitter has several sub systems, including: signal acquisition, amplification, filtering, and as the name dictates, transmitter. The receiver subsystem will receive the signal from the transmitter, perform any required analysis on the signal, and then display the results.

The transmitter is separate from the receiver, such that the transmitter can acquire the bioelectric signal and transmit to another device for remote viewing and analysis.

Existing biomedical transceivers are can be separated into two groups describing how they are powered; Radio Frequency (RF) and battery powered. In RF powered transceivers, an inductive link with external controller allows the transmission of power and commands [2]. A common application of the RF powered transceiver is the transcutaneous neural recording arrays. In battery-powered transceivers, an onboard battery is utilized power source [3]. This battery can be either disposable or rechargeable, depending on the device application. The use of a battery allows using higher frequencies for transmission and improved data rates can be achieved.

Another way to group biomedical transceivers is by their communication style. Biomedical transceivers can communicate either wirelessly or in the traditional wired connection. Not only can the device transmit the biomedical signal, but some devices have communication between the transmitter and receiver for not only biomedical information, but also any feedback or control signals. In this case, both subsystems are acting like transceivers.

1.2 Applications of biomedical signal transceivers

Biomedical signal transceivers can be very useful in the monitoring devices and biotelemetry. There are several applications for these devices and their design is as unique as the application. These applications also utilize wireless communications to improve the system and the ease of use.

A health monitoring system which acquires and transmits the vital signals of a patient remotely to a hospital or medical professional can be very useful. This application of biotelemetry can allow for a patient to leave the hospital or clinic, but still have their health monitored remotely. Various bioelectric signals can be recorded from the patient's body and transmitted such as EEG, ECG, body temperature and blood pressure. Biomedical signal transceivers do not have to be limited to just an overall health monitoring device. These transceivers can also have more specific functions that can allow for more in depth analysis, depending on the application.

An ECG monitoring system is a great example of an application of biomedical signal transceiver. When the device is developed wirelessly, patients can monitor their heart signal via a mobile device, while having the electrodes and transmitter attached to their body. Furthermore, a warning system can be designed that can inform the patient about any abrupt abnormality in the heart. As with the health monitoring system, these heart anomalies can also be reported remotely to medical professions who can more appropriately analyze the patient's condition in real time. Another application of biomedical signal transceivers is to monitor the drug and medication usages in the patients remotely.

2. Analog hardware design

One of the most important parts of any biomedical signal transceiver is the analog hardware. Using this circuitry the biomedical signal is acquired, filtered, and amplified to an appropriate level. Along with this circuitry, the power for the system needs to be addressed. Finally, safety for both the system circuitry and the patient must be understood and taken care of during design to protect the device as well as the users.

2.1 Electrodes

For all biomedical devices that operate outside of the human body (i.e. non-implantable devices), electrodes are critical components. It is through these electrodes that the bioelectric potentials of the body are collected and transmitted to the measurement and analysis device. In this sense, electrodes are the initial part of any biomedical device.

2.1.1 Electrode placement

The placement of the electrodes is dependent on the desired physiological signal. For example, to acquire an ECG signal, the electrodes may be placed in a triangle formation around the heart, creating the Einthoven's triangle. Each of the various bioelectric signals has a standard electrode placement on the body that must be understood and followed before acquiring signals. It is important to have the lead placement correct as noise and distortions will result from electrode misplacement. In some cases, only a small subset of the electrodes is required for signal acquisition. For example, in EEG recording the number of electrode may be from 1 to 128 electrodes. This is dependent on the application or use of the biometric signals by the device.

2.1.2 Electrode make-up and selection

An electrode is simply a mechanism that is used to make an electrical connection to a non-metallic surface. The electrodes have a common makeup, no matter what application or types of signals that are being acquired. Disposable electrodes have a very generic composition and purpose. Using an adhesive, the electrode is attached to the skin, which reduces the risk of noise artifact being introduced into by signal by electrode movement. Additionally, the electrode contains a gel that lowers the skins resistance and is therefore produces a better signal measurement. This allows for the metallic surface to conduct the signal onto the biomedical device.

There are several commercially available electrodes on the market today. The electrode performance will vary from company to company, and from part to part. It is essential to find an electrode that is appropriate for the application, all while keeping quality and price per electrode in mind.

The next step is to develop circuitry to prepare the analog signal for analysis. This will be accomplished by both amplifying and filtering the weak bioelectric signals. These steps are critical for all types of biometric signals.

2.2 Amplifier and filter design

When the bioelectric signals are acquired from the human body by the electrodes, the signals are very weak (small amplitudes). Because of their small amplitudes, these signals have little use to any biomedical sensor or system. However, if these signals are amplified to an appropriate level, they can be detected and read accordingly for analysis. The amount of amplification, termed gain, is determined by system specification and is dependent on the signal being measured, and other circuitry requirements. Another critical aspect of the signals that are acquired from the electrodes is the amount of noise in the signal. For proper signal analysis, these errors and noise need to be removed from the signal. The next sections go over the design of amplifiers and filters, all of which accumulates into the filter and amplifier circuitry design.

2.2.1 Amplification

To perform any sort of analysis on a bioelectric signal, the signal needs to be amplified to a level which an analog to digital converter (ADC) can sample the data with a high resolution. As well, the amplifier circuitry needs to include level shifting circuitry such that the signal is positive and has a similar dynamic range as the Analog to Digital conversion. The overall gain is defined by designer based upon the signal requirements.

The first stage in any amplification circuit is the instrumentation amplifier. This amplifier is a critical component for several different reasons, and has many applications outside of just biomedical devices. For one, the instrumentation amplifier acts as a buffer circuit by having large input impedance. This allows for very little current to be drawn from the source. By design, the instrumentation amplifier has a very large Common Mode Rejection Ratio (CMRR). The CMRR simply measures the tendency of the amplifier to reject a signal that is common between the two input pins. This is important for application in biomedical devices since the signal measurement is not coming from one electrode, but actually the difference between two electrodes (i.e. one lead). As well, the instrumentation amplifier will cancel out common noise between the two signals.

There are two ways to implement an instrumentation amplifier; a single IC package or a connection of several separate operational amplifiers (op-amps). Both are viable options, but the choice depends on the cost and efficiency of the choices. In most cases, it can be more efficient to use a single IC package instrumentation amplifier instead of the multiple op amp design. Figure 1 shows an example of cascaded op-amp design for the instrumentation amplifier.

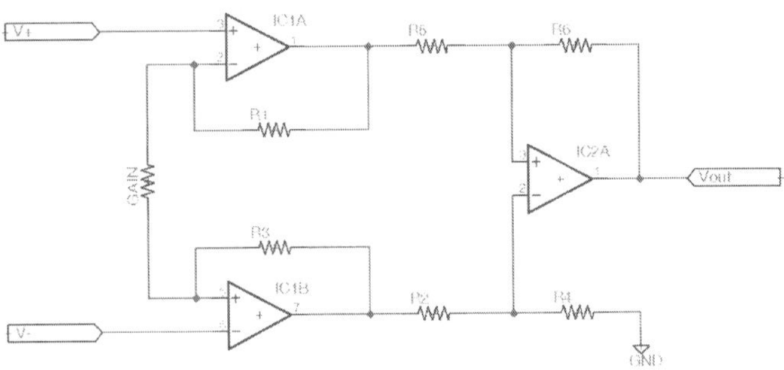

Fig. 1. Instrumentation amplifier layout, utilizing three op-amps

The next stages of the amplifier circuitry are very simple in nature. The amplifier stages only purpose is to increase the amplitude of the bioelectric signals via amplification. Typically, one will employ only non-inverting amplifier configuration so that the signal does not be become inverted or out of phase. The proper number of amplifier stages typically is user defined, but can also be determined based upon the filter configuration. Both of these topics will be covered in the following sections.

The final stage of the amplifier circuitry is a level shifting circuit. The purpose of the level shifting circuit is to shift the negative components of the signal to a positive level. This also shifts up the positive voltage components of the signal as well. This circuit is critical as an analog to digital converter (ADC) on a microcontroller cannot read negative voltages. Thus, the signal would not be accurately converted, and the bioelectric information would be lost. There are several ways to implement this circuit; for example, one can use a non-inverting summing amplifier, which is illustrated in Figure 2.

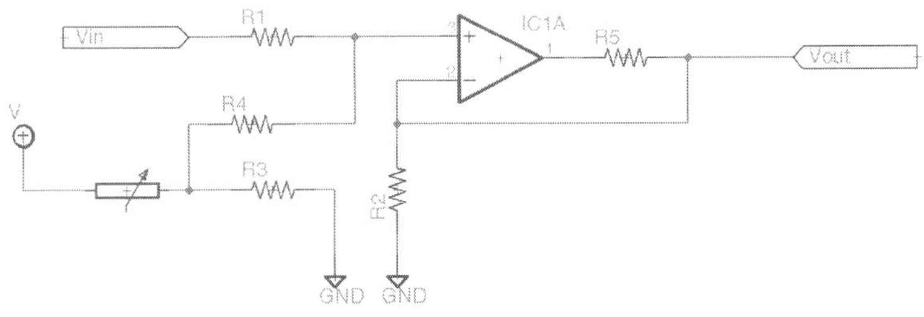

Fig. 2. Summing amplifier design

There are several other designs available, and they all require the use of an amplifier. The level shifting circuit in Figure 3 is a great example of this.

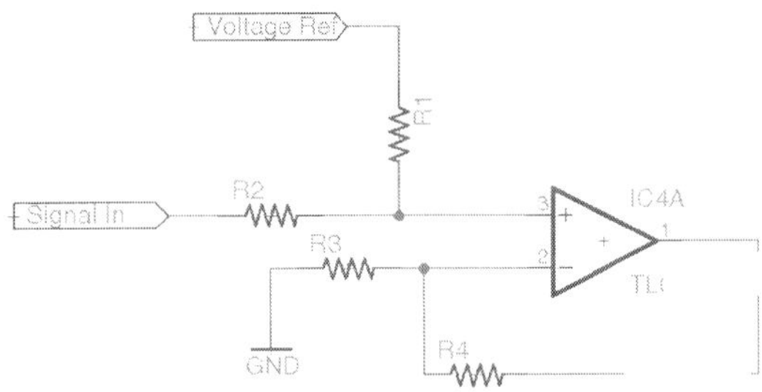

Fig. 3. Level Shifting Circuit

Both of these circuits will allow for the signal to be shifted to an adequate level. To do so, the resistor values will need to be designed such that the values that will allow for proper shifting. These values will also result in gain, if required. For example, if one does not want any gain from the level shifting circuit in Figure 3 (i.e. a gain of 1), simply follow the following guidelines:

$$R1 = R4$$
$$R2 = R3$$

If other values of gain (A) are required, the following equation should be considered:

$$A = (R1/R3)x(R3+R4)/(R1+R2)$$
$$R1 = R3$$
$$R2 = R4$$
$$A = (R4/R1)$$

This will allow to tune the circuit as required to shift the voltage. This level shifting circuit should be used if the exact value of shift is known; otherwise, the summing amplifier circuitry should be considered to allow for variance in the shift voltage. The potentiometer in summing amplifier allows the user to vary the voltage divider, which thus varies the shifting voltage level.

2.2.2 Amplifier selection

There are many op-amps on the market for use in the amplification of bioelectric signals. However, many of the more common amplifiers, such as the common 741 op amp, do not produce ideal response, especially for bioelectric signals. This is due to the 741 design, or any other op amp that utilizes Bipolar Junction Transistors (BJT) in the first stages of the amplifier. Unlike MOSFET (or other FETs) the BJT will draw current from the signal, thus affecting the signal. As well, there are leakage currents from the BJT that will also hinder the signal. Thus, it can be advantageous to utilize an op amp that uses BiMOS technology. BiMOS is circuit design that use both BJTs and MOSFETs. Similar, BiCMOS can also be used, which simply is BJTs and CMOS. To determine the proper op amp to use in biomedical device one needs to look into the various specifications for the given op amp.

2.2.3 Filters

Filters are the other critical component of the analog hardware design for a biomedical device. By removing noise and artifacts from the signal, a precise and more accurate signal can be utilized by the signal analysis code. However, there are a lot of options and configurations for filters, and it can be tricky to determine what is necessary for the application at hand.

Before designing a filter, one needs to determine the frequency range of the bioelectric signals that are being measured. This is critical so that one can determine the required frequency response of the analog filters. Once this is determined, then the filters can be designed.

One of the most important filters, no matter what the frequency range of the bioelectric signal is, is the 60 Hz (or 50 Hz outside of North America) notch filter, also known as a band stop filter. This filter removes the noise that is produced from the common AC wall outlet. There are several ways to design a notch filter, with both passive and active designs. The effectiveness of the filter depends on the design. The passive filter designs will not be as exact, and the cut off frequency will vary over time (passive components will vary over time). This can and will affect the signal integrity over time. If there is a substantial enough drift, actually information will be attenuated with the 60 Hz being freely passed. Active filters, even with their power requirements, are by far the best option for most biomedical device application. One very effective and efficient design is to utilize Texas Instruments' Universal Active Filter, the UAF42, in a notch filter configuration. This design is laid out in the data sheet for the component, which explains the proper design for a 60 Hz notch filter with the chip and selected resistor values. There are several other active filter design and options that can be utilized to attenuate the 60 Hz noise from the signal.

The next filter that needs to be designed is the high pass and low pass filters. With these two filters in the circuit, it creates a band-pass filter (the band will be the frequency range of the bioelectric signal). As mentioned before, it is critical that this range of frequencies

corresponds to the range of frequencies of the measured bioelectric signal. When designing the overall circuit, commonly the high pass filter is placed before the low pass filter.
High pass filter design is quite straightforward. Since a high pass filter will pass any frequency above the cut off frequency, the filter theoretically has an infinite frequency response. As such, if one was to design an active high pass filter, op amp utilized in the design may limit this response, as the op amp has a maximum frequency output. Therefore from a theoretical view, a passive filter will have the best response. In all practicality, this is not the case, but high pass active filters are still important to use, as they still can be effective. Depending on the bioelectric signal being measured, a simple RC passive filter can be sufficient. An example of a passive high pass filter is displayed in Figure 4.

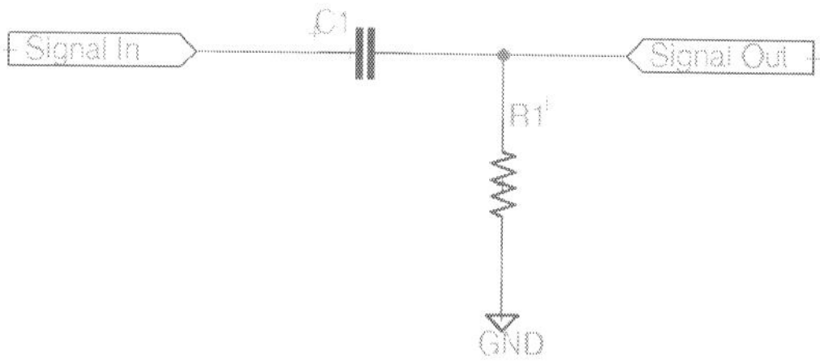

Fig. 4. Passive high pass filter

There are several possible common designs for the low pass filter. These include both active and passive filters. For these filters, there are several common types, including: Butterworth and Chebyshev. Each filter type has several configurations, with both active and passive designs. More commonly, for the low pass filter, an active configuration is utilized. As well, the Butterworth filter is typically used as it has an advantageous flat frequency response. There is also a choice of the filter order and configuration of the Butterworth Filter. Figure 5 shows a first order Butterworth low pass filter.

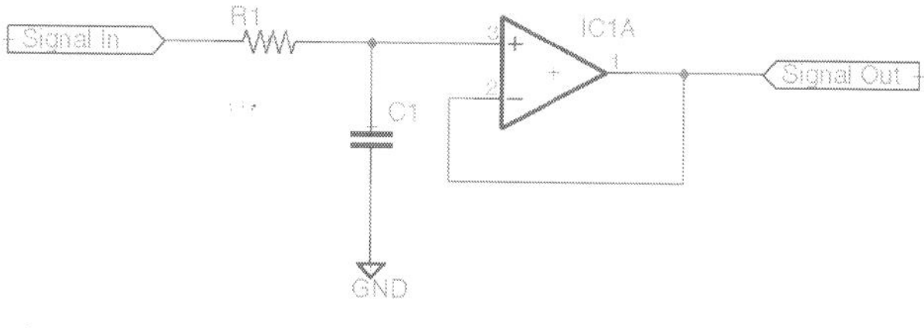

Fig. 5. First Order Butterworth Low Pass Filter

Typically, a filter with only a few orders will be utilized due to speed, cost, and space. A first order low pass Butterworth filter is perfectly acceptable choice for most applications. Another designer choice is the configuration of the filter. For active Butterworth filter, the Sallen-Key topology is an excellent choice. It allows for multiple orders, using only two op amps and several passive components. The design for the third order Butterworth filters is quite complex, and it involves calculating all values for the resistors and capacitors. There are several software packages that aide in the creation of these complex active filters.

2.2.3 Cascading filters and amplifiers

Now that both amplifiers and filters have been discussed and designed, the next step is the layout of the circuit in the most logical order. When designing circuitry that filters and amplifies a signal, there is a general rule of thumb to alternate stages of amplification and filtering. This is critical since one will introduce less noise into the circuitry as well as amplify less of the noise. This is why the design requires the cascading of op amps and filters to alternate. Now, depending on the amount of gain that is required for the bioelectric signal, the following order can be used:

- Instrumentation Amplifier
- High Pass Filter
- Gain Stage
- Low Pass Filter
- Gain Stage
- Notch Filter
- Level Shift

Naturally, the instrumentation amplifier will also have some gain. Most instrumentation op-amps have various levels of designable gain. To perform this type amplification, the de facto standard is to utilize a set of cascaded operational amplifiers. The need for cascaded stages will be explained later. When amplifiers are cascaded, one simply multiplies each of the gains together to determine the overall gain. Before designing the circuit, one needs to determine how much gain is actually necessary. The amount of gain will depend on what biometric signal is being measured, the ADC range, and other factors with that will vary from system to system.

2.3 Power

The voltage supply to the circuit components throughout the entire system is typically group together with the analog electronics design. Typically, there is a range of voltages are required through the system. For example, a microcontroller may require 5 V, a wireless transceiver may require 3.3 V, and the op-amps may require +/- 10 V. It is critical to design a system to effectively convert the input voltage to these different voltage values. It is also important to determine the total power that is required by the loads. There is a lot of DC - DC converters on the market, all of which have unique output power limits. In some cases it is perfectly acceptable to use voltage regulators instead of individual DC - DC converters.

2.4 Safety issues

With any electrical device that is being interfaced with a human, safety is a critical part of the hardware design. Not only do you have to be concerned about the damage a human can do to the device (i.e. ESD) but also the harm the device can make to human. In the case of a wireless transmitting biomedical device, over voltage protection is not as important to the device as opposed to when the device is connected directly to the computer. This is because the wireless transmitter acts as an isolated buffer between the patient and the monitoring computer or device. This way, the highest voltage in the device will be the source, typically a low voltage battery. Even at the low voltages of a battery, some protection is necessary for the device. Typically, this is performed using diodes that are designed into the circuit to only conduct when there is an over-voltage event. Naturally, these diodes are placed near the inputs, such that it is the first/last components before passing to the patient. This way, when the voltage is above the forward break down voltage (0.7 V for a silicon diode) the diode will then conduct. Since bioelectric signals have such small amplitude, the diodes do not disturb their signal.

3. Digital hardware design

3.1 Microcontroller and digital hardware design

The digital hardware system has three major parts: Microcontroller Unit (MCU), In System Programmer (ISP), and a Wireless Module (WM). The MCU includes a built in analog to digital converter (ADC). The ISP provides that capability to update the code on the MCU that is already a part of the board. Finally, the wireless module is involved in wireless data transmission. This communication is typically performed using Bluetooth. An illustration of this system is shown in Figure 6.

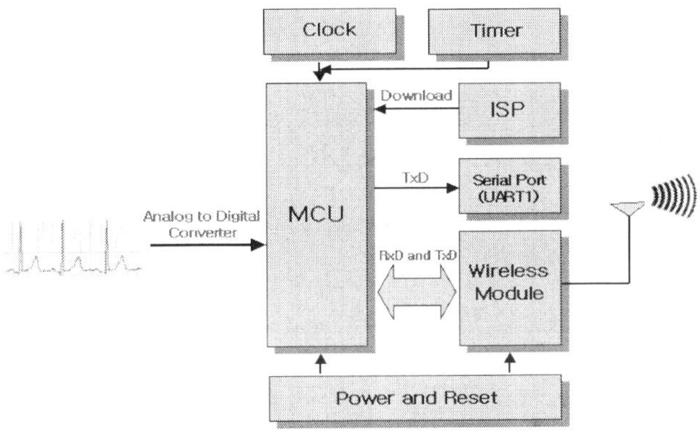

Fig. 6. Digital hardware block diagram

The MCU utilizes an 8-bit Reduced Instruction Set Computer (RISC), which has the advantages of simple commands, fast working speed, and low power consumption (2.7~5.5V). For example, the Atmel ATmega 128L has 16 Million Instructions per Second (MIPS) of performance. In addition, the ATmega MCU has 128 KB of In-System Programmable Flash with Read-While Writing capability. This is a type of flash memory that is 4 to 12 times faster than a general MCU. The ADC is responsible for converting continuous analog signals to digital signals. The ATmega MCU ADC has 8 channels and 10 bit resolution. This MCU also supports 16 different voltage input combinations and fast conversion time of 13~260us. Naturally, all MCUs are different, and these specifications will vary from MCU to MCU.

The ISP is the physical interface for programming the code on flash memory and EEPROM on the microcontroller. This hardware interface uses three signal lines: Master-Out-Slave-In (MOSI), Master-In-Slave-Out (MISO), and Clock (CLK). Once the reset pin on the microcontroller is set low, the code will updated via the ISP.

There are two possibilities to transmit the data from the microcontroller to a display device. One way to do this is via serial communication through the MAX232 IC. This IC will convert a TTL or CMOS signal into serial communication voltage level. This transmitting option requires a serial port and cable to transmit the data. In this sense, the communication is wired. Another option to transmit the data is via a wireless connection. This wireless communication is typically performed using a Bluetooth connection. This connection is created using a Bluetooth wireless module. In later sections, Bluetooth will be explored further. Other forms of wireless communication can be used, as per the system's requirements.

3.2 Wireless system characteristics

Wireless system (Bluetooth) uses a 2.4GHz band for short distance and low power consumption communication. Bluetooth is used for its high reliability and low cost. It is supported by AT-Command and has a transfer rate of approximately 1 Mbps to 3 Mbps. Another feature of Bluetooth is its ability to guarantee stable wireless communication, even under severe noisy environment, by use of Frequency Hopping Spread Spectrum (FHSS). Bluetooth utilizes a packet based protocol with a master slave configuration. This configuration allows a wireless system to connect and communication to up to 7 devices. The terminology of master and slave is very straight forward. One device has control over one or more devices. In this application, the wireless transmitter has control over the wireless receiver. During communication, the transmitter first selects and pools the slave. This is termed the "inquiry" stage of communication, as master is determining the devices that it can connect to. Once the master pools the slave, the slave responds to the communication. Then the communication enters the "paging" phase that allows for the devices to synchronize the clock and frequency between the master and the slave. Once the master and slave modules are paired, the master module provides information to slave module with the master module's address. Once this is complete, the communication between devices can begin. The specifications for Bluetooth 2.0 are listed in Table 1.

PART	Specification
Bluetooth Spec.	Bluetooth Specification 2.0 Support
Communication distance	10M
Frequency Range	2.4GHz ISM Band
Sensitivity	-83 dBm(Typical)
Input Power	3.3V
Current Consumption	48mA(Max)
Communication Speed	1,200bps ~ 230,400bps
Antenna	Chip Antenna
Interface	UART(TTL Level)

Table 1. Bluetooth 2.0 specifications

To perform the Bluetooth communication, a Bluetooth Module is utilized. This transceiver allows for communication between microcontroller and display device. For example, a WINiZEN Bluetooth RS232 wireless module is used for the Bluetooth communication. The data transmission and receiving power consumption of this Bluetooth module is 18 to 30mA for transmission and 21~33mA for reception. Data transmission/reception is achieved for up to 10 meter distances. The WINiZEN Bluetooth module is operated at low power (3.3 V), and has the dimensions of 18x20x12 (mm). This size can be visualized in Figure 7.

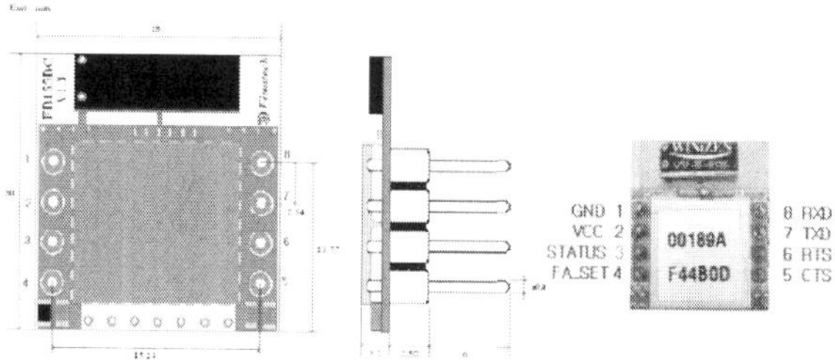

Fig. 7. Bluetooth Module Dimensions and Pin Assignments

The advantage of this, and any other small Bluetooth module, is the internal chip antenna that is used for short distance wireless communication. This is important since the transmitter or receiver device does not require an external antenna.

3.3 Firmware and data communication

The development of the firmware for the microcontroller is based upon the microcontroller that is being utilized in the design. As well, the code can be written in a verity of languages, typically Assembly and C, which again is dependent on the microcontroller selected. To continue the example microcontroller that was used in previous sections, Atmel ATmega microcontroller code was created using AVR Stdio4.0 and AVR ISP. The code was written in the C-language. AVR Stdio4.0 (Atmel Co., Ltd) which is a professional Integrated Development Environment (IDE) is used for writing, simulation, emulation and debugging. As a compiler, it also changes the firmware code from C-language to Hex code. An example firmware flow-charts for a biomedical signal transceiver is illustrated in Figure 8.

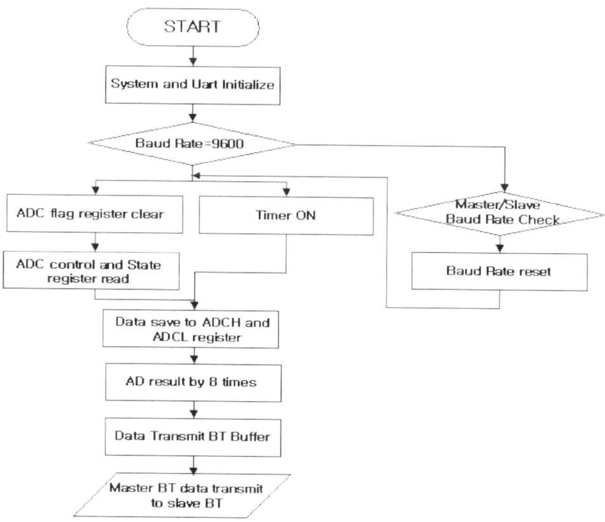

Fig. 8. Firmware Block Diagram

The digital hardware works as follows. Once data from analog hardware circuitry has been amplified, filter, and shifted, the signal is sent to the ADC on the microcontroller. After the signal has been sampled, the microcontroller then sends the digital signal to the Bluetooth module via UART communication protocol. Then, the biomedical signal is transmitted wirelessly through wireless Bluetooth module, utilizing the master-slave configuration.

4. ECG signal processing: A practical approach

As an example of biomedical signal processing in a transceiver device, in this section, ECG signal analysis for real-time heart monitoring will be discussed. Following the discussion on previous sections, this section particularly describes where real-time ECG monitoring using hand-held devices, such as, smart phones or custom-designed health monitoring system. ECG analysis is one of the very first areas of physiological measurement where computer processing was introduced successfully. ECG has been widely used as the diagnostic measurement for heart monitoring. Typically cardiologists used to interpret the ECG tracing for identifying abnormalities related to function of heart. With the advancement in biomedical signal processing, it is now reality that smart monitoring system can mimic the rules cardiologists applies in order to monitor heart health in real time. Signal Processing and machine learning techniques plays an important role in this purpose. Hence, this type of smart devices would be useful in monitoring patient's health in a more efficient way (Laguna et al., 2005).

In the previous sections, we have described a low-cost real-time biomedical signal transceiver/monitoring system which could also use ECG as one of the physiological parameter to monitor health.

In the following sub-sections, we will discuss the underlying ECG signal processing techniques used for identifying heart abnormalities. Typical steps are preprocessing of ECG, wave amplitude and duration detection, heart rate calculation, ECG feature extraction algorithms, and finally identifying the abnormalities. A typical block diagram is illustrated in following Figure 9 (Neuman, 2010).

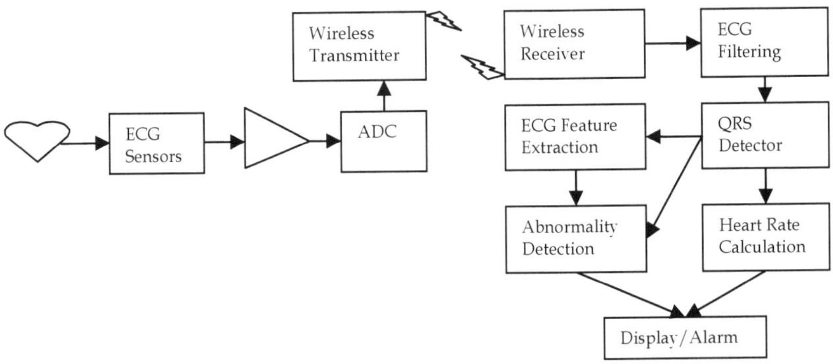

Fig. 9. Block diagram of biomedical signal transceiver for real-time acquisition, processing and heart condition monitoring system. The right portion of the system can be implemented in smart phone or PDA for smart health monitoring.

4.1 ECG digital filtering

ECG signal is usually corrupted with different types of noise. These are baseline wander introduced during data acquisition, power line interference and muscle noise or artifacts as discussed in the pervious sections. Prior to applying different signal processing techniques for extraction different ECG features which are of clinical interests, data needs to be filtered in order to reduce noise and artifacts. Some of these filtering techniques are discussed below with a practical approach where the methods can be easily implementable (Laguna et al., 2005, Clifford, 2006).

4.1.1 Power line interference

Appropriate shielding and safety consideration could be employed to reduce this particular type of noise in addition to analog filtering discussed in previous sections. After receiving signals at the receiver sides, it is preferred to get rid of this type of noise in the pre-processing step (Laguna et al.,2005). Typically, band-stop (notch) filtering with cutoff, Fc=50/60 Hz would suppress such noise. Figure 10 illustrates the magnitude and phase response of a digital second order Infinite Impulse Response (IIR) notch filter with cutoff frequency of 60 Hz.

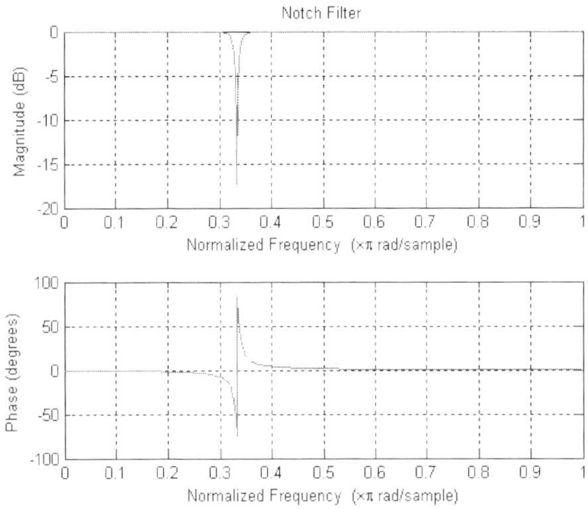

Fig. 10. Magnitude and phase response of an Infinite Impulse Response (IIR) notch filter to remove 60 Hz power line noise.

4.1.2 Baseline wanders correction

Due to the error in data collection process, baseline as well as dc offsets could be introduced. Removal of baseline wander is required prior to further processing. There are several techniques that have been widely used such as filtering and polynomial curve fitting method (Laguna et al. 2005, Clifford, 2006). Since all data processing starts with visual inspection, as for offline ECG analysis, we should inspect the data for baseline wander and dc bias. DC bias can easily removed by subtracting the mean from the original signal. As for

the baseline wander corrections, filtering method is most widely used. Here, we will describe the linear filtering method to remove the baseline wander in ECG signals.
The frequency of the baseline wander is usually below 0.5 Hz (Laguna et al. 2005). This information particularly helps in design a high-pass filter in order to get rid of baseline wander. The design of a linear time-invariant high pass filter requires several considerations, most importantly, the choice of cut-off frequency and filter order. The ECG characteristic wave frequencies are higher than baseline wander. Therefore, a carefully designed high pass filter with cut-off frequency, $F_c = 0.5$ Hz can effective remove the baseline. Baseline wander correction using a linear digital filter is shown in Figure 11. Instead of a high-pass filter we used band-pass filtering. We applied a sixth order butterworth filter with cutoff 0.7-40 Hz. To avoid distortion, zero phase digital filtering was performed by processing the data in both forward and reverse direction. This can be done using MATLAB command filtfilt.

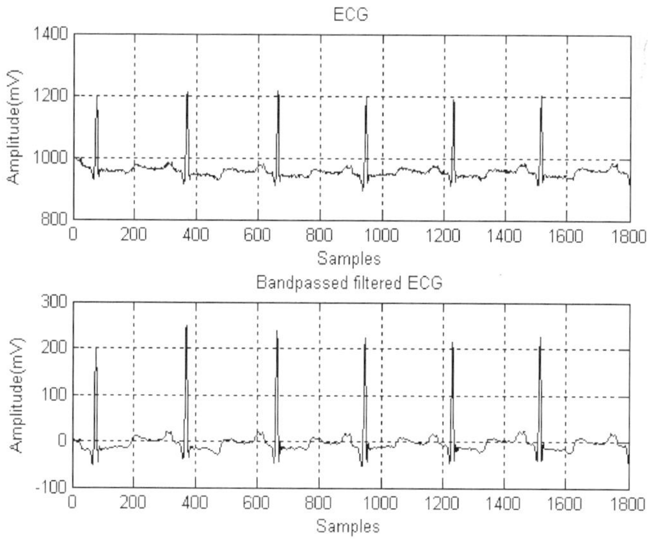

Fig. 11. ECG signal after band-pass filtering which effectively corrects baseline wander and reduces low frequency noise and high frequency artifacts. Prior to applying bandpass filter the DC components were removed from ECGs.

4.2 QRS detection

Detection of QRS complex is particularly most important in ECG signal processing. The information obtained from QRS detection, temporal information of each beat and QRS morphology information can be used for the improvement of performance for the other algorithms. In literature, many methods have been developed for detection of QRS complex. Most of these are based on filtering, nonlinear transformation and decision rules as well as using template matching method. In recent approaches, wavelet transform and empirical mode decomposition based algorithms have been developed. We will discuss a widely used and robust real-time QRS detection algorithm popularly known as Pam-Tompkins algorithm (Pan & Tompkins, 1985).

The Pan-Tompkins algorithm consists of several steps. This is a single channel detection method in order to achieve better performance. In order to attenuate noise, the signal is first passed through a digital band-pass filter composed of cascaded high-pass and low-pass filters (Pan & Tompkins, 1985). The band-pass filtering corrects the baseline wander, reduces muscle noise, 60 Hz power line interference, T-wave interference (Pan & Tompkins, 1985). The cutoff frequency of this band-pass filter is an important design parameter. Another reason of this filtering is to maximize the energy of QRS complex. Pan and Tompkins suggested choosing 5-15 Hz as desirable pass band. The next steps involve nonlinear transformation in order to highlight the QRS complex from baseline. These steps are differentiation, squaring followed by moving window integration. Derivative stage provides the slope information of QRS complex. Squaring operation intensifies the slope of the frequency response curve. It also helps to restrict the false positives caused by unusually high amplitude T waves. The signal produced by the moving window integration operation provides the slope and width of the QRS complex. The choice of window sample size is an important parameter. Generally, it should be chosen such a way that the window size is same as the QRS width. The window width can be determined empirically making sure that QRS complex and T waves do not merge together. For practical application, we choose window of 30 samples (150 ms, sampling frequency was 360 samples/s). Finally, an adaptive threshold will be applied to identify the location of QRS complexes (Pan & Tompkins, 1985).

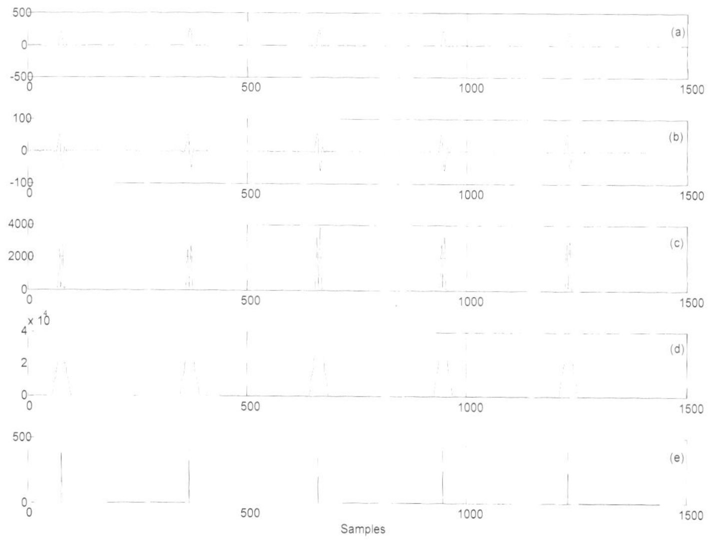

Fig. 12. Typical steps of Pan-Tompkins algorithm for detecting QRS complex: (a) band-pass filtered ECG signals; (b) after differentiation; (c) after performing squaring operation; (d) moving window integration; and (d) R peak detection.

The fiducial points of the QRS complex can be detected from the integration waveform. The time duration of the rising edge is equal to the QRS width. The maximum slope is the location of R wave peak. Q and S points are the start and end points of the rising slope respectively (Pan & Tompkins, 1985). The R peak detection is illustrated in Figure 12.

4.3 Heart rate computation and display

Heart rate is a vital sign to determine the patient's condition or well being. It can be easily computed from ECG (Neuman, 2010). Heart rate can be computed using various methods, for example, over one minute time period simply by counting the number of heart beats would give us the heart rate in beats per minute. However, if the QRS or R wave peak detector misses some beats that would adversely affect the heart rate and give wrong counts. The heart rate monitoring tool should avoid such wrong results. Therefore, it is more appropriate to measure the time duration between two successive R peaks known as R-R intervals and computing instantaneous heart rate directly from R-R interval. In clinical settings, heart rate is measured in beats per minute (bpm). So the formula for determining heart rate from RR interval is as following (Neuman, 2010).

$$Heart\,rate(bpm) = \frac{60{,}000}{RR\,interval\ (ms)}$$

Once the program computes the heart rate it can be presented on the display of the monitoring device. We have discussed a low cost biomedical signal transceiver, where ECG signal is one parameter for health monitoring. Using this wireless transceiver ECG signal can be transmitted to a hand-held device, such as, smart phone or PDAs. The smart phone will have applications capable of computing instantaneous heart rate or average heart rate of a pre-determined period of time and shown as a digital output in the display of the smart phone. The application would also be able to identify primary abnormalities such as premature atrial contraction (APC or PAC) or premature ventricular contraction (PVC) and present an auditory or visual alarm to the patient.

4.4 P and T wave detection

Once QRS locations are identified, two other fudicial marks in ECG, P and T wave peak can be detected using the R peak location information. For detecting T wave onset, peak and offset, we should define a search window in forward direction. The size of the search window can be function of heart rate calculated. For detecting P wave, a backward search is required. Search window size can be determined similarly (Laguna et al., 1994).

Laguna et al. (1994) proposed an automatic method of wave boundaries detection in multilead ECG. The algorithm includes a QRS detector for multilead ECG, P and T wave detection. Since, a robust method of QRS detector for single channel has already been discussed in previous sub-sections here we focus mainly on P and T wave detection. Moreover, this method is also based on the QRS detection method of Pan and Tompkins. In preprocessing steps, a second order linear bandpass filter (cutoff frequency of 0.8-18 Hz, -3dB) is applied to the signal to remove baseline wander and attenuate high frequency noise. This signal is called ECGPB. Then a low-pass differentiator (Pan & Tompkins, 1985) is applied to obtain the information about changes in slope. This differentiated signal is called

ECGDER. Then moving-window integration will be performed. In this case, Laguna et al. had chosen the window size of 95 ms. Since P and T waves usually have lower frequency components than the QRS complex, a digital low-pass filter (cutoff frequency of 12 Hz, -3dB) is applied to the ECGDER signal. This filtering reduces the remaining noise and highlights the P and T wave components and the signal is called (DERFI) (Laguna et al. 1994). Now a search window of 150 ms is defined which starts 225 ms before the R wave position. In this search window, the algorithm searches for maximum and minimum values. The P wave peak is assumed to be occurred at the zero-crossing of the maximum and minimum values (Laguna et al., 1994).

Similarly for T wave detection, a search window is defined which is a function of heart rate already calculated. In this search window, the algorithm searches for maximum and the minimum values. However, the T wave peak is assumed to be occurred at the zero-crossing of the maximum and minimum values. The T wave morphology varies hugely. The algorithm can also identify the type of T wave (for example, regular or inverted) by examining the relative position and values of the maximum and minimum values in the search window (Laguna et al., 1994).

5. References

B. Chi, J. Yao, S. Han, X. Xie, G. Li, Z. Wang, "Low-Power Transceiver Analog Front-End Circuits for Bidirectional High Data Rate Wireless Telemetry in Medical Endoscopy Applications," Biomedical Engineering, IEEE Transactions on , vol.54, no.7, pp.1291-1299, July 2007 doi: 10.1109/TBME.2006.889768

G. D. Clifford. Advanced Methods and Tools for ECG Data analysis. Cambridge, Massachusetts, 2006.

J. H. Schulman, P. Mobley, J. Wolfe, H. Stover, A. Krag, "A 1000+ Channel Bionic Communication System," Proceedings of the 28th IEEE EMBS Annual International Conference, New York City, USA, Aug. 30 - Sept. 3, 2006.

J. M. R. Delgado, "Electrodes for Extracellular Recording and Stimulation," in Physical Techniques in Biological Research, W.L. Nastuk, Ed., New York: Academic Press, 1964.

J. Pan and W. J. Tompkins, A Real-Time QRS Detection Algorithm" IEEE Transactions on Biomedical Engineering vol. 32(3), pp. 230-236, 1985.

J. Molina, Design a 60 Hz Notch Filter with the UAF42, Burr-Brown Application Bulletin,11/30/10 , <http://focus.ti.com/lit/an/sbfa012/sbfa012.pdf>

L. Sornmo, P. Laguna. Bioelectric Signal Processing in Cardiac and Neurological Applications. Elsevier Academic Press, 2005.

M. R. Neuman, "Vital Signs: Heart Rate," IEEE Pulse, November/December 2010, vol. 1(3), pp.51-55. 2010.

P. Laguna, R. Jane, and P. Caminal, "Automatic detection of wave boundaries in multilead ECG signals: validation with the CSE database," Computers and biomedical research , vol. 27(1), pp. 45, 1994.

R. R. Harrison, P. T. Watkins, R. J. Kier, R. O. Lovejoy, D. J. Black, B. Greger, F. Solzbacher, "A Low-Power Integrated Circuit for a Wireless 100-Electrode Neural Recording System," IEEE Journal of Solid State Circuits, Vol. 42, No. 1, Jan. 2007.

A. S. Sedra and A. C. Smith. Microelectronic Circuits. New York: Oxford UP, 2010.

5

Column Coupling Electrophoresis in Biomedical Analysis

Peter Mikuš and Katarína Maráková
Faculty of Pharmacy, Comenius University, Slovakia

1. Introduction

Biomedical analysis is one of the most advanced areas solved in analytical chemistry due to the requirements on the analyzed samples (analyte vs. matrix problems) as well as on the overall analytical process regarding automatization and miniaturization of the analyses. Separation methods for the biomedical analysis are requested to provide high resolution power, high separation efficiency and high sensitivity. This is connected with such conditions that analytes are present in the samples in very low (trace) amounts and/or are present in multicomponent matrices (serum, plasma, urine, *etc.*). These complex matrices consist from inorganic and organic constituents at (very) differing concentrations and these can overlap the analyte(s) peak(s) due to migration and detection interferences. In addition, a column overloading can occur in such cases. It can be pronounced especially for the microscale separation methods such as the capillary electrophoresis (CE). Hence, it is obvious that there is the need for the sample preparation: (i) preconcentration - lower limits of detection and quantification; (ii) purification of the sample and isolation of analytes - elimination of sample matrix; (iii) derivatization - improvement of physical and/or chemical properties of the analytes, before the CE analysis in these situations to reach relevant analytical information.

Sample pretreatment can be performed either off-line (before injection of analyzed sample into the analyzer) or on-line (after the injection). The conventional separation systems (single column) use mostly external (off-line) sample pretreatment, even though this analytical approach has many limitations. These are (i) a loss of the analytes, (ii) time consuming and tedious procedure, (iii) problematic manipulation with minute amounts of the samples, (iv) problematic for automatization, (v) decreased precision of the analyses, *etc.* On the other hand, on-line sample pretreatment has many advantages as (i) elimination of random and/or systematic errors caused by external sample handling, (ii) simplification of an overall analytical process (less number of an external steps), (iii) reduction of the total analysis time and (iv) possibility of the automatization and miniaturization of the analytical process (routine precise microanalyses). A significant enhancement of sensitivity and selectivity is one of the main benefits of the on-line sample pretreatment. An on-line pretreatment is crucial when there are only micro amounts of the samples for the analysis and/or when analytes/samples have lower stability.

The advanced single column electrophoretic techniques (transient isotachophoresis, field-enhanced sample stacking, dynamic pH junction, sweeping, in-capillary solid/liquid phase extraction-CE, in-capillary dialysis-CE, *etc.*), representing the CE with the on-line (in-column) sample preparation, were described and successfully applied for trace analytes and less or more complex matrices in many cases (section 2). The aim of this chapter is to demonstrate potentialities and practical applications of a column coupling electrophoresis as another group of the on-line sample preparation analytical approaches (section 3) enabling powerful combination of (i) electrophoretic techniques (ITP, CZE, IEF, CEC) (sections 3.1.1 and 3.2.1), (ii) electrophoretic and non electrophoretic (liquid chromatography, flow injection analysis, *etc.*) techniques (sections 3.1.2 and 3.2.2). In this way, it should be possible to create the most complex, flexible and robust tool filling the above mentioned requirements of the advanced analysis. Such tool and its modes are described in this chapter with regard to the theory, basic schemes, potentialities, for the capillary (section 3.1) as well as microchip (section 3.2) format. This theoretical description is accompanied with the performance parameters achievable by the advanced methods (section 4) and appropriate application examples in the field of the biomedical analysis (section 5). For a better understanding of the benefits, limitations and application potential of the column coupling electrophoretic methods the authors decided to enclose the short initial section with a brief overview of advanced single column electrophoretic techniques (section 2) that often take part also in the column coupling electrophoresis.

2. Advanced single column techniques

As it is known from the literature (Simpson et al., 2008; Bonato, 2003) CE has many advantages (high separation efficiency, versatility, flexibility, use of aqueous separation systems, low consumptions of electrolytes as well as minute amounts of samples). Beyond all the advantages, conventional CE has also some drawbacks, which limit its application in routine analytical laboratories. They include (i) relatively difficult optimization of conditions of analytical measurements, (ii) worse reproducibility of measurements (especially when hydrodynamically open separation systems are used where non selective flows, hydrodynamic and electroosmotic are acting) than in liquid chromatography, (iii) low sample load capacity and need for the external (off-line) sample preparation for the complex matrices (measurement of trace analyte besides macroconstituent(s) can be difficult without a sample pretreatment), and (iv) difficulties in applying several detection methods in routine analyses (Trojanowicz, 2009).

Some of these limitations can be overcome using advanced single column techniques. They provide (i) improved concentration LOD, (ii) automatization (external manipulation with the sample and losses of the analyte are reduced, analytical procedure is less tedious and overall analysis time can be shortened, labile analytes can be analysed easier) and (iii) miniaturization of the analytical procedure (pretreating of minute amounts of the sample is possible and effective), (iv) elimination of interfering compounds, according to the mechanism employed. However, the sample load capacity of these techniques is still insufficient (given by the dimensions of the CE capillaries). The advanced single column CE techniques usually suffer from lower reproducibility of the analyses due to the complex mechanisms of the separation which controlling can be difficult in practice. Moreover, the capillaries with embedded non electrophoretic parts (membranes, columns, fibers, monolits) are less versatile (Simpson et al., 2008).

2.1 Stacking electrophoretic pretreatment techniques

Stacking procedures are based on increasing analyte mass in its zone during the electromigration process via electromigration effects, enhancing sensitivity in this way. In all cases, the key requirement is that there is an electrophoretic component in the preconcentration mechanism and that the analytes concentrate on a boundary through a change in velocity. Then we can recognize (i) field-strength-induced changes in velocity (transient isotachophoresis (Beckers & Boček, 2000a), field-enhanced sample stacking (Kim & Terabe, 2003; Quirino & Terabe, 2000a), and (ii) chemically induced changes in velocity (dynamic pH junction (Britz-McKibbin & Chen, 2000), sweeping (Kitagawa et al., 2006; Quirino & Terabe, 1998, 1999; Quirino et al., 2000b)). In addition to these techniques, counter-flow gradient focusing (Shackman & Ross, 2007), electrocapture (Horáková et al., 2007), and many others can be considered as the techniques based on a combination of field-strength- and chemically induced changes in velocity offering new interesting possibilities in on-line sample preparation (mainly preconcentration).

Some of the stacking techniques (and their combinations) can provide besides (i) the preconcentration also other benefits such as (ii) an effective sample purification isolating solute (group of solutes) from undesired matrix constituents (Simpson et al., 2008) or they can be combined with (iii) chemical reaction of the analyte(s) (Ptolemy et al., 2005, 2006), simplifying overall analytical procedure in this way. The choice of on-line pretreatment method depends on the specific physical-chemical properties of the separated analytes (e.g. charge, ionization, polarity) and the sample matrices (mainly concentration). For example, an on-line desalting of a physiologic sample can be effectively accomplished by the electrokinetic removing of the fast migrating low molecular ions prior to the IEF focusing of the high molecular analytes (proteins) (Clarke et al., 1997).

2.2 Non electrophoretic pretreatment techniques

An on-line sample preparation can be carried out advantageously also combining the CE with a technique that is based on a non electrophoretic principles. Most of these approaches are based on (i) the chromatographic or extraction principles (separations based on chemical principles), but also other techniques, such as (ii) the membrane filtration, MF (separations based on physical principles), can be used. In this case, a non electrophoretic segment (*e.g.* extractor, membrane) is fixed directly to the CE capillary (in-line combination) (Petersson et al., 1999; Mikuš & Maráková, 2010).

In-line systems such as CEC/CZE (Thomas et al., 1999), SPE/CZE (Petersson et al., 1999) or MF/CZE (Barroso & de Jong, 1998) are attractive thanks to their low cost and easy construction. On the other hand, versatility of such systems is limited (in-capillary segment cannot be replaced). One of the main limitations of performing in-line sample preparation is that the entire sample must pass through the capillary, which can lead to fouling and/or even clogging of the separation capillary and significant decreasing of reproducibility of the analyses when particularly problematic samples (like biological ones) are used. It can be pronounced especially for the extraction techniques (created inserting a solid-phase column into capillary, where the whole analytical procedure is very complex and it includes conditioning, loading/sorption, washing, (labeling, if necessary), filling (by electrolyte), elution/desorption, separation and detection. In order to overcome these issues, on-line methods based on another way of coupling of two different techniques may be used as alternatives to the in-line systems.

3. Advanced column coupled techniques

Multidimensional chromatographic and capillary electrophoresis (CE) protocols provide powerful methods to accomplish ideal separations (Hanna et al., 2000; Křivánková & Boček,

1997a). Among them the most important ones are the integrated systems containing complementary dimensions, where different dimensions separate components on the basis of independent or orthogonal principles (Moore & Jorgenson, 1995; Lemmo & Jorgenson, 1993; Mohan & Lee, 2002). In such a multidimensional system, the peak capacity is the product of the peak capacities of each dimension (Guiochon et al., 1983). A key part in the instrumentation of the hyphenated techniques is an appropriate interface that enables to connect and disconnect two different stages (*e.g.* columns) reproducibly and flexibly according to the relevance and relation of the particular actions in the analytical process.

The column coupling arrangement, where two or more separation techniques are arranged into two or more separated stages, can be a very effective approach offering additional benefits to the advanced single column CE techniques and reducing some of their disadvantages. Nevertheless, the advanced mechanisms given in section 2 can also be adapted into the column coupling arrangement enhancing the effectivity and application potential of the resulting method. Two separate stages provide (i) sample preparation (preseparation, preconcentration, purification and derivatization) and (ii) analytical separation of on-line pretreated sample. The benefits of the column coupling configuration, additional to the advanced single column CE, involve (i) autonomic combination of various separation mechanisms that provide enhanced and well defined separation selectivity, and a possibility to replace easily one of the stages (ii) well defined and more effective elimination of the undesirable sample matrix components, (iii) significant enhancement of the sample load capacity (especially for the larger internal diameters of capillaries) resulting in the improved LOD, (iv) improved precision of the analyses due to well defined control of the separation mechanisms (Kaniansky et al., 1993; Kaniansky & Marák, 1990).

The most frequently used and the simplest column coupling configuration is the CE combined with another CE (CE-CE, CE-CE-CE) (Kaniansky & Marák, 1990). Hybrid column coupled techniques are based on the combination of a non electrophoretic technique with the CE, e.g. LC-CE (Pálmarsdóttir & Edholm, 1995), SPE-CE (Puig et al., 2007), dialysis-CE (Lada & Kennedy, 1997), FIA-CE (Mardones et al., 1999). They offer different separation mechanisms in comparison with the CE-CE, however, they have more demands on instrumentation. Additionally to the on-line combination of conventional column techniques (electrophoretic as well as non electrophoretic) the column coupling arrangement combining a conventional technique with an advanced one (section 2) is applicable too. These types of the column coupled techniques are discussed in detail and illustrated through the corresponding instrumental schemes for both the capillary (section 3.1) as well as microchip (section 3.2) format.

3.1 Capillary format

3.1.1 Hyphenation of electrophoretic techniques

The hyphenation of two electrophoretic techniques in capillary format (see Fig. 1) can effectively and relatively easily (simple and direct interface) solve the problems of the sample preparation and final analysis (fine separation) in one run in well defined way, i.e. producing high reproducibility of analyses, in comparison to the single column sample preconcentration and purification approaches (section 2). Moreover, the CE performed in a hydrodynamically closed separation system (hydrodynamic flow is eliminated by semipermeable membranes at the ends of separation compartment) with suppressed electroosmotic flow (EOF), that is typically used in the CE-CE configuration, has the advantage of (i) the enhanced precision due to elimination of the non selective flows (hydrodynamic, electroosmotic), and (ii) enhanced sample load capacity (30 μL sample injection volume is typical) due to the large internal diameter of the preseparation capillary (800 μm I.D. is typical) (Kaniansky & Marák, 1990; Kaniansky et al., 1993). The commercially available CE-CE systems have a modular composition that provides a high flexibility in arranging particular moduls in the separation unit. In this way, it is possible to create desirable CE-CE combinations such as (i) ITP-ITP, (ii) ITP-CZE, (iii) CZE-CZE, *etc.*, capable to solve wide scale of the advanced analytical problems (see Fig. 1). Although such combinations require the sophisticated instrument and deep knowledge in the field of electrophoresis, the coupled CE methods are surely the most effective way how to take/multiply benefits of both CE techniques coupled in the column-coupling configuration of separation unit. The basic instrumental scheme of the column coupled CE-CE system shown in Fig. 1 is properly matching with hydrodynamically closed CE modes where effective electrophoretic mobility is the only driving force of the separated compounds. On the other hand, when additional supporting effects such as counterflow, electroosmotic flow *etc.* must be employed, appropriate modifications of the scheme in Fig. 1 are made. Such modified instrumental schemes are attached into the sections dealing with IEF or CEC coupled techniques (3.1.1.3 and 3.1.1.5) that are principally applicable only in hydrodynamically open CE mode (Mikuš et al., 2006; Danková et al., 2001; Busnel et al., 2006).

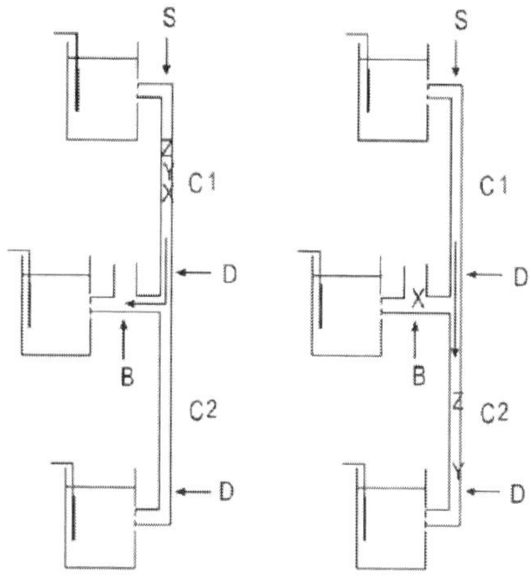

Fig. 1. CE-CE method in column coupling configuration of the separation units for the direct analysis of unpretreated complex matrices sample, basic instrumental scheme. On-line sample preparation: removing matrices X (ITP, CZE), preseparation (ITP, CZE) and/or preconcentration (ITP, stacking) and/or derivatization (with stacking) of analytes Y, Z in the first CE stage (column C1). Final separation: baseline separation of Y and Z in the second CE (ITP, CZE) stage (column C2). Reprinted from ref. (Tekeľ & Mikuš, 2005), with permission. C1 - preseparation column, C2 - analytical column, B - bifurcation block for coupling C1 and C2, D - positions of detectors.

3.1.1.1 ITP-CZE

Although all electrophoretic methods can be mutually on-line combined, the biggest attention was paid to the ITP-CZE coupling, introduced more than 20 years ago by

Kaniansky (Kaniansky & Marák, 1990). The analytical benefits of the ITP-CZE combination have been already well documented (Fanali et al., 2000; Danková et al., 2001; Kvasnička et al., 2001; Valcárcel et al., 2001; Bexheti et al., 2006; Beckers, 2000b; Křivánková et al., 1991; Křivánková & Thormann, 1993; Křivánková & Boček, 1997a).

An on-line combination of ITP with CZE appears to be promissing for alleviating some of the following practical problems (Kaniansky & Marák, 1990):

i. ITP is a separation technique with a well defined concentrating power while the separands migrate stacked in sharp zones, i.e., it can be considered as an ideal sample injection technique for CZE,
ii. In some instances the detection and quantitation of trace constituents separated by ITP in a large excess of matrix constituents may require the use of appropriate spacing constituents. Such a solution can be very beneficial when a limited number of the analytes need to be determined in one analysis. It becomes less practical (a search for suitable spacing constituents) when the number of trace constituents to be determined in one analysis is high,
iii. In CZE, high-efficiency separations make possible a multi-component analysis of trace constituents with close physico-chemical properties. However, the separations can be ruined, *e.g.*, when the sample contains matrix constituents at higher concentrations than those of the trace analytes.

A characteristic advantage of the ITP-CZE combination is a high selectivity/separability obtainable due to the CZE as the final analytical step. Hence, the ITP-CZE method can be easily modified with a great variety of selectors implemented with the highest advantage into the CZE stage enabling to separate also the most problematic analytes (structural analogs, isomers, enantiomers). The ITP-CZE methods with chiral as well as achiral CZE mode have been successfully applied in various real situations (Mikuš et al., 2006a, 2008a, 2008c; Danková et al., 2001; Marák et al., 2007; Kvasnička et al., 2001).

The most frequently used ITP-CZE system works in the hydrodynamically closed separation mode that is advantageous for the real analyses of multicomponent ionic mixtures because of the best premises for enhancing sample load capacity (enables using capillaries with very large I.D.). Such commercial system is applied with just one high-voltage power supply and three electrodes (one electrode shared by the two dimensions), see Fig. 1. The electric circuit involving upper and middle electrode (electric field No. 1) is applied in the ITP stage while upper and lower electrode (electric field No. 2) is applied in the CZE stage. For the separation ITP-CZE mechanism see chronological schemes in Fig.2. The focused zone in the first dimension (ITP) is driven to the interface (bifurcation point) by only electric field No. 1. The cut of the zone of interest in the ITP stage is based on the electronic controlling (comparation point) of the relative step heigth (R_{sh}, a position of the analyte between the leading and terminating ion, it is the qualitative indicator depending on the effective mobility of the analyte) of the analyte, see Fig. 3. The conductivity sensor (upper D in Fig. 1, D-ITP in Fig.2) serves for the indication of the analyte zone. This is very advantageous because such indication is (i) universal and (ii) independent on other comigrating compounds (sample matrix constituents migrating in the ITP stage) and therefore independent on sample composition. The electric circuit is switched and electric field No. 2 (upper and lower electrode) is applied in an appropriate time (this time is set electronically depending on requirements of the composition of the transferred plug) after the indication of the analyte zone passing through the upper D. From this moment the all ITP zones are directed to the CZE stage for the final separation and detection. It is possible to carry out one or more cuttings depending on the zones of interest and/or interfering matrix constituents present in the sample. The interface between the separation solutions in the ITP and CZE capillary is free (without any mechanical restraint) but mixing of the electrolytes is eliminated (with the exception of difusion) by suppressing all non selective flows (hydrodynamic, electroosmotic) in the system. This is advantageous by an easy construction and elimination of dead volumes in the separation system (Ölvecká et al., 2001; Kaniansky et al., 2003).

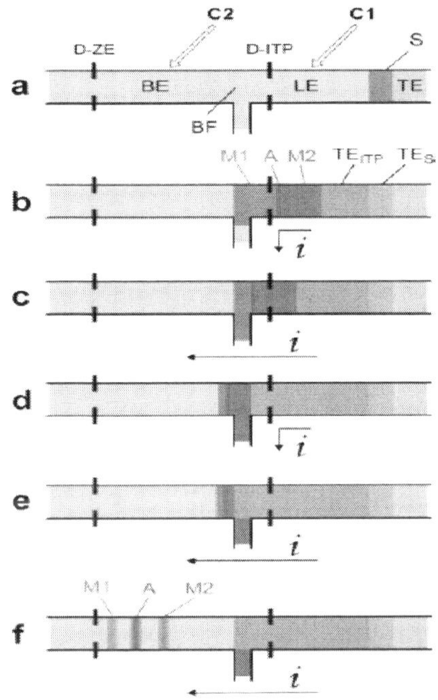

Fig. 2. ITP sample clean up for CZE with the closed separation system (without any supporting non selective flow). (a) Starting arrangement of the solutions in the capillaries; (b) ITP separation with the analyte (A) trapped into the boundary layer between the zones of front (M1) and rear (M2) spacers; (c) end of the run in the ITP capillary followed by an electrophoretic transfer of the analyte containing fraction to the CZE capillary (by switching the direction of the driving current); (d) removal of the sample constituents migrating behind the transferred fraction (by switching the direction of the driving current); (e) starting situation in the separation performed in the CZE capillary (the direction of the driving current was switched); (f) separation and detection of the transferred constituents in the CZE capillary. BF = bifurcation region; C1, C2 = the ITP and CZE separation capillaries, respectively; D-ITP, D-ZE = detection sensors in the ITP and CZE separation capillaries, respectively; TES = terminating electrolyte adapted to the composition of the sample (S); TITP = terminating electrolyte adapted to the composition of the leading electrolyte solution; A = analyte, i = direction of the driving current. Reprinted from ref. (Kaniansky et al., 2003), with permission.

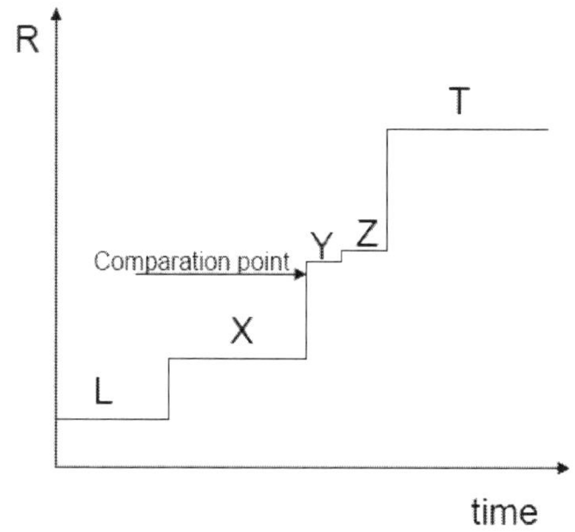

Fig. 3. Graphical illustration of the principle of the electronic cutting of the zone of interest in the ITP stage of the ITP-CZE combination. L = leading ion, T = terminating ion, X = matrix compound(s), Y, Z = analytes, R = resistance. Reprinted from ref. (Ölvecká et al., 2001), with permission.

The principle of this hyphenated technique consists from well-defined preconcentration (concentration LODs could be reduced by a factor of 10^3 when compared to conventional single column CZE) and preseparation (up to 99% or even more interfering compounds can be isolated (Danková et al., 1999)) of trace analytes in the first, wider, capillary (isotachophoretic step) and subsequently a cut of important analytes accompanied with a segment of the matrix, leading or terminator enters the second, narrower, capillary for the final separation by CZE (Fig. 2, Fig.3). The presence of this segment results from the fact that we do not want to lose a part of the analyzed zones and we must make a cut generously. The zone of this segment survives for a certain time during the CZE stage and this mean that ITP migration continues also in the second capillary for some time and it influences strongly the results of the analysis, especially the detection times of analytes used for identification of the analytes in CZE separations (Busnel et al., 2006; Gebauer et al., 2007; Mikuš et al., 2006a). From this is clear that it is important in an ITP-CZE combination to choose suitable electrolyte systems and find the optimum time to switch the current from the preseparation capillary to the separation capillary (Křivánková et al., 1995).

The ITP-CZE technique appeared to be very useful especially for the common universal detectors producing relatively low concentration LODs (UV-VIS photometric detector). It is because such method provides probably one of the most acceptable ratio simplicity-cost: universality-concentration LOD in comparison to other column coupling methods and detection systems. This suggestion is supported by many advanced applications of the ITP-CZE-UV method in the pharmaceutical and biomedical field (Marák et al., 2007; Mikuš et al., 2008a, 2008b, 2008c, 2009). Jumps in voltage (conductivity) between neighboring zones result in permanently sharp boundaries between zones (Fig. 3) that is extremely convenient for the conductivity detection in ITP. Although convenient to the detection of the ITP zones, conductivity detection technique has a limited applicability in the CZE separations (often measurements of small conductivity changes due to the zones on a relatively high conductivity background of the carrier electrolyte) (Ölvecká et al., 2001; Kaniansky et al., 2000).

3.1.1.2 ITP-ITP

The ITP-ITP combination represents the simplest possibility how to combine CE techniques. For the general instrumental scheme valid also for ITP-ITP, see Fig. 1. In the ITP–ITP mode both preseparation (wider) and analytical (narrower) capillaries are filled with (i) the same leading electrolyte (one-dimensional ITP) or (ii) different electrolytes (two-dimensional ITP) (Flottmann et al., 2006; Bexheti et al., 2006; Mikuš et al., 2006b; Kubačák et al., 2006a, 2006b, 2007). The ITP separation in a concentration cascade, introduced into conventional CE by Boček *et al.*, (Boček et al., 1978) enhances the detectabilities of the separated constituents from the response of the conductivity detection due to well-known links between the concentration of the leading electrolyte and the lengths (volumes) of the zones (Marák et al., 1990)
The first ITP stage of the ITP-ITP combination can apply all benefits as they are described for the ITP stage of the ITP-CZE combination in section 3.1.1.1. On the other hand, the ITP-ITP technique can take the highest advantage of the hyphenation with the MS detection (Tomáš et al., 2010). It is because of an intrinsic feature of ITP to produce pure analyte zones, i.e. those in which the analyte is accompanied only with counter ion, in the isotachophoretic steady state. In this way, the maximum response of the MS detector can be obtained for the analyte. Therefore, the ITP-ITP-MS hyphenation seems to be one of the most promissing methods for the fully automatized biomedical analyses such as pharmacokinetic studies, metabolomics, etc. An economic aspect of the ITP-ITP-MS method in comparison with the HPLC-MS method for the ionic compounds is apparent.

3.1.1.3 ITP-CEC

Another approach in the column coupled electrophoresis is the use of ITP sample focusing to improve the detection limits for the analysis of charged compounds in capillary electrochromatography (CEC). Besides this, the on-line isotachophoretic stage can serve also for a loadability enhancement (due to a large inner diameter of the ITP capillary). Both of these effects are then responsible for a dramatic reduction of the sample concentration detection limits through simultaneous acting of (i) large volume injection and (ii) analyte stacking (Mazereeuw et al., 2000).
In the ITP-CEC combination (Fig. 4), the open ITP mode must be applied because of the demands of the second stage (CEC) that is based on the EOF action. A coupled-column set-up can be used, in which counterflow ITP focusing is performed, and the separation capillaries are connected via a T-junction. For the schematic representation of the ITP-CEC procedure see Fig. 5. From the application point of view, the first ITP stage is advantageous especially for the injection of large volumes (tens of microliters) of diluted samples. When a very large sample is introduced, however, the focusing time of the sample often exceeds the migration time to the outlet of the ITP capillary. By applying a hydrodynamic counterflow (applicable in the hydrodynamically open CE systems) the ITP focusing will continue while extending the migration towards the outlet of the ITP capillary. Although the hydrodynamically open CE systems have the advantage of application of the supporting flows (counterflow, electroosmotic), it must be realized that

the reproducibility of cutting and also overall analysis is generally lower than in the hydrodynamically closed CE systems due to the fluctuations of the non selective flows in the separation system.

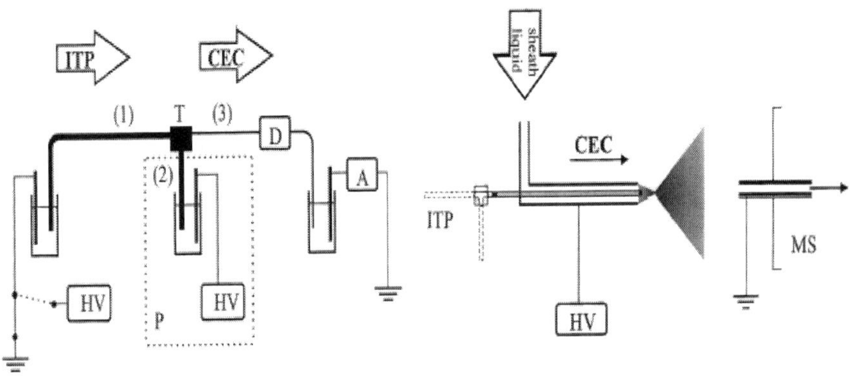

Fig. 4. Schematic representation of the ITP-CEC set-up. Right scheme: Schematic representation of the ITP-CEC-UV set-up with a (P) programmable capillary injection system, (D) UV-VIS absorbance detector, (A) amperometer and (T) laboratory made polyethylene T-piece. Untreated fused-silica capillaries of 220 μm I.D. (1 and 2) and 75 μm (3) are used. Left scheme: Schematic representation of the entire ITP-CEC-MS set-up. The electrospray needle with the sheath flow contains the CEC column, which is directly connected with the electrospray. The spray is directed towards the inlet capillary of the interface on the SSQ 710 mass spectrometer (MS). HV is the electrospray power supply. Reprinted from ref. (Mazereeuw et al., 2000), with permission.

The first ITP stage of the ITP-CEC combination can apply all benefits as they are described generally for the ITP stage of ITP-CZE combination in section 3.1.1.1. In ITP-CEC, the ITP sample clean-up effect is extremely important for enhancing reproducibility of CEC especially when injecting complex biological samples. The CEC stage of the ITP-CEC technique can take a high advantage of the hyphenation with the UV-VIS or MS detection, for the schemes of the experimental setups see Fig. 4. It is pronounced in the situations when the selectors interfering with the detection must be used in the separation system in order to establish the required selectivity. Immobilization of such selectors in the CEC column prevents their entering into the detector cell resulting in the elimination of the detection interferences. In this way, the maximum response of the UV-VIS or MS detector can be obtained for the analyte. Hence, the ITP-CEC combination seems to be a powerful tool for the on-line selective separation, sensitive determination and spectral identification of chiral compounds and various other isomers and structurally related compounds (i.e. "problematic" analytes) present in complex ionic matrices. The ITP-CEC-MS hyphenation seems to be one of the most promising methods for the fully automatized biomedical chiral analyses such as enantioselective pharmacokinetic studies, metabolomics, etc. (Mazereeuw et al., 2000).

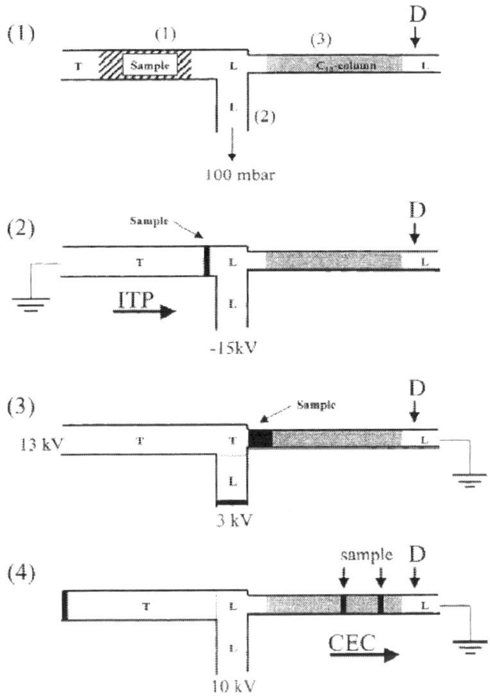

Fig. 5. Schematic representation of the ITP-CEC procedure (with a supporting non selective flow). The sample loading, ITP focusing step, sample zone transfer and CEC separation are shown in step 1, 2, 3 and 4, respectively. The set-up contains a (D) UV-VIS absorbance or MS detection, (T) terminator buffer and (L) leading buffer. Untreated fused-silica capillaries of 220 μm I.D. (1 and 2) and 75 μm (3) are used. Reprinted from ref. (Mazereeuw et al., 2000)., with permission.

3.1.1.4 CZE-CZE

CE separation system with tandem-coupled columns, i.e. CZE-CZE makes possible, within certain limits, splitting a CZE run into a sequence of the separation and detection stages (for the general instrumental scheme valid also for CZE-CZE, see Fig. 1). Therefore, the carrier electrolyte employed in the first (separation) stage of the run could be optimized with respect to the resolution of an analyte from complex (biological) matrix. In this way, a very significant "in-column" clean-up of the analytes from complex ionic matrices can be reached in the separation stage of the tandem by combining appropriate acid-basic (pH) and complexing (selectors) conditions. Due to this, the detection (*e.g.* spectral) data could be acquired in the detection stage of the tandem with almost no disturbances by matrix co-migrants (Danková et al., 2003).

The carrier electrolyte employed in the second (detection) stage could be chosen to reach favourable conditions in the acquisition of detection (*e.g.* spectral) data while maintaining the resolution of the analyte from matrix constituents as achieved in the separation stage

(Danková et al., 2003). Such two-dimensional systems reduce probability of component overlap and improve peak identification capabilities since the exact position of a compound in a two-dimensional electropherogram is dependent on two different separation mechanisms (Sahlin, 2007).

The CZE-CZE combination can be set to achieve a remarkable selectivity. On the other hand, it is considerably less sensitive than the ITP-CZE combination due to the absence of stacking capability of the basic CZE technique. It can be overcome, fortunately, replacing a basic CZE technique by an advanced one (*e.g.* stacking). The CZE-CZE technique is favorable for the hyphenation with various detection techniques (*e.g.* spectral, electrochemical) because it makes possible splitting of the CZE run into a sequence of the separation and detection stages (Danková et al., 2003).

3.1.1.5 IEF-CZE, -CGE

Arduous proteomics tasks require techniques with high throughput and high efficiency in order to screen a certain proteome expression and to monitor the effects of environmental conditions and time on the expression. There seldom is, at present, a single separation mode sufficient enough to deal with such complex samples. CE is a significant tool for the separation of proteins and peptides (Dolnik &. Hutterer, 2001). To finish complicated separation jobs, great efforts have been concentrated on the development of 2D CE (Yang et al., 2003b). IEF, CGE and CZE are the most effective electrophoretic techniques for zwitterionic compounds, therefore the on-line combination of these techniques is of the highest importance for the protein analysis with perspectives of their automatization and miniaturization (Kaniansky et al., 2000; Chen X. et al., 2002; Kvasnička et al., 2001).

When performing isoelectric focusing, one can fill the total volume of a capillary with sample solution. It can be expected that the detection sensitivity of the hyphenated system benefits from the concentration effect of the first dimension of IEF. This feature holds advantage over other CE modes such as CZE, CGE, micellar electrokinetic capillary chromatography (MECC), and capillary electrochromatography (CEC). Practically, IEF has a power to concentrate analytes up to several hundred folds in a capillary (Shen et al., 2000). Such a condensed and shortened analyte plug in a capillary is appropriate for sample injection to other CE modes. Therefore IEF is a proper candidate for the first dimension in a multi-dimensional CE system. Apparently, this will improve the sensitivity for mass detection. It is advantageous over those systems in which IEF was utilized as the second dimension. Nevertheless, the sensitivity of UV absorbance suffers from the necessity of the CAs involved in IEF. Of course, isotachophoresis (ITP) as a pretreatment tool for CZE separation also has a concentration effect (Kaniansky et al., 1999). ITP is carried out based on the mobility differences of ions and, IEF, based on different pIs of ampholytic molecules.

Capillary isoelectric focusing (IEF) and capillary zone electrophoresis (CZE) can be on-line hyphenated by a dialysis interface to achieve a 2D capillary electrophoresis (CE) system, i.e. IEF-CZE (Fig. 6), as it was demonstrated by Yang *et al.* (Yang et al., 2003b). The system was used with just one high-voltage power supply and three electrodes (one cathode shared by the two dimensions). The focused and preseparated (according to differences in the isoelectric points of the analytes) zones in the first dimension (i.e. the IEF) were driven to the dialysis interface by electroosmotic flow (EOF), besides chemical mobilization from the first anode to the shared cathode. Zero net charged analyte molecules focused in the first dimension are recharged in the interface (I_2 in Fig. 6) according to the pH of the altered buffer. The semi-permeable property of the interface ensures that macromolecules of ampholytic analytes remain in the separation channel. In the second dimension (i.e. the CZE), the preseparated zones were further separated (according to the ratios of charge and mass, i.e. electrophoretic mobility) and driven by an inverted EOF, which originated from the charged layer of a cationic surfactant adsorbed onto the inner wall of the capillary. It can be concluded that the 2D IEF-CZE system possesses higher resolving power than each of the single modes. This protocol of the 2D CE system endues the interface with durability and makes for convenient performance. To reduce the dead volume, it is necessary to match the inner diameter of the hollow fiber to that of the capillaries. The tangent surfaces of these units should be made even and smooth.

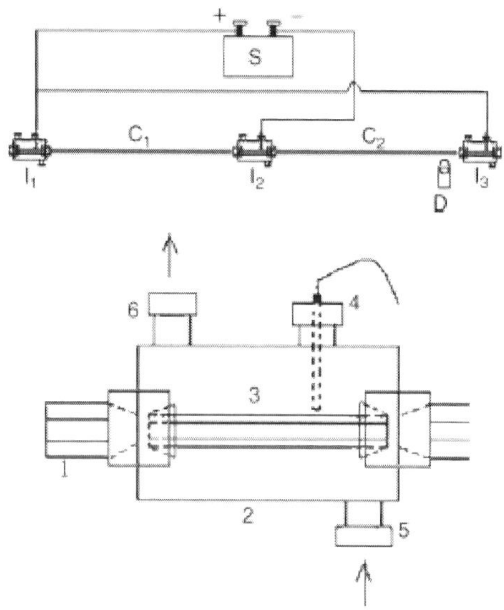

Fig. 6. Construction of 2D IEF-CZE. Upper scheme: general overview. S: high-voltage power supply; C1, C2: capillaries; I_1, I_2, I_3: interfaces; D: detector. Lower scheme: detail of dialysis interface. (1) capillaries; (2) buffer reservoir; (3) hollow fiber; (4) electrode; (5) buffer inlet; (6) buffer outlet. Reprinted from ref. (Yang et al., 2003b), with permission.

A two-dimensional capillary isoelectric focusing-capillary gel electrophoresis (IEF-CGE) system is another modification of the technique based on on-line combination of IEF with zone electrophoresis (Yang et al., 2003a). It also can be accomplished just with one high-voltage power supply and three electrodes. Chemical mobilization can be utilized to drive the sample zones of the first dimension. To actualize 2D IEF-CGE performance, coated and gel-filled capillaries are needed to eliminate the undesired EOF. In a gel-filled capillary the emergence of bubbles is tedious. From this point of view, it is valuable to exploit a more convenient and robust 2D CE system such as IEF-CZE (as illustrated above).

3.1.2 Hyphenation of electrophoretic and non electrophoretic techniques

Lately there were introduced into CE several hybrid on-line sample preparation techniques that are still in development as there is a big effort (i) to simplify usually a very complex instrumental arrangement and simultaneously (ii) to ensure the enhancement of the compatibility within and reproducibility of the procedure. The column coupled non electrophoretic stages include (i) chromatography (Pálmarsdóttir & Edholm, 1995; Pálmarsdóttir et al., 1996, 1997), (ii) SPE extraction (Puig et al., 2007), (iii) dialysis (Lada & Kennedy, 1997), and (vi) flow injection analysis (FIA) (Mardones et al., 1999). A great potential of the hybrid on-line sample preparation techniques is given by their complementarity that enables to cumulate positive effects and/or overcome the weak points of the individual sample preparation techniques. In addition, these techniques, likevise to CE-CE, can be simultaneously combined also with stacking effects or chemical reaction in order to enhance further overall analytical effect as it is demonstrated in the following sections. From the practical point of view, the following sections are starting with the on-line implementation of FIA because the flow injection principles and instrumental procedures/arrangements are widely applied also for the effective integration of other non electrophoretic techniques (SPE, LC, dialysis) with CE.

3.1.2.1 FI-CE

The concept of flow injection analysis (FIA) was introduced in the mid-seventies. It was preceded by the success of segmented flow analysis, mainly in clinical and environmental analysis. This advance, as well as the development of continuous monitors for process control and environmental monitors, ensured the success of the FIA methodology (Trojanowicz et al., 2009; Lü et al., 2009). A combination of CE with a flow injection (FI) offers a great scale of sample preparation and the most frequently it is used for the on-line implementation of chemical reactions. The technique of combined flow injection CE (FI-CE) integrates the essential favorable merits of FI and CE. It utilizes the various excellent on-line sample pretreatments and preconcentration (such as cloud point extraction, SPE, ionexchange, DPJ and head-column FESS technique, analyte derivatization) of FI, which has the advantages of high speed, accuracy, precision and avoiding manual handling of sample and reagents. Therefore, the coupling of FI-CE is an attractive technique; it can significantly expand the application of CE and has achieved many publications since its first appearance (Mikuš & Maráková, 2010).

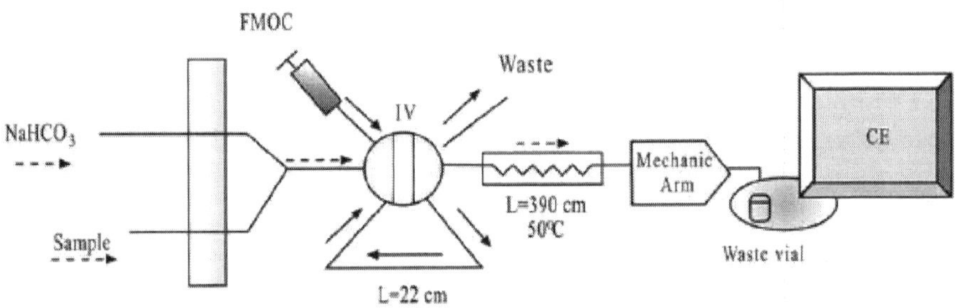

Fig. 7. Typical FI manifold used for the derivatization of the analytes and their on-line introduction into the CE system. Reprinted from ref. (Mardones et al., 1999), with permission.

A high potential of the FI-CE method in automatization of sample derivatization and subsequent separation was demonstrated by Mardones *et al.* (Mardones et al., 1999). The

derivatization reaction for carnitine as the model analyte was carried out on a FI system coupled with the CE equipment via a programmable arm (Valcárcel et al., 1998). The arrangement is shown in Fig. 7. The derivatization reagent (FMOC-Cl) is introduced directly into the loop of the injection valve (IV) when load position is selected, while the sample is introduced into the system and it is mixed with the buffer (carbonate). Then, valve is switched to the injection position allowing the mixing of sample-buffer and reagent solution. In this position the flow is stopped for a defined time in the reactor loop (390 cm), which is introduced into the thermostatic bath (50°C). Finally, the reaction mixture is introduced via the mechanic arm into the CE system.
The third generation of flow-injection (laboratory-on valve, lab-on-valve or LOV) allows scaling-down sample and reagent volumes to the 10-20 μL range, while waste production is typically 0.1-0.2 mL per assay (Solich et al., 2004). These facts make LOV an ideal tool for on-line coupling with CE systems (Kulka et al., 2006).

3.1.2.2 SPE-CE

The new trends in the coupling between SPE-CE are focused on several strategies, one of which involves developing new materials to increase the retention and selectivity of some analytes. In this sense the increasing use of materials such as immunoaffinity sorbents has been shown to overcome the problem of selectivity especially when complex samples are analysed. The use of molecular imprinted polymers (MIP) could be also an attractive alternative and further development is expected in this area in the near future. Carbon nanostructures also seem to be very promising materials which are in the first stages of development and so more research is expected in this field (Puig et al., 2007).

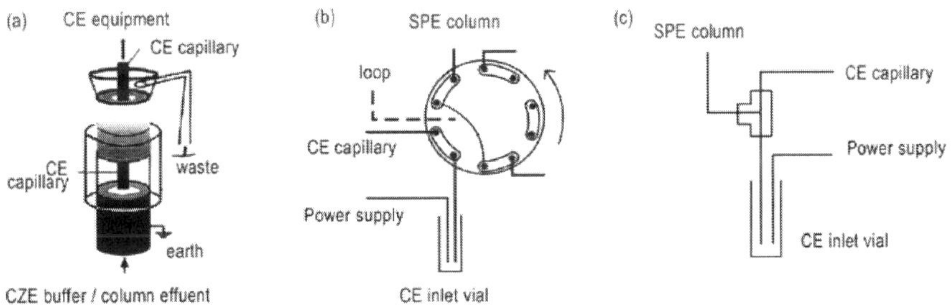

Fig. 8. Schematic diagram of the three types of interfaces for on-line SPE-CE coupling: (a) vial interface; (b) valve interface; (c) T-split interface. Reproduced with permission from (a) Stroink *et al.* (Stroink et al., 2003), (b) Tempels *et al.* (Tempels et al, 2007) and (c) Puig *et al.* (Puig et al., 2007).

Extraction techniques now play a major role for sample preparation in CE. These techniques can be used not only for reconstitution of the sample from small volumes but also for sample purification in complex matrices and desalting for very saline samples that would interfere with the electrophoretic process (e.g. FESS requires low conductivity sample). Considerable progress has been made towards the coupling of solid phase extraction (SPE) with a subsequent electrophoresis while coupling of liquid phase extraction (LLE) with electrophoresis is less used. Before coupling the SPE and CE, the appropriate SPE conditions for trapping and eluting the test compounds must be investigated. The breakthrough volumes, desorption efficiency and desorption volume must be studied too. Typical approaches of the on-line coupling of SPE with CE, advantageous by a high flexibility and variability of extraction volumes, are based on the use of a vial, valve or T-split interfaces. Schematic diagram of these types of interfaces for on-line SPE-CE coupling are shown in Fig.8.

An on-line SPE-CE approach based on a Tee-split interface was demonstrated by Puig et al. (Puig et al., 2007). The Tee-split interface is required for the on-line coupling of SPE-CE and to allow an injection volume that is suitable for CE analysis because the SPE elution volume is considerably larger than the maximum volume that can be injected into the CE capillary. Using this interface, a part of the SPE elution plug is injected while the rest of the sample is flushed to waste. Depending on the matrix, however, the sample must be appropriately pretreated prior to the injection into the first stage (i.e. SPE). As plasma is a relatively complex sample, the introduction of a pretreatment step (protein precipitation) prior to injection was necessary to prevent clogging of the SPE column.

For various specific purposes where chemical reaction and preconcentration must be involved simultaneously (*e.g.* in case of peptide mapping), the on-line coupling of microreactor (with an immobilized-enzyme), SPE preconcentrator and CE can be applied (Bonneil & Waldron, 1999). The problems related to the preconcentrator, such as reversal of EOF at low pH, can be eliminated by designing the on-line system in such a way that the preconcentrator is not part of the separation capillary, unlike most configurations reported in the SPE-CE literature. Consequently, the preconcentrator should not interfere with the separation process. Benefits of the on-line microreactor-SPE-CE system include (i) sensitivity (several hundred-fold preconcentration factor can be achieved) for the analyte products isolated in very small quantities from complex (biological) samples, (ii) avoiding conventional experimental steps that are quite long, labor intensive and require a lot of sample handling. Such system can be reused for several samples with acceptable reproducibility and relatively short analysis time. On the other hand, a loss of separation efficiency can be observed that is induced by the multiple-valve design of the system and dispersion of the desorption plug.

Another way of the integration of chemical reaction to the SPE-CE is the lab-on-valve (LOV) interface. The automatic minicolumn SPE preconcentration in LOV module coupled on-line with the CE equipment was proposed for the separation and quantification of mixtures of target analytes in very diluted samples (Jiménez & de Castro, 2008). This method can be applied with or without an on-line analyte derivatization depending on requirements. So that the complex derivatization-SPE-CE method integrates several different working principles such as (i) flow injection with chemical reaction, (ii) preseparation and preconcentration with non electrophoretic (extraction) principles, (iii) final separation with electrophoretic principles and detection of the separated zones. The usefulness of the LOV interface for the on-line coupling with a CE instrument interfaced by the appropriate manifold was reflected in excellent concentration LODs and linear dynamic ranges obtained.

Solid-phase microextraction (SPME) is interesting and alternative technique because it is simple, can be used to extract analytes from very small samples and provides a rapid extraction and transfer to the analytical instrument. Moreover, it can be easily combined with other extraction and/or analytical procedures, improving to a large extent the sensitivity and selectivity of the whole method (Lord & Pawliszyn, 2000; Ouyang & Pawliszyn, 2006; Saito & Jinno, 2003; Fang et al., 2006a, 2006b). Even though SPME is becoming an attractive alternative to using SPE, its use in combination with CE is still rather limited. Such coupling has not been widely used because of its inherent drawbacks regarding the low injection volumes typically required in CE (which are crucial to obtaining good separation efficiency) and also because the different sizes of the separation capillaries usually used for CE and the SPME fibers (Liu & Pawliszyn, 2006). Moreover, SPME suffers from limited choice of selectivity in comparison with SPE since only few stationary phases are avalaible (Puig et al., 2007).

3.1.2.3 LC-CE

When biological samples have to be analyzed, additional sample pretreatment prior to the SPE step may be needed to remove compounds that jeopardize an effective analyte concentration (or even block the SPE column) and the subsequent CE analysis. Sample pretreatment prior to SPE can be achieved by carrying out a preceding separation. Generally, sample analysis with on-line multidimensional separation systems can be performed using a comprehensive or a heart-cut approach. The comprehensive approach results in the analysis of the complete sample in all subsequent dimensions, whereas the heart-cut approach analyzes only a small part of the pre-separated sample in the second separation step. The comprehensive approach demands a slow preceding separation compared to the subsequent separation in order to accomplish analysis of the complete sample in all dimensions. Typical examples of such comprehensive systems are the on-line size exclusion chromatography (SEC)-CE systems and reversed phase LC-CE systems developed in the group of Jorgenson (Bushey & Jorgenson, 1990; Lemmo & Jorgenson, 1993; Moore Jr. & Jorgenson, 1995; Hooker & Jorgenson, 1997), which are coupled by various interfaces. These systems do not concentrate the chromatographic fractions prior to introduction into the CE system, which reduces the sensitivities of the total systems. Efforts to integrate such a focusing step would imply the need for an even slower preceding separation step to create time for sample trapping in a SPE column, washing and desorption of the concentrated fraction and sample introduction into the CE system. In practice, a comprehensive multidimensional system with a focusing step seems almost impossible, unless a number of columns are integrated into the system in a parallel fashion to enable "parking" of the LC fractions. In that case, the LC fractions are stored in the focusing step on various SPE columns and can be sent to the CE system at any convenient moment.

The heart-cut approach is less demanding and is best suitable for target analysis. In the case of a heart-cut approach for an on-line system, it is also easier to integrate a concentration step between the preceding and the final separation step because there are no time constraints. Stroink *et al.* (Stroink et al., 2003) coupled SEC-SPE with CE through a vial-type interface for the quantitative analysis of enkephalins in cerebrospinal fluid (CSF). The SEC dimension separated the sample in a protein and a peptide-containing fraction. This resulted in a relatively large volume of the peptide fraction (about 200μL), requiring a subsequent SPE step prior to CE analysis to obtain acceptable LODs.

Tempels *et al.* (Tempels et al., 2006) developed an on-line SEC-SPE-CE system with a Tee-split interface (Fig. 9) for the isolation, concentration and separation of peptides or other lower molecules in biological fluids (such as CSF). The SEC dimension served for the fractionation of the sample so that a fraction having required molecular weight could be easily selected (here, proteins were discarded). The small SPE column provided effective sample preconcentration using small desorption volumes (425 nL). The Tee-split interface enabled on-line injection of the concentrated analytes into the CE system without disturbing separation efficiency.

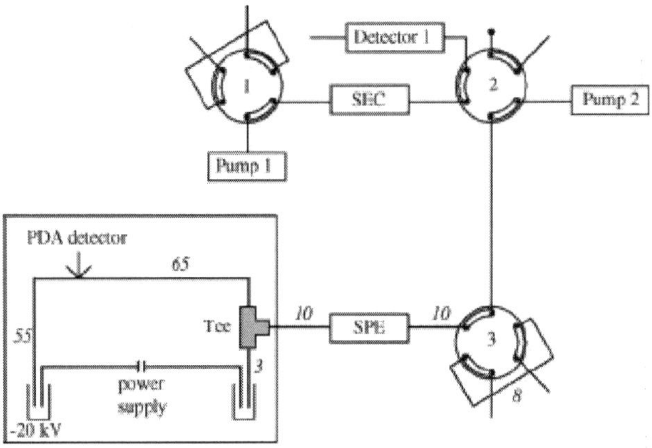

Fig. 9. Schematic diagram of the on-line SEC-SPE-CE system with the Tee-split interface. The on-line SEC-SPE-CE system was built in three distinct parts: a SEC, a SPE and a CE part. The SEC part consisted of a pump (pump 1), a valve (valve 1) for introduction of sample, a SEC column, and a UV detector (detector 1). The SPE part comprised a pump (pump 2), a micro valve (valve 3) for introduction of acetonitrile, and a SPE column. Valve 2 functioned as a selection valve to direct a fraction of solvent A towards the SPE column or to detector 1. The CE part of the complete system is framed. Lengths of capillaries are shown in italics (cm). The CE part consisted of a CE system with a build-in photodiode array detector. The CE and SPE parts were connected by a micro Tee with a void volume of 29 nL. The SEC part was filled with solvent A, whereas in the SPE and CE parts BGE was used. Reprinted from ref. (Tempels et al., 2006), with permission.

Although LC-CE coupling is technically much more difficult than CE-CE, because it has to be accompanied by collection, evaporation and reconstitution of fraction isolated by LC, some of these actions can be eliminated implementing an advanced CE stage (with a concentration capability) into LC-CE. Micro-column liquid chromatography (MLC) can be used on-line with an advanced (stacking) CE for sample purification and concentration allowing injection of microliter volumes into the electrophoresis capillary (Bushey & Jorgenson, 1990; Pálmarsdóttir & Edholm, 1995). By using the double stacking procedure with assistance of the backpressure almost complete filling of the electrophoresis capillary is possible without significant loss of CZE separation performance. The combined system has a much greater resolving power and peak capacity than either of the two systems used independently of each other.

3.1.2.4 Dialysis-CE

Microdialysis is a widely accepted sampling and infusion technique frequently used to sample small molecules from complex, often biological, matrices (Adell & Artigas, 1998; Chaurasia, 1999). In the microdialysis, small molecules are able to diffuse across the dialysis membrane into the probe, while large molecules, such as proteins and cell fragments, are excluded. This is the sample cleanup provided by the microdialysis.

On-line microdialysis-CE assays for neurotransmitters to date have been most successful for easily resolved analytes such as glutamate and aspartate (Thompson et al., 1999; Lada et al.,

1997, 1998). However, the efficiency and peak capacity of high-speed CE separations are often not high enough to resolve complex mixtures. Recently, improvements in injection technique and detection limits have improved separation efficiency (Bowser & Kennedy, 2001). In the microdialysis, the minimum volume required for analysis often determines the rate at which the dialysate can be sampled. On-line microdialysis-derivatization-CE-LIF assays as proposed by Lada *et al.* (Lada et al., 1997) (for the instrumental scheme see Fig. 10) eliminate fraction collection. The separation capillary was coupled to the reactor capillary via a flow-gated interface which allowed dialysate samples to be automatically injected onto the separation capillary. This elimination of fraction collection, combined with the high mass sensitivity of LIF or electrochemical detectors, makes sampling rates on the order of seconds possible (Thompson et al., 1999; Lada et al., 1997, 1998). The microdialysis-CZE-LIF system with on-line derivatization has the advantage of simultaneously obtained high relative recoveries and good temporal resolution with (in-vivo) microdialysis sampling for the real biological system (brain) (Lada et al., 1997).

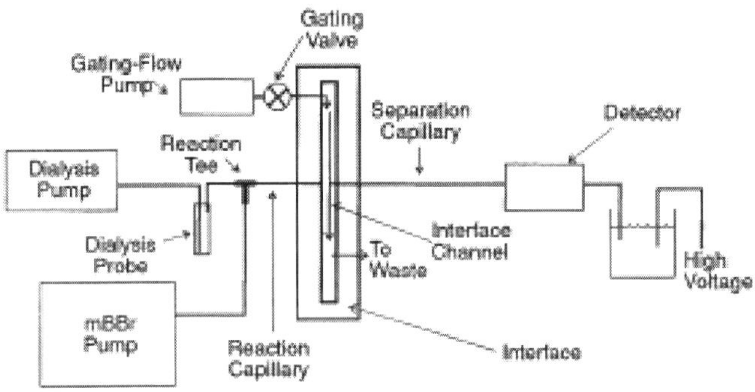

Fig. 10. Diagram of the microdialysis:CZE-LIF system with on-line derivatization. Reprinted from ref. (Lada et al., 1997), with permission.

3.2 Microchip format

Developments in the fields of microfluidics and microfabrication during the last 15 years have given rise to microchips with broad ranges of functionality and versatility in the areas of bioanalysis such as clinical applications (Li & Kricka, 2006) and chiral separations (Belder, 2006). Microfluidic devices such as microchips can provide several additional advantages over electromigration techniques performed in capillary format. The heat dissipation is much better in chip format compared with that in a capillary and therefore higher electric fields can be applied across channels of microchip. This fact enables, along with a considerably reduced length of channels, significant shortening of separation time (millisecond analysis time is possible to achieve, see e.g. (Belder, 2006)). Sample and reagent consumption is markedly reduced in microchannels. Hence, microchip capillary electrophoresis (MCE) can provide a unique possibility of ultraspeed separations of microscale sample amounts. Applicable are both electrophoretic (Gong & Hauser, 2006; Belder, 2006) as well as electrochromatographic modes (Weng et al., 2006).

In practice, however, the resolution achievable in MCE devices is often lower compared to that obtainable in classical CE utilizing considerably longer separation capillaries. In order to obtain sufficient resolution in MCE, different strategies have been used (Belder, 2006), such as (i) enhancing the selectivity of the system as much as possible (changing type and amount of selector, adding coselector, etc.), (ii) using of folded separation channels, the column length can be extended without enlarging the compact footprint of the device, (iii) using coated channels, internal coatings improve separation performance by the suppression of both analyte wall interaction and electroosmosis. A use/combination of above mentioned tools applicable in MCE gives a better chance for real-time process control and for multidimensional separations and makes the MCE to be powerful tool in real applications (pharmaceutical, biomedical, etc.). Sample pretreatment has been recognized as another significant barrier to higher levels of integration. Other accompanied problems in real applications of basic MCE are as follows: The detection volume of microfluidic devices due to the channel dimension and the sampling amounts is rather small, which would impact the detectable concentration. Fabricating a microchip with a large detection volume can be easily performed, but the separation efficiency is usually insufficient (Hempel, 2000). Another way is to inject a long sample band and then stack it into a narrow zone using on-line preconcentration techniques prior to separation (Chien, 2003). In such case, not only the preconcentration but also sample clean-up can be simultaneously carried out. Therefore, further considerable enhancement of analytical capabilities can be achieved in the MCE format using advanced single or multiple channel configurations.

Practically all of the advanced principles, effects and techniques described in previous sections (2 and 3.1) are applicable also in microchip format. The most effective advanced MCE approaches are briefly presented in this section.

3.2.1 Hyphenation of electrophoretic techniques

The column coupling (CC) configuration of the separation system is more compatible with microfluidic devices than capillary electrophoresis (Bergmann et al., 1996), since the manufacturing process is the same for simple and coupled channel chips (Huang et al., 2005). The on-line coupling of sample pretreatment systems to MCE have a great interest because it allows the automatization of the analytical process (from sample preparation to data treatment), which is a current trend in analytical chemistry (Ma et al., 2006; Cho et al., 2004). When we consider the sample amounts currently handled in conjuction with the separations on MCE it is clear that direct couplings of the sample pretreatment procedures to the separation stages of the analysis are almost inevitable (Kaniansky et al., 2003). For the above mentioned purposes the electrophoretic pretreatment methods are mostly used and it is important that they provide, mainly: (i) different separation mechanism in the pretreatment and separation stages of the analysis; (ii) an electrophoretically driven removal of the matrix constituents from the separation system on the pretreatment (to desalt the sample and reduce the number of the sample constituents); (iii) processing an adequate amount of the sample (to make the analyte detectable in the separation stage of the analysis); (iv) a nondispersive transfer of the analyte after the preteatment to the separation stage.

3.2.1.1 ITP-ZE

ITP-ZE (ZE, zone electrophoresis) performed on microchip is the most frequently used configuration similarly to the ITP-CZE in capillary format. It is because of the robustness and application potential of the microchip ITP-ZE. ITP and ZE, as the basic electrophoretic methods, differ in the sample loadabilities, spatial configurations of the separated constituents, concentrating effects, and in part in applicabilities for particular categories of the analytes they make tools that can be effectively on-line combined on the column coupling chip in two general ways (Kaniansky et al., 2000; Wainright et al., 2002; Bodor et al., 2002) (i) ITP, concentrating the sample constituents into a narrow pulse is intended, mainly, as a sample injection technique for ZE; (ii) ITP, while concentrating the analyte and some of the matrix constituents into a narrow pulse, serves mainly as a sample clean-up technique and removes a major part of the sample matrix from the separation system before the final ZE separation. For the separation mechanism of ITP-ZE in microchip format see Fig. 2, that is principally the same for the capillary and microchip format. MCE provided with the column-coupling (CC) configuration of the separation channels for the ITP-ZE separations is illustrated in Fig. 11. Different volumes of the sample channels (S1, S2) serve for a low or large volume injection depending on analyte and matrix concentration. At this scheme, the contact conductivity detector is used, nevertheless, other common detectors such as UV-VIS absorbance photometric detector, and especially LIF detector can be successfully applied, see e.g. (Belder, 2006).

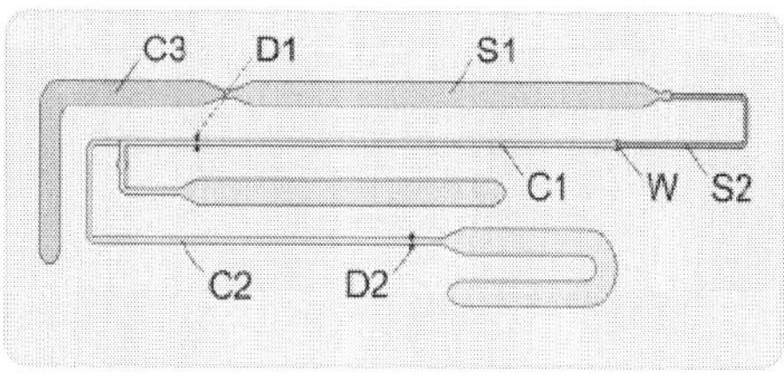

Fig. 11. MCE provided with the column-coupling (CC) configuration of the separation channels. CC poly(methylmethacrylate) chip provided with the conductivity detection cells. Details: C3 = terminating electrolyte channel; S1 and S2 = 9000 and 950 nL sample injection channels, respectively; W = an outlet hole from the chip channels to a waste container; C1 = first separation channel (3050 nL volume; 76x0.2x0.2 mm (length, width, depth)) with a platinum conductivity sensor (D1); C2 = second separation channel (1680 nL volume; 42x0.2x0.2 mm) with a platinum conductivity sensor (D2). Reprinted from ref. (Kaniansky et al., 2003), with permission.

3.2.1.2 ITP-GE

ITP-GE is proposed for the special category of separations where high molecular compounds are separated from each other in presence or absence of matrix constituents (Huang et al., 2005). A microchip for integrated ITP preconcentration with GE separation enables to decrease the detectable concentration of biopolymers such as sodium dodecyl sulfate (SDS)-proteins. Each channel of the chip is advantageously designed with a long sample injection channel to increase the sample loading and allow stacking the sample into a narrow zone using discontinuous ITP buffers. The preconcentrated sample is separated in GE mode in sieving polymer solutions. All the analysis steps including injection, preconcentration, and separation of the ITP-GE process are performed continuously, controlled by a high-voltage power source with sequential voltage switching between the analysis steps. Without deteriorating the peak resolution, the integrated ITP-GE system can result in a decreased detectable concentration of tens-fold compared to the GE mode only. The picture of the ITP-GE microchip and the protocol of the ITP-GE procedure on the microfluidic device are illustrated in Fig. 12.

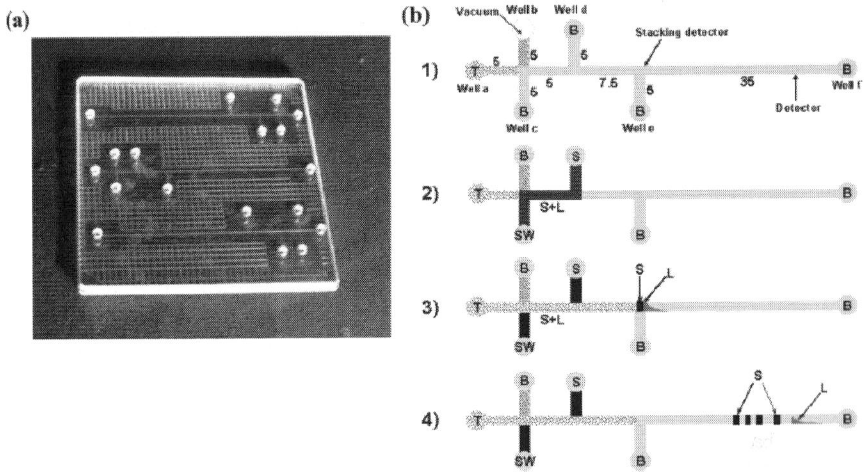

Fig. 12. (a) Glass microchip developed for ITP-GE separation, consisting of three separation elements; (b) protocol of the ITP-GE procedure on the microfluidic device. S: sample; SW: sample waste; B: background electrolyte; L: leading electrolyte; T: terminating electrolyte. 1) B and T loading; 2) S and L injection–S at ground, SW at high voltage; 3) stacking–T at ground, B (well 6) at high voltage; 4) separation–B (well 5) at ground, B (well 6) at high voltage. The electrodes not in use float. Channel lengths are expressed in mm. Reprinted from ref. (Huang et al., 2005), with permission.

3.2.1.3 ITP-ITP

Undoubtedly, the use of MCE can be extended advantageously to 2-D ITP separations (Ölvecká et al., 2001; Kaniansky et al., 2000). CE chip provided with the column-coupling (CC) configuration of the separation channels and corresponding scheme of the equipment for the ITP-ITP separations are the same as those ones for ITP-ZE illustrated in Fig.11. ITP-ITP with the tandem-coupled separation channels makes possible a complete resolution of various analytes, even the structurally related compounds (such as enantiomers). However, this can lead only to a moderate extension of the concentration range within which such analytes can be simultaneously quantified that is pronounced especially for the microfluidic devices such as MCE. The best results in this respect can be achieved by using a concentration cascade of the leading ions in the tandem coupled separation channels. Here, a high production rate, favored in the first separation channel, is followed by the ITP migration of the analytes in the second channel under the electrolyte conditions enhancing their detectabilities. This enables to separate structurally related analytes with their higher concentration ratios, and similarly, trace analyte besides higher concentration of matrix ions (Ölvecká et al., 2001).

3.2.1.4 ZE-ZE

In a ZE-ZE on-line combination, different separation mechanisms are implemented via appropriate compositions of the BGE solutions placed into the separation channels prior to the ZE run. Column switching provides means that significantly enhance resolving power attainable in the ZE separations performed on the CC chip. These, mainly include (i) on-column sample purification of the multicomponent and/or high salinity samples and (ii) different separation mechanism applicable in the coupled channels (2D features). Undoubtedly, a very reproducible transfer process, a well defined and highly efficient removal of the matrix constituents from the separation compartment and the use of different separation mechanisms in the channels are features that makes column switching ZE on the CC chip a very promising tool for a miniaturized analysis of multicomponenet samples. The ZE-ZE based MCE operating with a hydrodynamically closed separation system, makes a separation platform for highly reproducible migrations of separated constituents (Kaniansky et al., 2004; Sahlin, 2007; Hanna et al., 2000). The same instrumentation and channel arrangement as used for ITP-ZE, ITP-ITP or ITP-GE can be also applied for ZE-ZE (of course, with appropriate electrolyte systems).

3.2.2 Hyphenation of electrophoretic and non electrophoretic techniques

3.2.2.1 Extraction techniques

An interesting focus of research is the emergent development of microchips in the field of the chip-based SPE-CE. However, the research in this field is mainly centered in the manufacturing process, so the application of such microdevices is rather limited. In the coming years research in this field will focus on exploring the potential of chip-based SPE-CE for its application in the analysis of real samples (Puig et al., 2007, 2008). SPE is the most attractive way of coupling extraction with CE and, especially, MCE, particularly as it can provide significant improvements in sensitivity without the use of electrokinetic injection (Puig et al., 2007, 2008; Bertoncini & Hennion, 2004).

A potential of the affinity extraction in a chip format for a comprehensive proteomic analysis was demonstrated by Slentz (Slentz et al., 2003). This paper reports a system for three-dimensional chip electrochromatography (for the scheme of the chip, see Fig.13). The steps involved include (i) chemical reaction (enzymatic digestion), (ii) affinity extraction (selection of e.g. histidine-containing peptides), and (iii) CEC separation (reversed-phase capillary electrochromatography of the selected peptides). Fluidic manipulations including loading media, sample injection, and sample elution can be successfully performed by voltage manipulation alone.

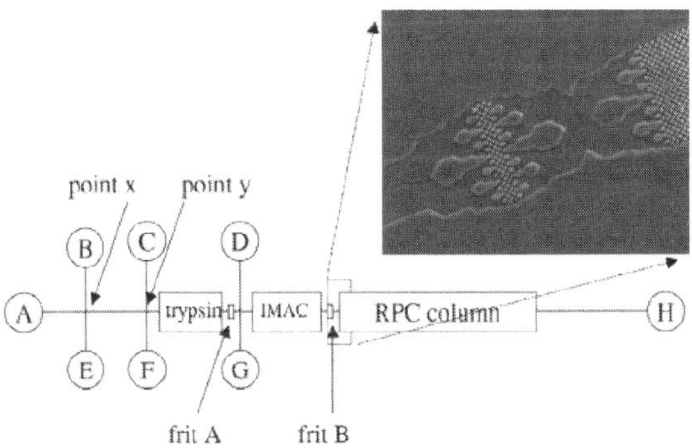

Fig. 13. Scheme of the column used and SEM of the microfabricated frit (frit B) and head of the collocated monolithic support structure (COMOSS) column. Reprinted from ref. (Slentz et al., 2003), with permission.

3.2.2.2 Membrane techniques

In bioanalytical applications, separation protocols based on molecular size are commonly required to extract small analytes from the sample matrix or clean up the macromolecular samples. Typical processes such as filtration (Broyles et al., 2003) and dialysis (Xu et al., 1998; Jiang et al., 2001) had been initially implemented upon microchips. Analytes can also be concentrated by inducing a velocity change due to their size by physically restricting their movement. This has traditionally been most easily performed with large molecules, such as proteins and DNA (Yu et al., 2008). Implementation of nanoporous media (nafion membrane, anionic hydrogel plug, *etc.*) in microchips (MCE is dominant in this field) has led to a number of interesting developments where the concentration of much smaller molecules is possible (Holtzel & Tallarek, 2007; Dhopeshwarkar et al., 2008; Long et al., 2006).

Porous membranes are ideal candidates for on-chip sample separation. Various researchers had attempted to integrate polymeric membranes to enhance the functionality of microfluidic devices. By sandwiching a dialysis membrane between two polycarbonate chips, Smith and co-workers (Xu et al., 1998) developed a microdialysis device to cleanup biosamples in ESI MS. In a similar approach, Lee and co-workers (Jiang et al., 2001; Gao et al., 2001) built some microfluidic devices with PVDF membranes for protein digestion, drug screening, and residue analysis of contaminants. Zhang and Timperman (Zhang Y. & Timperman, 2003) put a polycarbonate ultrafiltration membrane within the 3-D microchannel to act as a concentrator for fluorescein and FITC-labeled peptides. More recently, Bohn and co-workers (Kuo et al., 2003a, 2003b; Cannon et al., 2003; Tulock et al., 2004) reported several multilayer microfluidic structures with nanocapillary array interconnects; they studied the fluidic flow properties inside these devices and then utilized them for gated analyte injection and fraction collection in microchip electrophoresis. In most of the previous works, the membrane was insularly used as a dialyzer, a concentrator, or an injection valve.

On the other hand, the use of commercially available nanoporous membrane as a sample filter/concentrator prior to electrophoretic separation in a single microfluidic device has been shown by Long *et al.* (Long et al., 2006). These multilayer devices (Fig. 14) consist of a small piece of thin polycarbonate track-etched (PCTE) membrane (10 nm pore diameter) sandwiched between two PDMS monoliths with embedded microchannels and can work in two opposite operational modes. In the first, they can be used for selective injection and determination of small analytes from a complex sample matrix which contains particles or large molecules. For determination of small molecules, a "filter-CE" device layout shown in Fig. 14a can be used. Alternatively, they can be used for purification and preconcentration of macromolecular analytes by removing small interfering contaminants from the sample stream. For this purpose, "concentrator-CE" device shown in Fig. 14b can be utilized. Because of the membrane isolation, material exchange between two fluidic layers can be precisely controlled by applied voltages. Because the membrane is hydrophilic, the nanopores are filled with solutions by capillarity and can serve as an electrokinetic valve between two fluidic layers (present in upper and lower channels).

In another work, Foote *et al.* (Foote et al., 2005) fabricated a porous silica membrane incorporated into a microchip to perform on-line preconcentration of SDS-proteins before GE separation. Despite of significant improvement of sensitivity in this method, rather complicated microfluidic manipulations were necessary. Here, a microchip for integrated

ITP preconcentration with GE separation can be a simpler alternative to the membrane filtration-modified MCE devices for the decreasing of the detectable concentration of biopolymers as it was demonstrated in section 3.2.1.2.

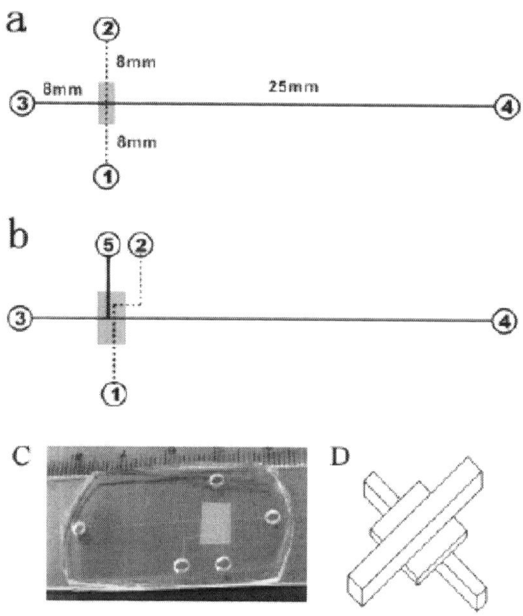

Fig. 14. Layout and dimensions of the "filter-CE" device (a) and "concentrator-CE" device (b), these multilayer devices consist of a small piece of nanoporous membrane (gray area) sandwiched between the upper (dotted line) and lower (solid line) PDMS layers. The microchannels were about 40 µm deep, 100 µm or 50 µm wide for upper and lower layers, respectively, and the size of the membrane was about 4 mm x 8 mm. (c) Photograph of the "concentrator-CE" device. (d) 3-D schematic diagram of the intersection region. The upper and lower channels are separated by a thin membrane. Reprinted from ref. (Long et al., 2006), with permission.

4. Performance parameters of column coupling electrophoresis

Limit of detection (cLOD) and limit of quantification (cLOQ) are usually calculated as the ratio of standard deviations of y-intercepts of regression lines (s_a) and the slopes of the regression lines (b) multiplied by factor 3.3 (cLOD) or 10 (cLOQ). The obtained values of cLOD and cLOQ by using electrophoretic methods in the column coupling arrangement clearly indicate significantly higher sensitivity in comparison to the single column CZE and therefore, favor the use of these hyphenated techniques (comparing with single column ones) in ultra trace quantitative determination of various analytes present in different multicomponent matrices.

Linearity of the calibration lines is indicated by the values of the corresponding correlation coefficient (r) and coefficient of determination (r^2). Column coupled techniques show acceptable linearity, in many cases better as it is in single column systems. Moreover, a linear dynamic range of the analytes can be considerably extended because of an elimination of major matrix constituents, higher sample load capacity, and sample preconcentration.
Precision (the repeatability) is usually expressed via relative standard deviation (RSD) of (i) peak areas measured within the concentration range of calibration line and/or (ii) migration times of analytes. Hydrodynamically closed separation systems contributed to high precisions of both the migration and quantitation data in comparison with the flow electrophoretic and non electrophoretic systems. It is because of a fluctuation of the flow velocity in the separation system contributing to a dispersion of the data.
Accuracy (expressed via relative error, RE) is evaluated through the recovery test of the analytes from relevant matrices (dosage form, urine, blood, etc.) at different concentration levels. Recovery is evaluated by spiking of blank complex matrix (dosage form, urine, blood, etc.) and water samples with an analyte at different concentration levels and comparing resulting peak areas of the analyte obtained in the different matrices (spiked complex matrix vs. spiked water). An on-line sample pretreatment can considerably enhance the recovery and accuracy of the method due to well controlled sample preparation procedure, minimization of the analyte losses, and effective elimination of the interfering matrix constituents.
The main performance parameters of particular column coupled methods are introduced in the Table 1 for a quick overview, what these electrophoretic techniques offer when using them in biomedical analysis.

Method (Detection)	**LOD (LOQ)**	**Linearity (r)**	**Precision[a] (RSD, %)**	**Recovery (%), (matrix)**	**Remarks**	**References**
Capillary arrangement						
ITP-CZE (DAD)	9.3 ng/mL (LOQ 28.3 ng/mL)	0.99989	-	104.7 (urine)	Robustness <6%	Mikuš et al., 2009
ITP-CZE (DAD)	6.5 ng/mL (LOQ 9.7 ng/mL)	0.99995-0.99998	0.58 - 2.79	99.25-100.15 (urine)	Robustness <2.3%	Mikuš et al., 2008b
ITP-CZE (DAD)	9.3 and 10.4 ng/mL (LOQ 28.2 and 31.5 ng/mL)	0.99989	-	98.9 - 99.5 (urine)	Robustness <6.5%	Mikuš et al., 2008a
ITP-CZE (DAD)	5.2 and 6.8 ng/mL (LOQ 7.7 and 10.1 ng/mL)	0.99965-0.99980	-	100.28 -101.16 (urine)		Marák et al., 2007
ITP-CZE (UV)	4.8, 1.1, 3.2 ng/mL (LOQ 16.0, 3.7, 10.7 ng/mL)	0.9994	3.95 - 4.54	94.4 - 96.8 (urine)	Robustness <5%	Mikuš et al., 2006
ITP-CZE (UV)	250 ng/mL (LOQ 830 ng/mL)	0.998	-	107.8 - 113.4 (serum)		Budáková et al., 2009

Method (Detection)	**LOD (LOQ)**	**Linearity (r)**	**Precision[a] (RSD, %)**	**Recovery (%), (matrix)**	**Remarks**	**References**
ITP-CZE (UV)	0.16 μM(blood) 0.11 μM (serum) 0.47 μM (urine)	-	3.5 - 11.4	-		Pantůčková et al., 2010
ITP-CZE (UV)	150 ng/mL	-	-	-	Elimination of matrix >95%	Kaniansky et al., 1993
ITP-CZE (DAD)	0.2 μM	0.9991 - 0.9998	3 - 5	-	Elimination of matrix 60-90%	Danková et al., 2001
ITP-CZE (UV)	0.3 μM	0.9996	7.27	-		Procházková et al., 1999
ITP-CZE (UV)	90-150 ng/mL	>0.998	8	-		Procházková et al., 1998
ITP-CZE (UV)	0.7 μM	> 0.999	<1	-		Křivánková et al., 1997b
ITP-CZE (DAD)	1.5 ng/mL	-	0.27 - 0.63	-	Elimination of matrix >99%	Danková et al., 1999
ITP-CZE (MS)	1 μM	-	-	-		Peterson et al., 2003
ITP-CZE (CON)	$2.5x10^3$ and $8.5x10^3$ng/mL					Budáková et al., 2007
ITP-ITP, ITP-CZE (CON)	4.8 - 20.5 μM (ITP-ITP) 3.7 - 14.6 μM (ITP-CZE) (LOQ 14.7- 45.7μM (ITP-ITP) 11.4- 42.6μM (ITP-CZE)	0.9979 - 0.9998 (ITP-ITP) 0.9986 - 0.9996 (ITP-CZE)	<4	95.3-97.4 (ITP-ITP) 96.5 - 97.7 (ITP-CZE) (urine)		Bexheti et al., 2006
ITP-ITP (CON)	1 – 8 μM (LOQ 2 -27 μM)	0.9980 - 0.9990	0.3 - 7.2	84.5 - 100.6 (serum)		Hercegová et al., 2000
ITP-ITP (CON)	100 μM	-	-	-		Mikuš et al., 2003
ITP-ITP (MS)	1.10^{-4} μM	-	<1	-		Tomáš et al., 2010
ITP-ITP (DAD)	2.7 -3.7 μM	0.9953 - 0.9970	-	-		Flottmann et al., 2006
ITP-ITP (CON)	LOQ $1.4x10^3$ and $5x10^2$ ng/mL					Sádecká & Netriová, 2005
ITP-CEC (UV, MS)	-	0.9849 - 0.9980	13.1	-		Mazareeuw et al., 2000

Method (Detection)	**LOD (LOQ)**	**Linearity (r)**	**Precision[a] (RSD, %)**	**Recovery (%), (matrix)**	**Remarks**	**References**
CIEF-tITP-CZE (UV)	-	-	5-10	-		Mohan & Lee, 2002
CZE-CZE (DAD)	3.5 μM (218nm) 0.4 μM (280nm)	0.9996 - 0.9998	-	93 – 98 (urine)		Danková et al., 2003
CZE-MEKC (UV)	-	-	1.7 - 4.0 (migration times)	-		Sahlin, 2007
Microdialysis-CZE (LIF)	0.02 and 0.04 μM	>0.9998	2.5 - 4.9 (peak heights)	~100 (caudate nucleus)		Lada & Kennedy, 1997
SPE-CE (UV)	-	-	0.5 - 5.2 (migration times)	-		Bonneil & Waldron, 2000
SPE-CE (UV)	100 ng/mL	0.9828 - 0.9879	8.1 - 11.9	57 – 90 (plasma)		Puig et al., 2007
SEC-SPE-CE (DAD)	100 ng/mL	>0.9950	10 (peak heights)	65 (cerebrospinal fluid)		Tempels et al., 2006
MLC-CZE (UV)	-	0.9998	0.7 - 3.5	-		Pálmarsdóttir & Edholm, 1995
Chips						
ITP-ZE (CON)				90-94 (serum)		Ölvecká et al., 2003
ITP-ZE (CON)	(LOQ 1.10^3-5.10^3 ng/mL)	0.9542 - 0.9999	6.7 - 11.8	-		Ölvecká et al., 2004
ITP-GE (LIF)	-	0.9992	-	-		Huang et al., 2005
ITP-ZE (LIF)	4.10^{-7} μM	-	-	-		Wainright et al., 2002
Membrane filtration-ZE (LIF)			14.6 (plasma) and 8.9 (cells)			Long et al., 2006

[a] RSD of peak areas

LOD=limit of detection, LOQ=limit of quantification, r=correlation coefficient, RSD=relative standard deviation, CON= conductivity detection, UV=spectral UltraViolet detection, DAD=diode array detection, LIF=laser fluorescence detection, MS=mass spectrometry, ITP=capillary isotachophoresis, CZE=capillary zone electrophoresis, CE=capillary electrophoresis, ZE=zone electrophoresis, CEC=capillary electrochromatography, MEKC=micellar eelctrokinetic chromatography, CIEF=capillary isoelectric focusing, CGE=capillary gel electrophoresis, GE=gel eelctrophoresis, SEC=size exclusion chromatography, CLC=column liquid chromatography, SPE=solid phase extraction.

Table 1. Performance parameters of column coupling electrophoretic methods

5. Applications of column coupling electrophoresis

The column coupled methods, described in previous sections (3 and 4) concerning the theory (principles, experimantal arrangement, benefits, limitations) and performance parameters (LOD, precision, recovery/accuracy, etc.), have been used in many applications. Capillary (CE) and microchip (MCE) formats were taken into consideration. CE and MCE determinations of various biologically active compounds in model (spiked samples) as well as real biological matrices, employing an on-line coupling of the electrophoretic methods with other electrophoretic or non electrophoretic methods, are listed in Table 2. In this table we tried to emphasize briefly the most important features and characteristics of the applications of column coupling electrophoresis in capillary as well as in chip arrangement. This table is further supported by the text where other relevant parameters and explanations are included for the real bioapplications and proteinic analysis.

Method (Detection)	Analyte	Matrix	Type of application	References
Capillary arrangement				
ITP-CZE (CON)	Valproic acid	Serum		Budáková et al., 2007
ITP-CZE (UV)	Lamotrigine	Serum	Biomedical (Theurapeutic drug monitoring)	Budáková et al., 2009
ITP-CZE (UV)	5-methyltetrahydrofolate	Blood, serum and urine	Biomedical	Pantůčková et al., 2010
ITP-CZE (UV)	Sulphanilate, 3,5-dinitrosalicylate	Urine (spiked)	Model	Kaniansky et al., 1993
ITP-CZE (DAD-spectral informations)	Orotic acid	Urine	Biomedical (biomarker analysis)	Danková et al., 2001
ITP-CZE (DAD-spectral informations)	Amlodipine	Urine	Biomedical (pharmakokinetic study)	Mikuš et al., 2009
ITP-CZE (DAD-spectral informations)	Amlodipine (enantiomers)	Urine	Biomedical (pharmakokinetic study)	Mikuš et al., 2008b
ITP-CZE (DAD-spectral informations)	Celiprolol	Urine	Biomedical (pharmakokinetic study)	Mikuš et al., 2008a
ITP-CZE (DAD-spectral informations)	Pheniramine (enantiomers)	Urine	Biomedical (metabolic study)	Marák et al., 2007
ITP-CZE (UV)	Pheniramine, dimethindene, dioxopromethazine (enantiomers)	Urine	Biomedical (metabolic study)	Mikuš et al., 2006

Method (Detection)	Analyte	Matrix	Type of application	References
ITP-CZE (UV)	Orotic acid	Urine	Biomedical (biomarker analysis)	Procházková et al., 1999
ITP-CZE (UV)	L-ascorbic acid	Serum, urine, stomach fluid	Biomedical	Procházková et al., 1998
ITP-CZE (UV)	Hippurate	Serum	Biomedical (biomarker analysis)	Křivánková et al., 1997b
ITP-CZE (DAD)	Tryptophan	Urine (spiked)	Model	Danková et al., 1999
ITP-CZE (UV)	2,4-dinitrophenyl labeled norleucine, tryptophan	Urine (spiked)	Model	Fanali et al., 2000
ITP-CZE (MS)	Angiotensin peptides	Aqueous	Model	Peterson et al., 2003
ITP-ITP, ITP-CZE (CON)	Amino bisphosphonate	Urine (spiked)	Model	Bexheti et al., 2006
ITP-ITP (CON)	Antirheumatic drugs	Serum (spiked)	Model	Hercegová et al., 2000
ITP-ITP (CON)	Cystine	Urine (spiked)	Model	Mikuš et al., 2003
ITP-ITP (MS)	Vitamins	Blood	Biomedical	Tomáš et al., 2010
ITP-ITP (DAD)	Homovanilic acid, vanillylmandelic acid	Urine (spiked)	Model	Flottmann et al., 2006
ITP-ITP (CON)	Naproxen and its metabolites	Urine		Sádecká & Netriová, 2005
ITP-CEC (UV, MS)	Cationic low molecular mass compounds (neostigmine, salbutamol, fenoterol)	Plasma, urine (spiked)	Model	Mazareeuw et al., 2000
CIEF-CGE	Hemoglobine			Yang et al., 2003a
CIEF-tITP-CZE	Tryptic digest proteins	Extract of proteins	Model	Mohan & Lee, 2002
CZE-MEKC (UV)	drugs	Urine		Zhang et al., 2010
CZE-CZE (DAD-spectral information)	Orotic acid	Urine	Biomedical (biomarker analysis)	Danková et al., 2003

Method (Detection)	Analyte	Matrix	Type of application	References
CZE-MEKC (UV)	Tryptic digest of bovine serum albumin	Extract of proteins	Model	Sahlin, 2007
Microdialysis-CZE (LIF-derivatization)	Glutathione and cystine	Rat caudate nucleus (in vivo)	Biomedical	Lada & Kennedy, 1997
SPE-CE (UV)	Tryptic peptides	Extract of proteins	Model	Bonneil & Waldron, 2000
SPE-CE (UV)	Cefoperazone and ceftiofur	Plasma (spiked)	Model	Puig et al., 2007
SEC-SPE-CE (DAD)	Peptides	Cerebrospinal fluid (spiked)	Model	Tempels et al., 2006
MLC-CZE (UV)	Terbutalin (enantiomers)	Plasma	Model	Pálmarsdóttir & Edholm, 1995
Chips				
ITP-ZE (CON)	Valproate	Serum		Ölvecká et al., 2003
ITP-ZE (CON)	Proteins	Aqueous	Model	Ölvecká et al., 2004
ITP-GE (LIF)	Sodium dodecylsulfate proteins	Aqueous	Model	Huang et al., 2005
ITP-ZE (LIF)	β–blockers	Urine	Biomedical	Kriikku et al., 2004
ITP-ZE (LIF)	Fluorescently labeled ACLARA eTag reporter molecules	Cell lysate (spiked)	Model	Wainright et al., 2002
ZE-ZE	Tryptic digest of proteins			Cong et al., 2008
ZE-ZE (LIF)	Gemifloxacin enantiomers	Urinary solution (spiked)	Model	Cho et al., 2004
Membrane filtration-ZE (LIF)	Reduced glutathione	Human plasma and red blood cells	Biomedical	Long et al., 2006
SPE-ZE (LIF)	Peptides	Extract of proteins	Model	Slentz et al., 2003

CON= conductivity detection, UV=spectral UltraViolet detection, DAD=diode array detection, LIF=laser fluorescence detection, MS=mass spectrometry, ITP=capilaary isotachophoresis, CZE=capillary zone electrophoresis, CE=capillary electrophoresis, ZE=zone electrophoresis, CEC=capillary electrochromatography, MEKC=micellar eelctrokinetic chromatography, CIEF=capillary isoelectric focusing, CGE=capillary gel electrophoresis, GE=gel eelctrophoresis, SEC=size exclusion chromatography, CLC=column liquid chromatography, SPE=solid phase extraction, EDTA=ethylendiaminotetraacetic acid.

Table 2. Applications of column coupling electrophoretic methods

5.1 Capillary arrangement

5.1.1 Analysis of drugs and biomarkers in clinical samples

ITP-CZE. In our recent works (Mikuš et al., 2006a, 2008a, 2008b, 2008c, 2009; Marák et al., 2007) we illustrated possibilities of ITP-EKC method combined with diode array detection (DAD) for the direct achiral (celiprolol, CEL, amlodipine, AML) as well as chiral (amlodipine, AML, pheniramine, PHM, dimethinden, DIM and dioxoprometazine, DIO) quantitative determination of trace drugs in clinical human urine samples, see an example in Fig.15. ITP, on-line coupled with EKC, served in these cases as an ideal injection technique (high sample load capacity, preseparation and preconcentration) producing analyte zone suitable for its direct detection and quantitation in EKC stage. Spectral DAD, used in our works, in comparison with single wavelength ultraviolet detection enhanced value of analytical information (i) verifying purity (i.e., spectral homogeneity) of drug zone (according to differences in spectrum profiles when compared tested and reference drug spectra) and (ii) indicating zones/peaks with spectra similar to the drug spectrum (potential structurally related metabolites). Very good selectivity was achieved by using a negatively charged carboxyethyl-β-cyclodextrin (CE-β-CD) as a chiral selector for enantioseparation and determination of trace (ng/mL) antihistaminic drugs (PHM, DIM, DIO) present in urine (Mikuš et al., 2006a, 2008c; Marák et al., 2007). Charged chiral selector provided significantly different affinity towards the analytes on one hand and sample matrix constituents on the other hand; enabling the analytes can be transferred into the analytical stage without any spacers and multiple column-switching even if accompanied by a part of sample matrix constituents detectable in analytical stage. This analytical approach enabled us to obtain pure zones of the drugs enantiomers (without the need of the sample pretreatment). DAD spectra of PHM metabolites were compared with the reference spectra of PHM enantiomers (Marák et al., 2007; Mikuš et al., 2008c) and a very good match was found which indicated the similarities in the structures of enantiomers and their metabolites detected in the urine samples. This fact was utilized for the quantitative analyses of PHM metabolites in the urine samples by applying the calibration parameters of PHM enantiomers also for PHM metabolites. Spectra obtained by DAD helped with the identification of analytes even having the similar structures but it was necessary that their peaks were resolved. The on-line coupled ITP-EKC technique was used also for the pharmacokinetic studies of CEL (Mikuš et al., 2008b) and AML (Mikuš et al., 2008a, 2009) in multicomponent ionic matrices. In order to control a reliability of the results, we utilized spectral data from DAD (evaluation of purity of separated analyte zone; confirmation of basic structural identity of the analyte). A great advantage of the ITP-EKC-DAD method was a possibility to characterize electrophoretic profiles of unpretreated (unchanged) biological samples and, by that, to investigate drug and its potential metabolic products with higher reliability.

The increase of the sensitivity, by applying ITP preconcentration before the final CZE separation, was necessary for a determination of orotic acid in human urine (Procházková et al., 1999; Danková et al., 2001). Procházková *et al.* showed, that this method was suitable for determination of orotic acid also in children's urine samples (conventional CZE method failed in this application) and they reached very high reproducibility of analyses (effective clean-up of the sample). Danková *et al.* increased in their work 3-4 times the amount of urine ionic constituents loadable on the ITP-CZE separation system in comparison with the work of Procházková *et al.* Moreover, DAD detection served in this work also for identification of the analyte by UV spectra, even though the analyte was present at very low concentration level.

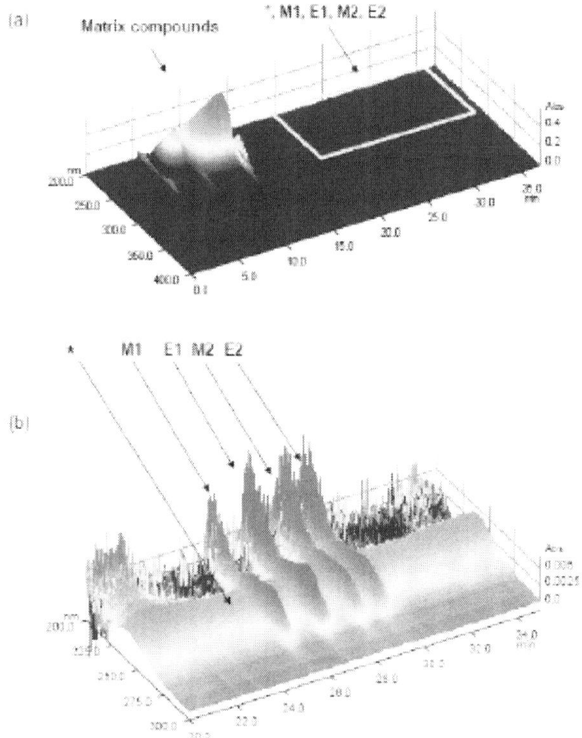

Fig. 15. ITP-EKC-DAD method for the direct sensitive determination of enantiomers in unpretreated complex matrices sample with spectral characterization of electrophoretic zones. 3D traces were obtained combining electrophoretic (EKC) and spectral (DAD) data where the spectra were scanned in the interval of wavelengths 200-400 nm. (a) 3D trace illustrating the whole EKC enantioseparation of pheniramine and its metabolites in the on-line pretreated clinical urine sample (spectra of matrix constituents, well separated from the analytes, are pronounced), (b) detail on the 3D spectra showing the migration positions of pheniramine enantiomers (E1 and E2) and their structurally related metabolites (M1 and M2). The spectrum of the little unknown peak marked with the asterisk differed from the pheniramine spectrum significantly and, therefore, it was not considered as a pheniramine biodegradation product. The urine sample was taken 8.5 hours after the administration of one dose of Fervex (containing 25 mg of racemic pheniramine) to a female volunteer and it was 10 times diluted before the injection. The separations were carried out using 10 mM sodium acetate - acetic acid, pH 4.75 as a leading electrolyte (ITP), 5 mM ε-aminocaproic acid - acetic acid, pH 4.5 as a terminating electrolyte (ITP), and 25 mM ε -aminocaproic acid - acetic acid, pH 4.5 as a carrier electrolyte (EKC). 0.1% (w/v) methyl-hydroxyethylcellulose served as an EOF suppressor in leading and carrier electrolytes. Carboxyethyl-β-CD (5 mg/mL) was used as a chiral selector in carrier electrolyte. Reprinted from ref. (Marák et al., 2007), with permission.

A comparison of two types of CE instrumentation, single CZE and commercially available ITP-CZE, used for the determination of hippuric acid in serum was demonstrated by Křivánková *et al.* (Křivánková et al., 1997b). Results obtained in the single-capillary methods (ITP and CZE) were comparable and were limited both by the sensitivity of the detector used and by the load capacity of the system. This work pointed out decreasing of concentration LOD (cLOD 7.10^{-7} M was two-orders of magnitude lower by using ITP-CZE method in comparison with single column CZE). The sample volumes that could be injected using this combined technique were up to 10^3 orders of magnitude higher in the case of natural biological samples than those that could be analyzed in a single capillary CZE technique. Excellent reproducibility of migration times (R.S.D. less than 1%) and resistance to changes in the matrix composition enabled the determination of HA in serum not only for patients suffering from renal diseases but also for healthy individuals.

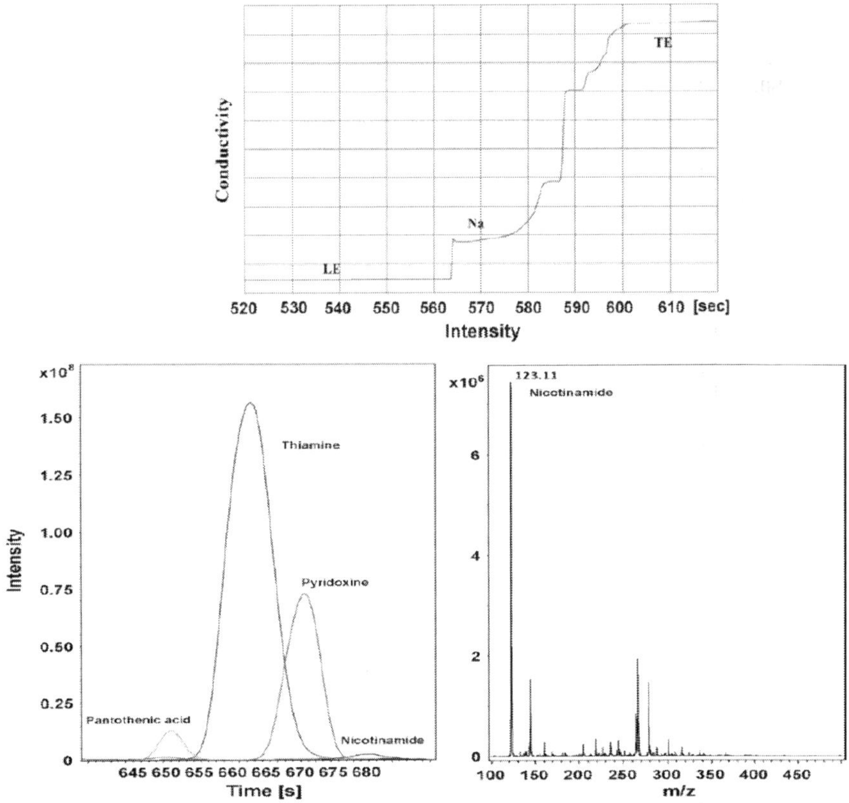

Fig. 16. (a) Conductivity trace of the analysis of 1µL undiluted blood. LE: 10mM ammonium acetate pH 7.8, TE: 20mM acetic acid pH 3.5. (b) Selected ion monitoring of the ions in the ITP zones of undiluted blood. Reprinted from ref. (Tomáš et al., 2010), with permission.

CZE-CZE. Danková *et al.* (Danková et al., 2003) showed also the analytical potentialities of CZE in the separation system with tandem-coupled columns to the spectral identification and determination of orotic acid (OA) in urine by diode array detection (DAD), coupled to the separation system via optical fibers. A very significant "in-column" clean-up of OA from urine matrix was achieved in the separation stage of the tandem by combining a low pH (2.8) with complexing effects of electroneutral agents [α- and β-cyclodextrins, poly(vinylpyrrolidone) and 3-(N,N-dimethyldodecylammonio)propanesulfonate]. Due to this, DAD spectral data of OA was acquired in the detection stage of the tandem with almost no disturbances by matrix co-migrants.

ITP-ITP. Tomáš *et al.* (Tomáš et al., 2010) have modified the commercial coupled column isotachophoresis system for direct connection to an ion trap mass spectrometer. Although identification of individual zones is possible with the help of standard substances, selected ion monitoring of the individual masses in the electrospray-MS signal provided additional means for identification. The instrumentation was tested for determination of vitamins in whole blood analysis (see Fig.16) and separation of tryptic peptides. The main advantage of large bore ITP system with fluoropolymer based columns which was used in this work was the possibility to inject crude samples, such as urine or blood, with minimum or no sample pretreatment. In many cases injections of 10μL or higher sample volumes result in sensitivities with cLOD in the range of 10^{-10} M.

Microdialysis-CE. A fully-automated method for monitoring thiols (glutathione and cysteine) in the extracellular space of the caudate nucleus of anesthetized rats (in vivo) using microdialysis coupled on-line with CZE with laser-induced fluorescence detection (dialysates were derivatized on-line) was investigated (Lada & Kennedy, 1997). This system allowed to obtain high relative recoveries (nearly 100%) and high temporal resolution (high mass sensitivity of CZE-LIF permits frequent sampling) simultaneously for multiple thiols present in the brain.

5.1.2 Analysis of proteins

ITP-CZE. Comprehensive ITP-CZE was successfully coupled to electrospray ionization orthogonal acceleration time-of-flight mass spectrometry using angiotensin peptides as model analytes (Peterson et al., 2003). ITP-TOF-MS alone was adequate for the separation and detection of high concentration samples. The problems (ion suppression and discrimination) can occur when lower analyte concentrations are analysed because mixed zones or very sharp peaks are formed. This problem was effectively overcome by inserting a CE capillary between the ITP and TOF-MS.

CZE-MEKC. Capillary zone electrophoresis at two different pH values has been developed to perform a comprehensive two-dimensional capillary electrophoresis separation of tryptic digest of bovine serum albumin using CZE followed by MEKC (Sahlin, 2007). Two-dimensional systems reduced probability of component overlap and improved peak identification capabilities since the exact position of a compound in a twodimensional electropherogram is dependent on two different separation mechanisms.

CIEF-CGE. An on-line two-dimensional CE system consisting of capillary isoelectric focusing (CIEF) and capillary gel electrophoresis (CGE) for the separation of hemoglobin (Hb) was reported by Yang *et al.* (Yang et al., 2003a). After the Hb variants with different isoelectric points (pIs) were focused in various bands in the first-dimension capillary, they were chemically mobilized one after another and fed to the second-dimension capillary for further separation in polyacrylamide gel.

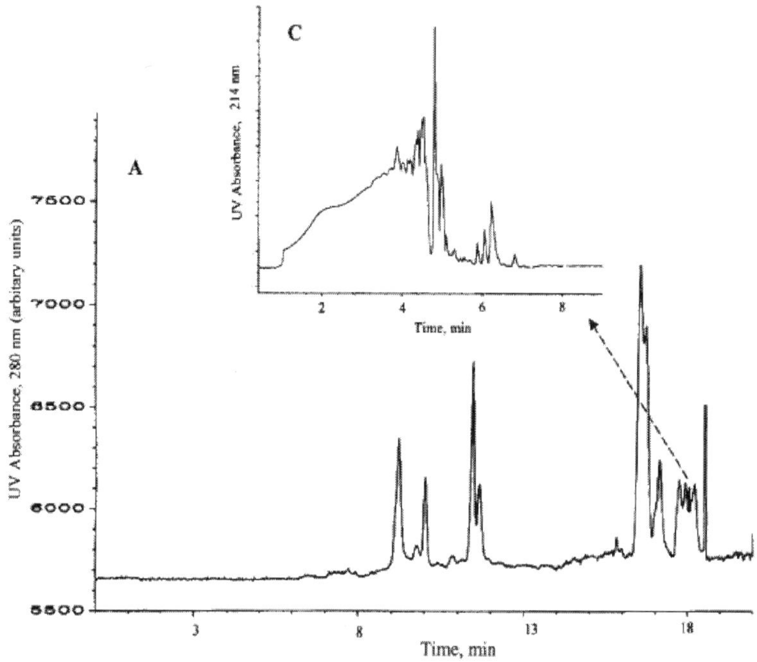

Fig. 17. (A) CIEF separation of cytochrome c digest in a single capillary setup. Capillary: HPC coating, 37 cm x 50 μm ID x 192 μm OD; sample, 0.1 mg/mL cytochrome c digest in 2% Pharmalyte pH 3-10 and 0.38% N,N,N',N',-tetramethylethylenediamine; anolyte, 0.1 M acetic acid at pH 2.5; catholyte, 0.5% w/w ammonium hydroxide at pH 10.5; electric field strength, 500 V/cm; hydrodynamic mobilization; detection, UVabsorbance at 280 nm, 7 cm from cathodic end. (C) Early fraction of acidic peptides (pI 3.6-3.9) analyzed by transient CITP-CZE in a 2-D separation system. Reprinted from ref. (Mohan & Lee, 2002), with permission.

CIEF-tITP-CZE. A microdialysis junction was employed as the interface for on-line coupling of capillary isoelectric focusing with transient isotachophoresis-zone electrophoresis in a two-dimensional separation system for the separation of tryptic proteins (Fig.17) (Mohan & Lee, 2002). This 2-D electrokinetic separation system combined the strengths of sample loading and analyte preconcentration in CIEF and CITP with high resolving power provided by isoelectric focusing and zone electrophoresis. Many peptides which have the same isoelectric point had different charge-to-mass ratios and thus different electrophoretic mobilities in zone electrophoresis. In comparison with chromatographic systems, electrokinetic separations require no column equilibration and offer further reduction in protein/peptide adsorption through the use of polymercoated capillaries.

SPE-CE. An on-line system allowing digestion of the protein, followed by preconcentration, separation and detection of the tryptic peptides of insulin chain B, cytochrome c and β-casein at sub-micromolar concentrations were developed by Bonneil and Waldron (Bonneil & Waldron, 2000) to minimise the sample handling. Despite fairly good reproducibility of the maps, the resolution and efficiency were poor compared to conventional CE. It was mainly because of backpressure generated by the preconcentrator, small internal volumes of the micro-tee, separation capillary and 60-nl injection loop, which led to inconsistent transfer of the elution plug into the separation capillary. To minimize the backpressure effect, elution plug injection should be made at the lowest pressure possible or by electroosmosis (the use of a separation buffer with moderate to high pH).

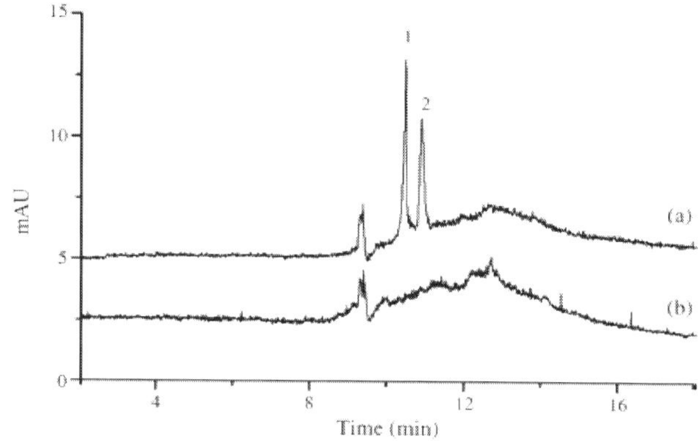

Fig. 18. Electropherogram of (a) CSF spiked with des-Tyr[1]-[d-Ala[2]-d-Leu[5]]-enkephalin (1) and [Met[5]]-enkephalin (2), each present at 0.5 μg/mL, and (b) unspiked CSF using the on-line SEC-SPE-CE system. Sample volume, 20 μL; split ratio, 1:40; analysis voltage, −20 kV. Reprinted from ref. (Tempels et al., 2006), with permission.

SEC-SPE-CE. An on-line coupled size exclusion chromatography (SEC) has been shown to be effective tool for removing potentially interfering proteins and permitted reproducible solid-phase extraction (SPE) and capillary electrophoresis (CE) in the analysis of peptides in biological fluids (enkephalins in cerebrospinal fluid-CSF), see Fig. 18 (Tempels et al., 2006). This method was shown to be effective enough for the determination of exogenous enkephalins (present in the low μg/mL range) in CSF or plasma, but for endogenous enkephalins (present in the low ng/mL range) sensitivity improvement would still be needed.

5.2 Microchip arrangement

5.2.1 Analysis of drugs and biomarkers in clinical samples

Membrane filtration-MCE. The multilayer MCE device consisting of a small piece of thin polycarbonate track-etched (PCTE) membrane (10 nm pore diameter) sandwiched between two PDMS monoliths with embedded microchannels serves for the speed microscale sample filtration (clean-up) and preconcentration of the complex samples composed of low and high molecular compounds (Long et al, 2006). This approach has been effectively applied in rapid determination of reduced glutathione in human plasma and red blood cells without any off-chip deproteinization procedure (Fig. 19).

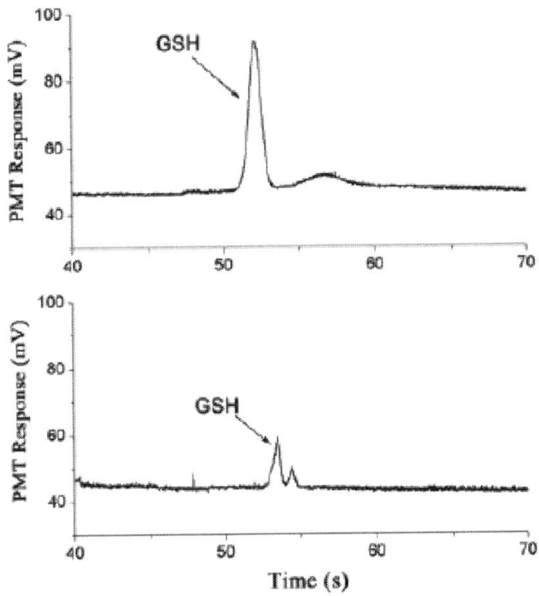

Fig. 19. Electropherograms of (a) human plasma and (b) red blood cell lysate injected across a 10 nm pore diameter membrane without any off-chip deproteinization procedure. The separation buffer was 100 mM TBE (pH 8.4). The injection time was 2 s, V_{inj} = 800 V, V_{sep} = 1500 V. Reprinted from ref. (Long et al., 2006), with permission.

5.2.2 Analysis of proteins

ITP-ZE. Ölvecká *et al.* (Ölvecká et al., 2004) demonstrated the potential of their CC chip for highly sensitive analysis of proteins using the online ITP–ZE combination method. The aim of the ITP step in this work was restricted mainly to the concentration of proteins before their ZE separation and conductivity detection. ITP and ZE cooperatively contributed to low- or sub-µg/mL concentration detectabilities of proteins and their quantitations at 1-5 µg/mL concentrations.

IEF-ZE. A two-dimensional electrophoresis platform, combining isoelectric focusing (IEF) and zone electrophoresis (ZE), was established on a microchip for the high-throughput and high-resolution analysis of complex samples (separation of the digests of bovine serum albimine and proteins extracted from *E. coli)* (Cong et al., 2008). During the separation, peptides were first focused by IEF in the first dimensional channel, and then directly driven into the perpendicular channel by controlling the applied voltages, and separated by ZE.

ITP-GE. A microchip for online combination of ITP with gel electrophoretic separation was developed to decrease the detectable concentration of SDS-proteins (Huang et al., 2005). Without deteriorating the peak resolution, this system provided a 40-fold increase of the sensitivity, saved analysis time and simplified the instruments for SDS-proteins analysis when compared to the gel electrophoresis mode (see Fig.20).

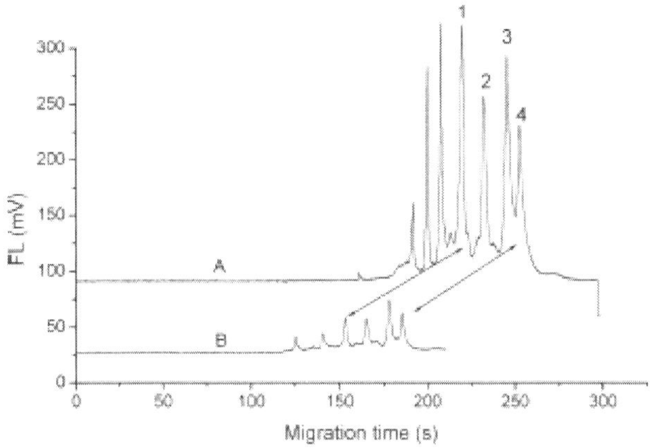

Fig. 20. ITP-GE (B) *versus* GE (A) mode of SDS-protein complexes analysis in the sieving matrix of 10% dextran on microchip. Peak identification: 1, carbonic anhydrase (124 μg/mL); 2, ovalbumin (20 μg/mL); 3, BSA (50 μg/mL); 4, conalbumin (60 μg/mL). Reprinted from ref. (Huang et al., 2005), with permission.

SPE-MCE. The study involved trypsin digestion, affinity extraction of histidine-containing peptides, and reversed-phase capillary electrochromatography of the selected peptides in a single polydimethylsiloxane chip was described by Slentz *et al.* (Slentz et al., 2003). Copper (II)-immobilized metal affinity chromatography 5μm-particles have been introduced into the chip. Frits have been fabricated in order to maintain the beads, with collocated monolithic support structures (COMOSS). They were able to trap particulate contaminants ranging down to 2μm in size. Fig. 21 presents the on-chip separation of fluorescein isothiocyanate-labeled bovine serum albumin digest (A) before and (B) after affinity extraction.

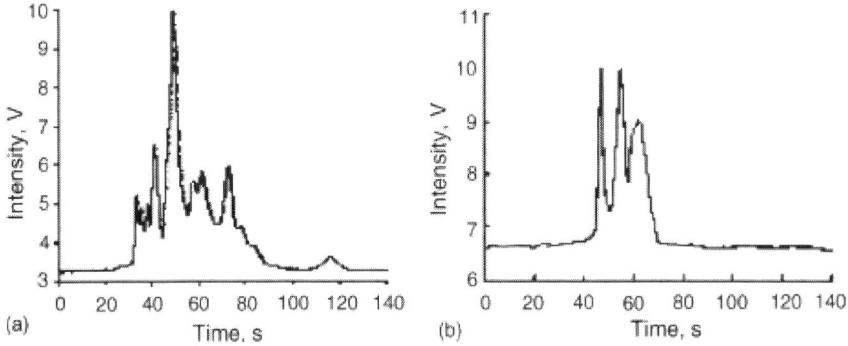

Fig. 21. On-chip separation of fluorescein isothiocyanate-labeled bovine serum albumin digest (A) before and (B) after affinity extraction. Reprinted from ref. (Slentz et al., 2003), with permission.

6. Conclusion

This thematic chapter of the scientific monograph indicates, as expected, that there is not available any universal method capable to solve all the analytical problems. On the other hand, this work clearly shows that the advanced on-line coupled systems are characterized by a capability to solve individual groups of very complex analytical tasks (trace analyte, structurally related analytes, high concentration ratio matrix:analyte, detection interferences, unstable substances, minute sample amounts, in-vivo applications, and various combinations of these problems). Moreover, they allow an elimination of external sample handling that is favorable for the automatization and miniaturization of the analytical procedure. All the categories of on-line column coupled methods provide one or more interfaces for the autonomic, flexible, and well defined/controlled performance of different analytical techniques. Nevertheless, the particular categories of on-line column coupled methods are differing from each other by their specific features and analytical potentialities. An on-line column coupling of CE-CE is advantageous especially because of a simple instrumentation and control of the analytical process, as well as good compatibility of combined separation (electrolyte) systems. On the other hand, an implementation of different separation mechanisms, reflected in an enhanced selectivity of the methods, and possibilities to process larger sample volumes can be counted among typical benefits of an on-line column coupling of CE with non electrophoretic techniques. Very interesting and promising alternative, compromising several analytical aspects, is the hydrodynamically closed CE-CE mode employing capillaries with higher internal diameters as employed in the conventional (hydrodynamically open) mode. Such closed mode has an advantage of higher sample load capacity and obtainable reproducibility of the measurements that are the parameters of a high importance for the real applications of the analytical method. On the other hand, hydrodynamically closed CE-CE systems are limited in the applicability of various supporting electrophoretic (e.g. electroosmotic flow) and non electrophoretic (e.g. pressure counterflow) effects and therefore the achieving of desired separation selectivity can be more difficult. Moreover, here are several critical parameters with respect to a deterioration of the separation efficiency such as capillary size (internal diameter), driving current/voltage, and electrolyte systems that must be very carefully selected and optimized. Therefore, the selection of the method will be determined by particular demands of the analysis. An appropriate selection of the method should then make possible to achieve favorable performance parameters (validation data) while maintaining all benefits of the given method. In such a case, the method can be fully accepted for a routine use in a given advanced application area.

Another future direction concerns the development of analytical microsystems, which is currently one of the major challenge in analytical chemistry and may play a role in the future of life science oriented research and development. The main incentives in miniaturization include a reduction of reagents and samples consumption, increased analytical performance, shorter analysis time, and high-throughput. The overall goal is progression towards a μ-total analysis system (μTAS), whereby chemical information is periodically transformed into an electronic or optical signal, where analysis is carried out on a micrometer scale using centimeter-sized glass or plastic chips. However, samples from biological extracts will always be complex and target analytes at trace-levels. With respect to the potentialities of the advanced CE separation systems, as illustrated also in this chapter, there is/will be thus a great current and future interest in adapting the advanced on-line electrophoretic and non electrophoretic techniques to a micrometer scale.

7. Acknowledgement

This work was supported by the grant of Comenius University No. UK/25/2011, and publication fund of the Faculty of Pharmacy Comenius University. The authors would like to give their great thanks to the Editors and Reviewers of InTech, namely Dr. Gaetano Gargiulo, Prof. Danjoo Ghista and Prof. Reza Fazel, for their valuable reviewing of this scientific monograph chapter. The authors also thank Mr. Davor Vidic and Ms. Romina Krebel for their excellent assistance during the whole publication process.

8. References

Adell, A. & Artigas, F. (1998). Chapter 1, In: *In Vivo Neuromethods*, A.A. Boulton, G.B. Baker, A.N. Bateson., (Eds.), Humana Press, ISBN 0896035115, Totowa, NJ.

Barroso, M.B. & de Jong, A.P. (1998). A new design for large, dilute sample loading in capillary electrophoresis. *Journal of Capillary electrophoresis*, Vol.5, No. 1-2, pp. 1-7, ISSN 1079-5383.

Beckers, J.L. & Boček, P. (2000a). Sample stacking in capillary zone electrophoresis: Principles, advantages and limitations. *Electrophoresis*, Vol.21, No. 14, pp. 2747-2767, ISSN 1522-2683.

Beckers, J.L. (2000b). Window optimalization in ITP superimposed on CZE. *Electrophoresis*, Vol.21, No. 14, pp. 2788-2796. ISSN 1522-2683.

Belder, D. (2006). Chapter 9: Chiral separations in microfluidic devices, In: *Chiral Analysis*, K.W. Busch, M.A. Busch (Eds.), 277-295, Elsevier B.V., ISBN 0444516697, Oxford, UK.

Bergmann, J.; Jaehde, U.; Mazereeuw, M.; Tjaden, U. R. & Schunack, W. (1996). Potential of on-line isotachophoresis-capillary zone electrophoresis with hydrodynamic counterflow in the analysis of various basic proteins and recombinant human interleukin-3. *Journal of Chromatography A*, Vol.734, No.2, pp. 381-389. ISSN 0021-9673.

Bertoncini, N.D. & Hennion, M.C. (2004). Immunoaffinity solid-phase extraction for pharmaceutical and biomedical trace-analysis—coupling with HPLC and CE—perspectives. *Journal of Pharmaceutical and Biomedical Analysis*, Vol.34, No.4, pp.717-736, ISSN 0731-7085.

Bexheti, D.; Anderson, E.I.; Hutt, A.J. & Hanna-Brown, M. (2006). Evaluation of multidimensional capillary electrophoretic methodologies for determination of amino bisphosphonate pharmaceuticals. *Journal of Chromatography A*, Vol.1130, No.1, pp. 137-144. ISSN 0021-9673.

Boček, P.; Deml, M. & Janák, J. (1978). Effect of a concentration cascade of the leading electrolyte on the seperation capacity in isotachophoresis *Journal of Chromatography A*, Vol. 156, No. 2, pp. 323-326. ISSN 0021-9673.

Bodor, R.; Kaniansky, D.; Masár, M.; Silleova, K. & Stanislawski, B. (2002). Determination of bromate in drinking water by zone electrophoresis-isotachophoresis on a column-coupling chip with conductivity detection. *Electrophoresis*, Vol.23, No. 20, pp. 3630-3637, ISSN 1522-2683.

Bonato, P.S. (2003). Recent advances in the determination of enantiomeric drugs and their metabolites in biological fluids by capillary electrophoresis-mediated microanalysis. *Electrophoresis*, Vol.24, No.22-23, pp. 4078-4094. ISSN 1522-2683.

Bonneil, E. & Waldron, K.C. (2000). On-line system for peptide mapping by capillary electrophoresis at sub-micromolar concentrations. *Talanta*, Vol. 53, No., 3, pp. 678-699, ISSN 0039-9140.

Bonneil, E. & Waldron, K.C. (1999). Characterization of a solid-phase extraction device for discontinuous on-line preconcentration in capillary electrophoresis-based peptide mapping. *Journal of Chromatography B*, Vol.736, No. 1-2, pp. 273-287. ISSN 1873-376X.

Bowser, M.T. & Kennedy, R.T. (2001). *In vivo* monitoring of amine neurotransmitters using microdialysis with on-line capillary electrophoresis. *Electrophoresis*, Vol.22, No.17, pp. 3668-3676, ISSN 1522-2683.

Britz-McKibbin, P. & Chen, D.D.Y. (2000). Selective focusing of catecholamines and weakly acidic compounds by capillary electrophoresis using a dynamic pH junction. *Analytical Chemistry*, Vol.72, No. 6, pp. 1242-1252, ISSN 1520-6882.

Broyles, B.S.; Jacobson, S.C. & Ramsey, J.M. (2003). Sample filtration, concentration, and separation integrated on microfluidic devices. *Analytical Chemistry*, Vol.75, No.11, pp.2761-2767, ISSN 0003-2700.

Budáková, L.; Brozmanová, H.; Kvasnička, F. & Grundmann, M. (2007). Determination of valproic acid by on-line coupled capillary isotachophoresis with capillary zone electrophoresis with conductometric detection. *Česká a slovenská farmacie*, Vol.56, No.5, pp. 249-253, ISSN 1210-7816.

Budáková, L., Brozmanová, H., Kvasnička, F., Grundmann, M. (2009). Determination of lamotrigine by isotachophoresis-capillary zone electrophoresis. *Chemické listy*, Vol.103, No.2, pp. 166-171, ISSN 1213-7103.

Bushey, M.M. & Jorgenson, J.W. (1990). Automated instrumentation for comprehensive 2-dimensional high-performance liquid-chromatography capillary zone electrophoresis. *Analytical Chemistry*, Vol.62, No. 10, pp. 978-984, ISSN 1520-6882.

Busnel, J.-M.; Descroix, S.; Godfrin, D.; Hennion, M.-C.; Kašička, V. & Peltre, G. (2006). Transient isotachophoresis in carrier ampholyte-based capillary electrophoresis for protein analysis. *Electrophoresis*, Vol.27, No. 18, pp. 3591-3598, ISSN 1522-2683.

Cannon, D.M.; Kuo, T.C.; Bohn, P.W. & Sweedler, J.V. (2003). Nanocapillary array interconnects for gated analyte injections and electrophoretic separations in multilayer microfluidic architectures. *Analytical Chemistry*, Vol.75, No.10, pp. 2224-2230, ISSN 0003-2700.

Chaurasia, C.S. (1999). In vivo microdialysis sampling: theory and applications. *Biomedical Chromatography*, Vol.13, No. 5, pp. 317-332, ISSN 1099-0801.

Chen, X.; Wu, H.; Mao, C. & Whitesides, G.M. (2002). A prototype two-dimensional capillary electrophoresis system fabricated in poly(dimethylsiloxane). *Analytical Chemistry*, Vol.74, No.8, pp. 1772-1778, ISSN 0003-2700.

Chien, R.L. (2003). Sample stacking revisited: A personal perspective. *Electrophoresis*, Vol.24, No.3, pp. 486-497, ISSN 1522-2683.

Cho, S.I.; Shim, J.; Kim, M.S.; Kim, Y.K. & Chung, D.S. (2004). On-line sample cleanup and chiral separation of gemifloxacin in a urinary solution using chiral crown ether as a chiral selector in microchip electrophoresis. *Journal of Chromatography A*, Vol.1055, No. 1-2, pp. 241-245, ISSN 0021-9673.

Clarke, N.J.; Tomlinson, A.J. & Naylor S. (1997). On-line desalting of physiologically derived fluids in conjunction with capillary isoelectric focusing-mass spectrometry. *Journal of the American Society for Mass Spectrometry*, Vol.8, No.7, pp.743-748, ISSN 1044-0305

Cong, Y.Z.; Zhang, L.H.; Tao, D.Y.; Liang, Y.; Zhang, W.B. & Zhang, Y.K. (2008). Miniaturized two-dimensional capillary electrophoresis on a microchip for analysis of the tryptic digest of proteins. *Journal of Separation Science*, Vol.31, No.3, pp. 588-594, ISSN 1615-9314.

Danková, M.; Kaniansky, D.; Fanali, S. & Iványi, F. (1999). Capillary zone electrophoresis separations of enantiomers present in complex ionic matrices with on-line isotachophoretic sample pretreatment. *Journal of Chromatography A*, Vol.838, No. 1-2, pp. 31-43, ISSN 0021-9673.

Danková, M.; Strašík, S.; Molnárová, M.; Kaniansky, D. & Marák, J. (2001). Capillary zone electrophoresis of orotic acid in urine with on-line isotachophoresis sample pretreatment and diode array detection. *Journal of Chromatography A*, Vol.916, No. 1-2, pp. 143-153, ISSN 0021-9673.

Danková, M.; Strašík, S. & Kaniansky, D. (2003). Determination of orotic acid in urine by capillary zone electrophoresis in tandem-coupled columns with diode array detection. *Journal of Chromatography A*, Vol.990, No. 1-2, pp. 121–132, ISSN 0021-9673.

Dhopeshwarkar, R.; Crooks, R.M.; Hlushkou, D. & Tallarek, U. (2008). Transient Effects on Microchannel Electrokinetic Filtering with an Ion-Permselective Membrane. *Analytical Chemistry*, Vol.80, pp.1039–1048, ISSN 0003-2700.

Dolnik, V. & Hutterer, K.M. (2001). Capillary electrophoresis of proteins 1999-2001. *Electrophoresis*, Vol.22, No. 19, pp. 4163–4178, ISSN 1522-2683.

Fanali, S.; Desiderio, C.; Ölvecká, E.; Kaniansky, D.; Vojtek, M. & Ferancová, A. (2000). Separation of enantiomers by on-line capillary isotachophoresis-capillary zone electrophoresis. *Journal of High Resolution Chromatography*, Vol.23, No.9, pp. 531-538, ISSN 1521-4168.

Fang, H.F.; Zeng, Z.R. & Liu, L. (2006a). Centrifuge microextraction coupled with on-line back-extraction field-amplified sample injection method for the determination of trace ephedrine derivatives in the urine and serum. *Analytical Chemistry*, Vol.78, No. 17, pp. 6043-6049, ISSN 0003-2700.

Fang, H.F.; Liu, M.M. & Zeng, Z.R. (2006b). Solid-phase microextraction coupled with capillary electrophoresis to determine ephedrine derivatives in water and urine using a sol-gel derived butyl methacrylate/silicone fiber. *Talanta*, Vol.68, No. 3, pp. 979-986, ISSN 0039-9140.

Flottmann, D.; Hins, J.; Rettenmaier, C.; Schnell, N.; Kuci, Z.; Merkel, G.; Seitz, G. & Bruchelt, G. (2006). Two-dimensional isotachophoresis for the analysis of homovanillic acid and vanillylmandelic acid in urine for cancer therapy monitoring. *Microchimica Acta*, Vol.154, No.1-2, pp. 49-53, ISSN 1436-5073.

Foote, R.S.; Khandurina, J.; Jacobson, S.C. & Ramsey, J.M. (2005). Preconcentration of proteins on microfluidic devices using porous silica membranes. *Analytical Chemistry*, Vol.77, No. 1, pp. 57-63, ISSN 0003-2700.

Gao, J.; Xu, J.D.; Locascio, L.E. & Lee, C.S. (2001). Integrated microfluidic system enabling protein digestion, peptide separation, and protein identification. *Analytical Chemistry*, Vol.73, No. 11, pp. 2648-2655, ISSN 0003-2700.

Gebauer, P.; Malá, Z. & Boček, P. (2007). Recent progress in capillary ITP. *Electrophoresis*, Vol.28, No.1-2, pp. 26-32, ISSN 1522-2683.

Gong, X.Y. & Hauser, P.C. (2006). Enantiomeric separation of underivatized small amines in conventional and on-chip capillary electrophoresis with contactless conductivity detection. *Electrophoresis*, Vol.27, No.21, pp. 4375-4382, ISSN 1522-2683.

Guiochon, G.; Beaver, L.A.; Gonnord, M.F.; Siouffi, A.M. & Zakaria, M. (1983). Theoretical investigation of the potentialities of the use of a multidimensional column in chromatography. *Journal of Chromatography A*, Vol.255, pp. 415-437, ISSN 0021-9673.

Hanna, M.; Simpson, C. & Perrett, D. (2000). Novel three-dimensional capillary electrophoresis system for complex and trace analysis. *Journal of Chromatography A*, Vol.894, No.1-2, pp. 117-128, ISSN 0021-9673.

Hempel, G. (2000). Strategies to improve the sensitivity in capillary electrophoresis for the analysis of drugs in biological fluids. *Electrophoresis*, Vol.21, No.4, pp. 691-698, ISSN 1522-2683.

Hercegová, A.; Sádecká, J. & Polonský, J. (2000). Determination of some antirheumatics by capillary isotachophoresis. *Electrophoresis*, Vol.21, No.14, pp. 2842-2847, ISSN 1522-2683.

Holtzel, A. & Tallarek, U. (2007). Ionic conductance of nanopores in microscale analysis systems: Where microfluldics meets nanofluidics. *Journal of Separation Science*, Vol.30, No.10, pp. 1398-1419, ISSN 1615-9314.

Hooker, T.F. & Jorgenson, J.W. (1997). A transparent flow gating interface for the coupling of microcolumn LC with CZE in a comprehensive two-dimensional system. *Analytical Chemistry*, Vol.69, No.20, pp. 4134-4142, ISSN 0003-2700.

Horáková, J.; Petr, J.; Maier, V.; Tesařová, E.; Veis, L.; Armstrong, D.W.; Gaš, B. & Ševčík, J. (2007). On-line preconcentration of weak electrolytes by electrokinetic accumulation in CE: Experiment and simulation. *Electrophoresis*, Vol.28, No.10, pp. 1540-1547, ISSN 1522-2683.

Huang, H.; Xu, F.; Dai, Z. & Lin, B. (2005). On-line isotachophoretic preconcentration and gel electrophoretic separation of sodium dodecyl sulfate-proteins on a microchip. *Electrophoresis*, Vol.26, No.11, pp. 2254-2260, ISSN 1522-2683.

Jiang, Y.; Wang, P.C.; Locascio, L.E. & Lee, C.S. (2001). Integrated plastic microftuidic devices with ESI-MS for drug screening and residue analysis. *Analytical Chemistry*, Vol.73, No.9, pp. 2048-2053, ISSN 0003-2700.

Jiménez, J.R. & de Castro, M.D.L. (2008). Lab-on-valve for the automatic determination of the total content and individual profiles of linear alkylbenzene sulfonates in water samples. *Electrophoresis*, Vol. 29, No. 3, pp. 590-596, ISSN 1522-2683.

Kaniansky, D. & Marák, J. (1990). On-line coupling of capillary isotachophoresis with capillary zone electrophoresis. *Journal of Chromatography*, Vol.498, pp. 191-204, ISSN 0021-9673.

Kaniansky, D.; Marák, J.; Madajová, V. & Šimuničová, E. (1993). Capillary zone electrophoresis of complex ionic mixtures with on-line isotachophoretic sample pretreatment. *Journal of Chromatography*, Vol.638, No.2, pp. 137-146, ISSN 0021-9673.

Kaniansky, D.; Marák, J.; Laštinec, J.; Reijenga, J.C. & Onuska, F.I. (1999). Capillary zone electrophoresis with on-line isotachophoretic sample pretreatment: sample clean-up aspects. *Journal of Microcolumn Separations*, Vol.11, No.2, pp. 141-153, ISSN 1520-667X.

Kaniansky, D.; Masár, M.; Bielčiková, J.; Iványi, F.; Eisenbeiss, F.; Stanislawski, B.; Grass, B. & Jöhnck, M. (2000). Capillary electrophoresis separations on a planar chip with the column-coupling configuration of the separation channels. *Analytical Chemistry*, Vol.72, No.15, pp. 3596-3604, ISSN 1520-6882.

Kaniansky , D.; Masár, M.; Bodor, R.; Žúborová, M.; Ölvecká, E.; Jöhnck, M. & Stanislawski, B. (2003). Electrophoretic separations on chips with hydrodynamically closed separation systems. *Electrophoresis*, Vol.24, No.12-13, pp. 2208 - 2227, ISSN 1522-2683.

Kaniansky, D.; Masár, M.; Danková, M.; Bodor, R.; Rákocyová, R.; Pilná, M.; Jöhnck, M.; Stanislawski, B. & Kajan, S. (2004). Column switching in zone electrophoresis on a chip. *Journal of Chromatography A*, Vol.1051, No.1-2, pp. 33 - 42, ISSN 0021-9673.

Kim, J.B. & Terabe, S. (2003). On-line sample preconcentration techniques in micellar electrokinetic chromatography. *Journal of Pharmaceutical and Biomedical Analysis*, Vol.30, No.6, pp. 1625-1643, ISSN 0731-7085.

Kitagawa, F.; Tsuneka, T.; Akimoto, Y.; Sueyoshi, K.; Uchiyama, K.; Hattori, A. & Otsuka, K. (2006). Toward million-fold sensitivity enhancement by sweeping in capillary electrophoresis combined with thermal lens microscopic detection using an interface chip. *Journal of Chromatography A*, Vol.1106, No.1-2., pp. 36-42, ISSN 0021-9673.

Kriikku, P.; Grass, B.; Hokkanen, A.; Stuns, I. & Sirén, H. (2004). Isotachophoresis of β-blockers in capillary and on a poly(methyl methacrylate) chip. *Electrophoresis*, Vol.25, No.10-11, pp. 1687-1694, ISSN 1522-2683.

Křivánková, L.; Foret, F. & Boček, P. (1991). Determination of halofuginone in feedstuffs by the combination of capillary isotachophoresis and capillary zone electrophoresis in a column-switching system. *Journal of Chromatography*, Vol.545, No.2, pp. 307-313, ISSN 0021-9673.

Křivánková, L. & Thormann, W. (1993). Options in electrolyte systems for on-line combined ITP and CZE. *Journal of Chromatography*, Vol.638, No.2, pp. 119-135, ISSN 0021-9673.

Křivánková, L.; Gebauer, P. & Boček, P. (1995). Some practical aspects of utilizing the on-line combination of isotachophoresis and capillary zone electrophoresis. *Journal of Chromatography A*, Vol.716, No.1-2, pp. 35-48, ISSN 0021-9673.

Křivánková, L. & Boček, P. (1997a). Synergism of ITP and CZE. *Journal of Chromatography B*, Vol.689, No.1, pp. 13-34, ISSN 1873-376X.

Křivánková, L.; Vrana, A.; Gebauer, P. & Boček, P. (1997b) On-line isotachophoresis-capillary zone electrophoresis versus sample self stacking capillary zone electrophoresis. Analysis of hippurate in serum. *Journal of Chromatography A*, Vol.772, No.1-2, pp. 283-295, ISSN 0021-9673.

Kubačák, P.; Mikuš, P.; Valášková, I. & Havránek, E. (2006a). Separation of dimetinden enantiomers in drugs by means of capillary isotachophoresis. *Česká a Slovenská Farmacie*, Vol.55, No.1, pp. 32-35, ISSN 1210-7816.

Kubačák, P.; Mikuš, P.; Valášková, I. & Havránek, E. (2006b). Chiral separation of feniramine in medicaments with the use of capillary isotachophoresis. *Farmaceutický Obzor*, Vol.75, No.2-3, pp. 48-51, ISSN 0014--8172.

Kubačák, P.; Mikuš, P.; Valášková, I. & Havránek, E. (2007). Chiral separation of alkylamine antihistamines in pharmaceuticals by capillary Isotachophoresis with charged cyclodextrin. *Drug Development and Industrial Pharmacy*, Vol.33, No.11, pp. 1199-1204, ISSN 0363-9045.

Kulka, S.; Quintás, G. & Lendl, B. (2006). Automated sample preparation and analysis using a sequential-injection-capillary electrophoresis (SI-CE) interface. *Analyst*, Vol.131, No.6, pp. 739–744, ISSN 1364-5528.

Kuo, T.C.; Cannon, D.M.; Chen, Y.N. & Tulock, J.J. (2003a). Gateable nanofluidic interconnects for multilayered microfluidic separation systems. *Analytical Chemistry*, Vol.75, No.8, pp. 1861-1867, ISSN 0003-2700.

Kuo, T.C.; Cannon, D.M.; Shannon, M.A.; Bohn, P.W. & Sweedler, J.V. (2003b). Hybrid three-dimensional nanofluidic/microfluidic devices using molecular gates. *Sensors and Actuators A-physical*, Vol.102, No.3, pp. 223-233, ISSN 0924-4247.

Kvasnička, F.; Jaroš, M. & Gaš, B. (2001). New configuration in capillary isotachophoresis-capillary zone electrophoresis coupling. *Journal of Chromatography A*, Vol.916, No.1-2, pp. 131-142, ISSN 0021-9673.

Lada, M.W. & Kennedy, R.T. (1997). In vivo monitoring of glutathione and cysteine in rat caudate nucleus using microdiolysis on-line with capillary zone electrophoresis-laser induced fluorescence detection. *Journal of Neuroscience Methods*, Vol. 72, No.2, pp. 153-159, ISSN 0165-0270.

Lada, M.W.; Vickroy, T.W.& Kennedy, R.T. (1998). Evidence for neuronal origin and metabotropic receptor-mediated regulation of extracellular glutamate and aspartate in rat striatum *in vivo* following electrical stimulation of the prefrontal cortex. *Journal of Neurochemistry*, Vol.70, No.2, pp.617-625, ISSN 0022-3042.

Lemmo, A.V. & Jorgenson, J.W. (1993). Two-dimensional protein separation by microcolumn size-exclusion chromatography-capillary zone electrophoresis. *Journal of Chromatography A*, Vol.633, No.1-2, pp. 213-220, ISSN 0021-9673.

Li, S.F.Y. & Kricka, L.J. (2006). Clinical Analysis by Microchip Capillary Electrophoresis. *Clinical Chemistry*, Vol.52, No.1,pp. 37–45, ISSN 0009-9147.

Liu, Z. & Pawliszyn, J. (2006). Online coupling of solid-phase microextraction and capillary electrophoresis. *Journal of Chromatographic Science*, Vol.44, No.6, pp. 366–374, ISSN 0021-9665.

Long, Z.C., Liu, D.Y., Ye, N.N., Qin, J.H. & Lin, B.C. (2006). Integration of nanoporous membranes for sample filtration/preconcentration in microchip electrophoresis. *Electrophoresis*, Vol.27, No.24, pp. 4927–4934, ISSN 1522-2683.

Lord, H. & Pawliszyn, J. (2000). Evolution of solid-phase microextraction technology. *Journal of Chromatography A*, Vol.885, No.1-2, pp. 153–193, ISSN 0021-9673.

Lü, W.J.; Chen, Y.L.; Zhu, J.H. & Chen, X.G. (2009). The combination of flow injection with electrophoresis using capillaries and chips. *Electrophoresis*, Vol.30, No.1, pp.83-91, ISSN 1522-2683.

Ma, B.; Zhou, X.; Wang, G.; Huang, H.; Dai, Z.; Qin, J. & Lin, B. (2006). Integrated isotachophoretic preconcentration with zone electrophoresis separation on a quartz microchip for UV detection of flavonoids. *Electrophoresis*, Vol.27, No.24, pp. 4904-4909, ISSN 1522-2683.

Marák, J.; Laštinec, J.; Kaniansky, D. & Madajová, V. (1990). Computer-assisted choice of electrolyte systems and spacing constituents for two-dimensional capillary isotachophoresis. *Journal of Chromatography A*, Vol.509, No.1, pp. 287-299, ISSN 0021-9673.

Marák, J.; Mikuš, P.; Maráková, K.; Kaniansky, D.; Valášková, I. & Havránek, E. (2007). Enantioselective analysis of pheniramine in urine by charged CD-mediated CZE provided with a fiber-based DAD and an on-line sample pretreatment by capillary ITP. *Electrophoresis*, Vol.28, No.15, pp. 2738-2747, ISSN 1522-2683.

Mardones, C.; Ríos, A.; Valcárcel, M. & Cicciarelli, R. (1999). Enantiomeric separation of D- and L-carnitine by integrating on-line derivatization with capillary zone electrophoresis. *Journal of Chromatography A*, Vol.849, No.2, pp. 609-616, ISSN 0021-9673.

Mazereeuw, M.; Spikmans, V.; Tjaden, U.R. & van der Greef, J. (2000). On-line isotachophoretic sample focusing for loadability enhancement in capillary electrochromatography-mass spectrometry. *Journal of Chromatography A*, Vol.879, No., pp. 219–233, ISSN 0021-9673.

Mikuš, P.; Kubačák, P.; Valášková, I. & Havránek, E. (2003). Capillary isotachophoresis of cystine in urine with on-line isotachophoresis sample pretreatment. *Pharmazie*, Vol.58, No.2, pp. 111-113, ISSN 0031-7144.

Mikuš, P.; Kubačák, P.; Valášková, I. & Havránek, E. (2006a). Analysis of enantiomers in biological matrices by charged cyclodextrin-mediated capillary zone electrophoresis in column-coupling arrangement with capillary isotachophoresis. *Talanta*, Vol.70, No.4, pp. 840-846, ISSN 0039-9140.

Mikuš, P.; Kubačák, P.; Valášková, I. & Havránek, E. (2006b). Comparison of capillary zone electrophoresis and isotachophoresis determination of dimethindene enantiomers in pharmaceuticals using charged carboxyethyl-beta-cyclodextrin as a chiral selector. *Methods and Findings in Experimenatal and Clinical Pharmacology*, Vol.28, No.9, pp. 595-599, ISSN 0379-0355.

Mikuš, P.; Maráková, K.; Marák, J.; Nemec, I.; Valášková, I. & Havránek, E. (2008a). Direct quantitative determination of amlodipine enantiomers in urine samples for pharmacokinetic study using on-line coupled isotachophoresis-capillary zone electrophoresis separation method with diode array detection. *Journal of Chromatography B*, Vol.875, No.1, pp. 266-272, ISSN 1873-376X.

Mikuš, P.; Maráková, K.; Marák, J.; Planková, A.; Valášková, I. & Havránek, E. (2008b). Direct determination of celiprolol in human urine using on-line coupled ITP-CZE method with fiber-based DAD. *Electrophoresis*, Vol.29, No.22, pp. 4561-4567, ISSN 1522-2683.

Mikuš, P.; Maráková, K.; Marák, J.; Kaniansky, D.; Valášková, I. & Havránek, E. (2008c). Posibilities of column-coupling electrophoresis provided with a fiber-based diode array detection in enantioselective analysis of drugs in pharmaceutical and clinical samples. *Journal of Chromatography A*, Vol.1179, No.1, pp. 9-16, ISSN 0021-9673.

Mikuš, P.; Maráková, K.; Marák, J.; Nemec, I.; Valášková, I. & Havránek, E. (2009). Pharmacokinetic study of amlodipine in human urine using on-line coupled isotachophoresis-capillary zone electrophoresis with diode array detection. *Current Pharmaceutical Analysis*, Vol.5, No.2, pp. 171-178, ISSN 1573-4129.

Mikuš, P. & Maráková, K. (2010). Chiral capillary electrophoresis with on-line sample preparation. *Current Pharmaceutical Analysis*, Vol.6, No.2, pp. 76-100, ISSN 1573-4129.

Mohan, D. & Lee, C.S. (2002). On-line coupling of capillary isoelectric focusing with transient isotachophoresis-zone electrophoresis: A two-dimensional separation system for proteomics. *Electrophoresis*, Vol.23, No.18, pp. 3160-3167, ISSN 1522-2683.

Moore, A.W. & Jorgenson, J.W. (1995). Comprehensive 3-dimensional separation of peptides using size-exclusion chromatography reversed-phase liquid-chromatography optically gated capillary zone electrophoresis. *Analytical Chemistry*, Vol.67, No.19, pp. 3456-3463, ISSN 0003-2700.

Ölvecká, E.; Masár, M.; Kaniansky, D.; Jöhnck, M. & Stanislawski, B. (2001). Isotachophoresis separations of enantiomers on a planar chip with coupled separation channels. *Electrophoresis*, Vol.22, No.15, pp. 3347-3353, ISSN 1522-2683.

Ölvecká, E.; Koníková, M.; Grobuschek, N.; Kaniansky, D. & Stanislawski, B. (2003). Direct determination of valproate in serum by zone electrophoresis-isotachophoresis on a column-coupling chip. *Journal of Separation Science*, Vol.26, No.8, pp. 693-700, ISSN 1615-9314.

Ölvecká, E.; Kaniansky, D.; Pollák, B. & Stanislawski, B. (2004). Separation of proteins by zone electrophoresis on-line coupled with isotachophoresis on a column-coupling chip with conductivity detection. *Electrophoresis*, Vol.25, No.21-22, pp. 3865-3874, ISSN 1522-2683.

Ouyang, G. & Pawliszyn, J. (2006). SPME in environmental analysis. *Analytical and Bioanalytical Chemistry*, Vol.386, No.4, pp.1059–1073, ISSN 1618-2642.

Pálmarsdóttir, S. & Edholm, L.H. (1995). Enhancement of selectivity and concentration sensitivity in capillary zone electrophoresis by online coupling with column liquid-chromatography and utilizing a double stacking procedure allowing for microliter injections. *Journal of Chromatography A*, Vol.693, No.1, pp. 131-143, ISSN 0021-9673.

Pálmarsdóttir, S.; Mathiasson, L.; Jönsson, J.A. & Edholm, L.H. (1996). Micro-CLC as an interface between SLM extraction and CZE for enhancement of sensitivity and selectivity in bioanalysis of drugs. *Journal of Capillary Electrophoresis*, Vol.3, No.5, pp. 255-260, ISSN 1079-5383.

Pálmarsdóttir, S.; Mathiasson, L.; Jönsson, J.A. & Edholm, L.H. (1997). Determination of a basic drug, bambuterol, in human plasma by capillary electrophoresis using double stacking for large volume injection and supported liquid membranes for sample pretreatment. *Journal of Chromatography B*, Vol.688, No.1, pp. 127-134, ISSN 1873-376X.

Pantůčková, P. & Křivánková, L. (2010). Analysis of 5-methyltetrahydrofolate in human blood, serum and urine by on-line coupling of capillary isotachophoresis and zone electrophoresis. *Electrophoresis*, Vol.31, No.20, pp. 3391-3399, ISSN 1522-2683.

Petersson, M.; Wahlund, K.G. & Nilsson S. (1999). Miniaturised on-line solid-phase extraction for enhancement of concentration sensitivity in capillary electrophoresis. *Journal of Chromatography A*, Vol.841, No.2, pp. 249-261, ISSN 0021-9673.

Peterson, Z.D.; Bowerbank, Ch.R.; Collins, D.C.; Graves, S.W. & Lee, M.L (2003). Advantages and limitations of coupling isotachophoresis and comprehensive isotachophoresis-capillary electrophoresis to time-of-flight mass spectrometry. *Journal of Chromatography A*, Vol.992, No.1-2, pp. 169-179, ISSN 0021-9673.

Procházková, A.; Křivánková, L. & Boček, P. (1998). Quantitative trace analysis of L-ascorbic acid in human body fluids by on-line combination of capillary isotachophoresis and zone electrophoresis. *Electrophoresis*, Vol.19, No.2, pp. 300-304, ISSN 1522-2683.

Procházková, A.; Křivánková, L. & Boček, P. (1999). Analysis of orotic acid in human urine by on-line combination of capillary isotachophoresis and zone electrophoresis. *Journal of Chromatography A*, Vol.838, No.1-2, pp. 213-221, ISSN 0021-9673.

Ptolemy, A.S.; Le Bilhan, M. & Britz-McKibbin, P. (2005). On-line sample preconcentration with chemical derivatization of bacterial biomarkers by capillary electrophoresis: A dual strategy for integrating sample pretreatment with chemical analysis. *Electrophoresis*, Vol.26, No.23-24, pp. 4206-4214, ISSN 1522-2683.

Ptolemy, A.S.; Tran, L. & Britz-McKibbin, P. (2006). Single-step enantioselective amino acid flux analysis by capillary electrophoresis using on-line sample preconcentration with chemical derivatization. *Analytical Biochemistry*, Vol.354, No.2, pp. 192-204, ISSN 0003-2697.

Puig, P.; Tempels, F.W.A.; Borrull, F.; Calull, M.; Aguilar, C.; Somsen, G.W & de Jong, G.J. (2007). On-line coupling of solid-phase extraction and capillary electrophoresis for the determination of cefoperazone and ceftiofur in plasma. *Journal of Chromatography B*, Vol. 856, No.1-2, pp. 365-370, ISSN 1873-376X.

Puig, P.; Borrull, F.; Calull, M. & Aguilar, C. (2008). Sorbent preconcentration procedures coupled to capillary electrophoresis for environmental and biological applications. *Analytica Chimica Acta*, Vol.616, No.1, pp. 1-18, ISSN 0003-2670.

Quirino, J.P. & Terabe, S. (1998). Exceeding 5000-fold concentration of dilute analytes in micellar electrokinetic chromatography. *Science*, Vol.282, No.5388, pp. 465-468, ISSN 0036-8075.

Quirino, J.P. & Terabe, S. (1999). Sweeping of analyte zones in electrokinetic chromatography. *Analytical Chemistry*, Vol.71, No.8, pp. 1638-1644, ISSN 0003-2700.

Quirino, J.P. & Terabe, S. (2000a). Sample stacking of cationic and anionic analytes in capillary electrophoresis. *Journal of Chromatography A*, Vol.902, No.1, pp. 119-135, ISSN 0021-9673.

Quirino, J.P.; Iwai, Y.; Otsuka, K. & Terabe, S. (2000b). Determination of environmentally relevant aromatic amines in the ppt levels by cation selective exhaustive injection-sweeping-micellar electrokinetic chromatography. *Electrophoresis*, Vol.21, No.14, pp. 2899-2903, ISSN 1522-2683.

Sádecká, J. & Netriová, J. (2005). Determination of naproxen and its metabolite, 6-O-desmethylnaproxen, in human urine by capillary isotachophoresis. *Journal of Liquid Chromatography & Related Technologies*, Vol.28, No.18, pp. 2887-2894, ISSN 1520-572X.

Sahlin, E. (2007). Two-dimensional capillary electrophoresis using tangentially connected capillaries. *Journal of Chromatography A*, Vol.1154, No.1-2, pp. 454-459, ISSN 0021-9673.

Saito, Y. & Jinno, K. (2003). Miniaturized sample preparation combined with liquid phase separations. *Journal of Chromatography A*, Vol.1000, No.1-2, pp. 53–67, ISSN 0021-9673.

Shackman, J.G. & Ross, D. (2007). Counter-flow gradient electrofocusing. *Electrophoresis*, Vol.28, No.4, pp. 556-571, ISSN 1522-2683.

Shen, Y.; Berger, S.J.; Anderson, G.A. & Smith, R.D. (2000). High-efficiency capillary isoelectric focusing of peptides. *Analytical Chemistry*, Vol.72, No.9, pp. 2154-2159, ISSN 0003-2700.

Simpson, S.L.; Quirino, J.P. & Terabe, S. (2008). On-line preconcentration in capillary electrophoresis Fundamentals and applications. *Journal of Chromatography A*, Vol.1184, No.1-2, pp. 504 - 541, ISSN 0021-9673.

Slentz, B.E.; Penner, N.A. & Regnier, F.E. (2003). Protein proteolysis and the multi-dimensional electrochromatographic separation of histidine-containing peptide fragments on a chip. *Journal of Chromatography A*, Vol.984, No.1, pp. 97 - 107, ISSN 0021-9673.

Solich, P.; Polasek; M., Klimundová, J. & Ruzicka, J. (2004). Sequential injection technique applied to pharmaceutical analysis. Trac-Trends in Analytical Chemistry, Vol.23, No.2, pp. 116–126, ISSN 0167-2940.

Stroink, T.; Schravendijk, P.; Wiese, G.; Teeuwsen, J.; Lingeman, H.; Waterval, J.C.M.; Bult, A.; de Jong, G.J. & Underberg, W.J.M. (2003). On-line coupling of size-exclusion chromatography and capillary zone electrophoresis via a reversed-phase C18 trapping column for the determination of peptides in biological samples. *Electrophoresis*, Vol.24, No.10, pp. 1126–1134, ISSN 1522-2683.

Tekeľ, J. & Mikuš, P. (2005). *Analysis of Substances in Biological Systems*, A. Jahnátková, (Ed.), pp. 135-171, Comenius University, ISBN 80-223-1988-0, Bratislava, Slovakia.

Tempels, F.W.A.; Wiese, G.; Underberg, W.J.M; Somsen, G.W. & de Jong, G.J. (2006). On-line coupling of size exclusion chromatography and capillary electrophoresis via solid-phase extraction and a Tee-split interface. *Journal of Chromatography B*, Vol. 839, No.1-2, pp. 30-35, ISSN 1873-376X.

Tempels, F.W.A.; Underberg, W.J.M.; Somsen, G.W. & de Jong, G.J. (2007). On-line coupling of SPE and CE-MS for peptide analysis. *Electrophoresis*, Vol.28, No.9, pp.1319–1326, ISSN 1522-2683.

Thomas, D.H.; Rakestraw, D.J.; Schoeniger, J.S.; Lopez-Avila, V. & Van Emon, J. (1999). Selective trace enrichment by immunoaffinity capillary electrochromatography on-line with capillary zone electrophoresis - laser-induced fluorescence. *Electrophoresis*, Vol.20, No.1, pp. 57-66, ISSN 1522-2683.

Thompson, J.E.; Vickroy, T.W. & Kennedy, R.T. (1999). Rapid determination of aspartate enantiomers in tissue samples by microdialysis coupled on-line with capillary electrophoresis. *Analytical Chemistry*, Vol.71, No.13, pp.2379-2384, ISSN 0003-2700.

Tomáš, R.; Koval, M. & Foret, F. (2010). Coupling of hydronynamically closed large bore capillary isotachophoresis with electrospray mass spectrometry. *Journal of Chromatography A*, Vol.1217, No.25, pp. 4144-4149, ISSN 0021-9673.

Trojanowicz, M. (2009). Recent developments in electrochemical flow detections—A review, Part I. Flow analysis and capillary electrophoresis. *Analytica Chimica Acta*, Vol.653, No.1, pp. 36–58, ISSN 0003-2670.

Tulock, J.J.; Shannon, M.A.; Bohn, P.W. & Sweedler, J.V. (2004). Microfluidic separation and gateable fraction collection for mass-limited samples. *Analytical Chemistry*, Vol.76, No.21, pp.6419-6425, ISSN 0003-2700.

Valcárcel, M.; Rios, A. & Arce, L. (1998). Coupling continuous sample treatment systems to capillary electrophoresis. *Critical Reviews in Analytical Chemistry*, Vol.28, No.1, pp. 63-81, ISSN 1040-8347.

Valcárcel, M.; Arce, L. & Rios, A. (2001). Coupling continuous separation techniques to capillary electrophoresis. *Journal of Chromatography A*, Vol.924, No.1-2, pp. 3–30, ISSN 0021-9673.

Wainright, A.; Williams, S.J.; Ciambrone, G.; Xue, Q.F.; Wei, J. & Harris, D. (2002). Sample preconcentration by ITP in microfluidic devices. *Journal of Chromatography A*, Vol.979, No.1-2, pp. 69-80, ISSN 0021-9673.

Weng, X.; Bi, H.; Liu, B. & Kong, J. (2006). On-chip chiral separation based on bovine serum albumin-conjugated carbon nanotubes as stationary phase in a microchannel. *Electrophoresis*, Vol.27, No.15, pp. 3129-3135, ISSN 1522-2683.

Xu, N.X.; Lin, Y.H.; Hofstadler, S.A. & Matson, D. (1998). A microfabricated dialysis device for sample cleanup in electrospray ionization mass spectrometry. *Analytical Chemistry*, Vol.70, No.17, pp. 3553-3556, ISSN 0003-2700.

Yang, C.; Liu, H.C.; Yang, Q.; Zhang, L.Y.; Zhang, W.B. & Zhang, Y.K. (2003a). On-line hyphenation of capillary isoelectric focusing and capillary gel electrophoresis by a dialysis interface. *Analytical Chemistry*, Vol.75, No.2, pp. 215-218, ISSN 0003-2700.

Yang, C.; Zhang, L.; Liu, H.; Zhang, W. & Zhang, Y. (2003b). Two-dimensional capillary electrophoresis involving capillary isoelectric focusing and capillary zone electrophoresis. *Journal of Chromatography A*, Vol.1018, No.1, pp. 97–103, ISSN 0021-9673.

Yu, C.J.; Chang, H.C. & Tseng, W.L. (2008). On-line concentration of proteins by SDS-CGE with LIF detection. *Electrophoresis*, Vol.29, No.2, pp. 483-490, ISSN 1522-2683.

Zhang, Y. & Timperman, A.T. (2003). Integration of nanocapillary arrays into microfluidic devices for use as analyte concentrators. *Analyst*, Vol.128, No. 6, pp. 537–542, ISSN 1364-5528.

Zhang, Z.X.; Zhang, X.W. & Li, F. (2010). The multi-concentration and two-dimensional capillary electrophoresis method for the analysis of drugs in urine samples. *Science China-Chemistry*, Vol.53, No.5, pp. 1183-1189, ISSN 1674-7291.

6

Design Principles for Microfluidic Biomedical Diagnostics in Space

Emily S. Nelson
NASA Glenn Research Center
USA

1. Introduction

The human body adapts to the space environment in a number of direct and indirect ways. With the near-removal of gravitational forces, body fluid tends to move headwards from the lower extremities. As the body adapts to this changed distribution of fluid, plasma volume in the blood decreases within days. This change increases the relative concentration of red blood cells in the blood, which may be a factor in the observed decrease in red blood cell generation. (For discussion of this and similar issues, see, e.g., (Blaber et al., 2010)). Newly modified concentrations of various dissolved gases, hormones, electrolytes, and other substances induce a cascade of inter-woven effects. Other direct effects of space include conformational changes in compliant tissue, including the shape of the heart. Muscles tend to atrophy without the challenge of gravitational loading. More troubling, key regions in the load-bearing skeleton, such as the hip and lumbar spine, can lose mass at a rate of 1.5-2.5% per month, at least for several months. Aside from the loss of gravitational loading, other environmental factors include radiation exposure (Akopova et al., 2005), altered light/dark cycles, and the psychological stress of living in a confined space in a dangerous environment with only a few people for months at a time. Biomedical research continues to expand our knowledge base and provide insights into the short- and long-term effects of spaceflight on the human body. Space medicine is concerned with the more immediate needs of astronaut patients who are living in low earth orbit right now. Both of these tasks require biodiagnostic tools that give meaningful information.

The retirement of the Space Shuttle removes the primary avenue for returning astronaut blood samples to earth for lab analysis. This requires a shift in focus from ground-based analysis of space-exposed samples to on-orbit analysis. While this is a significant challenge, it also provides an opportunity to use the International Space Station (ISS) to develop next-generation medical diagnostics for space. For long-duration spaceflight, we know that the crew will have to operate at an unprecedented level of autonomy. The need for compact, efficient, reliable, adaptable diagnostics will be critical for maintaining the health of the crew and their environment. The ISS can be used as a proving ground for these emerging technologies so that we can refine these tools before the need becomes urgent.

The demands placed on onboard diagnostics are not simple to meet. Minimal resources for power, storage, excess volume and mass are available. Assume that the entire medical supply kit for long-duration spaceflight will be roughly the size of a shoebox. Little or no supply chain is to be expected. Devices and their supporting reagents and additives must remain viable for several years. They must operate safely and reliably in an extreme envi-ronment. We would like to have testing capabilities that could respond to current needs as well as to evolving priorities. For blood analysis, we would like to perform routine chemis-try panels and cell counts as well as examine an array of biomarkers (some as yet unknown), which would aid in detecting radiative damage and assessing changes in bone, immune, cardiovascular, neurological, renal, and other functions. Aside from blood analysis, urine or saliva could provide useful diagnostic data while reducing invasiveness to the astronaut. Consequently, we would like to design towards a device that could accept other sample types including cell cultures, animal blood and urine, and environmental samples like potable water.

On earth, the Holy Grail for portable medical diagnostics is the development of a self-contained, robust, general-purpose assay system for analysis of bodily or environmental fluids. While this remains the goal, most research today focuses on bits and pieces of such a device, such as separation processes, onboard miniaturized sensors, or the development of highly specialized assays, e.g., detection of specific cancers. There are fewer investigations that focus on integration of sample introduction, processing, and detection with wide-ranging capability. But the pace of such development has progressed rapidly over the last decade. Most systems rely heavily on disposable components, which are a luxury for a spacebound tool. Devices that depend on bulky external infrastructure for optics, flow control or application of magnetic, electric, or optical fields are also ill-suited for space. Dynamic reconfiguration of device capabilities to accommodate different assays or sample types can be achieved with flow control and/or biochip-based reconfiguration, but these modular concepts remain more of an interesting oddity at present than a regularly employed strategy in biochip development. Complete integration, miniaturization, adaptability and breadth of capability are all essential features of a spaceworthy device.

On the commercial side, there are a handful of point-of-care devices that provide generalized blood analysis. None of these devices span the breadth of assays specified by the most current medical requirements (International Space Station Program, 2004). For a discussion, see (Nelson & Chait, 2010). For these devices, the design paradigm is a suite of disposable cartridges, coupled with a reusable reader. But for space travelers on extended missions, the volume and mass of the disposable components for these commercial systems are prohibitively large. Moreover, the shelf life is grossly inadequate.

For the past decade, NASA has invested in the development of next-generation medical diagnostics. In this chapter, we consider the benefit of squeezing down the resource requirements by limiting the use of disposable components. Instead, we emphasize the reuse of the microfluidic and detection infrastructure if cross-contamination can be avoided. The basic technology exists today to build a reusable microscale lab analysis tool that is versatile, resource-conscious, and miniaturized to an extent that beats the commercial devices by a very large margin. The primary obstacles are in development, specifically, the integration of all the functional components into a single device, the capacity for massive multiplexing and the broad availability of appropriate assays. Many excellent reviews on microfluidics are available in the literature, including (Arora et al., 2010; Bhagat et al., 2010; Chan, 2009; Chang & Yang, 2007; Cho et al., 2010; De Volder & Reynaerts, 2010; Di Carlo, 2009; Gossett et al., 2010; Huh et al., 2009; Hwang & Park, 2011; Kim & Ligler, 2010; Kist & Mandaji, 2004; Kuswandi et al., 2007; Lange et al., 2008; Lenshof & Laurell, 2010; Mogensen & Kutter, 2009; Mukhopadhyay, 2005; Pamme, 2006; Pamme, 2007; Salieb-Beugelaar et al., 2010; Sun & Morgan, 2010). Consequently, in this work, we will focus on the new directions that will reduce resource consumption, improve adaptability and expand breadth while increasing diagnostic value within the framework of a single device.

2. Requirements for spacebound devices

Diagnostics in space must be stingy with resources, such as volume, mass, power and reagent consumption. Ideally, biomedical devices should be highly adaptable to meet evolving needs of space medicine, biomedical research, plant, cell and animal biology, and environmental monitoring. Devices and their supporting reagents and additives must sustain performance during a multi-year lifetime in a low-gravity environment, characterized by radiation, low humidity and the lack of refrigeration. Efforts to reduce additives, expand capability, amplify ruggedness and simplify controls will ultimately be beneficial for all next-generation medical devices, whether for use on earth or in space.

2.1 Resource consumption

In 2010, a prototype microfluidic device purified water and mixed it with salt crystals on orbit to deliver medical-grade saline solution in an approach described by (Niederhaus et al., 2008). This technique could maintain the availability of saline for medical or lab use on the Space Station, while eliminating the need to consume limited storage space in resupply vehicles. But in general, additives, including reagents, buffers, and clean water, are very limited. No dedicated hardware can be expected for cleaning or storage. Every pipette, lancet, cleansing wipe, and other supplies used for device operation or maintenance must be considered as part of an assay system's resource "load" and scrutinized for potential savings. From the standpoint of resource efficiency, the microdevices fabricated by embedding polymer microchannels on paper by Whitesides and co-workers are noteworthy (Martinez et al., 2010). A droplet of blood is applied to a snippet of paper, which uses capillary action to draw the sample through the device to colorimetric sensor pads. The overall system is extremely small, requires no power or other infrastructure for qualitative measurement, and can easily perform several blood tests simultaneously. Expanding its capabilities to dozens or hundreds of tests per sample is a major challenge, but this direction is progressing through the use of multi-layer microsystems (Martinez et al., 2010). However, this approach is unlikely to provide cell counts without major redesign.

One fundamental design choice is the use of a disposable cartridge, which accepts the sample and contains the microfluidic network necessary for processing the sample, versus a reusable system, which would ideally reuse all of the microfluidic infrastructure. In the latter case, only the sample itself and supporting additives would remain as biological waste. Those additives include the fluids required for flushing or cleaning the reusable device to remove all detectable traces of the sample and reagents. In contrast, the disposable cartridges encapsulate the biosample within its borders, simplifying the process of disposal while potentially eliminating the risk of cross-contamination. And, certainly, the disposable components could be designed to be more resource-conscious than current commercial designs. But even so, systems based on disposable cartridges will likely require more upmass for resupply than a reusable system would require. ("Upmass" is a term used to describe the mass occupied by something placed in a spacebound vehicle.) Close examination of the resources required by the device, the availability of flushing fluids and of upmass, the tolerance for risk, and the diagnostics requirements of the mission will determine the best approach for any specific space mission.

A device designed for reusability can be more easily re-engineered to operate with a disposable, bioencapsulating cartridge than vice versa. Consequently, in this work, we will examine the less studied problem of a reusable biomedical analyzer.

There are many avenues for scaling down a biodiagnostic system's footprint:

- *Reduce the scale at which the device operates.* Operating volumes on the scale of several hundred nL have been proven. The need for effective pre-filtering is however essential.
- *Include onboard sensors and fluidics.* Optical and electrochemical detection are at this point reasonably mature. Fluidic components such as micropumps and valving can be integrated with electronics for speedy communication and improved ruggedness.
- *Exploit shared resources,* such as a PC for signal processing and display. USB ports can also be used to supply power that is adequate for well-designed systems.
- *Scale back the size of the disposable portion.* Examples include a disposable insert for sample retrieval following separation by capillary electrophoresis (Mohanty et al., 2006) or portions of a microperistaltic pump (Liu et al., 2003).
- *Incorporate modularity,* introduced into the system virtually through dynamic programmability, or physically by using quick disconnects or swapping out chips for different sample types or detection strategies (see §2.2).
- *Use systems that can perform massive multiplexing,* i.e., process dozens to hundreds of diagnostic tests from a single sample (see §2.2 and §4.2).

2.2 Flexibility, adaptability and modularity

For space biodiagnostics, we would like to perform garden-variety blood and urine analysis, as well as more specialized tests. All testing will involve counting particulates, such as cell, platelet, bacterial, and crystal counts, as well as detecting concentrations of dissolved substances in the sample, including gases, electrolytes, small molecules, and a range of large and small proteins (see §4.2). Due to the sheer number of assays to be processed, one key requirement will be the capacity for massive multiplexing on an individual sample. ("Multiplexing" simply refers to the capability of performing multiple measurements on the same sample.) The multiplexing should avoid "hard coding" an assay suite to the system to permit adaptability. Finally, we would like to extend the range of sample types to more broadly address the needs of physiological, biological and environmental analysis.

Mix-and-match modules with simple connection strategies are one way to embed flexibility into a resource-conscious assay system. In one example, the development of "Zero Insertion Force" sockets allowed reconfiguration of the fluidic and electrical connectivity with up to 60 independent electrical connections joined to a variety of microfluidic systems (Dalton & Kaler, 2007). For space diagnostics, a module for cell separation and counting could be coupled to a serum analysis module. The latter could be designed to operate on nL-scale volumes of well-filtered fluid. The blood pre-processor for cell separation and analysis could then be swapped out with a urine pre-processing stage, which would separate out solids content, while sending well-filtered urine on to the nanoscale detection device.

Alternatively, dynamic flow control could be used to route the sample through different pathways to appropriate processing stations onboard a single chip. The basic principles of programmability that have become so integral to information technology are available for fluidic networks as well. In this case, the assay suite and the flow path can be specified at runtime, which can be effective at conserving reagents and streamlining operations. The rudiments of a Java interface were developed for operations on arbitrary portions of one biochip design, including metering, transporting, mixing, and purging (Urbanski et al., 2006). A device for studying protein precipitation included a Labview-driven system for quickly creating complex mixtures using 32 stock reagents in a 5 nL reactor (Hansen et al., 2004). The metering precision of 83.4± 0.6 pL ensured minimal reagent consumption. These approaches could add significant capability to a resource-conscious, adaptable biodiagnostic system.

Both of the strategies discussed above assume that reconfiguration requires the sample to access different sets of fluidic pathways, such as various reagent reservoirs, mixing devices, incubation chambers and/or detection stages. In §4.2, we will discuss other approaches to massive multiplexing through assay design.

2.3 Lifetime

Devices and their supporting consumables must remain viable in a space habitat for years in an environment characterized by radiation exposure and low humidity, without dedicated hardware for sterilization or guaranteed access to refrigerated storage. This is a significantly higher bar than the requirements on shelf life for earthbound devices. Moreover, little or no supply chain will exist for maintenance or replenishment. Therefore, NASA must find a solution with the right combination of physical and biochemistry, device and sensor design, and materials and fabrication choices to operate under the demanding conditions of long-duration spaceflight.

Like most commercial systems, the widely used i-STAT blood analyzer employs single-use assay cartridges. Its cartridges are rated by the manufacturer at a 4-6 month shelf life when refrigerated at 2-8°C. NASA researchers found that some of the more common assays for blood chemistry retained their effectiveness for up to 12 months (Smith et al., 2004). No such testing is available for the single-assay cTNI cartridge, which detects troponin. This is problematic since the biochemical reagents in immunoassays are less stable over time than chemical reagents. Additional packaging to reduce the effects of gas diffusion and radiation exposure is likely to be the maximum effort that NASA could reasonably consider to extend the lifetime of commercial devices. See §4.2 for further discussion on assay design.

Few studies explore the impact of long-term exposure to space radiation on shelf life. One of the only studies to address this issue is considered in a preliminary fashion by (Fernandez-Calvo et al., 2006). High doses of low-energy gamma radiation were not found to be significantly deleterious on antibody activity, which was contained in stabilizing solutions. However, the duration of exposure was not reported in this work, and shelf life was not addressed. Furthermore, the study does not address the type of radiation of most concern, i.e., that of large energetic particles, such as high-energy protons and neutrons emitted in solar flares. More work in this area would be valuable.

Biochips must maintain geometric stability over their lifetime in space. Polymer chips are easy to manufacture, but are softer than silicon and glass, and may be more vulnerable in this regard. Cleaning and maintenance functions also impact this aspect of chip lifetime, particularly if disassembly is involved (Xie et al., 2005). Another concern is the degradation of seals, coatings, and sensing components, such as electrodes. Shelf life is certainly an issue for microscale electrodes (Shen et al., 2007; Zhang et al., 2007). Degradation could also affect overall containment in addition to sensing performance, and it could introduce fouling contaminants into the microfluidic network. The latter is of most concern when the contaminant is introduced downstream of filtration. One solution is to use techniques that isolate degradable sensors like electrodes from contact with fluids in the device (Nikitin et al., 2005).

Operational lifetime will be a function of the underlying (bio)chemistry, the biochip design, and the environment in which the sensor operates. In the literature on biochips, operational lifetime is occasionally reported, particularly for reusable immunoassays with expensive antigens or other biological recognition elements, since binding kinetics can degrade with cycling. Some studies report adequate function with some reusability (Chen et al., 2003; Yuan et al., 2007), depending on storage conditions. In spaceflight, devices must be stable for several years with hundreds to thousands of uses.

2.4 Gravitational independence

Mars exploration requirements prompted the development of biochip-based solutions for detection of organic acids using capillary electrophoresis (Skelley et al., 2005), which integrated power, pneumatic control and optics. Some microdiagnostics for biology have been tested in specially outfitted aircraft in parabolic flight campaigns. In this reduced gravity environment, a sequence of roughly 40 parabolic trajectories are traversed. At the peak of each parabola, 20-25 seconds of microgravity can be attained. Such testing provides insight into behavior on the Space Station, in which the net quasisteady acceleration is typically on the order of a few μg (where 1 μg=1x10-6g), although there can be much larger vibrational and transient disturbances (Nelson, 1994). Microfluidic devices that have undergone parabolic flight testing include electrophoretic separation of amino acids in an aqueous environment (Culbertson et al., 2005), an immunoabsorbent assay (Maule et al., 2003), and more recently, a blood analyzer on a reusable microfluidic platform (Chan et al., 2011).

We should not expect large variations in biochemistry (e.g., the biokinetic constants that describe binding processes) over short periods in reduced g. However, we should anticipate altered heat and mass transport due to differences in fluid behavior. Gravity and other accelerations act on density differences to drive processes such as sedimentation, bubble migration and natural (buoyancy-driven) convection. As we decrease the size of fluidic channels, we create a system with an increased surface-to-volume ratio, which in turn changes the relative importance of the forces that drive fluid transport. Macroscale systems, such as separation of plasma from whole blood through centrifugation, are governed by volumetric forces such as gravity and centrifugal acceleration acting through density variation to produce the separation. In microfluidics, surface forces, such as friction and surface tension, become more important. Nevertheless, we must also consider the altered competition of intermolecular forces leading to observed binding kinetics between neighboring surfaces and the bulk liquids in microfluidics devices. Both molecular orientation changes and direct molecular attraction/repulsion through surface coatings could potentially influence overall assay results if bulk transport is affected in microgravity.

In microgravity, particles are less likely to sediment in any static system, but bubble management can become more challenging. Processes that require large liquid/vapor interfaces to generate bulk flows in liquid will operate in an even less intuitive manner in microgravity. In space, surface-tension forces dominate liquid/vapor interface behavior without the application of other forces, creating blobs of liquid in unconfined space, or fully wetted surfaces with an interior bubble in enclosures. To be prudent, processes that can create bubbles must be analyzed for microgravity operation before use in space. In some cases, bubble generation is fundamental to the technique (Satoh et al., 2007; Furdui et al., 2003) and in other cases, bubbles can be an unintended consequence, e.g., of hydrolysis (Lancaster et al., 2005). Metabolic processes or biochemical reactions can create dissolved gases. Temperature and/or pressure variation can thermodynamically drive dissolved gases out of solution. Over time, liquid evaporation and gas diffusion through seals or porous materials can cause gaseous pockets to form in a liquid-filled device. Wherever there is a discontinuity in the fluid path, the potential for bubble generation exists. The location at which the sample meets the microfluidic device is one such juncture.

These considerations are of interest because bubbles can effectively clog the pathways of a microfluidic device and/or interfere with the detection process. The consequences are more serious for a device in space because bubbles are less inclined to migrate to specific locations, such as the top of the device, for easy removal. One strategy is to prime the biochip system on earth so that all bubbles are removed before leaving for space. For short-term usage in carefully designed systems, this may provide adequate bubble control, but for long-duration flight, it is probably insufficient. Application of a large pressure gradient is a brute-force method to clear the fluidic channels of bubbles. As the channel dimensions decrease in size, the pressure gradients needed to drive bubbles out of the device increases, particularly for microfluidic channels with torturous geometry. A recent parabolic flight experiment demonstrated that a net pressure difference of about 10 kPa was sufficient to clear even large bubbles of air through channels with a cross-section of 200x120 μm^2 (Chan et al., 2011), although this device was intentionally designed to avoid channel features that could become bubble traps. Wetting properties in microchannels can be affected by surfactants, which can reduce the resistance to flow caused by bubbles (Fuerstman et al., 2007). Another strategy is to propel bubbles out of the system through the use of gradients in wetting properties of the walls, created through active control of an electrical field (§3.2.1). For our purposes, unless a device employs electrowetting for other purposes, it is not worth including it if application of pressure is adequate.

While the density ratio of most vapors to aqueous solutions is on the order of 1000:1, the density variation between typical biological liquids and particles is just a few percent, so the effect of gravity is less significant than for bubbly liquids. However, even at the scale of 10-100 μm, buoyancy and drag can affect particle behavior in electromagnetic sorting (Furlani, 2007) and microvortex cell trapping (Hsu et al., 2008), indicating that microgravity sensitivity should be examined during the design of biodiagnostics.

3. Hardware design

This section focuses on chip design, flow actuation, separation, mixing, and transport to the detection stage for space applications. To operate in the real world, devices must respond to the properties of real samples, so we begin with a discussion of sample properties.

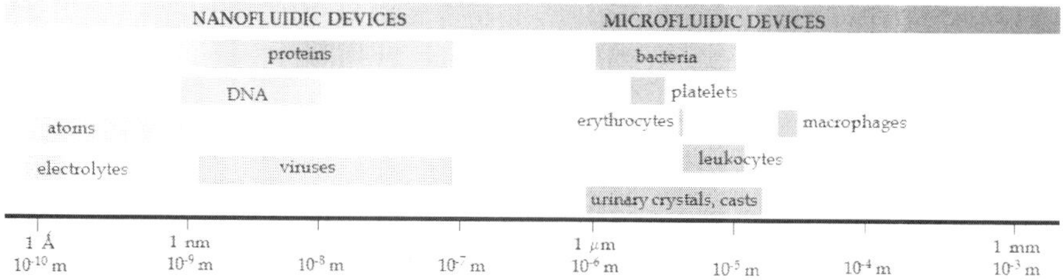

Fig. 1. Length scales of components commonly found in blood and urine samples.

3.1 Sample characteristics

Blood is a mixture of ~55% plasma by volume with ~45% solids content, comprised of red blood cells (erythrocytes), white blood cells (leukocytes) and platelets (thrombocytes, which are the least dense type of cell). The number density of leukocytes is typically 100-800 times less than that of erythrocytes. These cells form the raw material for measurement of hematocrit (volumetric fraction of erythrocytes in blood), counts of erythrocytes, leukocytes, platelets and hemoglobin content. Leukocytes are further distinguished into

	Shape	size (μm)	deform-ability	density (kg/m³)	count (number/μL)	suscepti-bility (SI)
erythrocytes	biconcave, discoid	diameter ~8.5 thickness ~2.3	high	1100	3.5-5.5x10^6	-9.22x10^{-6} * -3.9x10^{-6} **
leukocytes	Spherical	diameter ~6-15	low	1070	3.5-11x10^3	-9.2x10^{-6}
platelets	platelike or irregular	1-3	high	lower	1.5-4.5x10^5	

Table 1. Properties of blood cells. Data from (Furlani, 2007) and (Wikipedia, 2011). *deoxygenated, **oxygenated

five basic subtypes. The number density of these white blood cell subtypes vary widely in the blood, as do their size and structure. The least populous subtype, basophils, are found in concentrations of 40-900 cells/μL (Wikipedia, 2011), so that the required sample volume may be larger than a single drop of blood to derive meaningful statistics. More detailed subtyping on rarer white blood cells can provide even more specific diagnostic information, such as the presence of particular cancers or other pathologies. There is much diagnostic value in such information, so significant effort is placed on separating white blood cells and specific subtypes from whole blood. Fortunately, blood cells differ significantly in size, shape, deformability and electrical properties, as shown in Table 1 for healthy adults. As a rheological fluid, the viscosity of whole blood is a function of shear rate and other environmental factors. Its viscoelastic behavior derives primarily from erythrocyte deformability. Blood viscosity is also dependent on its composition and can be correlated to hematocrit and fibrinogen content. Depending on shear rate, the mean whole blood viscosity in healthy people varied from 3.2 to 5.5 mPa·s in one study. With blood cells removed, plasma viscosity decreased to 1.4 mPa·s (Rosenson et al., 1996). As with whole blood, plasma viscosity can be correlated to composition, specifically to fibrinogen, total serum protein and triglycerides (Rosenson et al., 1996). Plasma is primarily composed of water, but also contains essential salts; ionic species such as calcium, sodium, potassium and bicarbonate; and larger molecules such as amino acids, lipids, and hormones and other proteins. Serum is produced from blood plasma by adding anticoagulant, such as ethylenediaminetetraacetic acid (EDTA). Serum is desirable for most assays, with some exceptions such as clotting assays (Hansson et al., 1999).

Platelets are normally platelike in shape, but when activated, they become rounder and long filaments protrude from their surface (Fig. 2(b)). In this state, platelets readily clump together, or aggregate, forming connections via two key proteins, fibrinogen and von Willebrand Factor (vWF). The latter is contained in endothelial cells of blood vessel linings as well as in granules inside platelets. The combination of shear stress and vWF are key players in platelet activation. Shankaran and co-workers identified two stages: one in which the presence of high fluid shear and vWF sensitize the platelet to shear. At later times, platelets can become activated at much lower shear stresses and without the presence of vWF (Shankaran et al., 2003). The process is only weakly dependent on local platelet concentration, indicating that it is fluid shear acting on individual cells, and not cell collisions, that govern the process. Following exposure to a threshold fluid shear stress

τ= 75 dynes/cm^2, they found that a suspension of isolated platelets with viscosity μ=1.1 mPa·s was significantly more likely to become activated (similarly for whole blood at τ=83 dynes/cm^2, μ=3.8 mPa·s). Even a few seconds of exposure can be sufficient to sensitize platelets (Dayananda et al., 2010). The viscosity of the fluid medium is important because it is the shear *stress*, not the shear *rate* reported in many studies, that governs the behavior. (In a homogeneous fluid, shear stress is the shear rate multiplied by viscosity.) Clearly, the microfluidic design must avoid such levels of shear stress. But given the dependence on shear stress history, the sample should avoid wall proximity to limit the potential for adhesion. This is a strong argument for rigorously avoiding fluid separations (recirculating flow cells), which may occur near sharp bends, corners, and steps. It also suggests that sample dilution can be beneficial by lowering fluid viscosity and reducing protein and cell concentration.

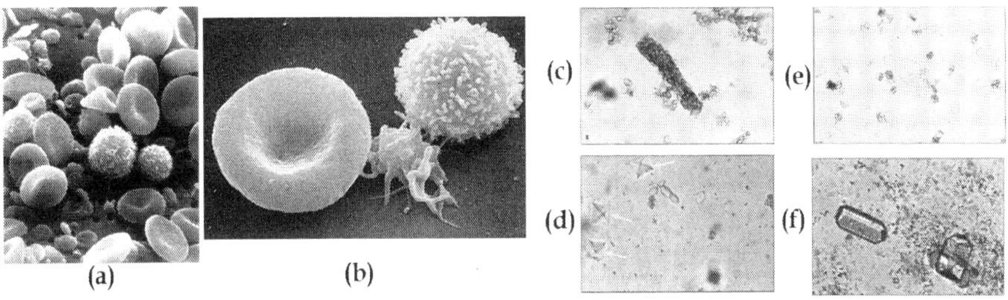

Fig. 2. Solids found in blood and urine samples: (a) blood cells; (b) erythrocyte, activated platelet, and leukocyte; (c) urinary erythrocyte cast; (d) calcium oxalate crystals (arrows) (e) uric acid crystals; (f) triple phosphate crystals with amorphous phosphate.
(a)-(b) reprinted from the National Cancer Institute, Frederick, Md.; (c)-(f) reprinted from the National Institutes of Health Clinical Center Department of Laboratory Medicine, Bethesda, Md.

Urine separation presents a different set of challenges. Although the solids content is far less than blood, the size and other properties of the particulates vary more widely. These can include cells, casts (which include blood and tissue cells that have passed through the renal system, retaining the renal tubule's shape, Fig. 2(c)), proteins, and a wide array of crystals (Fig. 2(d)-(f)). Size, electromagnetic properties, rigidity, and staining propensities are also quite variable. Obtaining well-filtered urine should be straightforward with branching techniques (§3.2.2). Examination of urinary sediment can also yield critical diagnostic information, but it is somewhat more challenging to accommodate in a microfluidic context. Typically, a urine sample of 10-15 mL is centrifuged at ~2000-3000 rpm for five minutes to concentrate the solids content. Pure fluid is withdrawn until ~0.2-0.5 mL remains. A drop of this fluid is then examined under a microscope (Simerville et al., 2005). To examine urinary sediment in the space environment, an effective microfluidic concentrator would be required as well as a means of staining and imaging the concentrated sample.

Saliva is of interest to space biodiagnostics because of its ready availability and marginal invasiveness to the astronaut, particularly since wound healing proceeds more slowly in space (Delp, 2008). Saliva's non-Newtonian viscoelastic behavior is a result of its high mucin concentration, which makes it a challenging fluid for microfluidic applications. In one study, pre-processing the saliva via filtration through a 0.2 μm membrane was found to remove 92% of total proteins and 97% of the mucins, so that treated saliva could be analyzed in a microfluidic sensor (Helton et al., 2008). However, sensor fouling still remained an issue. Another study used a commercially available sorbent within a microdevice as a preparatory stage for microscale capillary electrophoresis to concentrate hydroxyl radicals while removing undesirable saliva components (Marchiarullo et al., 2008). While these pre-processing stages are not compatible with reusability, they may provide an avenue to pre-processing saliva for use in a reusable device.

Other sample types of interest include examination of potable water for toxin and bacterial content, animal fluids and cell cultures, for which the strategies discussed above are applicable. Throughout the rest of this document, the term "analyte" or "target" refers to the component of the sample that is to be analyzed. An "assay" is simply a test performed on a sample to yield information on the desired target.

3.2 Chip design

For a reusable device, the potential for cross-contamination is a major concern. Designs should therefore minimize residence time of the sample near the walls to minimize the opportunity for adsorption. In general, channels of uniform height without sharp bends, steps, expansions or contractions will have less opportunity to form stagnation zones that could increase sample residence time near the walls. A continuous, uniform flow rate also limits the potential for fluid eddies that could bring the sample into contact with the wall. (On the other hand, devices with unavoidable and persistent stagnation zones could benefit from periodic disruption by pulsatile flow (Corbett et al., 2010.)) Unless a competing design presents substantial advantages and minimal compromises in operation and lifetime, this should be the baseline design of a reusable microfluidic device.

In general, passive processes are preferred for space applications in order to reduce power consumption. The most robust system will have no moving parts, simple geometries, and simple flow controls. Meeting this goal may involve relatively simple design tradeoffs in separation and mixing processes (§3.2.2), but it is more difficult for flow actuation (§3.2.1).

From §3.1, it is clear that for reusable microfluidics, it is advantageous to avoid sample contact with walls. Consequently, droplet-based processing will not be included in this discussion. Sheathing, which surrounds a sample by flowing streams of inert liquid such as buffer, is one means of separating the sample from the chamber walls. This strategy is routinely employed in flow focusing (§3.3). If the sheathing fluid does not mix effectively with the sample, one study showed that the sheathing fluid could even be recycled in an automated fashion (Hashemi et al., 2010). Another microfluidic device encapsulated plugs of aqueous analyte in oil to prohibit sample contact with the biochip surface (Urbanski et al., 2006). Oil and water are examples of two fluids that are immiscible, i.e., they do not mix, but instead maintain a sharp interface.

3.2.1 Flow actuation and control

Fluids handling requires effective means of actuating (initiating) flow, priming, pumping, metering, separating, mixing, and flushing. There are many options for initiating fluid motion in microfluidics. Capillary forces are sufficient to draw blood into a glass micropipette. While this technique could be used to introduce blood into the device, it is generally insufficient to pump fluid through a microfluidic device (with some notable exceptions (Martinez et al., 2010).) Mechanically, the simplest way to drive flow is through a hydrodynamic pressure difference, produced by connecting the inlet and exit ports to fluid reservoirs of different heights (Shevkoplyas et al., 2005; Simonnet & Groisman, 2006). A 1-m difference in water column height between two reservoirs translates to an overall pressure drop of 10 kPa, which is sufficient to drive flow in an uncomplicated microdevice. This might also be an option on the lunar and Martian surfaces, after taking into account their reduced gravity to roughly 1/6th and 2/3rd earth gravity, respectively.

Pressure-driven flow can also be actuated with syringe pumps. Although they represent an unacceptable penalty on mass, volume and power resources for space diagnostics, they provide reliable, precise control over the flow rate on earth. A manually operated syringe for driving flow is feasible for space operations, but flow control would be more difficult.

Mechanical micropumps include centrifugal, peristaltic, reciprocating and rotary pumps. Displacement pumps apply forces to move boundaries, which in turn move fluid. One example of this class is peristaltic pumping, in which three or more pumping chambers are squeezed in a deliberate sequence with an actuating membrane. Reciprocating pumps initiate flow in a pressure chamber through actuation of a diaphragm. Rotary pumps move fluids by means of rotating, meshing gears. All of these standard techniques for actuating fluid have counterparts at the microscale, but there are also additional options available. Below we describe some of the more intriguing microfluidic flow actuators that could be suitable for space.

Microfluidic networks built on a rotating disk can operate without internal moving parts, using centrifugal force as the sole means of flow actuation (Madou et al., 2006). Many such systems conform to the size of compact discs and can even be used in a conventional CD drive. The current convention is a disposable "lab-on-a-CD" with single-use membranes acting as valves, but this design could conceivably be made reusable with appropriate valving, extraction and flushing functions. Recent innovations with such devices on larger-scale samples (Amasia & Madou, 2010) could make this technique a design choice worth considering for urinary solids concentration.

Bubbles can be used as a type of displacement pump, since they displace liquid during controlled growth. Hydrolysis can be used to generate bubbles with precision to drive flow in a microfluidic channel (Furdui et al., 2003). Deliberate creation of bubbles within a microfluidic device for space, however, should be considered with caution, since bubble management is not a trivial matter.

Other electrically based methods include electrocapillary or electrowetting micropumps, which use an electrical field to dynamically modify the surface charge, thereby controlling the local surface tension. Surface-tension gradients can be generated in a manner that mimics peristaltic pumping. Electrokinetic pumps use electrophoresis and electroosmosis to drive flow. All can be effective in microdevices, since they can be designed to operate at low power and without moving parts. There are a variety of commercial and research-level micropumps and microvalves based on these principles. These techniques represent a viable alternative to micromechanical actuation, but bubble control, surface stability and gravitational independence must be demonstrated over a long lifetime.

Timing, valve control, and well-controlled mixing over a long lifetime are going to be essential features of a successful device. If tight precision on metering, mixing and splitting is needed, one solution with easy computer interfacing may be found using solenoid actuators that pneumatically control elastomeric valves. One such device reliably manipulated sample volumes down to 5.7 nL (Urbanski et al., 2006).

3.2.2 Microfluidic channel design

The microfluidic network must accept the sample and supporting fluids, perform sample pre-processing such as separation or concentration, provide a means of mixing the sample and reagents or other additives, and transport the fluid to the detection region. For reusable devices, they must also have associated flushing operations performed in them.

Mixing can be achieved passively by introducing texture to walls, placing obstacles in the flow, splitting and recombining fluid streams, or introducing curvature. When two miscible fluid streams are introduced into a single microfluidic channel, the fluids will mix spontaneously via molecular diffusion as they traverse downstream. However, this can require a very long distance because diffusion is a very slow process. Complete mixing over a shorter length can be achieved if additional incentives are introduced, such as convective motion. Convective mixing is added through geometry by channel bending, twisting, and flattening (MacInnes et al., 2007). However, these convoluted flow paths come at the price of increased flow resistance, which imposes increased power requirements (Hsu et al., 2008).

Modification of wall geometry was used to improve immunoassay performance through mixing enhancement (Golden et al., 2007). In this case, antibodies were immobilized at the bottom sensor surface. The target protein was captured from the sample stream as it bound with the antibodies, resulting in a layer of increasingly target-poor solution next to the sensor downstream. By adding grooves at the top of their channel, they promoted mixing over the entire cross-section of the channel. Increased mixing resulted in better delivery of fresh analyte to sensor surface. Other studies have examined in detail the effect of such surface modifications on flow profiles (Howell et al., 2005). Surface patterning can provide effective mixing, but it adds complexity to the fabrication process, and may slightly increase the necessary driving force to move fluid through the system. Most critically for reusable devices, they must be evaluated for fouling potential in the vicinity of the patterning.

Diamond-shaped obstacles force the flow to break up and recombine, providing good mixing at low power over a broad range of flow conditions (Bhagat et al., 2007). The sharp leading edge acts to separate the fluid streams. The design also provides a potential location for a stagnation zone just downstream of the sharp corner at the widest portion of the diamond. In the laminar flows that are typical of microfluidics, such expansions can generate flow separations if the expansion angle exceeds 7° (Panton, 1984). Substituting a slimmer biconvex shape could reduce this proclivity, but it would also reduce the intensity of mixing. The mixing becomes less vigorous by decreasing the span of the obstruction and hence the amount of fluid lateral motion. By eliminating the separated zone next to the obstacle, we have limited the region of increased mixing to strictly downstream of the obstruction. This option increases geometric complexity only slightly, although it introduces new walls into the system. For reusable systems, the fouling potential must be evaluated on the surfaces of the obstruction and weighed against gains in mixing efficiency.

Another technique for passive mixing without tortuosity, splitting, obstructions or surface roughness is through the introduction of curved channels. As fluid rounds the bend, centrifugal forces drive Dean flow, evidenced in secondary flow structures in the form of two counter-rotating vortical structures along the flow direction that span the channel cross-section. Frictional drag on a given particle is proportional to its effective radius in the flow direction and the net acceleration acting on the particle. Through this mechanism, the mere presence of the curved channel can serve to drive size-based particle separation (Di Carlo, 2009). Any relative motion between the particle and its carrier fluid should also serve to provide additional fluid mixing. This design is attractive for reusability because it enhances mixing without requiring geometric features that introduce fouling potential. In a recent example, a spiral architecture was a core design principle of a reusable blood analyzer prototype for space (Chan et al., 2011).

Electrokinetics-based techniques in mixing (Chang et al., 2007) generally require more attention to lifetime for space applications, since their function is dependent on surface properties and treatments, which can degrade over time (Mukhopadhyay, 2005). Valve functions can be lost due to contamination during usage, although surface geometry can be an aid in this regard (Nashida et al., 2007). Finally, these techniques may not have the same level of control as micromechanical metering (Urbanski et al., 2006).

Careful filtration reduces the likelihood of introducing fouling contaminants to the system, which minimizes clogging and simplifies post-test cleaning. Filtration may be necessary at multiple length scales in sequential stages, based on the constituents in the sample and the assay under consideration. By removing unnecessary components from the sample, it can have the added benefit of improving the signal-to-noise ratio due to nonspecific response in the detection stage. On the other hand, filtration could also remove large molecules, such as some proteins, that may be the target of a particular assay.

Filtration techniques range from brute-force mechanical trapping to elegant biomimetic capture. For filtration in reusable devices, continuously flowing techniques are preferred to mechanical trapping. All separations exploit variations in size, density, deformability, biokinetic and electromagnetic properties among the blood components. In the systems in Fig. 3, blood cells are preferentially directed into specific channels, but are not trapped nor are they subjected to vigorous mechanical forces that could cause cell lysis, or rupture.

Plasmapheresis is the process by which plasma is separated from whole blood. Fig. 3(a) demonstrates the utility of simple bifurcations to extract pure plasma (Yang et al., 2006). Processing time could be reduced by adding pulsatile flow (Devarakonda et al., 2007), but the increased complexity and fouling potential may be of concern for space diagnostics. Another design option is to send the entire fluid stream through a constriction followed by an expansion. In this case, a cell-free layer develops next to the downstream walls, the extent of which is a function of the length and width of the constriction, as well as the flow rate (Faivre et al., 2006). Gentle contraction and expansion flows may serve to further segregate the cells from the walls while providing a plasma-rich region nearer to the wall close to the branch points.

Prototypes for separation often use inorganic analogs for blood cells as a starting point. Although a reasonable analog for leukocytes can be found in appropriately sized and weighted rigid spheres, erythrocytes are neither spherical nor rigid. Studies that carefully design geometries and flow rates to separate out differently sized spherical particles are likely to miss the mark when extrapolating to real-life blood cell separation. Dense suspensions of rigid particles in flowing fluid tend to have a high concentration of the smallest particles immediately adjacent to the boundaries. However, hydrodynamic forces acting on deformable, biconcave erythrocytes drive them to the fastest-moving region of flow, although they are smaller than leukocytes. Consequently, in bifurcating flow (Fig. 3(b)), erythrocytes preferentially choose the higher velocity bifurcation (Yang et al., 2006).

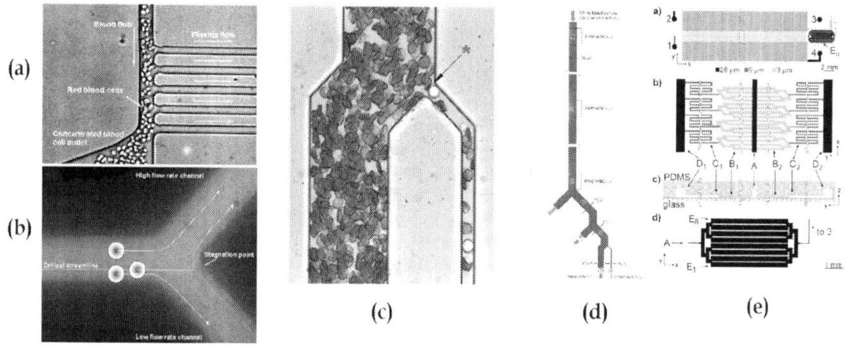

Fig. 3. Continuous flow separation techniques: (a) plasmapheresis through branching channels, (b) erythrocytes exhibit a preference for the faster moving stream, (c) detail of branching technique for leukocyte enrichment from whole blood using the network of (d) leukopheresis geometry for 34x enrichment; (e) leukopheresis geometry for 4000x enrichment. (a)-(b) reproduced with permission from **(Yang et al., 2006)**, copyright 2006, The Royal Society of Chemistry; (c)-(d) reproduced with permission from **(Shevkoplyas et al., 2005)**, copyright 2005, American Chemical Society; (e) reproduced with permission from **(VanDelinder & Groisman, 2007)**, copyright 2007, American Chemical Society.

Blood flow exhibits Poisseuille (parabolic) velocity profiles in microchannels. Erythrocytes favor the faster-moving flow at the center of the channel rather than the slower-moving fluid near the walls. As these cells migrate to the center of the channel, cell/cell collisions tend to drive leukocytes toward the channel walls. The design in Figs. 3(c) and (d) ensured that all of the collisional energy among blood cells was dedicated to driving leukocytes to the walls, providing efficient locations for siphoning off cells (Shevkoplyas et al., 2005). This clever biomimetic technique operated effectively without sample dilution and with simple process control for minimal resource consumption. The lack of dilution and the reliance on collisions may impact fouling potential, however.

Excellent performance in leukocyte separation from whole blood was demonstrated in the device in Fig. 3(e), without fouling over an hour in continuous use (VanDelinder et al., 2007). In a single pass, the ratio of white to red blood cells at the outlet showed a 4000-fold increase. The simpler design shown in Fig. 3(d) showed more modest leukocyte enrichment of 34 times (Shevkoplyas et al., 2005). However, both designs beat "buffy coat" preparation produced by single-spin centrifugation, which provides 10-20 times enrichment. The geometrically complex design of Fig. 3(e) features channels of varying height which intersect at right angles, and requires flow control. Contrast this to Fig. 3(d) which exhibits uniform height, minimal branching at gentle angles, and is driven by a single pressure drop over the entire system. Either design provides adequate enrichment for simple leukocyte differentiation. Space biodiagnostics favors devices that provide adequate function with minimal resources and simple geometries.

Another common method of enrichment uses an array of micropillars strategically placed in the channel (Chang et al., 2005). The physical obstructions preferentially slow down leukocytes without stopping them completely, thus providing enrichment. Many other separation techniques also rely on hydrodynamic principles to separate cells from blood. Electrokinetic, electroosmotic, dielectrophoretic and magnetic forces can also be used for active separation, discussed in depth elsewhere (Lenshof et al., 2010; Salieb-Beugelaar et al., 2010).

3.2.3 Materials choices and fouling considerations

Most prototype biochips are created from materials that are easy and inexpensive to manufacture, particularly polydimethylsiloxane (PDMS). However, such polymers readily absorb small molecules that can interfere with fluorescence measurements (Toepke & Beebe, 2006) as well as nonspecific proteins (Mukhopadhyay, 2005). To mitigate this unfortunate property, surface treatments such as plasma exposure can be used to create a hydrophilic surface. This treatment also improves surface bonding. A great deal of effort is devoted to design of low-fouling surface coatings, but they may not survive in microdevices requiring use over a long lifetime (Balagadde et al., 2005; Mukhopadhyay, 2005). In addition, the non-negligible permeability of polymers to gases imposes the need for good strategies for fluids priming, flushing and bubble control, since liquids within a polymer device will evaporate over time.

More promising materials include silicon and glass, which are less surface-active and less permeable to gases. They maintain integrity over a longer lifetime, and geometric details can be more tightly controlled, especially with silicon. They are, however, more expensive to manufacture (Han et al., 2003). In order to use a glass biochip safely on the Space Station, it must have containment that filters particulates down to 50 μm (International Space Station, 2002). Silicon presents some unusual design possibilities by providing bounding walls that can be dynamically charged to change wetting and adsorption properties. In one design, which also included a low-fouling polymer layer, a controlled electrostatic attraction pulled proteins from solution onto the wall reversibly (Cole et al., 2007). This technique could potentially be used to concentrate urinary protein for detection, filtration, or flushing (with the usual caveats for addressing lifetime and cross-contamination issues).

Regardless of materials choice, it is beneficial to minimize contact between the sample and the wall or sensor to reduce the potential for fouling. To avoid wall interaction entirely, one strategy is to encapsulate the aqueous sample in an immiscible fluid (Urbanski et al., 2006). Aside from fabrication challenges and gas permeability, another concern is the degradation of biochip components, such as electrodes (Chen et al., 2003; Shen & Liu, 2007; Shen et al., 2007; Zhang et al., 2007), which may interfere with detection performance, release contaminants into the device, or affect containment. In some cases, electronics can be placed outside of the channel to prohibit contact between the sample and the sensor (Nikitin et al., 2005). Processes that employ electrical or magnetic fields to drive, mix or separate fluid streams can also be designed to avoid contact of the control elements with the sample.

Materials choices, surface treatments and coatings, the type of reagents and samples can all influence device lifetime and performance. Silicon and glass are good working materials for producing a long-lived, reusable microfluidic device. Polymers are less suitable candidates for space diagnostics due to higher gas permeability, greater potential for fouling, and reduced geometric integrity. Electrodes and other biochip components must not degrade over a lifetime of several years and hundreds to thousands of uses.

3.3 Detection strategies

The primary functions of biodetection are to count particles, detect and/or quantify concentrations of dissolved compounds and visualize particulates. Detection techniques can be based on direct sensing or may require an intermediate step for labeling, binding, or chemical reaction. To minimize reagent usage, reduce sample residence time and fouling potential, reusable design has a strong bias towards detection schemes requiring short incubation periods, fast reaction kinetics, and short detection times.

Since there are many comprehensive reviews cited in §1 and elsewhere that cover the field in great depth, we will focus on optifluorescent detection, which provides great versatility in designing assays using a single detection modality, for both cell counting and massively multiplexed biomarker detection. The popularity of this technique has prompted development of multi-channel laser systems, which increase the multiplexing potential. The capability to differentiate many targets simultaneously is enhanced by recent developments in assay development, discussed in §4.2.

An impressive differentiation of all 5 leukocyte subtypes was recently achieved by Tai and co-workers (Shi et al., 2011). Their approach is based on strategic choice of three fluorescent dyes which stain proteins, nucleic acids, and cytoplasm contents. The resultant fluorescent signatures are sufficient for a two-channel laser detection system to discriminate among all the cell types. This approach was tested on 5μL human blood samples, spiked with purified basophils due to their rarity in whole blood. The differences in the cell's internal structures cause the uptake of the dyes to be proportionally different for each cell type. A scatter plot of red vs. green fluorescence intensity produces 5 distinct regions, which correlate to the 5 cell types. Data points in each cluster are counted to enumerate the number of cells in each category. The resulting measurement agreed well with a commercial assay system in terms of cell subtype percentages as well as overall leukocyte count. In operation, the blood sample will be acquired through a needle integrated with a disposable cartridge, which interfaces with their portable microcytometer. They deliberately designed the system to avoid the need for diluents, which keeps the chip size small. By encapsulating the sample within the chip, the biohazardous waste from sample acquisition and processing is contained and the possibility for cross-contamination minimized or eliminated.

In some cases, visual examination of microstructural detail can add enormous insight into the physical, biological and physiological processes of interest. The International Space Station hosts the Light Microscopy Module, which can perform high-resolution color video microscopy, brightfield, darkfield, phase contrast, differential interference contrast, spectrophotometry, and confocal microscopy. Options include custom-designed laser tweezers for sample manipulation and remote control from earth at NASA Glenn Research Center. Experiments using the device began in March 2011 as this is being written. No results are yet available, but human blood will be one of the early samples examined. These capabilities bring the power of a state-of-the-art terrestrial imaging facility to the Space Station, continuing NASA's shift in focus from ground-based analysis of space-exposed samples to *in situ* analysis in microgravity.

To facilitate ease of use and expand capabilities for bioanalysis, Todd and co-workers are developing an observation platform to interface with the Light Microscopy Module, which adds a substage illuminator and epi-illumination (Todd, 2009). Onboard controllers and actuators can be used to exchange fluids between two small chambers on the platform to initiate a process, fix biological samples or retrieve suspended cells. This device could be used for cell counting and detailed visual examination of cell and plant cultures, animals and human blood, urine, and water samples.

4. Operational design

To function effectively in a space habitat as a general-purpose laboratory, a reusable microfluidics-based biodiagnostic must include strategies for sample acquisition (§4.1), incorporation of new assays (§4.2), and effective flushing/cleaning operations (§4.3).

4.1 Sample acquisition and transport to the microfluidic device

As with any biological diagnostics, protocols for sample acquisition must be established to ensure reliable, repeatable measurements, including skin cleansing to remove potential contaminants as well as efficient, non-contaminating sample acquisition and transport to the microfluidic channels of the biochip. To reduce invasiveness to the astronaut, acquisition of capillary blood is preferred to a venous blood draw. Resource-conscious fingerprick devices for space are under development (Chan, 2009). Biohazardous waste from sharp needles can be reduced through the use of microneedles, which are also better at reducing invasiveness and pain. But they require a means of transporting the sample to the chip in a sterile, bio-contained fashion. For our purposes, the flow driver for sample transport could be integrated into either the lancet/needle side or the device side of the system, depending on which design is most compact or practical. Actuation drivers can be placed on the biodiagnostic device, acquisition device, or both, to supplement capillary forces in bringing the sample onto the biochip. Since there is a discontinuity in the fluid path at the junction of the sample transport device and the chip, acquisition is a key element in device design for bubble-free operation.

Acquisition and transport of a urine sample in space can be a messy procedure. From the standpoint of reusables, the best option would be integration of sample collection with the urine collection system on the spacecraft. Since urine has a much lower solids content than blood, acquisition of a well-filtered fluid sample should be simpler than for blood. Examination of urinary sediment would require a means of concentration. Branching techniques as used for plasmapheresis in §3.2.2 could be considered. More efficient concentration could be achieved with micro- (or milli-) centrifugation (Amasia et al., 2010).

Following sample acquisition, any nondisposable components will require cleaning to return it to a clean state. It may be impractical to clean some components, particularly those at the smallest scale. In this case, the next best goal is to minimize the disposable part of the system.

4.2 Assay design

Assay development is going to be one of the limiting factors in realizing the full capabilities of a massively multiplexed biodiagnostic device. Techniques that require no additional staining, labeling or binding agents are particularly attractive for space use, but a general-purpose system will not be able to avoid the use of additives. For example, opportunities to exploit autofluorescence are only available for a few targets. The biokinetics of some immunoassays are reversible in principle, but performance degrades after a number of binding and unbinding cycles, although gains have been recently made (Choi & Chae, 2009). The least attractive option for space diagnostics is to introduce single-use reagents into the system, but it is unavoidable considering the need for a reasonable range on the assay suite.

The sensitivity and specificity of a given assay will be a function of (bio)chemistry, sensing modality, design and calibration standards, and the fluid matrix in which the target is embedded (Vesper et al., 2005a; Vesper et al., 2005b), as well as the fabrication process. In designing a system that can be used for blood, urine and other sample types, some system efficiencies can be realized through the existence of common assays. For example, measurement of glucose is specified in the crew health requirements for both urine and blood. Moreover, from a medical standpoint, diagnostic value may be improved when both serum and urine data are available, e.g., for osmolality (Pagana & Pagana, 2005).

When reagents are needed, wet chemistry is the most widely used approach for blood analyzers. Stability can be improved by reconstituting dried reagents at runtime (Chen et al., 2005), microencapsulation techniques (Sahney et al., 2006), and stabilizers, particularly in the case of immunoassays (Guire, 1999; Park et al., 2003). Dry chemistry is likely to have the best payoff in the stability of biological recognition elements, such as antibodies. This is the approach taken in urinalysis test strips, e.g., Chemstrips, that have a shelf life of one year after opening the package. Reconstitution of soluble reagents or tethered molecules at runtime is unlikely to present any microgravity-related issues.

Aptamers are bioengineered molecules, usually based on nucleic acids, which may have similar binding affinity to the more conventional antibody. These biorecognition elements may be more stable than antibodies, and have great potential for assay design through the ability to place chemical agents at highly specific binding sites (Cho et al., 2009). Work is progressing rapidly in this area, in part through the support of NASA (Yang, 2008), but these reagents are much less broadly available than antibodies.

Magnetic beads are functionalized by immobilizing antibodies or other biorecognition elements on the bead surface. When exposed to the target, there is a strong affinity for binding. This technique can be used to separate components from the bulk fluid efficiently. These processes can be exquisitely sensitive and are well-suited to sorting rare cell types; and they are discussed comprehensively elsewhere (Furdui & Harrison, 2004; Pamme, 2006). With beads as a reagent carrier, the microfluidic system becomes much more adaptable and resource-conscious. The same microfluidic channels can be re-used, and the set of micron-scale beads introduced at runtime determine which assays are performed. The ability to discriminate among assay signals at the detection stage then becomes the chief bottleneck. At this time, 8-color fluorescence systems have become available commercially, which expands capacity greatly if appropriately fluorescing compounds can be matched to targets. Recent work moves towards expanding the number of fluorescing sensing stations on each magnetic bead, which can also increase capacity (Chan, 2009; Hu et al., 2011). Unfortunately, much of the current work is geared to genomics and proteomics.

Nanostrips are ingenious new reagents that are conceptually similar to the standard urinalysis test strip, but the strip is shrunk a billion-fold down to the micron scale (Chan, 2010). As with urinalysis test strips, each nanostrip can have multiple sensor locations, each of which responds to a different target. The embedded reagents may be antibodies or aptamers tagged to fluorescent molecules that are designed for protein detection, or fluorescent dyes that react with other targets in the sample, such as electrolytes. These small, rectangular nanostrips are similar in size to blood cells, simplifying detection and analysis protocols. A dual-channel laser system measures the fluorescence signatures of both nanostrips and blood cells. For the nanostrips, one channel is dedicated to identifying the strip, so that the system can determine which set of targets is being measured. Essentially, the concentration of dye on each sensor pad creates a bar code for identifying the strip type. The other channel is used for the actual measurement. Quantitative measurements are obtained through analysis of fluorescence intensity at each sensor location. Since the identification channel can easily discriminate many levels of fluorescence intensity to add further differentiation, a set of 5-part nanostrips could theoretically measure thousands of targets from a single sample. At present, nanostrips of up to 7 parts have been fabricated. As with the other systems discussed, a major bottleneck is assay development. Some effort in nanostrip delivery and data analysis techniques will also be needed. But the beauty of this approach is that another limiting factor may become the user's ability to take advantage of nanostrip capacity.

4.3 Flushing and cleaning protocols

The first step in developing flushing protocols is to define what constitutes an adequately clean device. Sterility is a very high standard, especially in an environment like the Space Station without access to an autoclave or common sterilizers, such as bleach or glutaraldehyde. But sterilization between each blood sample is probably unnecessary. High-throughput systems for blood analysis, such as the Shenzhen Mindray Bio-Medical Electronics Co. BC-2800, can run continuously for several days before its tubing and other components must undergo even a routine cleaning with an enzymatic detergent. However, there are few commercial examples of a reusable portable device for guidance in developing cleaning protocols. The simplest strategy for cleaning a microdevice is to flush the system with saline. To assess effectiveness, quantitative measures can be used for comparison, such as fluorescence or color, against pre-test levels (Balagadde et al., 2005) or to some specified reduction, such as 10^{-6} times the reference signal (Verjat et al., 1999).

For a reusable multipurpose analyzer, we must also think in terms of the assays we require the device to handle, the sample components that could be fouling agents, and estimated concentration levels for the sample. The presence of some nonspecifically adsorbed protein X on the wall may not matter much if we are counting cells. We are neither measuring protein X, nor is the attachment or detachment of protein X from the wall likely to interfere significantly with the cell counting. It could compromise the measurement entirely if the target of interest is protein X or if the target is a rare protein Y, which adsorbs to the wall, or displaces protein X, or protein X desorbs independently and has the unfortunate ability to add noise to the measurement of protein Y. In other words, the standards for cleaning the device must be more exacting for measurement of a rare protein than for, say, albumin, which is the most common protein in blood.

Recently, the subject of reusability in biomicrofluidics has received more attention in the literature. Microfluidic devices have begun to report reusability, with applications from the culturing of human lung carcinoma cells with a few re-uses (Jedrych et al., 2010) to the detection of pathogens in livestock with up to 75 assays (Kwon et al., 2010). Self-assembled monolayers can be deposited on the channel wall as capture agents for proteins. Although the binding of proteins to these monolayers is reversible, the degradation of performance with multiple binding/unbinding events has been substantial. Recent efforts in this area have reported that the use of densely packed, short-chain monolayers in conjunction with controlled surface roughness can increase device lifetime to 50 uses (Choi & Chae, 2009). Another fascinating development has been in the area of Surface Acoustic Wave devices, in which an acoustic wave propagates along a solid/liquid interface for detection of binding events. In a device that was designed to produce a wave with a substantial surface-normal component, the force resulting from the surface oscillation was sufficient to remove non-specifically bound proteins from the surface. Also, the steady streaming motion in the fluid driven by the oscillating boundary prevented reattachment (Sankaranarayanan et al., 2010). Another recent work describes the use of nanomechanical resonant sensors in reusable microfluidic channels for the simultaneous detection of interleukin-8 and vascular endothelial growth factor in serum (Waggoner et al., 2010). Continuing efforts in promoting reusability are yielding insights, but much work remains to be done in this area.

Finally, the cleanliness requirements may also vary depending on the end user. Diagnostic data used to treat an individual for a medical condition may require higher standards than biological or biomedical research. All of these areas are ripe for further exploration.

5. Conclusions

In this work, we have explored the principles that can guide the design of a reusable biomedical device for space. The requirements that drive development for space demand far more attention to resource-conscious operation than a similar system designed for earth. However, the efficiencies provided by these considerations can also be of benefit to terrestrial devices by driving down costs and opening up new applications through reduced resource consumption, improved ruggedness, breadth of capability and enhanced adaptability. Some of the essential features for reusability are:

- Continuous flow through the device to minimize sample residence time
- Simple geometries without sharp bends, steps or expansions that could create separation zones or act as bubble traps
- Minimization of sample contact with the wall through low-fouling surfaces and coatings, sample encapsulation, and dilution to reduce sample concentration.

Operation in the extreme environment of space leads to additional design considerations:

- Dry chemistry offers substantial advantages to meet the extended reagent shelf life needed for Exploration class missions
- Bubble control and solids behavior may be different in a reduced gravity environment relative to earth and must be assessed for any spacebound device
- The load on mission resources can be reduced by minimizing the mass, volume, power, and consumables of the system through hardware miniaturization, using shared resources, dynamic reconfiguration capabilities, and the flexibility to accommodate a range of assays on an array of sample types.

Reusable devices are coming closer to maturity for some areas of biological and biomedical research, but there are few examples that are targeted towards a fully integrated blood and urine analyzer for routine medical diagnostics, as well as for a wide range of biomedical research needs. Nevertheless, the basic technology for such a device exists right now. The primary stumbling blocks are integration of sample processing and onboard detection in a single device, the capacity for massive multiplexing and the availability of a broad assay suite. Optifluorescent detection methods are well-suited to reusable design and can accommodate a wide range of assays. Nanostrips can provide massive multiplexing while maintaining a simple, reusable geometry. These approaches hold genuine promise for reaching the much sought-after Holy Grail for portable biodiagnostics: a self-contained, robust, general-purpose assay system for analysis of bodily or environmental fluids.

6. Acknowledgements

The funding for this work was provided by the Human Research Program at NASA Johnson Space Center. Their support is gratefully acknowledged.

7. References

Akopova, A. B., Manaseryan, M. M., Melkonyan, A. A., Tatikyan, S. S., & Potapov, Y. (2005). Radiation measurement on the International Space Station. *Radiation Measurements*, Vol.39, No.2, pp. 225-228.

Amasia, M. & Madou, M. (2010). Large-volume centrifugal microfluidic device for blood plasma separation. *Bioanalysis*, Vol.2, No.10, pp. 1701-1710.

Arora, A., Simone, G., Salieb-Beugelaar, G. B., Kim, J. T., & Manz, A. (2010). Latest developments in micro Total Analysis Systems. *Analytical Chemistry*, Vol.82, No.12, pp. 4830-4847.

Balagadde, F. K., You, L. C., Hansen, C. L., Arnold, F. H., & Quake, S. R. (2005). Long-term monitoring of bacteria undergoing programmed population control in a microchemostat. *Science*, Vol.309, No.5731, pp. 137-140.

Bhagat, A. A. S., Bow, H., Hou, H. W., Tan, S. J., Han, J., & Lim, C. T. (2010). Microfluidics for cell separation. *Medical & Biological Engineering & Computing*, Vol.48, No.10, pp. 999-1014.

Bhagat, A. A. S., Peterson, E. T. K., & Papautsky, I. (2007). A passive planar micromixer with obstructions for mixing at low Reynolds numbers. *Journal of Micromechanics and Microengineering*, Vol.17, No.5, pp. 1017-1024.

Blaber, E., Marcal, H., & Burns, B. P. (2010). Bioastronautics: The influence of microgravity on astronaut health. *Astrobiology*, Vol.10, No.5, pp. 463-473.

Chan, C. P. Y. (2009). Ingenious nanoprobes in bioassays. *Bioanalysis*, Vol.1, No.1, pp. 115-133.

Chan, E. (2009). Reusable Handheld Electrolytes & Lab Technology For Humans: rHEALTH Sensor. NASA SBIR NNX09CA44C.

Chan, E. (2010). Nanoscale test strips for multiplexed blood analysis. NASA SBIR NNX10CA97C. The DNA Medicine Institute, Boston, MA.

Chan, E. Y., Bae, C., Phipps, W., Bishara, A., McKay, T. L., Weaver, A., Zimmerman, J., & Nelson, E. S. (2011). Performance of the rHEALTH biomedical sensor on reduced gravity parabolic flights. *18th International Academy of Astronautics Humans in Space Symposium*. April 11-15, 2011. Houston, TX.

Chang, W. C., Lee, L. P., & Liepmann, D. (2005). Biomimetic technique for adhesion-based collection and separation of cells in a microfluidic channel. *Lab on A Chip*, Vol.5, pp. 64-73.

Chang, C. C. & Yang, R. J. (2007). Electrokinetic mixing in microfluidic systems. *Microfluidics and Nanofluidics*, Vol.3, No.5, pp. 501-525.

Chen, G., Bao, H. M., & Yang, P. Y. (2005). Fabrication and performance of a three-dimensionally adjustable device for the amperometric detection of microchip capillary electrophoresis. *Electrophoresis*, Vol.26, No.24, pp. 4632-4640.

Chen, H. M., Lin, M. L., & Chen, S. H. (2003). Fabrication of piezoelectric biochips with self-assembled alkanethiol layer and hydrocoating. *Journal of the Chinese Institute of Chemical Engineers*, Vol.34, No.1, pp. 151-160.

Cho, E. J., Lee, J. W., & Ellington, A. D. (2009). Applications of aptamers as sensors. *Annual Review of Analytical Chemistry*, Vol.2, pp. 241-264.

Cho, S. H., Godin, J. M., Chen, C. H., Qiao, W., Lee, H., & Lo, Y. H. (2010). Review Article: Recent advancements in optofluidic flow cytometer. *Biomicrofluidics*, Vol.4, No.4, pp. 043001-1 to 043001-23.

Choi, S. & Chae, J. (2009). Reusable biosensors via *in situ* electrochemical surface regeneration in microfluidic applications. *Biosensors & Bioelectronics*, Vol.25, No.2, pp. 527-531.

Cole, M. A., Voelcker, N. H., & Thissen, H. (2007). Electro-induced protein deposition on low-fouling surfaces. *Smart Materials and Structures*, Vol.16, pp. 2222-2228.

Corbett, S.C., Ajdari, A., Coskun, A.U. and Nayeb-Hashemi, H. (2010). Effect of pulsatile blood flow on thrombosis potential with a step wall transition. *ASAIO Journal*, Vol.56, No.4, pp.290-295.

Culbertson, C. T., Tugnawat, Y., Meyer, A. R., Roman, G. T., Ramsey, J. M., & Gonda, S. R. (2005). Microchip separations in reduced gravity and hypergravity environments. *Analytical Chemistry*, Vol.77, pp. 7933-7940.

Dalton, C. & Kaler, K. V. I. S. (2007). A cost effective, re-configurable electrokinetic microfluidic chip platform. *Sensors and Actuators B-Chemical*, Vol.123, No.1, pp. 628-635.

Dayananda, K. M., Singh, I., Mondal, N., & Neelamegham, S. (2010). von Willebrand factor self-association on platelet GpIb alpha under hydrodynamic shear: Effect on shear-induced platelet activation. *Blood*, Vol.116, No.19, pp. 3990-3998.

Delp, M. D. (2008). Unraveling the complex web of impaired wound healing with mechanical unloading and physical deconditioning. *Journal of Applied Physiology*, Vol.104, No.5, pp. 1262-1263.

Devarakonda, S. B., Han, J., Ahn, C. H., & Banerjee, R. K. (2007). Bioparticle separation in non-Newtonian fluid using pulsed flow in micro-channels. *Microfluidics and Nanofluidics*, Vol.3, No.4, pp. 391-401.

De Volder, M. & Reynaerts, D. (2010). Pneumatic and hydraulic microactuators: a review. *Journal of Micromechanics and Microengineering*, Vol.20, No.4, Article No.043001.

Di Carlo, D. (2009). Inertial microfluidics. *Lab on A Chip*, Vol.9, No.21, pp. 3038-3046.

Faivre, M., Abkarian, M., Bickraj, K., & Stone, H. A. (2006). Geometrical focusing of cells in a microfluidic device: An approach to separate blood plasma. *Biorheology*, Vol.43, No.2, pp. 147-159.

Fernandez-Calvo, P., Nake, C., Rivas, L. A., Garcia-Villadangos, M., Gomez-Elvira, J., & Parro, V. (2006). A multi-array competitive immunoassay for the detection of broad-range molecular size organic compounds relevant for astrobiology. *Planetary and Space Science*, Vol.54, pp. 1612-1621.

Fuerstman, M. J., Lai, A., Thurlow, M. E., Shevkoplyas, S. S., Stone, H. A., & Whitesides, G. M. (2007). The pressure drop along rectangular microchannels containing bubbles. *Lab on A Chip*, Vol.7, No.11, pp. 1479-1489.

Furdui, V. I. & Harrison, D. J. (2004). Immunomagnetic T cell capture from blood for PCR analysis using microfluidic systems. *Lab on A Chip*, Vol.4, No.6, pp. 614-618.

Furdui, V. I., Kariuki, J. K., & Harrison, D. J. (2003). Microfabricated electrolysis pump system for isolating rare cells in blood. *Journal of Micromechanics and Microengineering*, Vol.13, No.4, pp. S164-S170.

Furlani, E. P. (2007). Magnetophoretic separation of blood cells at the microscale. *Journal of Physics D-Applied Physics*, Vol.40, No.5, pp. 1313-1319.

Golden, J. P., Floyd-Smith, T. M., Mott, D. R., & Ligler, F. S. (2007). Target delivery in a microfluidic immunosensor. *Biosensors & Bioelectronics*, Vol.22, No.11, pp. 2763-2767.

Gossett, D. R., Weaver, W. M., Mach, A. J., Hur, S. C., Tse, H. T. K., Lee, W., Amini, H., & Di Carlo, D. (2010). Label-free cell separation and sorting in microfluidic systems. *Analytical and Bioanalytical Chemistry*, Vol.397, No.8, pp. 3249-3267.

Guire, P. E. (1999). Stability issues for protein-based in vitro diagnostic products. *IVD Technology*. Accessible at http://www.ivdtechnology.com/article/stability-issues-protein-based-vitro-diagnostic-products.

Han, A., Wang, O., Graff, M., Mohanty, S. K., Edwards, T. L., Han, K. H., & Frazier, A. B. (2003). Multi-layer plastic/glass microfluidic systems containing electrical and mechanical functionality. *Lab on A Chip*, Vol.3, pp. 150-157.

Hansen, C. L., Sommer, M. O. A., & Quake, S. R. (2004). Systematic investigation of protein phase behavior with a microfluidic formulator. *PNAS*, Vol.101, No.40, pp.14431-14436.

Hansson, K. M., Vikinge, T. P., Ranby, M., Tengvall, P., Lundstrom, I., Johansen, K., & Lindahl, T. L. (1999). Surface plasmon resonance (SPR) analysis of coagulation in whole blood with application in prothrombin time assay. *Biosensors & Bioelectronics*, Vol.14, No.8-9, pp. 671-682.

Hashemi, N., Howell, P.B., Erickson, J.S., Golden, J.P., & Ligler, F.S. (2010). Dynamic reversibility of hydrodynamic focusing for recycling sheath fluid. *Lab on A Chip*, Vol.10, No.15, pp. 1952-1959.

Helton, K. L., Nelson, K. E., Fu, E., & Yager, P. (2008). Conditioning saliva for use in a microfluidic biosensor. *Lab on A Chip*, Vol.8, No.11, pp. 1847-1851.

Hsu, C. H., Di Carlo, D., Chen, C.C., Irimia, D. & Toner, M. (2008). Microvortex for focusing, guiding and sorting of particles. *Lab on A Chip*, Vol.8, No.12, pp. 2128-2134.

Hu, J., Xie, M., Wen, C. Y., Zhang, Z. L., Xie, H. Y., Liu, A. A., Chen, Y. Y., Zhou, S. M., & Pang, D. W. (2011). A multicomponent recognition and separation system established via fluorescent, magnetic, dualencoded multifunctional bioprobes. *Biomaterials*, Vol.32, No.4, pp. 1177-1184.

Huh, Y. S., Chung, A. J., Cordovez, B., & Erickson, D. (2009). Enhanced on-chip SERS based biomolecular detection using electrokinetically active microwells. *Lab on A Chip*, Vol.9, No.3, pp. 433-439.

Hwang, H. & Park, J. K. (2011). Optoelectrofluidic platforms for chemistry and biology. *Lab on A Chip*, Vol.11, No.1, pp. 33-47.

Howell, P. B., Mott, D. R., Fertig, S., Kaplan, C. R., Golden, J. P., Oran, E. S., & Ligler, F. S. (2005). A microfluidic mixer with grooves placed on the top and bottom of the channel. *Lab on A Chip*, Vol.5, No.5, pp. 524-530.

International Space Station. (December 18, 2002). Payload flight equipment requirements and guidelines for safety - critical structures. SSP 52005 Revision C.

International Space Station Program. (June 3, 2004). International Space Station Crew Health Care System (CHeCS) Functional Requirements Document. Draft 2.0. NASA Johnson Space Center, Houston, TX,

Jedrych, E., Ziolkowska, K., Chudy, M., & Brzozka, Z. (2010). Microfluidic device for cell culture. *Przeglad Elektrotechniczny*, Vol.86, No.10, pp. 33-35.

Kim, J. S. & Ligler, F. S. (2010). Utilization of microparticles in next-generation assays for microflow cytometers. *Analytical and Bioanalytical Chemistry*, Vol.398, No.6, pp. 2373-2382.

Kist, T. B. L. & Mandaji, M. (2004). Separation of biomolecules using electrophoresis and nanostructures. *Electrophoresis*, Vol.25, No.21-22, pp. 3492-3497.

Kwon, H. J., Lee, C. H., Choi, E. J., Song, J. Y., Heinze, B. C., & Yoon, J. Y. (2010). Optofluidic device monitoring and fluid dynamics simulation for the spread of viral pathogens in a livestock environment. *Journal of Environmental Monitoring*, Vol.12, No.11, pp. 2138-2144.

Kuswandi, B., Nuriman, Huskens, J., & Verboom, W. (2007). Optical sensing systems for microfluidic devices: a review. *Analytica Chimica Acta*, Vol.601, pp. 141-155.

Lancaster, C., Kokoris, A., Nabavi, M., Clemmens, J., Maloney, P., Capadanno, J., Gerdes, J., & Battrell, C. F. (2005). Rare cancer cell analyzer for whole blood applications: Microcytometer cell counting and sorting subcircuits. *Methods*, Vol.37, No.1, pp. 120-127.

Lange, K., Rapp, B. E., & Rapp, M. (2008). Surface acoustic wave biosensors: a review. *Analytical and Bioanalytical Chemistry*, Vol.391, No.5, pp. 1509-1519.

Lenshof, A. & Laurell, T. (2010). Continuous separation of cells and particles in microfluidic systems. *Chemical Society Reviews*, Vol.39, No.3, pp. 1203-1217.

Liu, C., Guo, M., Chen, X., and Cheng, J. (2003). Low voltage driven miniaturized pump with high back pressure. *Proceedings of the SPIE - The International Society for Optical Engineering* 4982, 344-355.

MacInnes, J. M., Vikhansky, A., & Allen, R. W. K. (2007). Numerical characterisation of folding flow microchannel mixers. *Chemical Engineering Science*, Vol.62, No.10, pp. 2718-2727.

Madou, M., Zoval, J., Jia, G., Kido, H., Kim, J., & Kim, N. (2006). Lab on a CD. *Annual Review of Biomedical Engineering*, Vol.8, pp. 601-628.

Marchiarullo, D. J., Lim, J. Y., Vaksman, Z., Ferrance, J. P., Putcha, L., & Landers, J. P. (2008). Towards an integrated microfluidic device for spaceflight clinical diagnostics Microchip-based solid-phase extraction of hydroxyl radical markers. *Journal of Chromatography A*, Vol.1200, No.2, pp. 198-203.

Martinez, A. W., Phillips, S. T., Whitesides, G. M., & Carrilho, E. (2010). Diagnostics for the developing world: Microfluidic paper-based analytical devices. *Analytical Chemistry*, Vol.82, No.1, pp. 3-10.

Martinez, A. W., Phillips, S. T., Nie, Z. H., Cheng, C. M., Carrilho, E., Wiley, B. J., & Whitesides, G. M. (2010). Programmable diagnostic devices made from paper and tape. *Lab on A Chip*, Vol.10, No.19, pp. 2499-2504.

Maule, J., Fogel, M., Steele, A., Wainwright, N., Pierson, D. L., & McKay, D. S. (2003). Antibody binding in altered gravity: implications for immunosorbent assay during space flight. *Journal of Gravitational Physiology*, Vol.10, No.2, pp. 47-55.

Mogensen, K. B. & Kutter, J. P. (2009). Optical detection in microfluidic systems. *Electrophoresis*, Vol.30, pp. S92-S100.

Mohanty, S. K., Kim, D., & Beebe, D. J. (2006). Do-it-yourself microelectrophoresis chips with integrated sample recovery. *Electrophoresis*, Vol.27, No.19, pp. 3772-3778.

Mukhopadhyay, R. (2005). When microfluidic devices go bad - How does fouling occur in microfluidic devices, and what can be done about it? *Analytical Chemistry*, Vol.77, No.21, pp. 429A-432A.

Nashida, N., Satoh, W., Fukuda, J., & Suzuki, H. (2007). Electrochemical immunoassay on a microfluidic device with sequential injection and flushing functions. *Biosensors & Bioelectronics*, Vol.22, No.12, pp. 3167-3173.

Nelson, E. S. (1994). An examination of g-jitter and its effects on materials processes. *NASA Technical Memorandum* 103775.

Nelson, E. S. & Chait, A. (2010). Portable diagnostics technology assessment for space missions Part 2: Market survey. *NASA Technical Memorandum* 2010-215845/PART2.

Niederhaus, C. E., Barlow, K. L., Griffin, D. W., & Miller, F. J. (May 1, 2008). Medical grade water generation for intravenous fluid production on Exploration missions. *NASATechnical Memorandum* 2008-214999.

Nikitin, P. I., Gorshkov, B. G., Nikitin, E. P., & Ksenevich, T. I. (2005). Picoscope, a new label-free biosensor. *Sensors and Actuators B-Chemical*, Vol.111-112, pp. 500-504.

Pagana, K. D. & Pagana, T. J. (2005). *Mosby's Manual of Diagnostic and Laboratory Tests*. C.V. Mosby.

Pamme, N. (2006). Magnetism and microfluidics. *Lab on A Chip*, Vol.6, No.1, pp. 24-38.

Pamme, N. (2007). Continuous flow separations in microfluidic devices. *Lab on A Chip*, Vol.7, No.12, pp. 1644-1659.

Panton, R. L. (1984). *Incompressible flow*. John Wiley & Sons, Inc.

Park, J.-W., Kurosawa, S., Aizawa, H., Wakida, S.-I., Yamada, S., & Ishihara, K. (2003). Comparison of stabilizing effect of stabilizers for immobilized antibodies on QCM immunosensors. *Sensors and Actuators B-Chemical*, Vol.91, pp. 158-162.

Rosenson, R. S., McCormick, A., & Uretz, E. F. (1996). Distribution of blood viscosity values and biochemical correlates in healthy adults. *Clinical Chemistry*, Vol.42, No.8, pp. 1189-1195.

Sahney, R., Anand, S., Puri, B. K., & Srivastava, A. K. (2006). A comparative study of immobilization techniques for urease on glass-pH-electrode and its application in urea detection in blood serum. *Analytica Chimica Acta*, Vol.578, No.2, pp. 156-161.

Salieb-Beugelaar, G. B., Simone, G., Arora, A., Philippi, A., & Manz, A. (2010). Latest developments in microfluidic cell biology and analysis systems. *Analytical Chemistry*, Vol.82, No.12, pp. 4848-4864.

Sankaranarayanan, S. K. R. S., Singh, R., & Bhethanabotla, V. R. (2010). Acoustic streaming induced elimination of nonspecifically bound proteins from a surface acoustic wave biosensor: Mechanism prediction using fluid-structure interaction models. *Journal of Applied Physics*, Vol.108, No.10, pp. 104507-1 to 104507-11.

Satoh, W., Shimizu, Y., Kaneto, T., & Suzuki, H. (2007). On-chip microfluidic transport and bio/chemical sensing based on electrochemical bubble formation. *Sensors and Actuators B-Chemical*, Vol.123, No.2, pp. 1153-1160.

Shankaran, H., Alexandridis, P., & Neelamegham, S. (2003). Aspects of hydrodynamic shear regulating shear-induced platelet activation and self-association of von Willebrand factor in suspension. *Blood*, Vol.101, No.7, pp. 2637-2645.

Shen, J., Dudik, L., & Liu, C. C. (2007). An iridium nanoparticles dispersed carbon based thick film electrochemical biosensor and its application for a single use, disposable glucose biosensor. *Sensors and Actuators B-Chemical*, Vol.125, No.1, pp. 106-113.

Shen, J. & Liu, C. C. (2007). Development of a screen-printed cholesterol biosensor: Comparing the performance of gold and platinum as the working electrode material and fabrication using a self-assembly approach. *Sensors and Actuators B-Chemical*, Vol.120, No.2, pp. 417-425.

Shevkoplyas, S. S., Yoshida, T., Munn, L. L., & Bitensky, M. W. (2005). Biomimetic autoseparation of leukocytes from whole blood in a microfluidic device. *Analytical Chemistry*, Vol.77, No.3, pp. 933-937.

Shi, W., Guo, L.W., Kasdan, H., Fridge, A., & Tai, Y-C. (2011). Leukocyte 5-part differential count using a microfluidic cytometer. To be presented at *IEEE 16th International Conference on Solid State Sensors, Actuators and Microsystems*. Beijing, China. June 5-9, 2011.

Simerville, J. A., Maxted, W. C., & Pahira, J. J. (2005). Urinalysis: A comprehensive review. *American Family Physician*, Vol.71, No.6, pp. 1154-1162.

Simonnet, C. & Groisman, A. (2006). High-throughput and high-resolution flow cytometry in molded microfluidic devices. *Analytical Chemistry*, Vol.78, No.16, pp. 5653-5663.

Skelley, A. M., Scherer, J. R., Aubrey, A. D., Grover, W. H., Ivester, I. H., Ehrenfreund, P., Grunthaner, F. J., Bada, J. L., and Mathies, R. A. (2005). Development and evaluation of a microdevice for amino acid biomarker detection and analysis on Mars. *PNAS* 102[4], 1041-1046. National Academy of Sciences.

Smith, M. D., Davis-Street, J. E., Calkins, D. C., Nillen, J. L., & Smith, S. M. (2004). Stability of i-Stat EC6 cartridges: Effect of storage temperature on shelf life. *Clinical Chemistry*, Vol.50, pp. 669-673.

Sun, T. & Morgan, H. (2010). Single-cell microfluidic impedance cytometry: a review. *Microfluidics and Nanofluidics*, Vol.8, No.4, pp. 423-443.

Todd, P. (2009). Observation Chambers for Dynamic Microscopic Flow Visualization. NASA SBIR 09.01-9992. Space Hardware Optimization Technology, Greenville , IN.

Toepke, M. W. & Beebe, D. J. (2006). PDMS absorption of small molecules and consequences in microfluidic applications. *Lab on A Chip*, Vol.6, No.12, pp. 1484-1486.

Urbanski, J. P., Thies, W., Rhodes, C., Amarasinghe, S., & Thorsen, T. (2006). Digital microfluidics using soft lithography. *Lab on A Chip*, Vol.6, pp. 96-104.

VanDelinder, V. & Groisman, A. (2007). Perfusion in microfluidic cross-flow: Separation of white blood cells from whole blood and exchange of medium in a continuous flow. *Analytical Chemistry*, Vol.79, No.5, pp. 2023-2030.

Verjat, D., Prognon, P., & Darbord, J. C. (1999). Fluorescence-assay on traces of protein on re-usable medical devices: cleaning efficiency. *International Journal of Pharmaceutics*, Vol.179, No.2, pp. 267-271.

Vesper, H. W., Archibold, E., & Myers, G. L. (2005a). Assessment of trueness of glucose measurement instruments with different specimen matrices. *Clinica Chimica Acta*, Vol.358, No.1-2, pp. 68-74.

Vesper, H. W., Archibold, E., Porter, K. H., & Myers, G. L. (2005b). Assessment of a reference procedure to collect and analyze glucose in capillary whole blood. *Clinical Chemistry*, Vol.51, No.5, pp. 901-903.

Waggoner, P. S., Tan, C. P., & Craighead, H. G. (2010). Microfluidic integration of nanomechanical resonators for protein analysis in serum. *Sensors and Actuators B-Chemical*, Vol.150, No.2, pp. 550-555.

Wikipedia. Accessed March 28, 2011. Reference ranges for blood tests. http://en.wikipedia.org/wiki/Reference_ranges_for_blood_tests#Hematology

Xie, J., Miao, Y. N., Shih, J., Tai, Y. C., & Lee, T. D. (2005). Microfluidic platform for liquid chromatography-tandem mass spectrometry analyses of complex peptide mixtures. *Analytical Chemistry*, Vol.77, No.21, pp. 6947-6953.

Yang, S., Undar, A., & Zahn, J. D. (2006). A microfluidic device for continuous, real time blood plasma separation. *Lab on A Chip*, Vol.6, No.7, pp. 871-880.

Yang, X. (2008). Thioaptamer diagnostic system. NASA SBIR X10.01-9543 AM Biotechnologies, Houston, TX.

Yuan, J., Oliver, R., Li, J., Lee, J., Aguilar, M., & Wu, Y. (2007). Sensitivity enhancement of SPR assay of progesterone based on mixed self-assembled monolayers using nanogold particles. *Biosensors & Bioelectronics*, Vol.23, No.1, pp. 144-148.

Zhang, L., Zhang, Q., Lu, X., & Li, J. (2007). Direct electrochemistry and electrocatalysis based on film of horseradish peroxidase intercalated into layered titanate nano-sheets. *Biosensors & Bioelectronics*, Vol.23, No.1, pp. 102-106.

7

Biotika®: ISIFC's Virtual Company or Biomedical pre Incubation Accelerated Process

Butterlin Nadia[1], Soto Romero Georges[1], Guyon Florent[1] and Pazart Lionel[2]
[1]*University of Franche-Comté, ISIFC*
[2]*Hospital University Centre of Besançon, CHU*
France

1. Introduction

This chapter concerns a new concept of innovation in healthcare technology. ISIFC is the internal engineering school of University of Besançon (France) and is accredited by the French Ministry of National Education. The « Institut supérieur d'ingénieurs de Franche-Comté » (ISIFC) graduates 216 biomedical engineering students since 2004 for the prevention, diagnosis and treatment of disease, for patient rehabilitation and for improving health. Its originality lies in its innovative course of studies, which trains engineers in the scientific and medical fields to get both competencies. The Institute therefore collaborates with the University Hospital Centre of Besançon (CHU), biomedical companies and National Research Centres (CNRS and INSERM). The teaching team consists mainly in lecturer-researchers and researchers as well as biomedical and health industry professionals. It's an innovative engineering French school, which tries to understand the expectation of the specific healthcare and medical devices markets. It trains engineers in 3 years (2400 hours per student) with a double culture, medical and technical, who will work for 80% in biomedical industry, 10% in healthcare centre and 5% in research laboratory. They master all the life cycle of a medical device from the idea to the launch of the market. They can lead to improve product functionality, usability, safety and quality. We prepare our students to:

- Medical and biological instrumentation in general, with a special interest for Microsystems. The course's main targets are design enhancement and the development of equipment for clinical, medical and biological investigation (biochips, automated devices for biological analysis, probes, endoscopes, artificial organs and systems for physiological assistance etc…).
- The analysis, design and development of biomechanical systems. They thus receive special training on mechanical design, manufacturing engineering, and special training on materials used in surgery (metal, polymer, ceramic, composite…) as well as their different use in biological environments, ie tissues and human organs (biocompatibility). The main applications are orthopaedics (prosthesis and orthesis).

Our students play a significant role in emergence of combination products (e.g. biologic and device or drug and device).

1.1 11 months' work experience

Training periods and projects in laboratories, in health services or in companies enable ISIFC trainees to acquire practical experience, and to communicate with all the actors of the biomedical sector.

During the second year, all the students are invited to have a 6 weeks work experience (February and March) at the hospital. It enables future engineers to fully grasp the integration of biomedical equipments within a health service, from a technical and human point of view.

During their third year (master degree), students are challenged through a development project. It lasts 3 months (December to February), and the project is addressed individually. Projects may be done at a private company or at a public research department.

A working period in a company premises concludes the 3-year course. It lasts from 16 weeks up to 24 weeks (March to September). Industrial trainee engineers take on missions that are usually assigned to junior engineers within a firm.

The ISIFC engineers' specificities are their good knowledge in regulatory affairs and in the quality aspects of the technologies of health, their analysis of benefits/risks for the patient and the pre clinical investigations they can manage. In it is added strategies of tradition from Franche-Comté as mechanical/biomechanical, medical instrumentation and microtechniques.

ISIFC engineers master regulatory and clinical affairs. At the end of the training, they are able to elaborate the technical file indispensable for the CE mark and FDA and so for the launch of the European and American market. They can design and create medical devices.

In fact, ISIFC School is an important partner for medical device technology development and evaluation process. ISIFC is also a tool of effectively surveying prospective device users. These users are healthcare professionals, patients, elderly people or people with disabilities, researchers and industrials.

1.2 Why Biotika®?

To stimulate greater academia/business interactions, in 2006, ISIFC created Biotika®, a virtual company (without legal status) specialized in design engineering of innovative medical devices. ISIFC created an environment for innovation in healthcare to stimulate commercialization of new medical device, to reduce costs and to deliver faster. Marketing, regulatory and clinical affairs, service support, accounting and inventory are concerned (no manufacturing and no production engineering). This company was built on the basis of a training module at the end of 2nd year (75 hours per student) and in the beginning of the third and last year (100 hours per student). It's not only an educational entrepreneurship exercise to encourage students during their university programme. The purpose is to make discover to the pupils engineers the various facets of their future job with a real professional overview and to establish real new innovative businesses enhancing the research academic researchers or supporting real start up activities. Biotika® is guaranteeing quality throughout its organization and is systemising quality within the organization (according ISO 13 485). The idea is to sensibilize the students to the innovation, the entrepreneurship, the quality approach, and the project management with specific angles to the regulatory affairs, clinical investigations, the financing of the innovation, the industrial and intellectual properties and the market studies.

The goal of this chapter is to show how was built inside ISIFC a "catalyst" and performing tool for the innovation and the partnership research. Biotika® is in fact a cell of pre incubation of technological projects for the health, stimulating proof of concept and development of new ideas arising from patients, physicians, surgeons, universities and industrials.
An experience feedback of 5 years will be described. The virtual company works on development projects and transfers of medical devices, and is in fact real cell pre incubation. The chapter describes its collaboration in the creation of start up Cisteo MEDICAL (incubator Franche-Comté**)**. It gives three examples, financial supported by OSEO and Besançon University valorisation maturing process. Different applications domains are concerned: maxillofacial surgery, dental surgery, oncology, palliative care, gastroenterology and cardiovascular diagnosis. Very recently, Biotika® obtains financial support from the French Agency of Research (ANR program Emergence) with innovative saliva substitute technique for maxillofacial surgery.

2. General Biotika® principle

The nature of this innovative concept is based on the originality of the ISIFC School. It's the heart of an innovative process to accelerate device deployment in the market. It's required strong interactions among academia, life sciences, technology, engineering and industry.
The pupils-engineers recruited in Biotika® (about 20 a year) work one-two days a week on real projects and according ISO13485 standard. Three permanent members pilot the virtual company. They are punctually assisted by university experts, secretary finance and by a technician in electronics. The CEO of Biotika® is guiding in reality ISIFC and is also associate professor in optoelectronics. The Human Resources manager is in fact an associate professor in electronics and educational responsible of this training unit. The QA and regulatory affairs manager is a half time teacher but also Quality manager in a biomedical industry Statice Santé, ISIFC partner. The director of CIC-IT (Clinical Investigation Center-Innovation Technology) of Besançon Hospital collaborates regularly with Biotika®.
Every year, a new project is developed. The students participate with the staff to the choice of the new maturation. This general brainstorming (4 hours) is just after their six weeks hospital internship.
Different scenarios are possible:

- development of a medical device new to the market
- major upgrade of an existing medical device after a regulatory affairs modifications or after device deployment in the market and first users feedbacks
- re-design of a device prototype and regulatory affairs optimisations.

3. Biotika® partnership arrangement and network

Biotika®, pre-incubation cell of technology projects for the health of the ISIFC is in fact a tool catalyst for innovation and research partnerships. All of partners are important and we have a complementary network. They need to interact with and to learn from each other.
The three permanent members of the ISIFC Biotika® (CEO, Director human resources and Director Quality / Regulatory Affairs) are full time university assistant professor. The director of the Besançon CIC IT, physician of CHU, participates regularly for validation and clinical trials.
The three categories of general customers are: patients, healthcare professionals (nurses, biomedical hospital engineers, physicians and clinical researchers) and industrials.

Four categories of customers have significant influence in the decision to innovate in the company. Firstly there are ISIFC students. The second category is prescribers (physicians, manage care organization and hospitals). The third category consists of the payers and policy makers. The last but not least category is the Biotika® permanent staff (teacher and researcher).

Biomedical engineering students recruited Biotika® work every year on real projects, detected during hospital internship and serving clinicians and patients. It's in close collaboration with research laboratories of the UFC and businesses Franc-Comtois.

Due to ISIFC links to established research laboratories in the field of engineering, micro-technologies or health (about 30 laboratories and research centres are worldwide known and associated to National Research Centres such as CNRS and INSERM), each student benefits from the most recent scientific and technological innovation and has access to up to date equipment available in these units. We work particularly with the scientific group specialized in engineering and innovative method for health (GIS) [FEMTO-ST 6174 CNRS Institute (with the French label Carnot "ability to conduct research with industrial partners), IFR 133 INSERM institute and LIFC informatics research laboratory].

The University of Franche-Comté established a Valorisation Administration in 1997 in order to develop in the institution a culture of partnership with the socio-economic environment, and to support laboratories in the valorisation process of their research results. To support this move, a SAIC (Department of Industrial and Commercial Activity), which is a valorisation management tool, was set up in 2004. An annual maturation process, called "Maturation Franche - Comté" was set up at the University of Franche-Comté thank to the ANR 2005 program. Biotika® has succeeded 5 times to benefit of this kind of financial process (Fibrotika in 2006, Physiotika® in 2008 and 2009, S-Alive in 2010, AgiMilk in 2011).

The Clinical Investigation Centre - Technological Innovations of Besançon (INSERM CIT 808) is located in and managed by Besancon University Hospital and INSERM as co-manager. The Clinical Investigation Centre is approved by INSERM and the DHOS for two activities: biotherapies (CIC-BT approved in 2005 and reconducted in 2010) and Technological Innovation (CIC-IT approved in 2008). The CIC-IT is already implied in medical devices development through ANR and OSEO programmes and translational research. The institute collaborates with the environmental platform MicroTech-hosted by the Health institute of technology transfer of Franche-Comte (Institut Pierre Vernier).

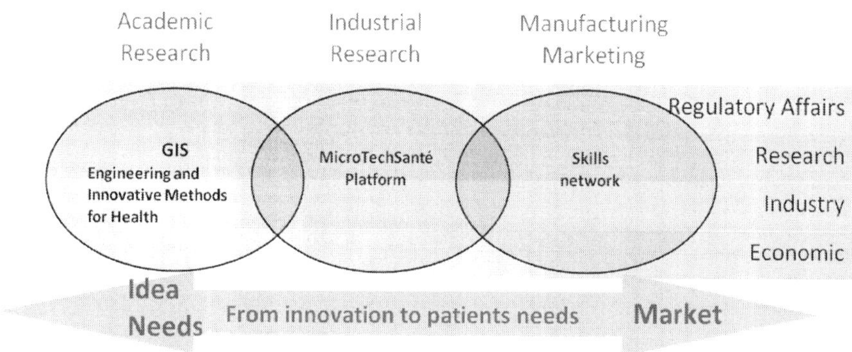

Fig. 1. MicroTech platform principle

Our virtual firm collaborates with the incubator in Franche Comté. Christophe Moureaux, a senior engineer, joined the incubator in December 2009 to set up a company (Cisteo MEDICAL) dedicated to the development and manufacture of new medical devices combining established material, associated motor units, sensors and embedded energy, in partnership with the ISIFC and Biotika® and the University Hospital of Besançon. This start up is now supported by OSEO. The further development of the devices pre incubated by Biotika® will be provided later with Cisteo MEDICAL by consortium.
Biotika®, virtual firm, develops real active partnerships with industrial actors: Cisteo MEDICAL but also Alcis, Covalia, Statice and Technologia. This industrial partnerships' list is undergoing constant. Franche-Comté lies at the heart of Europe, a region in the east of France. The border between Franche-Comté and Switzerland is 230 km long. It's an important factor of our biomedical industrial network's success.

4. Virtual company structure

The "virtual company" works with French collective agreements 3018 but without legal status. The legal status is in fact a university status. The activity is only on 2 days per week and only during 7 months per year. It's in fact an innovative educational concept with focus on real medical devices' conception. The trademarks are INPI registered.
In 2006, students enrolled and whose names are designated in part N°16 in thanks, created all together and in total autonomy (but after validation of management) all communication tools. For example, they create their company name and logo (fig. 2) which were INPI registered in 2007. Now, it's the same process for new products' names. Physiotika® in 2008, S-Alive® in 2009 and Agimilk® in 2010 names were INPI registered.

Fig. 2. Logo of our virtual company is INPI registered

The Biotika®'s website is http://biotika.adeisifc.fr/
The webmaster is a student.

5. Management principle

5.1 Innovative principle

Further to the hospital training course (6 weeks), the new members of Biotika® decide together on new projects they want to develop. The objective is to innovate, that means to develop at least one innovative medical device per year. Since its creation, 8 projects were pre incubated. We want essentially to work for patients who are affected in terms of their quality of life and a significant reduction in their disability.

5.2 Steps principle

Principle is described on figure below. We have five steps and two phases during half year 4 and half year 5:

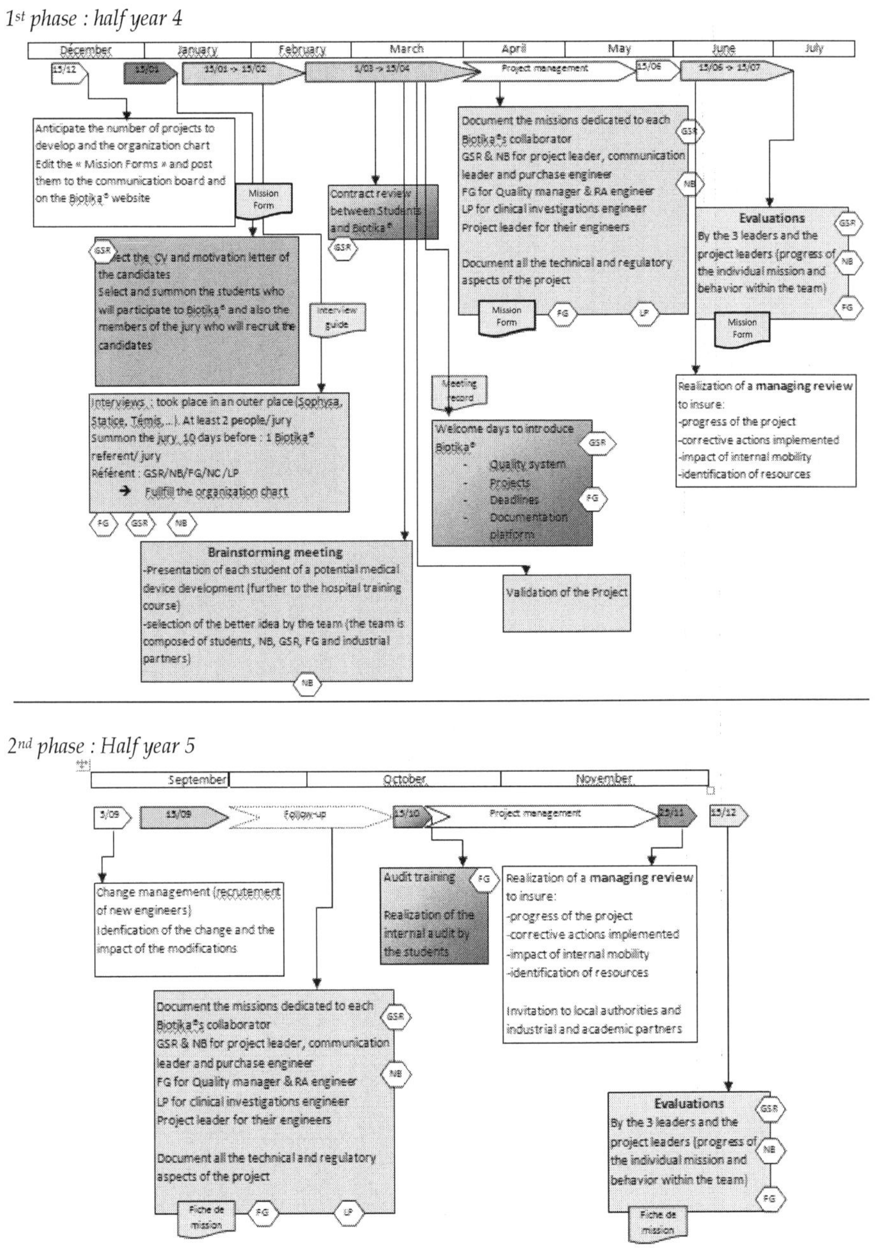

Fig. 3. Management principle during the two semesters, half year 4 and 5

- Detection of needs (after hospital internship) Definition of functional specifications, bibliographic research, relevant economic and clinical benefit / risk
- Research evidence, experiments and simulations of feasibility, design demonstration models of preclinical protocols and files for CE marking, removal of the first scientific obstacles
- Research funding, confidentiality agreements and partnership
- Launch of joint development and validation of preclinical
- Transfer to real companies in the manufacture of prototypes and pre-industrial to industrial

6. Organizational structure

Biotika® team for 2006 was initially made up of thirteen people, including eleven ISIFC engineering students (see list in Part 16, Acknowledgements). Every year, Biotika® staff is completely renewed. All the posts (except management) are attributed to the new pupils-engineers of the 2nd year of ISIFC. They are really interviewed by professional people.
In 2007, the team organization changed. It consisted of eighteen people, including fourteen engineering students ISIFC sometimes with double missions. A department Quality / Regulatory Affairs / Marketing / Communication was created. Technical Director (half part time Human Resources Director) droved three different projects (CP 1-3) and the purchasing manager logistics. Most of them worked in project team (a team leader with R&D engineers by project). Some of them worked with transverse missions or with specific responsibilities (purchase, communication, regulatory affairs, quality, marketing, supplier quality assurance, clinical investigations).

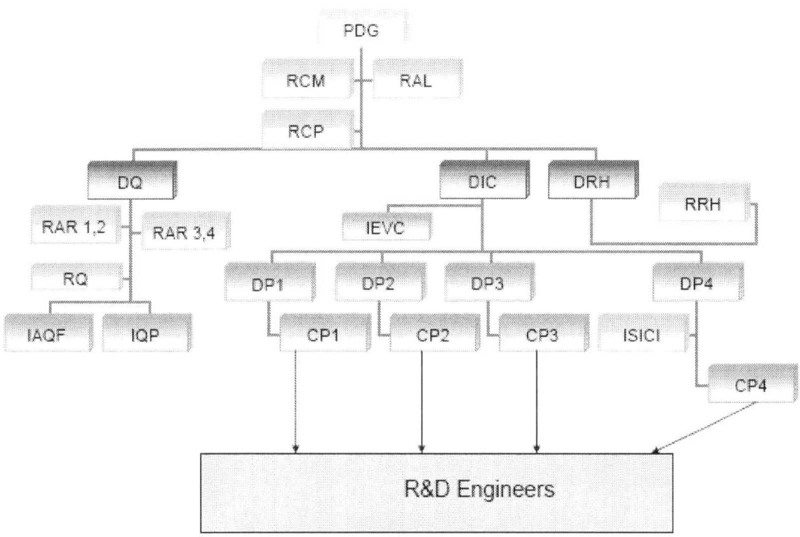

Fig. 4. Biotika® 2008 team

In 2008, the Biotika®'s team (Fig. 4) was composed of 30 persons, including twenty-one students ISIFC engineers. The direction of Biotika® included additional permanent members: a doctor of hospital university CIC-IT department (Dr. Lionel Pazart) as director clinical investigations (DIC), four project managers (DP1 to DP4, Georges Soto Romero, Fabrice Richard, Sébastien Thibaud and Sébastien Euphrasie are all teachers and researchers of FEMTO-ST CNRS laboratory). Each tutorial provides a close with the respective project manager. The new interviews of the virtual firm are outsourced over Statice Santé Company and Témis Institute. It tooks place in Besancon in April 2008 to allocate to each its place within the virtual company and to fill a number of new missions related to the following positions:

- Four project leaders, CP1 to CP4
- Research and Development Engineers,
- Logistics & Purchasing Manager, RAL
- Communications project manager, RCP
- Communication / Marketing, RCM
- Quality Manager, RQ
- Regulatory affairs Manager, RAR
- Quality assurance manager with suppliers, RAQF
- Product qualification engineer, IQP
- Information system engineer-collaborative platform and internal communication, ISIC
- Clinical testing and validation engineer, IEVC.

The offices of Biotika® are located in the premises of ISIFC in Besançon. Their members have access to the technological and logistical resources of FEMTO-ST, University of Franche-Comté, ISIFC, Besancon Hospital and CIC-IT. A platform of engineering collaborative allows a technical partnership with schools of Morteau and Dole. We work nearby the IUT (University Institute of Technology) in mechanical engineering as well as the AIP Primeca of Besançon. Thus, all pieces are manufactures in Franche Comté region.
A PLM tool is used to share the different documents generated by the students during the R&D process.

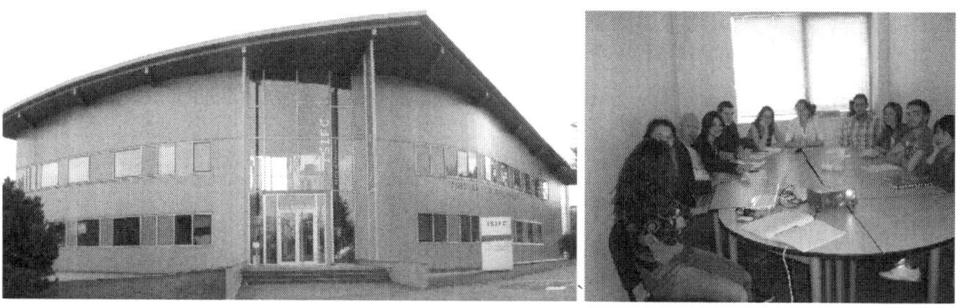

Fig. 5. ISIFC/Biotika® building located on TEMIS Park and managing revue meeting

Now, managing director uses a cross matrix described bellow.

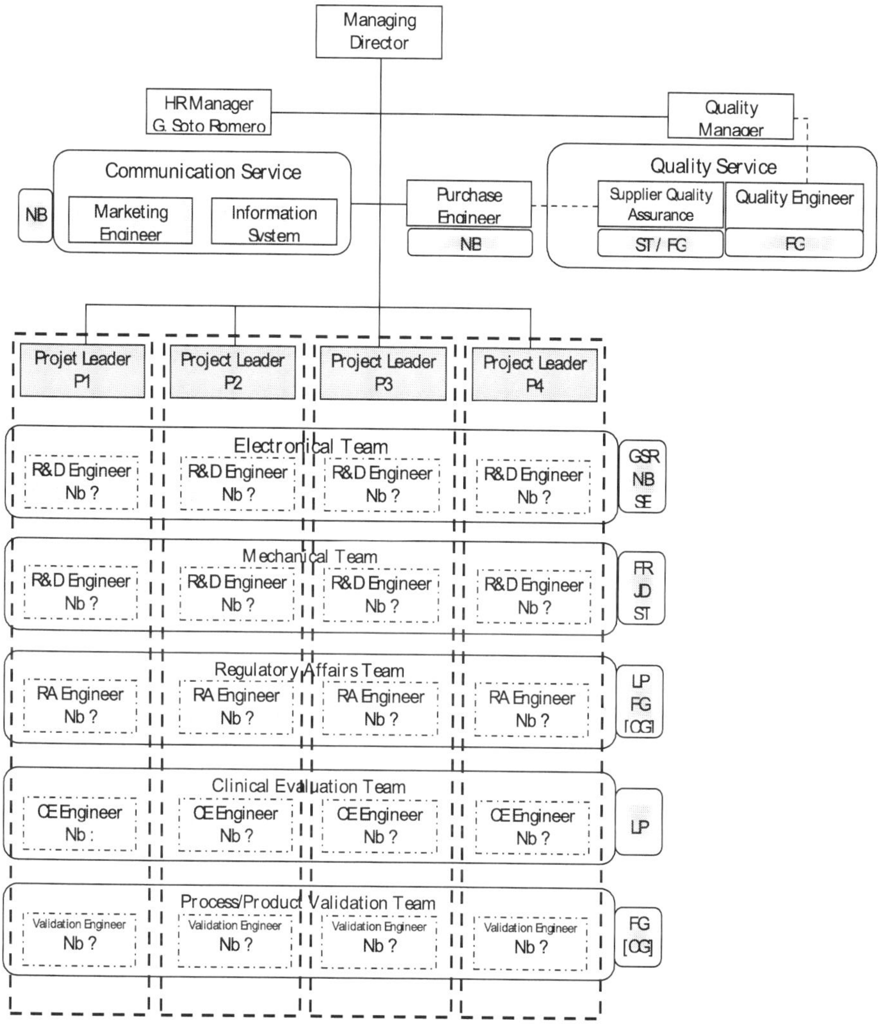

The legend is for the permanent staff:
NB : N. Butterlin, GSR : G. Soto Romero, FG : F. Guyon, LP : L. Pazart, ST : S. Thibaut, SE : S. Euphrasie, JD : J. Duffaud, FR : F. Richard, [CG] : C. Garcia.
The general organization is composed of permanent staff and there is one project manager by project. All the others functions are assumed by students. Their number depends on complexity and project. There are mechanical and electronical R&D engineers' teams.

Fig. 6. Crossed matrix, organization chart functional

7. Innovative active training

7.1 Missions of the training module

This is, in a virtual firm, to create and maintain a dynamic coaching and collaborative work that gives students opportunities for implementation of academic knowledge in biomedical engineering. The purpose is to provide students and this during their training, a scenario first real experience "tutored" and participative management style. They discover in their future learning progressive industrial activities.

This allows students in terms of autonomy, initiatives and recovery:

- To highlight their individual skills (know-how and skills: passion for work and for other people especially patients....),
- To correct their shortcomings and provide a true assessment of skills
- To involve them fully in the development of image with:
  - Companies in the biomedical sector,
  - Hospital centres,
  - Local, regional, national and international institutions of higher education or secondary technical and regional operators,
  - Students from Faculty of Medicine,
  - Patients associations.
- To have ideas for innovation
- To be able to develop innovative medical devices

After the module, they know that innovation takes a lot of time, a lot of energy, a lot of creativity and needs strong interactions between mentors, mentees and many others.

7.2 Resources available

This module is expected late in the second year (semester N°4) and the beginning of the third (semester N°5). It is built on a base of 7 European Credit Time System (ECTS) or 175 hours in terms of teaching model. It is divided into two parts: a form of 3 ECTS in semester 4 (Number of Hours: 8 h classes, Individual Project Time 67h) and 4 ECTS in semester 5 (Number of Hours: 8h classes, Individual project Time 92h). These hours are: controlling and monitoring of the "virtual firm", the organization and implementation of recruitment in offshore locations, the organization of "events" such as progress meetings, quality audits technical and internal customer visits and / or suppliers, participation in trade shows ...), organization and implementation of talks progress and interviews. It must include a plan for internal training in innovation, clinical trials, programming microcontrollers or finite elements, internal auditing, first aid, ...

The "budget schedule" of compensation for the part of teachers entrepreneurship varies from year to year: it partly depends on the training plan (action contractors) and "consulting" done by specialists from Biotika®. A "system standby" (on the model of hospital guards) is being implemented for the management team and rewarded accordingly. The "maximum budget" available for payments of permanent staff and / or individual contractor is calculated on the basis of

1 group / 24 students and 1 group TP / 5 students.

A teaching group of at least 6 people for the management team and technical supervision is necessary for steering Biotika®. It consists of permanent members of the ISIFC who are at least one specialist in quality (DQ), a specialist in research and R & D (PDG), a human resources manager himself a technical expert (DRH and DT) and a specialist in investigations clinical

DIC. The four students project managers (P1 to P4) act as intermediaries between students recruited technical and management Biotika® staff. The support by "consultants" in optics, mechanical and electronic designs, marketing and business plan (participation of university companies' management school of Besançon), medicine allows students to have recruited ad hoc support. The supervision of the training module Biotika® Entrepreneurship is thus a specific and custom framing increased. It's a real experimental innovative educational program.

7.3 Activities associated with the module

For each project developed, it is:

Design and implement a technology demonstration vehicle (or functional model) of a biomedical device. So get models' skills students ISIFC "for trade shows, national day" Celebrate Science "forum of students, JPO ...

Introduce a quality approach in designing a medical device in collaboration with technicians and / or operators, according to the standard ISO 13485.

Conduct a market analysis and research prior art product.

Conduct a comprehensive study in order to obtain the CE mark.

Conduct research and transfer of technological device designed to a manufacturing process in collaboration with secondary schools, technical platforms and / or regional IUT.

Implement corrective action following audits to ensure the quality policy of the company.

Learn self-assessment and / or evaluate its partners know how to respond to questioning skills assessments.

Learn to understand the needs of businesses in terms of qualifications, with a good-looking management of the student's career.

8. Building the appropriate team and managing people

Every year, Biotika® renews its staff (excluding permanent management) and no period of recovery is possible! A real campaign is organized. The process is conducted with multiple conversations between individuals. It's after Internet publication by firm's website posting. The candidates are selected by pre-processing of curriculum vitae and cover letters in French and English. Lasting about one month, ten recruiters are necessary for the recruitment operation. This year, 47 candidates are examinated for 23 jobs. Between recruiters, they are: manufacturers (and in fact also ISIFC engineer graduated), consultants, permanent Biotika®'s staff. The recruitment locations are offshore (business partners or local business incubator). All aspects of a job interview are discussed and a response to each application is made (the call to service or not, positive / negative). The final allocation of posts is based on current skills but also detected (refining the professional project of the student). This is the moment to initiate a real active support success.

In March as is explained in Figure 3, each student turnover, innovative projects are proposed and discussed by staff Biotika® (permanent and students). Then, the final choice is made by all staff but with a constraint: only one has to be new and innovative. The other projects will be developed in continuity with the previous team and with at least one of them, specifically oriented biomechanics.

House training specific to programming microcontroller is available to all. A second phase of internal training is then carried out by Internal Audit.

Individual interviews with each student assessments, both technical and position are made in late June and late November by the N +1 and permanent managers. The rating and credits obtained allow validation as an engineer graduated from ISIFC. A review of activities, such general meeting and open house, are presented every year in late November to the major partners.

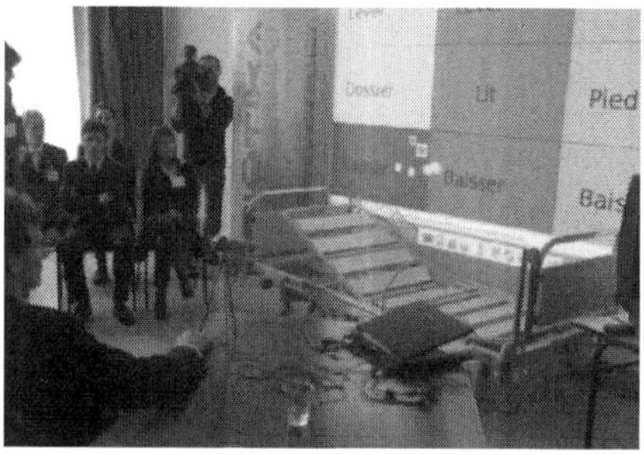

Fig. 7. Managing revue meeting.

9. Patenting, trademarks and copyrights

The patenting and intellectual properties are very important for the general manager of Biotika®. The university valorisation framework supports Biotika®'s projects by different processes:

- Negotiating and writing the consortium agreements,
- Implementing conventions (recruitment, managing expenditure and receipts, sub-contracting),
- Following ANR programme implementation
- Closing conventions and producing administrative items justifying expenses.

Valorisation University Department ensures in particular that the results of the project are protected, if necessary by submitting a patent, as well as commercial valorisation by identifying the partners likely to take out user licenses.

The INPI is the national institute for intellectual and industrial properties registrations. The original and innovative concept of our "ISIFC's virtual firm" can't patent. But the mark and logo of Biotika® are INPI registered on four classes: N° 09, 10, 41 and 42 with specifications detailed bellow:

- Class N° 09: Devices and instrumentations for scientific research in biomedical engineering domain.
- Class N° 10: Devices and instrumentations for surgeons, physicians and biomedicines. Beds for healthcare, endoscopes, fibro scopes, saliva automatic distributors....
- Class N° 41: teaching and professional training services for biomedical engineering students.

The community law requires a use of the brand «in the life of the business" that means according to the community case law «the exercise of an economic activity ", " the offer of the goods and the services on a market " or " the exercise of a commercial activity aiming at an economic advantage ". The name of the class 41 thus asks question: does the training service proposed by the ISIFC raise of the life of the affairs? Yes, because we consider that the training is paying and that there is a "market" of engineering schools (competition to recruit the bests "pupils-customers")

- Class N° 42: Scientific and technologic services for biomedical engineering domain (medical devices, instrumentation). Research studies and developments services are included.

Biotika® INPI registered 4 Soleau letters and 3 marks and worked on 4 anteriority studies.

10. Documentary and communications system

Within Biotika®, which remains a young company, all the staff is involved in the communication strategy of the company. By this approach, the management team expects from every student that he learns to communicate with various interlocutors (MD, senior engineers and customers). But also, because of the renewal of all the staff from one year to the next, the written traceability of all the activities, the technical choices on each project and the whole life of the company must be guaranteed by each staff member.

External communication:

> This requirement justifies our choice of using, more than a web domain (biotika-isifc.com) in which we can store our website, a new communication and networking platform, Agora Project. We found in it a reliable an easy handling tool for collaborative engineering.
>
> Agora project allows sharing all useful information with our different partner, such as Morteau and Dole schools (mechanical drawings, printed circuits board designs). In that case, Agora is used as a powerful external communication tool.

Internal communication:

Agora project is also an internal communication tool, used as same as an intranet. Memorandums, agendas and meeting reports are uploaded and shared with all the staff.

The quality system of Biotika® requires a lot of data records. We can use Agora Project as a distant storage server, and a HR resource tool (for new staff members, holidays planning, etc).

Best results :

This network based communication system help to increase our productivity. Also, our students were able to contribute on scientific production (papers, posters) related with each project and with the firm. In the other hand, they could participate on several meetings like Micronora (3 times since 2006) and MEDTEC France (2 times since 2010).

11. Quality management system

11.1 Quality policy

In addition to train students for the workplace, Biotika® has its own goals as a company whose virtual goal is to improve the lives of patients:

- Develop and implement innovative medical devices,
- Establish a quality system for the company according to ISO 13485,
- Conduct a technical file on each product,
- Assume the investigations and clinical trials for a CE
- Ensure internal / external communication of the company, market analysis
- Managing the company in its entirety: budget, employment contracts, quality audit, meetings with industry, intellectual property, ...

- To transfer the concept to an academic or industrial partner able to guarantee production (mission partnership, quality file) or create a real business.

The quality process unfolds within any organization Biotika® (structure documentary records in relation to the requirements of ISO 13485). Every years, actions are validated through an internal audit carried out in the end of annual activity.

Quality Policy of Biotika®

BIOTIKA® aims at developing medical devices and improving the industrial and academic partnership. Also Biotika® makes a commitment:

- To implement a case study
- To reach the missions defined at the beginning of the project
- To give a new approach of the entrepreneurship
- To implement the engineer's sciences learned during the year
- To allow the students to integrate the industry dimension
- To transfert the knowledge to the following promotion and so to maintain a dynamic within ISIFC
- To facilitate the professional insertion
- To implement the partnership with local schools
- To insure the recognition of BIOTIKA® by the professional of the biomedical area and by the local authorities

As managing director, me, Nadia Butterlin, I make a commitment to give all the resources necessary for the good functioning of BIOTIKA®. In order to meet all biomedical industry aspects, I named a quality manager who is in charge of the Quality Management System according to the ISO 13485 standard.

Nadia Butterlin
Managing Director

Fig. 8. Quality policy of Biotika®

11.2 Processes and mapping

At the beginning, the main important step was to identify the customers and their expectations. It was not simple to define the main customers to satisfy. The direction decided to satisfy in first the student themselves.

One of the first actions initiated by the student was also to identify the processes which would have an impact of the customer's satisfaction. For them, there were 2 main activities:

- **Communication** : in order to become known Biotika®
- **Design** : in order to develop the innovative medical device chosen

To monitor these 2 processes, a management process is there to define the policy, to engage the corrective and preventive actions, to audit the system in place and to review at an adequate frequency the aptitude of Biotika® to meet customer's requirements during managing review.

And to support the realization processes, some activities were precised as:

- Documentation management
- Purchasing actions
- Incoming inspection
- Measuring instruments monitoring
- Regulatory survey

The students after the processes identification decided to map them in order to define the interfaces between each process.

Another important action was to define the documentation (describe all the procedures of the quality system) and the record necessary to prove that the activities are implemented according the quality system in place.

An internal audit is performed every year and two management reviews are led to insure that the system of quality management is conform to the ISO13485 standard. The implemented actions are reviewed and also the objectives. The evaluation of the "employees" validates the obtaining of the engineering degree of ISIFC.

You can find below the map which is also in the Quality Manual

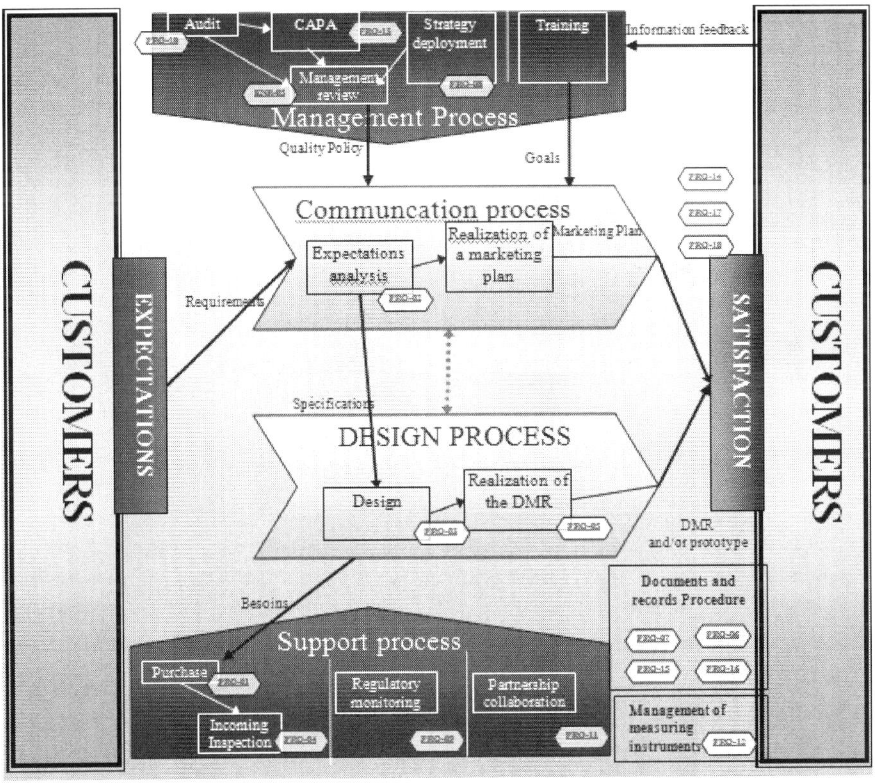

Fig. 9. Quality Map

12. Maturing projects' story

Within Biotika®, two products were developed in 2006: a bed voice-activated and an automated flexible endoscope. This year, there are five different projects.

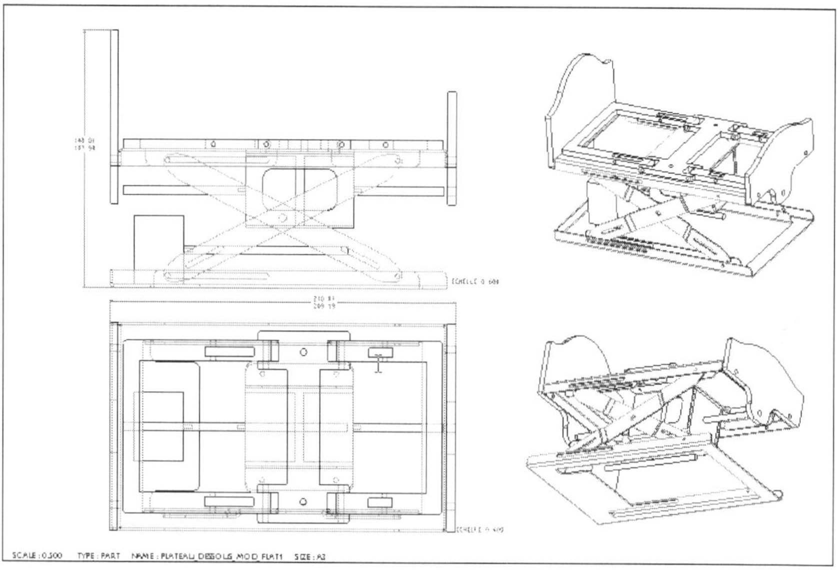

Fig. 10. Manufacturing plans exhibited at Micronora 2006

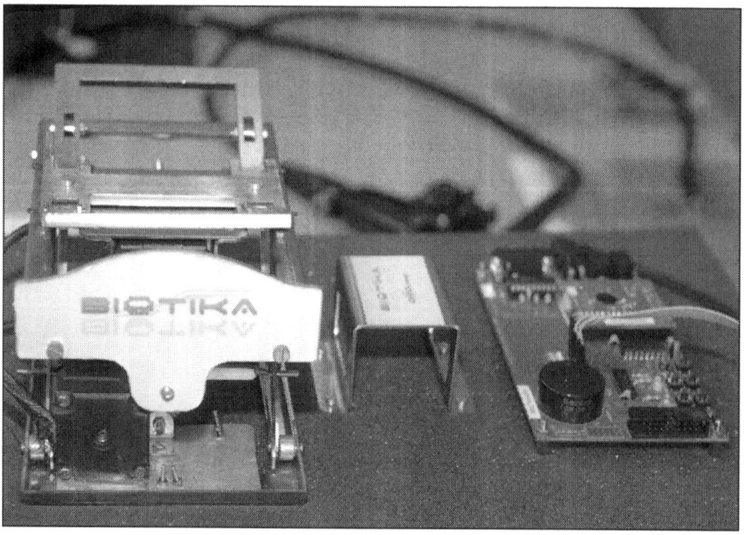

Fig. 11. Working model exhibited at Micronora 2006

12.1 Hospital bed with voice recognition

The concept is based on the instrumentation of a motorized hospital bed to a patient or the caregiver to control the position of the bed by voice recognition. Instructions, recorded in advance, allow engines to operate the corresponding control. Possible instructions are "up" and "down". They can then be combined with "whole", "head" and "feet". To ensure the functionality of the bed, an alternative means by remote control manual has been planned.
A working model shown in Figure 10 and based on the principles outlined above was performed.

12.2 Automated flexible endoscope

The concept is based on remote instrumentation, using a joystick and miniature motors, displacement of the head of a video endoscope (a variety of flexible endoscope) which is used in the exploration of some cavities body and the taking of samples. To date, this shift is based on mechanical action at the end of an endoscope through knobs. A wheel provides the lateral movement of the endoscope head and the other the vertical displacement, which makes the system cumbersome. However, this system has many disadvantages for the user. Originally intended to be manipulated with one hand (while the second deals with the insertion and withdrawal of the endoscope), this is not the case in reality. Indeed, it is found to be extremely difficult to use simultaneously, with ease and precision, the two control knobs with one hand.
There are two solutions to the practitioner:

- Use both hands to control, requiring the presence of a third hand for insertion and withdrawal of the endoscope (nurse)
- Or use only one of two dials (most accessible) with one hand and rotate the 90 ° endoscope to access the other direction.

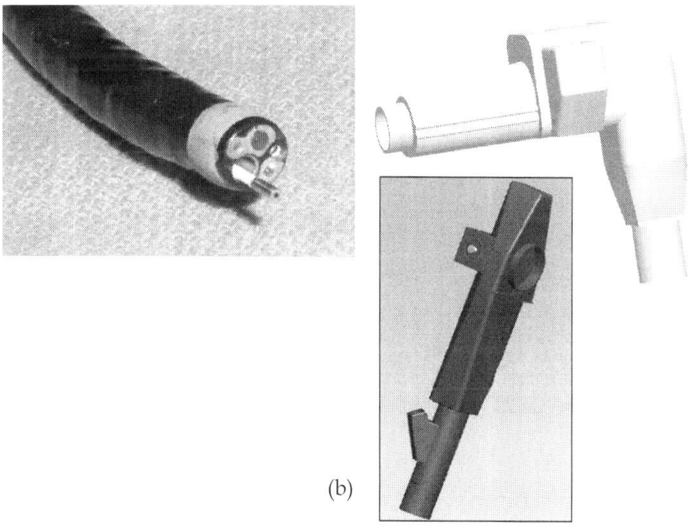
(a) (b) (c)

Fig. 12. (a) Head of the endoscope control ,(b) Model of the proposed handle with joystick, (c) handle being designed

If, to maintain total control of the procedure, experienced practitioners have mastered the second method presented above, this is not true of young interns who need lots of practice before they can act alone. This problem of handling the endoscope, it is clear: an increase in the time of the intervention, a greater risk of irritation or perforation of the walls for patients (especially during this period of learning internal) and an increase in the learning period of the endoscopic technique.

This study on improving the ergonomics of flexible endoscopes has led to Biotika® proposes as a solution to automate the order.

A feasibility study was undertaken in partnership with the Division of Gastroenterology CHU Besançon and Dr. Stéphane Koch. A first demonstrator has been realized in 2006.

In 2007, the new team has developed the product automated endoscope, Fibrotika renamed, and worked in parallel on two new projects: Visiotika, a device for visual control interface for controlling the environment for people paralyzed and S-Alive dispensing device of artificial saliva for patients with xerostomia (destruction of the salivary glands).

12.3 Fibrotika: Following the project automated flexible endoscope

In 2007, Biotika® decided to continue the project renamed Fibrotika automated flexible endoscope. The goal is to move from a demonstration model named by students Simulscopie at a pre-prototype used for preclinical trials. The tests are scheduled at the University Hospital in late 2008 (R&D internship, L.Debar). Contacts with companies specialized in the design and manufacture of endoscopes have been established. The ability to add sensors at the end of the sheath of the endoscope to create a force feedback on the action of the command, and the development of a simulator test to measure efficacy are studied. Anteriorities' research results and the important fund needs are the two major reasons to stop the maturation process of Fibrotika inside Biotika®.

12.4 S-Alive ®

This project involves the development of a new distributor of artificial saliva for patients with Xerostomia (dry mouth sensation) and / or Asialia or oral dryness (lack of or decrease in production of saliva). These patients can not produce saliva following a destruction of the salivary glands usually secondary to radiation therapy. The result is pain everyday that degrade the live of these patients. There are currently sprays and gels to fill the lack of saliva, but these solutions do not allow the patient to receive the saliva continuously.

The anticipated benefits for patients are: greater autonomy, improved quality of life, particularly in the context of social life and greater discretion with respect to the other people and finally an increased efficiency on oral complications and comfort due to direct and regular administration of the substitute on the oral mucosa and dental tissue.

The main investigator of this project is Dr. Edouard Euvrard (INSERM CIT 808 - IBCT INSERM UMR 645). The hospital coordinator manager is Professor Christophe Meyer. He supervises research program and he's Head of the Department of Oral and Maxillofacial Surgery at the University Hospital of Besançon. They are responsible for the definition of specifications (including the physiopathologic aspects) and the surgical acts during pre-clinical studies in animals. They are responsible for writing up intermediary reports and the final report. The study will take place in the department of maxillo-facial surgery of Besançon CHU. The CIC-IT will carry out the necessary administrative steps (writing and submitting a file to the committee for the protection of persons in the East of France, for example), conducting the study and the statistical analysis of the results.

In 2007, project begun with an ISIFC hospital internship. In 2008 and 2009, several steps were taken by Biotika®: defining specifications and technical, pre-record risk analysis, designing a virtual model in CAD with SolidWorks and SpaceClaim, then building a demonstrator incorporating a miniature peristaltic pump alarm with a battery and for filling (PCB feasibility demonstrator, see bellow).

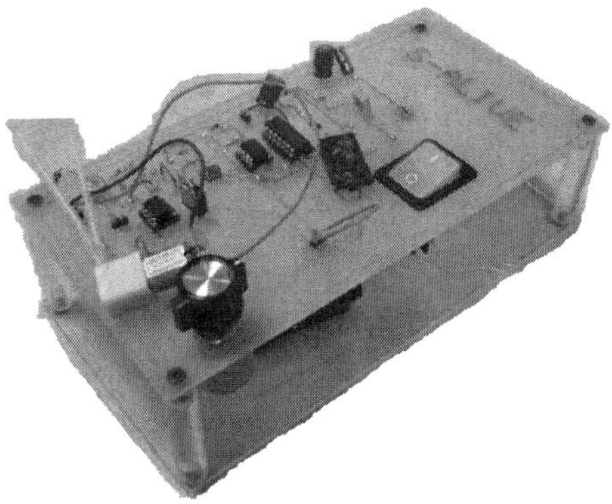

Fig. 13. Feasibility experimental demonstrator

A first patent search (December 2006) led to the submission of a Soleau envelope (Dr. Edouard Euvrard INPI N°305818, December 6, 2007). Recently, with new patent search of March 2010 (ARIST), five competing patents were identified: they are mostly North American with one from France. These patents were not considered a threat to our device by ARIST. Such a device is not currently on the market and the priority analysis shows that freedom to operate and patentability is possible for our idea.

Before the S-Alive ANR project, which has just started, the valorisation framework had already contributed to the realisation of a pre-study, with en amount of 25.000 € through an innovating project maturation fund in 2010. This OSEO-Maturation project names "Substitution of the insufficiency or absence of saliva in patients suffering from xerostomia" and is coordinated between ISIFC/Biotika®, Besancon University Hospital, Department of Maxillo-Facial Surgery, CIC-IT, EA4267 Biologic separative sciences and pharmaceutics laboratory and Vetagro-Sup animal's school and its external providers (Cisteo MEDICAL and Statice Santé firms). A market analysis is also planned for, as well as the realisation of prototype tests on animals to evaluate the risks associated with using this type of device.

12.5 Visiotika

This project aims to enable completely paralyzed patients, such as those suffering from Locked-In Syndrome, to regain some autonomy by giving them the ability to control their environment through their eyes. Currently, such solutions exist but are extremely expensive. Biotika 2007 has made such a device at low cost by simply using common materials. Thus, Visiotika consists of a webcam connected to a laptop quite commonplace, free software easy to use and infrared connections for connecting the PC to control the elements. The motivation is to enable patients to purchase this device for their home. The eye movements of patients captured by the camera can act on the software as you would with a computer mouse. The information is then sent via IR wavelengths to different parts of the patient's environment. Visiotika can control a TV and the hospital bed set up by previous team. It can be easily adapted to other applications, such as the opening of electric shutters, turn on and off the lights...This project is in stand by for the moment.

13. Physiotika® project 's description

Physiotika®, was developed to measure pulse wave velocity, a strong predictor of cardiovascular risk. This innovative device measures pulse wave velocity by using two infra-red probes, placed on two artery sites.
Increased arterial stiffness is associated with an increased risk of cardiovascular events. For example, in patients with chronic renal disease, this risk appears to be far greater than in the general population. Several methods are available to determine arterial stiffness, and pulse wave velocity (PWV) appears to be the most accurate. The current gold standard to measure PWV is through applanation tonometer (AT).
Non-invasive and predictive of adverse cardiovascular outcomes, this device is technically challenging and expensive. However, Physiotika®, a non-invasive method, uses the principle of reflectance PhotoPlethysmoGraphy to detect cardiovascular pulse waves. This is a common optical technique used to monitor peripheral pulsation.
The Physiotika® device described bellow is composed of

- specialized software program (1)
- housing containing a microcontroller (convert the analogical signal into a numeric signal) (3)
- USB cable to connect the housing to the laptop (2)
- two infra-red probes (carotid and radial) (4 and 5)
- neck support to secure the carotid probes (6)
- wrist support to secure the radial probe (7)

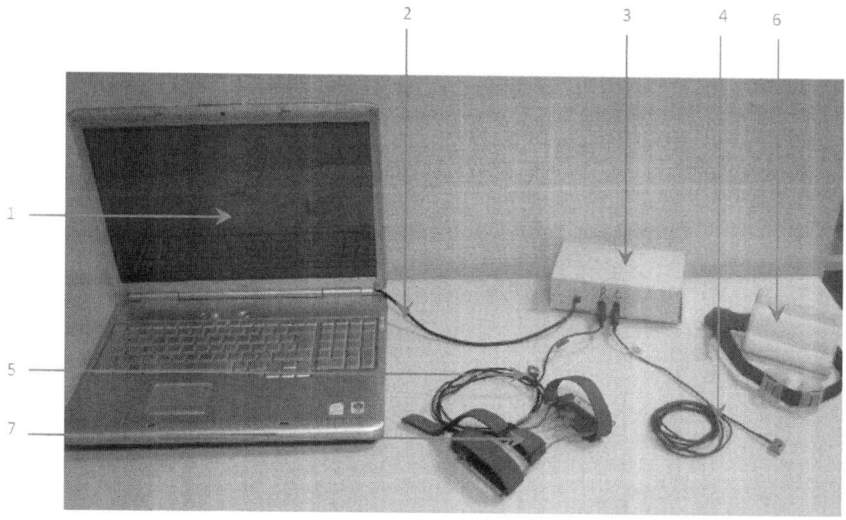

Fig. 14. The Physiotika® device

Three different Biotika® teams (managed firstly by J.Imbert, secondly by C.Soulaine and V.Journot and lastly by B.Jacob) have shown that this new device is able to measure a valid index of PWV, as compared to the AT technique in healthy subjects. This project has been technically established but requires continued validation in a clinical population. This year, we decide to extract this project from Biotika® and to transfer 3 prototypes to researcher partners for new international experimentations (in Venezuela and Colombia) and new campaigns of data's collect.

14. Pre-clinical validations process and regulatory affairs

In fact, Biotika® is able to conduct:

- Technical and preclinical studies
- Technical and preclinical trials
- Technical and preclinical validations

An important vigilance is conducted in these phases.

When we are developing or modifying a medical device, it needs to perform clinical but also animal trials to obtain scientific datas that demonstrate the safety and effectiveness of the new device. When the device is a class I or class IIa classification, it's possible to prove these by bibliographic data. Biotika®'s team can demonstrate scientific and technical concepts and also it can clinical validate the device with simulations and animals trials. We use medical and computing data Center and data research Bases of the University. The clinical investigation works out a contractual arrangement with the teaching and research Hospital of Besançon University (Centre d'Investigation Clinique, CIC). The CIC sponsor (Doctor Lionel Pazart) is responsible for selecting investigators, submits research protocol and human care assurance.

14.1 Example of Physiotika® Investigations

This example of investigations are conducted by a student, J.Picouley, during her 3 months R&D intership. It was just after Biotika 2009 exercise and a previous 2008 R&D internship (N.Mathias).

It was located in the Clinical Renal Investigation Unit at the Kingston General Hospital Satellite Dialysis Clinic, in Kingston (Canada). Trisha Parsons, Assistant Professor, School of rehabilitation therapy at Queen's University was the tutor of this intership. It's an important collaboration with Nicolas Tordi, general coordinator of Physiotika® project. N.Tordi is professor at the University of Franche-Comté and works with ISIFC. The purpose of this study was to determine the test-retest reliability on healthy volunteers and to perform a pilot assessment of the response to change during dialysis. Preliminary results suggest that the Physiotika® device may offer a reliable, low-cost alternative for the clinical assessment of PWV.

Renal failure is associated with an increased prevalence of cardiovascular morbidity and mortality. Arterial stiffness, as determined by pulse wave velocity, is predictive of adverse cardiovascular outcomes such as left ventricular hypertrophy, heart failure, hypertension, and cardiovascular related mortality in the population with kidney disease.

The current gold standard method for assessing arterial stiffness is through the use of applanation tonometry. This method is highly skill dependent and results in difficulty pooling data from different examiners. Given the logistic considerations with subject recruitment, it has been postulated that an alternative method of determining pulse wave velocity using infra-red technology, may provide greater inter-tester reliability.

14.2 S-Alive example

The animals' laboratory, Vetagro Sup in Lyon, works with us for animals trials. If the trial doesn't involve significant risk for patients, a patient consent forms is only necessary to collect clinical datas for human use. The trials and validations campaign conduct to the risk management report in accordance with regulatory expectations.

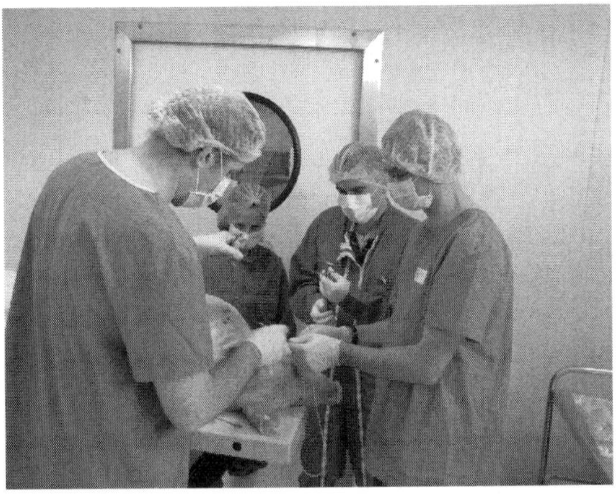

Fig. 15. Professor C.Meyer, Doctors E.Euvrard and L.Pazart , S-Alive mean coordinators and Biotika®'s partners. First tests on animal monitored by Vetagro Sup.

S-alive project is an active implantable medical devices [AIMD] requiring surgery. Our device will be part of the class IIb Rule 8 (EC Directive 2007/47). Sole responsibility of AIMD's manufacturer is subjected to obtaining the CE mark in "essential conformity" with health and safety requirements set by EU directives (93/42 / CE for medical devices 90/385/EEC). And in this context, the most complex issue in order to obtain the CE mark will remain "the risk management analysis" according to EN ISO 14971:2007 which is mandatory provision. Biotika®'s team participates to the product development with Hospital of Besançon and Cisteo MEDICAL company. The ANR's purposes program is to qualify "the risk / benefit ratio" by referencing all possible risks associated with the physical characteristics of the device, its use before and during manufacture, predictable external influences, medical or surgical procedures, ionizing radiation (sterilization due to radiation), a fault or aging of the device.

15. Conclusion

In the scope of a new module, the ISIFC launched in May 2006 its own virtual company, named by students Biotika®. Virtual means that this company has no real legal status. It is a sort of pedagogic model but on the other hand, the situation scenario for the ISIFC student engineers is itself indeed real. They are currently working-in real conditions-on the development of new medical devices or on modernization of medical products. The needs of these innovative medical devices were identified by the students during their second-year (6 weeks) work experience in hospital. Every year, this activity takes place between March to December. The end-year students were recruited following an imitation job interview and each of them was entrusted with a mission (engineer or project manager) in one of the company's four departments; R&D, Quality-regulatory affairs, Clinical investigations and Public relations-marketing. Every two days per week and for seven months, the personal of Biotika® works on development of innovative medical devices and on the preparation of CE marking or FDA. Biotika® developed **eight products since 2006.**

Biotika® works on medical devices development projects and on research for patients and clinicians. It became in 5 years a real academic pre incubation cell. Firstly, Biotika® was awarded a financial prize of 15.000€ by the OSEO Agency and Valorisation Department of the Besançon University (maturation funds). It was in June 2006. The youth chamber JCE allowed to our virtual firm participating in European competition for the innovative company in category INNOVACT Community (Reims, October 2006). We participate every year to industrial meetings such as MEDTEC FRANCE and MICRONORA.

We obtained:

- In 2009 a real partnership with Besançon University Hospital's CIC-IT
- In 2010 a real partnership with Cisteo MEDICAL, start-up created in Besançon
- By 5 times, financial support given by OSEO/UFC Valorisation Department

These supports in maturation of innovative projects were intended for the pain and salivary disorders treatment, and for the gastroenterology and cardiovascular diagnosis.

- 5 clinical trials
- 9 R&D and hospital ISIFC internships

Recently, the selection to the ANR (National Agency for Research) is going to allow developing industrial prototypes of technical substitution of saliva for the maxilla facial cancer research with Besançon University Hospital, EA 4267 Laboratory, Cisteo MEDICAL start up and Lyon animals' school. For this 2010 ANR campaign, only 30 projects are selected and obtained 2 years financial support for 271 national candidates.

For the moment, no Biotika®'s product is still marketed. Two patents are in the course of writing, 4 Soleau Letters are INPI registered. The main difficulty is not due to unavailability of the students, in contrary! They are principally due to their irregular presence (discontinuity in the time) and by students coming from different promotion. And for the development of innovative projects, it needs real industrial partnership for a potential transfer. Furthermore because the staff is completely renewed, the transfer between the 2 teams is a critical process and requires a documentary system exemplary.

Very recently, we obtain funds from Franche Comté Economic Chamber (Intelligence Agency) and from University for a real LNE/GMED ISO 13 485 certification. The first audit will be in November 2011.

Three options are selected for Biotika® 2012:

- keep our original and innovative ISIFC's university Biotika® virtual company concept and move every year new ideas and technology to other partner companies (for conventions).
- actually create a company with the status "Thurs Young Enterprise University" (Biotika® 2011 engineering students involved will graduate in July 2012).
- create a "junior company"with 1901 association legal status and for convention with the engineering school ISIFC which currently has 144 students.

Biotika® is in fact a university structured process for helping patients, clinicians and researchers turn a good idea into a viable medical device business.

Biotika® is not a real firm but it's a real innovative education program for graduate excellent biomedical engineers able to develop real innovative medical device.

16. Acknowledgments

The "virtual CEO" would like to thank especially, in agreement with its management team, the eleven co-creators of Biotika. These student engineers / contractors, graduated in 2007, are now working for the real tasks of development and marketing of medical devices for patient care. Firstly, they were: Khalid Azzouzi, Anthony Bataillard, Amandine Botella, Jérémy Degrave, Florent Demonmerot, Emmanuel Gantou, Cyril Gamelon, Mathieu Guillaume, Marie-Claire Leve, Davy Ung and Yohann Viennet. Thank course the young and dynamic who is now provided by all engineering students/Biotika® engineers of ISIFC: the last but not least 2011 Biotika® team (23 students)! But, I particularly want to express my gratitude to 2007, 2008, 2009 and 2010 teams which represent a total of 89 different students. I would have been able to list all their names! Sébastien Thibaud, Sébastien Euphrasie, Nadège Bodin Courjal from FEMTO-ST institute and Jacques Duffaud (ISIFC studies director) and Christophe Moureaux are our scientific experts. Magaly Roy and Mohamed El Hamdaoui are always presents for helping our virtual firm and in fact our students. Sincerely thanks to them. I don't forget our major Besançon's hospital Collaborator Dr Lionel Pazart and his colleagues and physicians and/or researchers: Professors R.Aubry, E.Euvrard, S.Koch, C.Meyer, A.Menget, G.Thiriez, J.Regnard and N.Tordi. This chapter would not have been possible without the enormous support from Georges Soto Romero and Florent Guyon.

17. References

O. Blagosklonov, G. Soto-Romero, F. Guyon, N. Courjal, S. Euphrasie, R. Yahiaoui and N. Butterlin, *Virtual Firm as a Role-Playing Tool for Biomedical Education*, Proceedings of the 28th IEEE EMBS'06, Engineering in medicine and biology conference, New York city, USA, Paper SaC 14.3, pp 5451-5452, August 30-Sept 3, 2006

N. Butterlin, *Biotika students put to the test at a virtual school*, Reference innovation N°5, pp 64-67, November-December 2006, (invited paper)

N. Butterlin, G. Soto-Romero, J. Duffaud, O. Blagosklonov, ISIFC, *Dual Biomedical Engineering School*, Proceedings of the 29th Conference of the IEEE Engineering in Medicine and Biology Society, Lyon, paper FrC12.1, pp3098-3101, August 23-26 2007

N. Butterlin, G. Soto-romero, F. Guyon , *L'entreprise virtuelle Biotika de l'ISIFC ou les grands principes d'une ingénierie pédagogique innovante en relation directe avec les entreprises*, EdP Sciences: J3eA 8, 1024 (2009), DOI: 10.1051/j3ea:2008065, Access Jan. 2009, Aavilable from http://www.j3ea.org/10.1051/j3ea:2008065

A. Moreau-Gaudry, L. Pazart, *Développement d'une innovation technologique en santé : le cycle CREPS, Concept-Recherche-Essais-Produit-Soins*, IRBM 31 (2010)12-21, Biomedical Engineering and Research, Elsevier Masson, Access Feb. 2010 , Available from http://wwwsciencesdirect.com

8

Nano-Engineering of Complex Systems: Smart Nanocarriers for Biomedical Applications

L.G. Guerrero-Ramírez[1] and Issa Katime[2]
[1]Departamento de Química, Universidad de Guadalajara, Centro Universitario de Ciencias Exactas e Ingenierías. Guadalajara Jalisco,
[2]Grupo de Nuevos Materiales y Espectroscopia Supramolecular, Facultad de Ciencia y Tecnología (Campus Leioa),
[1]México
[2]Spain

1. Introduction

The latest research in the area of polymeric materials focus on the design of increasingly complex devices that have a specific objective (Dubé et al., 2002). The knowledge of a world beyond our simple fire vision of research that, in turn, have generated a more complete knowledge about the surrounding environment and the development of new sciences that attempt to explain the behavior of micro scale.
Among the new sciences of the XXI century are to nanotechnology, which is still being developed. The transition from micro to nano scale will provide significant improvements in the understanding of matter and its applications (Katime et al., 2004). Nanotechnology is the study, design, creation, synthesis, manipulation and application of materials, devices and functional systems through control of matter at the nano scale and the exploitation of phenomena and properties of matter at the nano scale.
Nanotechnology requires a new interdisciplinary approach to both research and in fabrication processes (Katime, 1994). We consider two routes: the first is the miniaturization of microsystems and the second mimics nature by building structures from atomic levels molecular (Thomson, 1983). Because of the latter need emerges nanotechnology to biomedicine, science that is now channeled to the study of biological systems, largely based on the science of polymers to achieve this goal (Mendizábal et al., 2000).
One of the areas in the twentieth century has been supplemented to the science of polymers is biomedicine within it, biomaterials have the most diverse types of devices, and that demonstrate the advantages over other materials traditionally used (Lee et al., 1996). Because of its versatility, polymeric hydrogels are a special type of biomaterials whose use has expanded rapidly in many areas of medicine (Lee & Wang, 1996). When designing a synthetic polymer is generally aimed at satisfying a need, in other words, it seeks to confer a characteristic end product that helps solve the problem for which it was designed.
There is a direct relationship between the properties of a hydrogel (or a polymer in general) and its structure, so that both features cannot be considered in isolation, since the method of synthesis has a decisive influence on them. Therefore, when evaluating the properties of the hydrogels is to be referred to the structural parameters that condition

them[8]. In the field of polymers, the term biocompatibility concerns two different aspects, but those are directly related: (a) The high tolerance have to show the tissues to the foreign agent, mostly when the polymer is to be implemented, and (b) chemical stability, and especially physics polymer material during the time that is in contact with the body. There is no single definition of smart polymer; however we can say that is one that to an external stimulus undergoes changes in its physical and/or chemical. The first time I coined the term "smart polymer" was in a newspaper article of the year 1998 (Nata & Yamamoto, 1998). This paper described how a group of researchers from the University of Michigan using Electro-rheological fluids (ER) to create smart materials. These fluids have the potential to change viscosity almost instantly in response to an electrical current. The fact revealed the existence of a new type of material with the ability to modify its properties in a given time and adjust to changes in conditions. Two years later, in 1990, Hamada et al., Published an article in which phase transitions glimpsed a photo-induced gel (Mamada et al., 1990). A year later in 1991 appeared a review article on functional conducting polymers, which envisioned its potential application as intelligent materials (Kwon et al., 1991).

Currently there are several processes which can yield polymeric nanoparticles with a high yield of reaction, however, which allows the production of nanoparticles with high control of its features is the microemulsion polymerization. Microemulsion polymerization is a method with interesting perspectives and a type of polymerization alternative to existing processes to produce polymer latex of high molecular weight but with particle sizes smaller than those obtained in emulsion, which vary from 10 to 100 nm (Escalante et al., 1996; Candau & Buchert, 1990).

Microemulsions are fluid phases, microstructure, isotropic, optically transparent or translucent, at thermodynamic equilibrium, containing two immiscible fluids (usually water and oil) and surfactants (Candau & Zekhinini, 1987). Unlike emulsions are milky, opaque and thermodynamically unstable. The biggest difference between emulsion and microemulsion is given by the amount of surfactant needed to stabilize the system, which is much higher for the case of microemulsions ($\approx$ 10% of the total mass). This restricts the potential use of microemulsions in most applications due to the requirement of a formulation as cheap as possible, characterized by a high proportion monomer/surfactant (Katime et al., 2001).

Hoar and Schulman were the first to introduce the concept of microemulsion and to postulate the first mechanism for the formation of a microemulsión (Corkhill et al., 1987). The reason for the formation of a stable microemulsion is to be found in the analysis of the energies present in dispersion, a fact which can be expressed in terms of Gibbs free energy necessary for the formation of a microemulsion (Hoar & Schulman, 1943).

The nano-hydrogels commonly exhibit volume changes in response to changing environmental conditions (Katime & Mendizábal, 1997). The polymer network can change its volume in response to a change in the environment such as temperature, pH, solvent composition, electrical stimulation, the action of electric fields, etc (Bokias et al., 1997). The combination of molecular interactions such as van der Waals forces, hydrophobic interactions, hydrogen bonds and electrostatic interactions, determine the degree of swelling of hydrogel at equilibrium. If a gel contains ionizable groups, is a pH sensitive gel, since the ionization is determined by the pH in terms of equilibrium ionization (Kurauchi et al., 1991). The variation of pH of the swelling induces changes in the degree of ionization of electrolytes and, therefore, a change in the degree of swelling of the hydrogel. Moreover, the temperature is one of the most significant parameters affecting the phase behavior of the gels. Recent studies show that it is possible to produce hydrogels with a particular transition temperature or even develop hydrogels with various transition temperatures (Kurauchi et al., 1991).

One of the most studied polymers, which respond to temperature changes in the external environment, is poly (N-isopropyl acrylamide) (PNIPA). This polymer undergoes a strong transition in water at 32°C, from a hydrophilic state below this temperature to a hydrophobic state above it. Currently the development of polymeric complexes have bioactive properties, that are able to interact with cellular mechanisms has grown considerably because of the many applications that can take the coupling of biological receptors within the polymer matrices. One of the biological receptor that has attracted interest from the scientific community is folic acid receptor Saunders & Vincent, 1999. The protein encoded by this gene is a member of the folate receptor family (FOLRF). The members of this family of genes have a high affinity for folic acid and reduction of various folic acid derivatives, in addition to mediate the delivery of 5-methyl tetrahydrofolate inside cells. This gene is composed of 7 exons, exons 1 to 4 encode the 5 'UTR and exons 4 through 7 encode the open reading frame. Due to the presence of 2 promoters, there are multiple transcription start sites and alternative splicing of exons, there are several variants of the transcript derived from this gen (Choi et al., 1988).

The importance of folate receptor is that in various diseases this gene is overexpressed on the cell surface that makes it easy to capture through the cellular process of receptor-mediated endocytosis RME (Tannock & Rotin, 1989). Folic acid, in addition to high specificity towards the tumor tissue, offers potential advantages, including its small size, which carries favorable pharmacokinetics, reduced immunogenicity allowing repeated administration, high availability and safety (Vert, 1986). Devices for controlled release of drugs are an especially important application that exploits the collapse-swelling properties of the polymers in response. In this field are particularly important hydrogels containing poly (N-isopropyl acrylamide) (PNIP), which generate matrices that can exhibit thermally reversible collapse above the LCST of the homo polymer is taken as base (Stubbs et al., 2000).

The collapse in the structure of the matrix is accompanied by loss of water and any co-solute, as it may be a therapeutic agent or active ingredient. Drug expulsion and loss of water takes place at the initial stage of gel collapse, followed by a slower release of drug that diffuses from the gel visibly shrunken and physically compacted (Rivolta et al., 2005). A useful synthesis allows delivery systems be prepared to respond to a pre-designated value of pH and/or temperature to release some kind of drug. For drug delivery applications the response of the nanogels should be nonlinear with different levels of expectation and response, that is where the key is to develop materials that should show strong transitions to a small stimulus or change in the environment. One way to accomplish this is by defining the structures of micro and nano-scale.

2. Nano-engineering of nanometric systems

One of the main challenges in designing a delivery system directed or specific control variables is necessary for the device you are thinking about getting this necessary features for use depending on which system to be used. The case of the current treatments for cancer therapy devices required to recognize a biological marker on the surface of tumor cells, so

that this device can act as a mechanism Tipi "Trojan horse", which tumor cell invaginates the vehicle as if it were a necessary nutrient for cellular functions. Having recognized the growing problem: How can the vehicle be able to release their cargo within the cell cytoplasm? To answer this question it is necessary to consider some facts: a) new research has shown that folic acid specific ligand is over expressed in cancer cells and can be also referred to as a tumor marker. Also, as already mentioned in this work that the folate receptor is one of the 25 receptors that mediate the endocytosis process mediated by receptors (Mathur & Scranton, 1996) (previously described), b) the pH inside the tumor cell has a decrease to a value of 4.5 (Katime et al., 2009) and c) the average body temperature is near 36°C (Katime et al., 2008).
Focusing on these facts we can say that the design of a nanostructure that can be used to treat diseases like cancer must submit specificity, sensitivity to pH and temperature.

2.1 pH-sensitivity

If a gel contains ionizable groups, is a pH sensitive gel, since the ionization is determined by the pH in terms of ionization equilibrium. The variation of pH of the swelling induces changes in the degree of ionization of electrolytes and, therefore, a change in the degree of swelling of the hydrogel. Table 1 shows the functional groups that can induce changes in the polymer network to changes in pH.

Stimulus	Hydrogel Type	Release Mechanism
pH	Acidic or basic hydrogel	Change in pH-swelling-release of drug
Ionic Strength	Ionic hydrogel	Change in ionic strength-change in concentration of ions inside the gel-change in swelling-release of drug
Chemical species	Hydrogel containing electron-accepting groups	Electron-donating compounds-formation of charge-transfer complexes-change in swelling-release of drug
Thermal	Thermo-responsive hydrogel	Change in temperature-change in polymer-polymer and water-polymer interactions-change in swelling-release of drug
Enzyme substrate	Hydrogel containing immobilized enzymes	Substrate present-enzymatic conversion-product changes swelling of gel-release of drug
Electrical	Polyelectrolyte hydrogel	Applied electric field-membrane charging-electrophoresis of charged drug-change in swelling-release of drug
Magnetic	Magnetic particles dispersed in microspheres	Applied magnetic field-change in pores in gel-change in swelling-release of drug

Table 1. Effect of Different External Stimuli on the release of Bioactive Molecules from Smart Nanohydrogels (Katime 2010).

Therefore, the understanding to the sensitivity to a change in pH for drug transport vehicle is based on the incorporation of ionizable groups within the polymer matrix. These groups will be responsible for ensuring, through its characteristics, the change in size in the pores of the polymer network with some variation of pH. Studies by Katime and colleagues (2009) show that depending on the type of ionizable structure, a polymer gel can change their swelling properties - collapse before a stimulation of pH, specifically the gels with more basic properties studied in recent years are those who owe their acid-base properties to the presence of pyridine rings in its structure molecular (Katime et al., 2005).

Pyridine is a cationic ionizable group has a pKa value of 5.2, so this functional group appears to be a strong candidate to obtain pH-sensitive cationic gels having a pH of swelling (pH_s) around 5 (Figure 1).

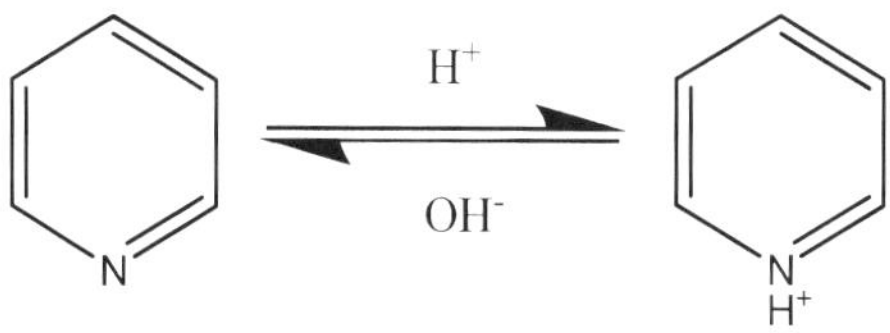

Fig. 1. Ionizing process of the pyridine ring.

One way to achieve the inclusion of pyridine functional groups is the copolymerization with vinyl monomers derived from the ionizable group, as is the case of 4-vinylpyridine (4VP) and 2-vinylpyridine (2VP). Polymerization and crosslinking leads to the obtaining of intersecting networks pyridine ring and ortho position respectively, with the carbonate skeleton of the network.

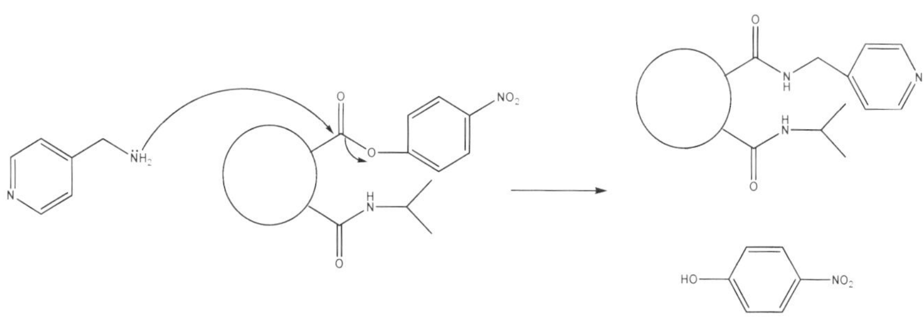

Fig. 2. Synthetic procedure proposed by Katime and coworkers to obtain microgels with ionizable pyridine groups.

Loxley and Vincent (1997) synthesized microgels by copolymerizing 2-vinylpyridine and styrene, and found its swelling at pH values lower than 4531, while Fernandez-Nieves et al. (2000) studied the volume phase transition of microgels obtained from the direct polymerization of 2 vinyl pyridine, finding a pH of swelling of 4.032. Snowden et al. for their part, have been studied extensively in recent years cationic copolymer microgels of P (NIPA-co-4VP), and have found pH-sensitive properties of swelling with pH change 5.5. These microgels 4VP derivatives, obtained by different synthesis methods have also been recently studied by Vincent et al. (2005), also found pH-sensitive properties, although the pH of swelling were determined to be lower (~ pH 3.5-4.0). More recently, several studies show that 4-aminomethyl pyridine (4AMP) coupled in post polymerization reactions to a crosslinked polymer network, can govern the collapse-swelling transition at a pH of 4.53-36

(Figure 2), by use of molecules with "good leaving groups" allowing the incorporation of 4AMP within the polymer network (Guerrero-Ramírez, 2008).

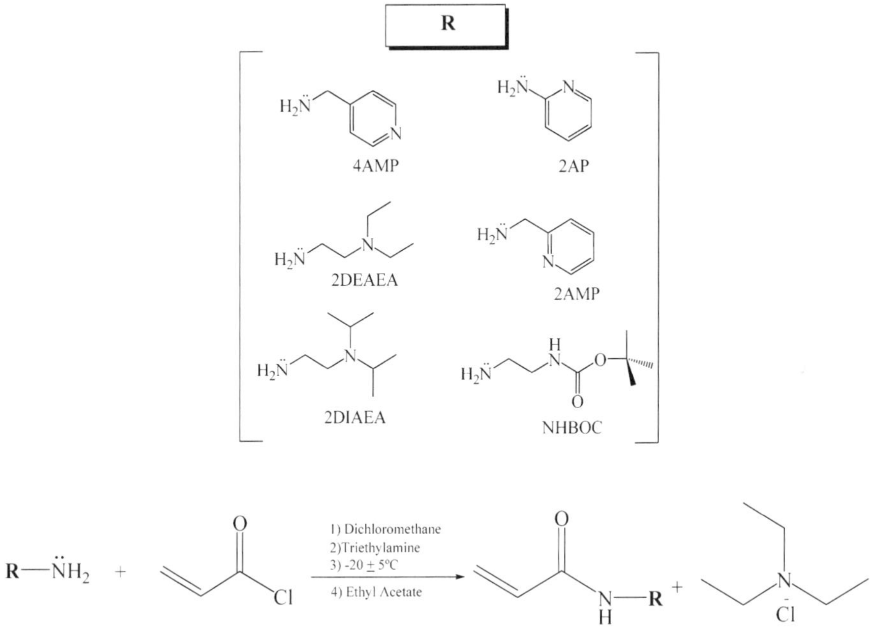

Fig. 3. Schematic procedure proposed by Katime et al. (2010) for the synthesis of amine-based monomers.

Katime et al. (2010) have proposed the synthesis of vinyl monomers from amines for potential use in modification reactions that result in the ownership of pH sensitivity for polymeric gels (Agüero et al., 2010). The synthesis of monomers is a simple procedure that involves a nucleophilic substitution reaction by the use of a "good leaving group (Figure 3). Such reactions have a yield above 80%, which generates a good alternative to the inclusion of these compounds to drug transport vehicles.

2.2 Temperature sensitivity

Temperature is one of the most significant parameters affecting the phase behavior of the gels. Recent studies show that it is possible to produce hydrogels with a particular transition temperature or even develop hydrogels with various transition temperatures (Guerrero-Ramírez et al., 2008). One of the most studied polymers, which respond to temperature changes in the external environment, is poly(N-isopropyl acrylamide) (PNIPA). This polymer undergoes a strong transition in water at 32°C, from a hydrophilic state below this temperature to a hydrophobic state above it. Above the phase transition, as shown schematically in figure 4, is based on the entropic gain associated water molecules to the side chain isopropyl substituent.

The temperature at which this happens (called lower solution critical temperature or LCST) corresponds to the region in the phase diagram in which the enthalpic contribution of water bound to the polymer chain is less than the entropic gain of the system as whole and, therefore, depends largely on the ability to form hydrogen bonds and the chemical nature of constituent monomer units. Consequently, the LCST of a polymer can be adjusted to measure the variation in the content of hydrophilic or hydrophobic co-monomers.

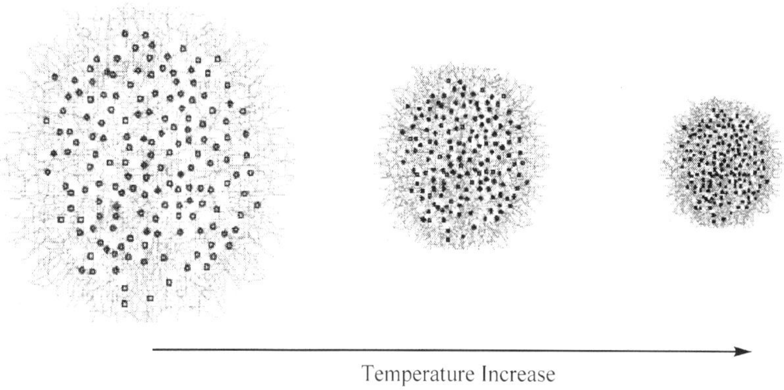

Fig. 4. Temperature behavior of typical pNIPA hydrogel.

3. Synthetic mechanisms

A nanogel is polymer network that is ranged between 10 to 100 nm of particle size. The nanogeles can present well defined structures as a spherical structure or heterogeneous structure (non-defined structure). The synthesis of nanohydrogels besides the usual elements in any polymerization such as solvent, monomer or monomers and the initiator, it requires a crosslinking agent, who will be responsible for the crosslininked structure (Hervias et al., 2008; Guerrero-Ramírez et al., 2008; Guerrero-Ramírez et al., 2008; Bruck & Mueller, 1988; Agüero et al., 2010). For this purpose the synthetic procedure can be done using a large number of monomers that are classified divided in three different categories (Murray & Snowden, 1995): a) Monomer with no lateral ionizing groups, b) Monomers with ionizable functional groups and, c) Zwitterionic monomers.

There are several methods for preparing crosslinked hydrogels. One of this methods that is widely use is by a chemical reaction, this method is a copolymerization and crosslinking reaction between one or more monomers and multifunctional monomers which is present in very small quantities. Initiation systems that can be used are those used in conventional polymer synthesis: thermal decomposition of an initiator, temperature, ionic initiators, gamma radiation or redox.

Also it is possible to obtain crosslinking by the polymerization of a concentrated solution which can cause self-crosslinking through the elimination of hydrogen atoms in the polymer backbone, followed by combinations of radicals. The choice of the crosslinking agent is essential to optimize the properties of the hidrogel (Orrah et al., 1988).

There are different ways to reach a successful synthetic procedure: within which are precipitation polymerization, emulsion, microemulsion and nanoemulsion. Each is aimed at obtaining polymeric materials with different characteristics.

Among these, the microemulsion polymerization is offered more versatility because through it is possible to obtain very small particles (10-150 nm) by synthetic variation of different parameters within which we can find the surfactant system The oil phase, the aqueous phase, monomer ratio, the amount and type of crosslinking agent, the amount and type of initiator and the addition of compounds capable of reducing ionic micellar space.

Recently there have been reports of the synthesis of microgels using a new polymerization technique, microemulsion polymerization, which allows for smaller particle sizes (15-40 nm) than those obtained by emulsion polymerization (Zhang et al., 2002).

Microemulsion polymerization is an alternative to existing processes to produce latex containing polymer of high molar mass but with particle sizes smaller than those obtained by emulsion polymerization (Kudela, 1987; Krane & Peppas, 1991). Microemulsions are fluid phases, microstructured, isotropic, optically transparent or translucent, at thermodynamic equilibrium, containing two immiscible fluids (usually water and oil), contrary to emulsion which are milky, opaque and thermodynamically unstable. An important difference between emulsion and microemulsion is that the amount of surfactant needed to stabilize the micromulsions (> 10% wt) is much greater than that used in the emulsions (1 to 2% wt). This greatly restricts the potential use of microemulsions in most applications, since it is required to use a formulation as cheap as possible (Franson & Peppas, 1991). However, since by microemulsion polymerization it is possible to obtain monodisperse spherical microgels with diameters less than 50 nm (Downey et al., 1999; Tanaka et al., 1984; Osada et al., 1989) there is a promissory future for this technique.

The most important part of a microemulsion is the surfactant. Usually mixtures of surfactants are used to take advantage of each of them and their sinergy (Pelton, 2000). Surfactants are organic compounds that are amphiphilic because they have hydrophobic groups (tails) and hydrophylic groups (heads). Therefore, they are soluble in both organic solvents and water.

There are four types of surfactants: a) Anionic, b) Cationic, c) Non ionic and, d) Amphoteric. Increasing the concentration of surfactant causes the formation of microstructures, which are aggregates of colloidal dimensions that exist in equilibrium with individual surfactant molecules. The concentration at which these microstructures (micelles) are formed is the critical aggregation concentration (CAC).

The micellization phenomena is a cooperative process in which a large number of surfactant molecules associate to form a closed aggregate. When forming the micelles, the critical aggregation concentration is called critical micelle concentration (CMC). The critical micelle concentration depends on the number, length, type, branching or substitution of the hydrophobic chain and the nature of the polar group. The effects favoring micellization produce a decrease in the critical micelle concentration and viceverse.

The type of micelles that are formed depends on the properties of the surfactant and dissolution. The micellization is a cooperative process in which a large number of surfactant molecules associate to form a closed aggregate in which the nonpolar parts of the surfactant are separated from the water. The micellization process occurs through a series of conflicting effects: 1) effect that tend to favor the formation of a micelle and the hydrophobic effect, which increases with the size of the hydrocarbon chain of surfactant, and 2) effect that tend to oppose the formation of a micelle, as the repulsion between the hydrophilic groups, particularly important in ionic surfactants.

The presence of alcohol, which is sandwiched between the surfactant molecules at the interface, or the addition of electrolytes to produce a screen effect that reduces the intermolecular electric field, reduces the repulsive forces favoring the micelización (Zhu et al., 1989).

The critical micelle concentration depends on the number, length, nature, saturation, branching or substitution of the hydrophobic chain and the nature of the polar group. The effects that favor the micellization produce a decrease in critical micelle concentration and vice versa.

When is added to the medium a salt or an ionic monomer, latex stabilization is achieved (Antonietti & Bremser, 1990). It is known that the addition of an electrolyte to an aqueous solution produces a variation in the cloud point, i.e. the point at which the solubility changes. When this addition causes a migration of surfactant molecules into the oil phase, increasing the packing of it at the interface, it favors the formation of the microemulsion, due to an increase in the solubility by the presence of salt (salting out). If instead there is a decrease in the cloud point, there is a decrease in solubility by the presence of the salt (salting in). These phenomena are usually related to changes in the water structure around the ions which modify the interactions between water and the surfactant (Funke et al., 1998). Ions such as Na^+ and K^+ decrease the of the surfactant polar head, while ions such as $SCN^-$and I^-, favor the solvation of the surfactant making it more water soluble (Kazakov et al., 2002). In general, the introduction of an electrolyte with salting out effect causes a change in the hydrophilic-lipophilic (HLB) balance of the surfactant, shifting the optimum HLB to form a microemulsion towards higher values. Regarding the preparation method, there is a difference between these two types of dispersions, which focuses on the order of addition of components. In the emulsion case the addition order is very important, contrary to what happens in the formation of microemulsions, where it is not important.

3.1 Inverse microemulsion polymerization

The inverse microemulsion polymerization is based on training, pre-polymerization, microemulsion system of water in oil, which include micromicelas containing monomers to react. Within this group, with globular structure and those with bicontinuous structure.

The inverse microemulsion polymerization of monomers soluble in water is a particularly suitable method for preparing high molecular weight polymers and fast reaction rates (Nata & Yamamoto, 1998), due to high local concentration of monomer within each particle as the growth of radical separate particles prevents termination by combination.

According to studies by Candau, throughout the reaction there is an excess of surfactant stabilizing micells (Candau & Leong, 1985). Two populations are shown as typical colloidal aggregates: a particle with a diameter of about 50 nm and a micelle. It has also been observed that the number of particles increases continuously throughout the polymerization reaction due to excess surfactant, which makes the amount of micelles is at all times well above the particle, allowing for entry of radicals nucleation into micelles. According to the kinetic mechanism for the inverse microemulsion polymerization is depicted in figure 5, the radicals are absorbed into the micelles. They react with the monomer to spread and form a polymer particle. This particle is growing due to the contribution of monomer from other micelles that act as reserve deposits. Eventually the system is reduced to two populations of polymer particles and a water swollen micelles.

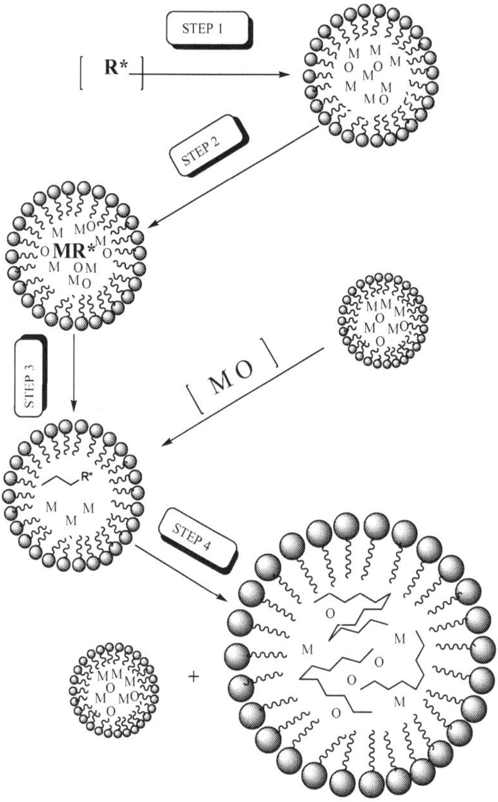

Fig. 5. Kinetic mechanism for the inverse microemulsion polymerization.

4. Bioactive nanosystems

Currently the development of polymeric complexes have bioactive properties, i.e. that are able to interact with cellular mechanisms has grown considerably because of the many applications that can take the coupling of biological receptors within the polymer matrices. Among these recipients are: acetylcholine receptor, cytokine receptor, insulin receptor T cell receptor, recipient of transforming growth factor beta, receptor phosphotyrosine phosphatase, receptor guanylyl cyclase, muscarinic receptor, M1 muscarinic receptor, muscarinic receptor M2, muscarinic receptor M3, M4 muscarinic receptor, nicotinic receptor, mineralocorticoid receptor.

But a biological receptor that has attracted interest from the scientific community is folic acid receptor (Candau & Zekhinini, 1986). The protein encoded by this gene is a member of the folate receptor family (FOLRE). The members of this family of genes have a high affinity for folic acid and reduction of various folic acid derivatives, in addition to mediate the delivery of 5-methyl tetrahydrofolate inside cells. This gene is composed of 7 exons, exons 1 to 4 encode the 5 'UTR and exons 4 through 7 encode the open reading frame. Due to the presence of 2 promoters, there are multiple transcription start sites and alternative splicing of exons, there are several variants of the transcript derived from this gene.

The importance of folate receptor is that in various diseases this gene is overexpressed on the cell surface that makes it easy to capture through the cellular process of receptor-mediated endocytosis EMR (Bleiberg et al., 1998). Folic acid, whose chemical structure is shown in figure 6, is a natural vitamin required for transfer reactions in many metabolic processes and is now a promise in the vectorization of anticancer drugs. Several investigations in recent decades have concluded that folic acid receptors have a preferential expression in ovarian, endometrial, lung, kidney, colon, among others, but are very limited in the normal tissues (Boggs et al., 1996; Castro et al., 2005; Alléman et al., 1993; Coney et al., 1991). This specific folate-cancer cell has been used for the design of anticancer using folic acid as the ligand molecule to the director of their tumoral cells (Weitman et al., 1992; Garin-Chesa et al., 1993; Ross et al., 1994; Anderson et al., 1992).

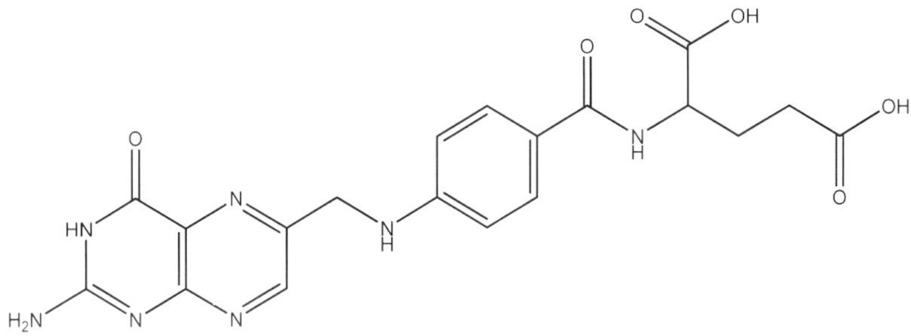

Fig. 6. Molecular structure of folic acid.

Folic acid, in addition to high specificity towards the tumor tissue, offers potential advantages, including its small size, which carries favorable pharmacokinetics, reduced immunogenicity allowing repeated administration, high availability and safety. Moreover, folic acid is stable at very different temperatures and in a variety of solvents, and in slightly acidic or basic media, unlike antibodies that require careful handling to avoid distortion. Another point to note is that it is cheaper than the aforementioned monoclonal antibodies. All this, combined with its relatively simple chemical conjugation, makes it an interesting and promising molecule specific antitumoral therapies (Bronstein, 2004).

To determine at which pH these folate conjugates are subject to when passing into the intracellular environment, in studies it has been measured indirectly the pH of individual endosomes containing folate conjugates and it was found that although this value can vary considerably (4.7-5.3), the average pH is 5.0 (Brannon-Peppas, 1997; Tannock & Rotin, 1989; Vert, 1986; Stubbs et al., 2000; Katime et al., 2006). This pH is markedly different of the physiological pH of the blood stream and of any healthy tissue (pH = 7.4).

5. Membrane cell transport: receptor-mediated endocytosis (RME)

Endocytosis is a cellular process by which the cell introduces large molecules or particles, and does so by including them in an invagination of the cytoplasm membrane, forming a vesicle that eventually breaks off and enters the cytoplasm. When endocytosis leads to the capture of particles is called phagocytosis, and when only portions of liquid are captured is called pinocytosis. Pinocytosis traps substances indiscriminately, while receptor-mediated endocytosis only includes those molecules that bind to the receptor being this type of endocytosis very selective. The RME allows cells to take specific macromolecules called ligands, such as proteins that bind insulin (a hormone), transferrine (a protein that binds to iron), cholesterol carriers and low density lipoproteins.

1) The RME requires specific membrane receptors to recognize a particular ligand and link to it, 2) ligand-receptor complexes migrate along the surface of the membrane structures called coated pits. Just inside the cytoplasm, these pits are lined with a protein that can polymerize into a cage-shaped structure (membrane vesicle), and 3) The vesicles move within the cytoplasm, taking the ligand from the extracellular fluid to within the cell. The materials bound to the ligand, such as iron or cholesterol, are introduced into the cell, then the empty ligand returns to the surface.

Devices for controlled release of drugs are an especially important application that exploits the collapse-swelling properties of the polymers in response. In this field are particularly important hydrogels containing poly (N-isopropyl acrylamide) (PNIPA), which generate matrices that can exhibit thermally reversible collapse above the LCST of the homopolymer is taken as base (Mathur & Scranton, 1996).

The collapse in the structure of the matrix is accompanied by loss of water and any co-solute, as it may be a therapeutic agent or active ingredient. Drug expulsion and loss of water takes place at the initial stage of gel collapse, followed by a slower release of drug that diffuses from the gel shrunk visibly and physically compact.

When the polymer matrix has been incorporated into a co-monomer to respond when the polymer changes state, swelling of the gel can be exploited as a release mechanism to change as a result of the expansion of the polymer. The smart nanogels have the potential to be used with a variety of drug loading and release of active ingredients as well as features and release can be adapted to a wide range of different environments (Bruck & Mueller, 1988; Alléman et al., 1993; Bleiberg et al., 1998).

A useful synthesis allows delivery systems be prepared to respond to a pre-designated value of pH and/or temperature to release some kind of drug. For drug delivery applications the response of the nanogels should be nonlinear, i.e., with different levels of expectation and response, that is where the key is to develop materials that should show strong transitions to a small stimulus or change in the environment. One way to accomplish this is by defining the structures of micro and nano-scale.

5.1 Smart nanocarriers

Smart copolymeric nanoparticles can be synthesized using a microemulsion polymerization process using a reported method (Guerrero-Ramírez et al., 2008). The microemulsion solution was introduced in a mechanical reactor at 25 ± 1°C operated at 131 rpm and nitrogen was bubbled to maintain an inert atmosphere during the whole reaction. The monomers N (4-methyl pyridine) acrylamide (NPAM) and tert-butyl 2 acrylamidoethyl carbamate (2AAECM) are not commercial products, they were synthesized by a nucleophilic substitution reaction from the precursors, modified 4AMP and BOC, respectively. To obtain NPAM monomer, 4AMP reagent was previously prepared and reacted with acryloil chloride at -5°C under vigorous stirring to produce a nucleophilic substitution by the amino functional group and releasing HCl to the average reaction. The 2AAECM synthesis procedure involves several steps: the first was to obtain a di-tert-butyl dicarbonate (BOC) modified by reaction with ethylenediamine at -19°C using dichloromethane as a reaction medium and when all the BOC reactive was added the reaction was maintained for 16 hours at 25°C. Then, dichloromethane was evaporated and the diprotected amine formed as a secondary product was separated due is insoluble in water, so water was added to precipitate system. Diprotected amine was separated by filtration and the resulting solution was saturated with NaCl and extracted with ethyl acetate. Then the solution was dried by adding anhydrous sodium sulphate and the final product was obtained by rotoevaporation. Finally, the resulted product of the reaction was reacted with acryloil chloride to produce an active monomer (2AAECM).

This kind of particles can be used to load, transport and deliver active drugs. These characteristics permits that smart nanocarriers be use against different diseases including cancer or tuberculosis.

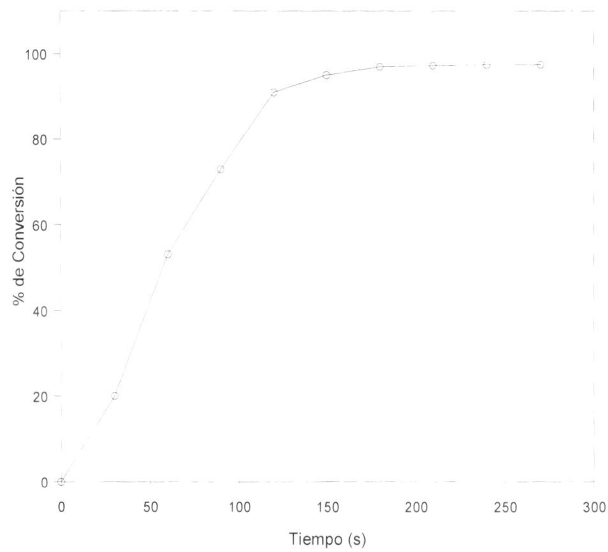

Fig. 7. Polymerization kinetics for COP23 sample obtained using a gravimetric method.

In the case of anti-cancer therapies it is also necessary the functionalization with folic acid, as it has been described, this director molecule is widely used as a biological cellular marker due to it is overexpressed in a number of human tumors, including cancer of lung, kidney and blood cells.

Dissolution of folic acid is prepared by mixing it with 1-(3-dimethylaminopropyl)-3-ethyl carbodiimide hydrochloride (EDC) and tryethylamine, at 25°C, using magnetic stirring for one hour to produce activated folic acid. This mixture is dropped into a dispersion of nanogels in water to incorporate the guide molecule. The purification and the isolating procedure of the final product is carried out by dialysis using a phosphate buffer solution of pH = 7.4, and then distilled water. All of this procedure is performed in a dark environment to avoid degradation of the folic acid molecule.

The total reaction time for obtaining this type of system is estimated at an average of 3 minutes. Figure 7 can be seen that reaction times higher than the 3 minutes are not a significant change in conversion rate. As low curing times, with conversions above 97%, produce nanoparticles more efficiently.
An important fact is that in samples where the amount of initiator used in the synthesis is increased, decreased reaction time. For this system has not been given this trend, because as mentioned, the average reaction times for all cases are set at 3 minutes.
The particle size of several samples of smart nanogels have been synthesized, for all formulations, small particle sizes. Table 1 shows this behavior, in the same way, the remarkable effect of initiator concentration on particle size has a tendency that increasing the initiator concentration, particle size decreases. On the other hand, the particle size of the nanogels synthesized with different concentrations of crosslinking agent and different amounts of salt added, show that the particle diameter decreases nanogel depending on the content of crosslinking agent. As can be seen when the concentration of crosslinker increases, the particle diameter decreases. However, there is a concentration limit, both as crosslinking initiator, from which particle size can not decrease nanogel more.

Sample code	%crosslinker	%initiator	%KNO_3	Dp (nm)
COP20	5	1	0	45
COP21	5	2	0	43
COP22	5	3	0	40
COP23	5	4	0	38
COP24	5	5	0	36
COP25	4	5	0	40
COP26	3	5	0	42
COP27	2	5	0	41
COP28	1	5	0	41
COP29	5	3	0	42
COP30	5	3	0	40
COP31	5	3	0	42
COP32	5	3	0	41
COP33	5	3	0	40
COP34	5	3	2	35
COP35	5	3	4	33
COP36	5	3	6	30
COP37	5	3	8	28
COP38	5	3	10	28

Table 1. Particle sizes of smart nanogels obtained by QELS.

The addition of a soluble salt such as potassium nitrate (KNO_3) produced a reduction of space inside the micelles because the salt creates a series of charges in the continuous phase. They produce a reduction in size of the micelle by the action of electrostatic forces external to that micelle, thereby limiting the size of the particles. This effect can be seen in the same table, so that when the concentration of KNO_3 increases, the particle size is reduced, and when the concentration of KNO_3 is greater than or equal to 5% (based on the total amount of monomers). Particle size has no appreciable change and remains constant.
The micrograph of a nano-synthesized samples is presented in figure 8, this figure shows the spherical nature of the obtained nanoparticles.

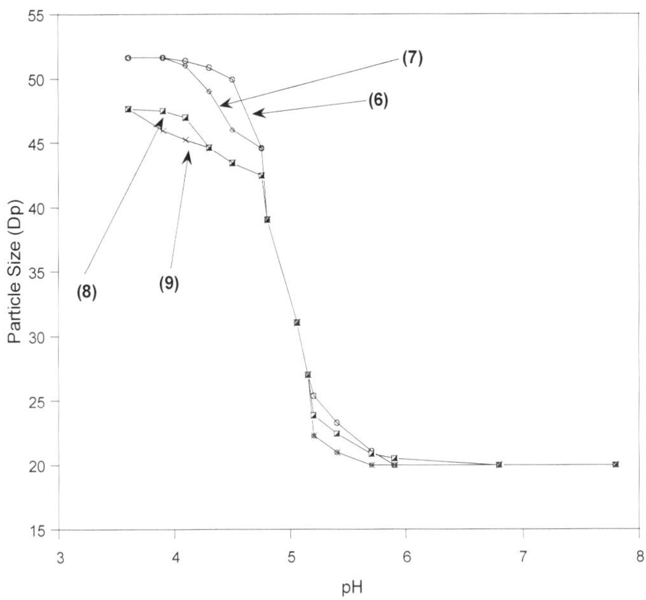

Fig. 8. Variation of particle size of the nanogels. Samples COP25(6), COP26 (7), COP 28 (8) and COP29 (9).

Moreover, when these particles are subjected to changes in pH values can be clearly seen as the inclusion of molecules ionizing groups within the skeleton of the system allow the nanogel have an answer "smart" to these variations. This can be seen in Figure 8, which shows that at pH values lower than 4.5 the nanogel is in the swollen state while values close to 5 the gel collapses.
Because these nanoparticles are designed primarily for use in cancer therapy, the choice of the active ingredient can be transported by this system must comply with the desired characteristics of an anticancer drug. For this reason we have chosen the 5-fluorouracil (5FU). 5FU is a drug that blocks the methylation reaction of acid to convert deoxyuridylic thymidylic acid, by inhibiting an enzyme that is important for the synthesis of thymidine.

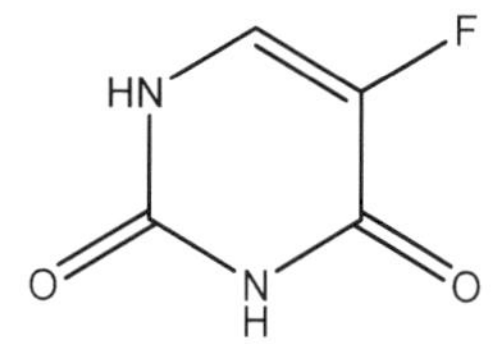

Fig. 9. Chemical structure of 5-fluorouracil (5FU).

5-fluorouracil is involved in DNA synthesis and inhibits the formation of RNA. Both actions are combined to promote a metabolic imbalance that ultimately kills the cell. The inhibitory activity of the drug, by analogy with uracil nucleic acid affect the growth of neoplastic cells, preferably taking advantage of the molecule of uracil for nucleic acid biosynthesis. The effects of DNA and RNA deprivation are more affected cells grow and multiply without control over the normal. Its effectiveness is that it binds irreversibly to the enzyme thymidylate synthase, essential for the synthesis of thymine nucleotides. Thymine is one of four nitrogenous bases that make up the DNA, and lack means that DNA cannot replicate, which inhibits cell division and therefore tumor growth. 5FU structure shown in figure 9.

6. Study of the release kinetics measured by HPLC

To keep track of the release rate of 5FU from the NIPA copolymer nanogels NPAM-2AAECM-HPLC was previously required a calibration with standards of 5-FU. 5FU standards were prepared at concentrations of 0, 10, 20, 30, 40, 50, 60, 70, 80, 90 and 100 ppm, and injected into a liquid chromatograph, using the method described in the experimental section. After obtaining the chromatograms of standards, chromatographic peaks were integrated to obtain the area under the curve, the data obtained for this calibration is shown in table 2.

STD	Concentration (ppm)	Peak area (A.U.)	Retention time T_R (minutes)
1	100	37366	6,58
2	90	33256	6,58
3	80	30749	6,56
4	70	26572	6,55
5	60	22294	6,53
6	50	17353	6,51
7	40	14176	6,51
8	30	11406	6,51
9	20	7615	6,51
10	10	3751	6,51

Table 2. Data obtained for calibration standards of 5-FU.

Before performing the action for the release of 5FU, the nanogels of NIPA-NPAM-2AAECM were loaded with the drug. Recall that the swelling of our nanogels depends on the pH of the medium in which it is, so a simple yet effective to carry the burden of these the nanogels is to introduce a known amount of nanogel in a concentrated solution of 5FU (known concentration) to a pH below 4.5 which guarantees that the nanogel will be swollen in the middle. The set is kept under constant magnetic stirring for 2 hours. After the loading time, changing the pH of the medium to a value greater than 6, which ensures that the nanogel will be collapsed. Thus, when the nanogel collapses, 5FU is retained in the polymer network and water solution ejected from the macromolecular matrix.

To quantify the total burden of nanogels was necessary to take a sample of the remaining load, as the difference in concentration, both initial (before loading) and final (after loading), will indicate the amount 5FU retained in the nanogel.

In the first instance, two experiments were conducted 5FU release two different pH values. The first experiment was performed at pH 7.4, in a release time of 2 hours. In this experiment, there should be no release from the nanogel, since, as mentioned above, the nanogel above a value of 5 on the pH scale is collapsed. However, in this experiment we can see that there is little sign of 5FU in the chromatogram obtained by HPLC, which indicates that in the release medium are molecules of 5FU. This can be attributed to the release of 5-FU molecules absorbed on the surface of nanogel, since the concentration at which 5FU is in the release medium is very small. This behavior can be seen in figure 10.

Furthermore, this experiment was to perform the release at pH 4 during a time of 2 hours, which in our case ensures that the polymer network is in a swollen state, allowing the contents within the nanogel 5FU out release to the environment by diffusion effects. As expected, the chromatogram of this test presents a significant peak of 5FU in a retention time of 6.7 minutes, characteristic of this compound. The chromatogram of this test is shown in figure 11. The total area of this peak has a value of 16,890 A.U.

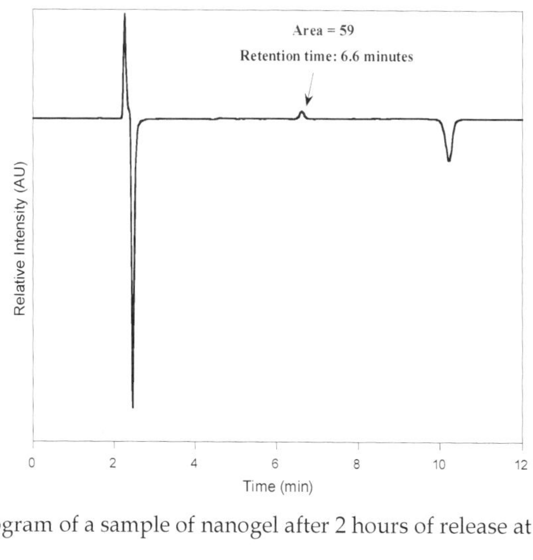

Fig. 10. Chromatogram of a sample of nanogel after 2 hours of release at pH 7.4.

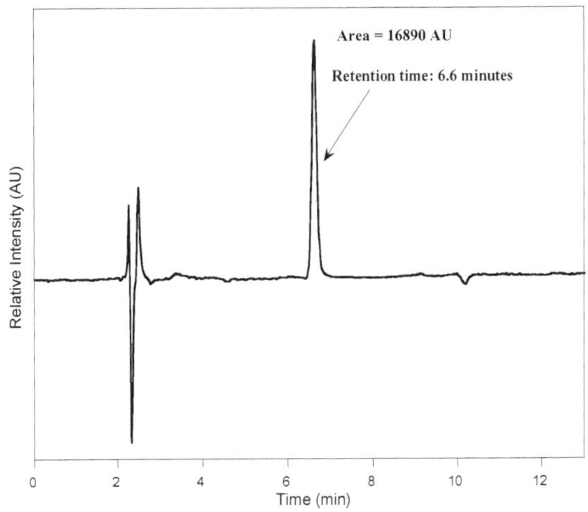

Fig. 11. Chromatogram of a sample of nanogel after 2 hours of release at pH 4.

7. Conclusions

We have synthesized a new pH- and T-responsive smart copolymeric nanohydrogel by inverse microemulsion polymerization. The size particle was determinate by QELS showing an average value of 33 nm. The success of the synthesis was confirmed by FTIR, ^{1}H NMR and DSC. A versatile and successful synthetic strategy to obtain potential nanodevices for targeted drug delivery has been designed. NPA-based copolymeric microgels have been employed as reactive substrate for specific derivatization that led to a smart biomedical function. These precursor microgels were easily chemically modified by aminolysis reaction with amino derivatives to achieve two purposes: firstly, to introduce linkage sites for bonding with the tumor guiding molecule folic acid, which is coupled to the folate receptors in the surface of tumor cells and once internalized by receptor-mediated endocytosis, swell as result of the difference of pH and secondly, to get a specific swelling behavior that determines the capability of the microgels for intelligent therapy. The functionalization with 4-MP leads to an interesting pH-driven swelling transition. This pH-selective swelling potentially leads to an exclusive release of antitumoral drug into the cancer cells. The networks drastically swell when external pH varies from neutral to pH values around 5. There are some facts that influence this swelling behavior, such as copolymer composition.

8. Acknowledgements

The financial support from the Ministerio de Ciencia y Tecnología of Spain is gratefully acknowledged.

9. References

Agüero L., Guerrero-Ramírez L.G. & Katime I., 2010, "New Family of Functionalized Monomers Based on Amines: A Novel Synthesis that Exploits the Nucleophilic Substitution Reaction", *Materials Sciences and Applications,* 1, 103-108, ISSN: 2153-1198.

Alléman E., Doelker E. & Gurny R., 1993, "Drug-loaded nanoparticles-preparation methods and drug targeting issues", *Eur. J. Pharm. Biopharm.*, 39(1), 13-20, ISSN: 0939-6411.

Anderson R. G., Kamen B. A., Rothgber K.G. & Lacey S.W., 1992, "Potocytosis: sequestration and transport of small molecules by caveolae", *Science,* 255, 410, ISSN: 0036-8075

Antonietti M. & Bremser W., 1990, "Microgels: model polymers for the crosslinked state", *Macromolecules,* 23, 3796-3805, ISSN: 0024-9297.

Bleiberg H., Hulstaert F., Buyse M. & De Keyser P., 1998, "Tropisetron in the prevention of acute and delayed nausea and vomiting over six courses of emetogenic chemotherapy, *Anti-cancer drugs,* 9(9), 773 ISSN: 0959-4973.

Boggs L.J., Rives M. & Bike S.G., 1996,"Characterization and rheological investigation of polymer microgels used in automotive coatings", *J. Coat Technol,* 68(855), 63, 63-74, ISSN: 0361-8773

Bokias G., Hourdet D., Ilipoulos I., Staikos G. & Audebert R., 1997, "Hydrophobic Interactions of Poly(*N*-isopropylacrylamide) with Hydrophobically Modified Poly(sodium acrylate) in Aqueous Solution" *Macromolecules,* 30, 8293, ISSN: 0024-9297.

Bronstein L.M., 2004, *Encyclopedia of Nanoscience and Nanotechnology.* Nalwa H.S. (editor), vol 7, 193-214, ISSN: 1550-7033. Indiana University, Bloomington (USA)

Bruck S. D. & Mueller E. P., 1988, "Radiation Sterilization of polymeric implant materials", *J. Biomed. Mater. Res.*, 22 (A2), 133-144, ISSN: 1549-3296.

Candau F. & Buchert P., 1990, "Rheological Studies on inverse microlatices", *Colloids Surf.*, 48, 107-122, ISSN: 0927-7757.

Candau F., Leong Y.S. & Fitch R.M., 1985, "Kinetic Study of the Polymerization of Acrylamide in inverse microemulsion", *J. Polym. Sci. Part. A: Polym. Chem.*, 23, 193-214, ISSN: 1099-0518.

Candau F., Zekhinini Z. & Durand JP., 1986, "Copolymerization of water-soluble monomers in Non-ionic Bicontinous Microemulsion", *J. Colloid Interf. Sci.*, 114(2), 398-408, ISSN: 1095-7103

Candau F. & Zekhinini Z., 1987, "Copolymerization of acrylamide and sodium acrylate in microemulsions", *Prog. Colloid and Sci.*, 73, 33-36, ISSN: 0340-255X

Castro López V., Hadgraft J. & Snowden M.J., (2005), "The use of colloidal microgels as a (trans)dermal drug delivery system", *Int. J. Pharm.*, 292, 137-147. ISSN: 0378-5173.

Choi H.S., Kim J.M., Lee K.J. & Bae Y.C., 1988, "Volume phase transition behavior of *N*-isopropyl acrylamide-*N*-cyanomethyl acrylamide copolymer gel particles: The effect of crosslinking density", *J Appl. Polym. Sci.*, 72(8), 1091-1099. ISSN: 1097-4628.

Coney L.R. Tomaselti A., Carayannopoulos, L. Frasca, V., Kamen B.A., Colnaghi M. I. & Zurawski V.R., 1991, "Cloning of a tumor-associated antigen-MOV18 and MOV19 Antibodies recognize a folate-binding protein", *J. Cancer Res.*, 51, 6125-6132. ISSN: 1538-7445

Corkhill P.H., Jolly A.M., Ng C.O. & Tighe B.J., 1987, "Synthetic hydrogels. 1. Hydroxyalkyl acrylate and methacrylate copolymers-water binding-studies", *Polymer,* 28, 1758-1766. ISSN: 0032-3861

Orrah D.J., Semlyen J.A. & Ross-Murphy S.B., 1988, "Studies of cyclic and linear Poly(Dimethylsiloxanes). 27. Bulk Viscosities above the Critical Molar Mass for Entanglement", *Polymer,* 29, 1452-1454, ISSN: 0032-3861.

Downey J.S., Frank R.S., Li WH. & Stover H.D.H, 1999, "Growth mechanism of poly(divinylbenzene) microspheres in precipitation polymerization", *Macromolecules,* 32, 2838-2844, ISSN: 1520-5835.

Dubé D., Francis M., Leroux J.C., Francoise M. & Winnik D., 2002, "Preparation and tumor cell uptake of poly(N-isopropylacrylamide) folate conjugates", *Biocojugate Chem.,* 13, 685-692. ISSN: 1520-4812.

Escalante I. I., Rodríguez-Guadarrama L.A.; Mendizábal E., Puig J., López R.G. & Katime I., 1996, "Synthesis of Poly(butyl methacrylate) in Three-Component Cationic Microemulsions", *J. Appl. Polym. Sci.,* 62(9), 1313-1323. ISSN: 1097-4628

Franson N.M. & Pepas N.A., 1983, "Influence of copolymer composition on Non-Fickian water transport through glassy copolymers", *J. Appl. Polym. Sci.,* 28, 1303-1310. ISSN: 1097-4628.

Funke W., Okay O. & Joos-Müller B., 1998, "Microgels - Intramolecularly crosslinked macromolecules with a globular structure", *Adv. Polymer Sci.,* 136, 139-234 ISSN: 1436-5030.

Garin-Chesa P., Camell I., Saigo P., Lewis J., Old L. & Retting W., 1993, "In vitro detection of occult bone marrow metastases in patients with colorectal cancer hepatic metastases", *Am. J. Pathol.,* 42, 557, ISSN: 0887-8005.

Guerrero L.G., Hervías X., Nuño-Donlucas S., Cesteros L.C., Sanz L. & Katime I., 2008, *"Synthesis of nano-structured copolymeric hydrogels based on N-Isopropyl acrylamide (NIPA) by Microemulsion Polymerization", Nanospain Congress, Braga Portugal.*

Guerrero L.G., Nuño-Donlucas S., Cesteros L.C., Sanz L. & Katime I., 2008, "Study of drug release on smart nano-sized hydrogels based on N-isopropyl acrylamide by High Performance Liquid Chromatography", Nanospain Congress, Braga Portugal

Guerrero-Ramírez L.G., Nuño-Donlucas S.M., Cesteros L.C. & Katime I., 2008, *Material Chemistry & Physics,* 112(3), 1088-1092, ISSN: 0254-0584.

Guerrero-Ramírez L.G., Nuño-Donlucas S.M., Cesteros L.C. & Katime I., 2008, *J. Physics Conference Series,* J. Phys.: Conf. Ser., 127, 012010, ISSN: 1742-6596.

Hoar T.P. & Schulman J.H., 1943, "Transparent water in oil dispersions: the oleopathic hydromicelle", *Nature,* 102, 2252, ISSN: 1476-4687.

Katime I., Katime O. & Katime D., 2004 "*Los materiales inteligentes de este milenio: Los hidrogeles macromoleculares. Síntesis, propiedades y aplicaciones*". Servicio Editorial de la Universidad del País Vasco. Bilbao. ISBN: 84-8373-637-3

Katime I., Arellano J., Mendizábal E. & Puig J., 2001, "Synthesis and characterization of poly(n-hexyl methacrylate) in three-component microemulsion", *Eur. Polym. J.,* 37(11), 2273-2279, ISSN: 0014-3057.

Katime I. & Mendizábal E., 1997, "Influence of physico-chemical parameters on the kinetics of microemulsion polymerization", *Recent. Res. Devel. Polymer Sci.,* 1, 271-289, ISBN: 81-7736-157-0

Katime I., Quintana J.R., Valderruten N. & Cesteros L.C., 2006, *Macromol. Chem. Phys.,* 207, 2121-2127, ISSN: 1521-3935.

Katime I., *Química Física Macromolecular,* 1994, Servicio Editorial UPV/EHU, Bilbao. ISBN: 84-7585-583

Kazakov S., Kaholek M., Teraoka I. & Levon K. 2002, "UV-induced gelation on nanometer scale using liposome reactor", *Macromolecules,* 35,1911-1920, ISSN: 1520-5835.

Krane A.R. & Peppas N. A., 1991, "Gel Syneresis as a Method to Release Drugs at Prescribed intervals", *Polymer News*, 16, 230-240. ISSN: 0032-3918.

Küdela V., *Encyclop. Polym. & Technol.*, 1987, Kroschwitz J.I. (editor), 7, 783, Wiley, New York. ISBN: 9780471440260.

Kurauchi K., Shiga T. & Yokada H. A., 1991, "*Polymer Gels: Fundamentals and Biomedical applications*", De Rossi D. , Kajiwara K., Osada Y. & Yamauchi A. (eds.) Plenum Press, New York, 237

Kwon I.C., Bae Y.H. & Kim S.W., 1991, "Electrically erodible polymer gel for controlled release of drugs", *Nature*, 354(6351): 291-293. ISSN: 1476-4687.

Brannon-Peppas L., 1997, "Polymers in Controlled Drug Delivery", *Medical Plastics and Biomaterials*, 4, 34-44. ISSN: 1083-5466.

Lee R.J, Wang S. & Low P.S., 1996, "Measurement of endosome pH following folate receptor-mediated endocytosis", *Biochim. Bioph. Acta*, 1312, 237-242. ISSN: 0005-2736.

Lee R.J. & Low P. S., 1994, "Delivery of liposomes into cultured KB cells via folate receptor-mediated endocytosis", *J. Biol. Chem.*, 269(5), 3198-3204. ISSN: 0021-9258.

Mamada A., Tanaka T., Kungwatchakun D., Irie M., 1990, "Photoinduced Phase-Transition of Gels", *Macromolecules*, 23(5) 1517-1519. ISSN: 1520-5835.

Mathur A. M. & Scranton A. B., 1996, "Characterization of hydrogels using nuclear magnetic resonance spectroscopy", *Biomaterials*, 17, 547-557, ISSN: 0142-9612.

Mendizábal E., Flores J., Puig J., Katime I., Lopez-Serrano F. & Alvarez J., 2000, "On the modeling of microemulsion polymerization. Experimental validation", *Macromolecular Chemistry and Physics*, 201(12), 1259-1265, ISSN: 1022-1352.

Murray M.J. & Snowden M.J., 1995, "The preparation, characterization and applications of colloidal microgels", *Adv. Colloid Interf. Sci.*, 54, 73-91, ISSN: 0001-8686.

Naka Y. & Yamamoto Y., 1998, "Preparation of poly(aryleneethynylene)-type copolymers containing flexible linking methylene units. Optical properties of the copolymers suggesting occurrence of energy transfer between π-conjugated local units", *J. Polym. Sci. Part A: Polym. Chem.*, 36(13), 2209-2214, ISSN: 1099-0518.

Osada Y., Umeawa K. & Yamauchi A., *Macromol Chem.*, 1989, 189, 3859. ISSN: 1521-3935.

Pelton R., 2000, "Temperature-sensitive aqueous microgels", *Adv. Colloid Interf. Sci.*, 85(1), 1-33, ISSN: 0001-8686.

Pérez L., Sáez V., Heráez E. & Katime I., 2008, "Synthesis and characterization of pH-sensitive microgels by derivatization of NPA-based reactive copolymers", *Materials Chemistry and Physics*, 112 (2), 516-524, ISSN: 0254-0584

Pérez L., Sáez V., Heráez E. & Katime I., 2009, "Novel pH and Temperature Responsive Methacrylamide Microgels", *Macromolecular Chemistry and Physics*, 210, 1120-1126, ISSN: 1022-1352.

Pérez L., Sáez V., Heráez E., Rodríguez E. & Katime I., 2005, "Synthesis and characterization of reactive copolymeric microgels", *Polym. Int.* 54, 963-971, ISSN: 1097-0126.

Rivolta, C.M., Moya, Christian M. & Esperante S.A., *Medicina (B. Aires)*. 2005, "The thyroid as a model for molecular mechanisms in genetic diseases", 65(3), 257-267, ISSN: 1669-9106.

Ross J.F., Chaudhuri, R.K. & Ratnam M., *Cancer*, 1994, "Differential regulation of folate receptor isoforms in normal and malignant-tissues in vivo and in established cell-lines-physiological and clinical implications", 73, 2432-2443, ISSN: 1097-0142.

Saunders B.R. & Vincent B., 1999, "Microgel particles as model colloids: theory, properties and applications", *Adv. Colloid Interf. Sci.*, 80(1), 1-25, ISSN: 0001-8686.

Stubbs M. , MeSheedy P.M.J., Griffiths J.R. & Bashford C.L., 2000, "Causes and consequences of tumour acidity and implications for treatment", *Mol. Med. Today*, 6(1), 15-19, ISSN: 1357-4310

Sudimack J. & Lee R.J., 2000, "Targeted drug delivery via the folate receptor", *Adv. Drug Deliv. Rev.*, 41(2), 147-162., ISSN: 0169-409X.

Thompson S. Gandhi M.V., 1988, "Smart materials know when to change properties". *Metal Progress*, 134(3), 22-25, ISSN: 1335-8987.

Tanaka H., Touhara H., Nakanishi K. & Watanabe N., 1984, "Computer experiment on aqueous solution. IV. Molecular dynamics calculation on the hydration of urea in an infinitely dilute aqueous solution with a new urea-water pair potential ", *J. Chem. Phys.*, 80(10), 5170-5176. ISSN: 0021-9606.

Tannock L. & Rotin D., 1989, "Acid pH in Tumors and Its Potential for Therapeutic Exploitation", *Cancer Res.*, 4, 4373-4384, ISSN: 1538-7445.

Thomson R.A.M., 1983 *"Chemistry and Technology of water-soluble polymers"*, Finch A. (Editor). Plenum. New York

Vert M., 1986, *Crit. Rev. Ther. Drug Carrier Syst.*, 2, 291-297, ISSN: 0743-4863.

Weitman D. & Etlinger J.D., 1992, "A monoclonal antibody that distinguishes latent and active forms of the proteasome (multicatalytic proteinase complex)", J. Biological Chem., 267(10), 6977-6982, ISSN: 0021-9258

Zhang X.Z., Yang Y.Y. & Chung T.S., 2002, "The influence of cold treatment on properties of temperature-sensitive Poly(N-isopropylacrylamide) hydrogels", *J. Colloid Interface Sci.*, 246(1), 105-108, ISSN: 0021-9797.

Zhu Z., Xue R. & Yu Y.C., 1989, "Toughening of epoxy-polyamide adhesives with rubbery reactive microgels", *Angew. Makromol. Chem.* 171, 65-77, ISSN: 0003-3146.

9

Targeted Magnetic Iron Oxide Nanoparticles for Tumor Imaging and Therapy

Xianghong Peng[1,2], Hongwei Chen[3],
Jing Huang[3], Hui Mao[2,3] and Dong M. Shin[1,2]
[1]Department of Hematology and Medical Oncology,
[2]Winship Cancer Institute,
[3]Department of Radiology,
Emory University School of Medicine, Atlanta, GA
USA

1. Introduction

Nanoparticles and nanotechnology have been increasingly used in the field of cancer research, especially for the development of novel approaches for cancer detection and treatment (Majumdar, Peng et al. 2010; Davis, Chen et al. 2008). Magnetic iron oxide (IO, i.e. Fe_3O_4, γ-Fe_2O_3) nanoparticles (NPs) are particularly attractive for the development of biomarker-targeted magnetic resonance imaging (MRI) contrast agents, drug delivery and novel therapeutic approaches, such as magnetic nanoparticle-enhanced hyperthermia. Given the unique pharmacokinetics of nanoparticles and their large surface areas to conjugate targeting ligands and load therapeutic agents, biodegradable IO nanoparticles have many advantages in targeted delivery of therapeutic and imaging agents. IO nanoparticles possess unique magnetic properties with strong shortening effects on transverse relaxation times, i.e., T_2 and T^*_2, as well as longitudinal relaxation time, i.e., T_1, at very low concentrations, resulting in contrast enhancement in MRI. Together with their biocompatibility and low toxicity, IO nanoparticles have been widely investigated for developing novel and biomarker-specific agents that can be applied for oncologic imaging with MRI. In addition, the detectable changes in MRI signals produced by drug-loaded IO nanoparticles provide the imaging capabilities of tracking drug delivery, estimating tissue drug levels and monitoring therapeutic response in vivo. With recent progress in nanosynthesis, bioengineering and imaging technology, IO nanoparticles are expected to serve as a novel platform that enables new approaches to targeted tumor imaging and therapy. In this chapter, we will review several aspects of magnetic nanoparticles, specifically IO nanoparticles, which are important to the development and applications of tumor-targeted imaging and therapy. An overview of general approaches for the preparation of targeted IO nanoparticles, including common synthesis methods, coating methodologies, selection of biological targeting ligands, and subsequent bioconjugation techniques, will be provided. Recent progress in the development of IO nanoparticles for tumor imaging and anti-cancer drug delivery, as well as the outstanding challenges to these approaches, will be discussed.

2. Preparation of IO nanoparticles

Typical IO nanoparticles are prepared through bottom-up strategies, including coprecipitation, microemulsion approaches, hydrothermal processing and thermal decomposition (**Figure 1**) (Gupta and Gupta 2005; Laurent, Forge et al. 2008; Laurent, Boutry et al. 2009; Xie, Huang et al. 2009). The advantages and disadvantages of these conventional nanofabrication techniques are important and need to be taken into account in designing and developing a nanoparticle construct for specific cancer models and applications.

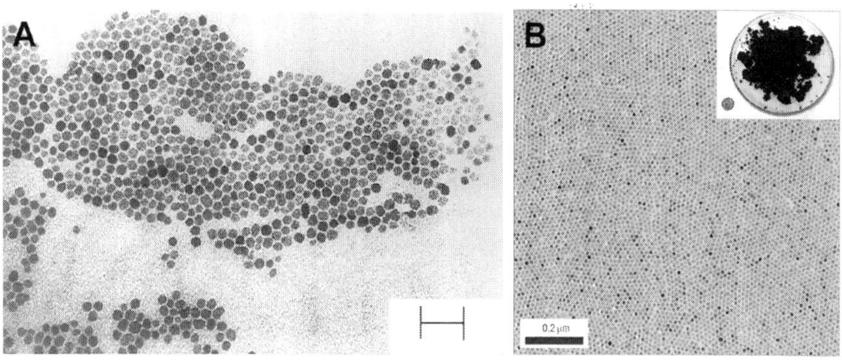

Fig. 1. (A) Fe_3O_4 NPs synthesized by coprecipitation method, the scale bar is 30 nm; (B) Fe_3O_4 NPs prepared by thermal decomposition of iron oleate $Fe(OA)_3$. (Reproduced with permission from Kang, Y. S., S. Risbud, et al. (1996). "Synthesis and characterization of nanometer-size Fe_3O_4 and gamma-Fe_2O_3 particles." Chemistry of Materials 8(9): 2209-2211and Park, J., K. J. An, et al. (2004). "Ultra-large-scale syntheses of monodisperse nanocrystals." Nature Materials 3(12): 891-895.

Coprecipitation is the most commonly used approach due to its simplicity and scalability. It features coprecipitating Fe(II) and Fe(III) salts in the aqueous solution by adding bases, usually NH_4OH or NaOH (Massart 1981). The resulting IO nanoparticles are affected by many synthetic parameters, such as pH value, concentrations of reactants, reaction temperature etc. In addition, small molecules and amphiphilic polymeric molecules are introduced to enhance the ionic strength of the medium, protect the formed nanoparticles from further growth, and stabilize the colloid fluid (Kang, Risbud et al. 1996; Vayssieres, Chaneac et al. 1998). Though this method suffers from broad size distribution and poor crystallinity, it is widely used in fabricating IO-based MRI contrast agents (such as dextran-coated IO nanoparticles), because of its simplicity and high-throughput (Sonvico, Mornet et al. 2005; Muller, Skepper et al. 2007; Hong, Feng et al. 2008; Lee, Li et al. 2008; Agarwal, Gupta et al. 2009; Nath, Kaittanis et al. 2009). A modification of the coprecipitation method is the reverse micelle method, in which the Fe(II) and Fe(III) salts are precipitated with bases in microemulsion (water-in oil) droplets stabilized by surfactant. The final size and shape of the nanoparticles can be precisely tuned through adjusting the surfactant concentration or the reactants concentration (Santra, Tapec et al. 2001; Zhou, Wang et al. 2001; Lee, Lee et al. 2005; Hong, Feng et al. 2009). The disadvantages of this method are its low yield and poor crystallinity of the product, which limit its practical use. A hydrothermal method is also considered a promising synthetic approach for IO nanoparticles towards biomedical applications, which is performed in a sealed autoclave with high temperature (above solvent boiling points) and autogenous high pressure, resulting in nanoparticles with narrow size distribution (Daou, Pourroy et al. 2006; Liang, Wang et al. 2006; Taniguchi, Nakagawa et al. 2009).

High quality IO nanoparticles with perfect monodispersity and high crystallinity can be fabricated by the state of the art thermal decomposition method. Iron precursors, usually organometallic compounds or metal salts (e.g. $Fe(acac)_3$, $Fe(CO)_5$, and $Fe(OA)_3$), are decomposed in refluxing organic solvent in the presence of surfactant (e.g. oleic acid, and oleic amine) (Hyeon, Lee et al. 2001; Sun and Zeng 2002; Park, An et al. 2004; Sun, Zeng et al. 2004; Park, Lee et al. 2005; Lee, Huh et al. 2007). In this method, the size and morphology of the nanoparticles can be controlled by modulating the temperature, reaction time, surfactant concentration and type of solvent. Using smaller nanoparticles as growth seed, Hyeon and co-workers prepared 1-nm IO nanoparticles through additional thermal decomposition growth (Park, Lee et al. 2005). The obtained nanoparticles are usually hydrophobic, dispersible in organic solvent, which requires further phase transfer procedures to make them water-soluble. Recently, several studies have demonstrated that directly thermal decomposing iron precursors in strong polar solvents (e.g. DMF, 2-pyrrolidone) resulted in hydrophilic IO nanoparticles, which could be readily dispersed in water, as preferred in biomedical applications (Liu, Xu et al. 2005; Neuwelt, Varallyay et al. 2007; Wan, Cai et al. 2007).

Coating materials play an important role in stabilizing aqueous IO nanoparticle suspensions as well as further functionalization. Appropriate coating materials can effectively render the water solubility of the IO nanoparticles and improve their stability in physiological conditions. The coating of IO nanoparticles can be achieved through two general approaches: ligand addition and ligand exchange (Gupta, Gupta 2005; Xie, Huang et al. 2009). In ligand addition, the stabilizing agents can physically adsorb on the IO nanoparticle surface as a result of various physico-chemical interactions, including electrostatic interaction, hydrophobic interaction, and hydrogen bonding, etc. Besides physical adsorption, coating materials with abundant hydroxyl, carboxyl, and amino groups can readily and steadily absorb on the surface of the bare IO nanoparticle core, as the active functional groups are capable of coordinating with the iron atoms on the surface to form complexes (Gu, Schmitt et al. 1995). Even for nanoparticles with pre-existing hydrophobic coating, newly added amphiphilic agents could also stick on the surface physically or chemically to complete phase transfer. Various materials, including natural organic materials (e.g. dextran, starch, alginate, chitosan, phospholipids, proteins etc.) (Kim, Mikhaylova et al. 2003; Peng, Hidajat et al. 2004; Kumagai, Imai et al. 2007; Muller, Skepper et al. 2007; Nath, Kaittanis et al. 2009; Zhao, Wang et al. 2009) and synthetic polymers (e.g. polyethylene glycol (PEG), poly(acrylic acid) (PAA), polyvinylpyrrolidone (PVP), poly(vinyl alcohol) (PVA), poly(methylacrylic acid) (PMAA), poly(lactic acid) (PLA), polyethyleneimine (PEI), and block copolymers etc.) (Lutz, Stiller et al. 2006; Narain, Gonzales et al. 2007; Mahmoudi, Simchi et al. 2008; Hong, Feng et al. 2009; Yang, Mao et al.

2009; Yang, Peng et al. 2009; Hadjipanayis, Machaidze et al. 2010; Huang, Bu et al. 2010; Namgung, Singha et al. 2010; Vigor, Kyrtatos et al. 2010; Wang, Neoh et al. 2010) have been demonstrated to successfully coat the surface of IO nanoparticles through ligand addition. Alternatively, ligand exchange refers to the approach of replacing the pre-existing coating ligands with new, higher affinity ones. One such example is that of dopamine (DOP)-based molecules, which can can substitute the original oleic acid molecules on the surface of IO nanoparticles, as the bidentate enediol of DOP coordinates with iron atoms forming strong bonds (Huang, Xie et al. 2010; Xie, Wang et al. 2010). Dimercaptosuccinic acid (DMSA) and polyorganosiloxane could also replace the original organic coating by forming chelate bonding (De Palma, Peeters et al. 2007; Lee, Huh et al. 2007; Chen, Wang et al. 2010). After ligand addition and ligand exchange, surface-initiated crosslinking might be performed for further coating stabilization, yielding nanoparticles with great stability against agglomeration in the physiological environment (Lattuada and Hatton 2007; Chen, Wang et al. 2010).

3. Surface modification and functionalization of IO nanoparticles

Surface modification and functionalization play critical roles in the development of any nanoparticle platform for biomedical applications. However, the capacity of the functionalization may be highly dependent on the diversity and chemical reactivity of the surface coating materials as well as the functional moieties used for biological interactions and targeting. Commonly used functional groups, i.e., carboxyl -COOH, amino $-NH_2$ and thiol -SH groups, are ideal for covalent conjugation of payload molecules or moieties. However, there is an increased application of non-covalent interactions, such as hydrophobic and electrostatic forces, to incorporate the payload molecules.

Recently developed theranostics IO nanoparticles, i.e., multifunctional nanoparticles capable of both diagnostic imaging and delivery of therapeutics, often consist of small molecules (e.g, chemotherapy drugs, optical dyes) or biologics (e.g., antibodies, peptides, nucleic acids) to achieve effective targeted imaging and drug delivery. These functional moieties have high affinity and specificity for biomarkers, such as cell surface receptors or cellular proteins, which can enhance specific accumulation of IO nanoparticles at the target site. Major techniques for the functionalization of IO nanoparticles include the selection of biomarker-targeting ligands and the conjugation of targeting ligands on the nanoparticle surface (**Figure 2**). Targeting moieties can be obtained via screening of synthetic combinatorial libraries and subsequent amplification through an in vitro selection process (Yang, Peng et al. 2009; Hadjipanayis, Machaidze et al. 2010; Lee, Yigit et al. 2010). The selection process usually starts with a random moieties library generated through chemical synthesis, and polymerase chain reaction (PCR) amplification or cloning of the identified targeting moiety through transfected/infected cells. Purification is acheived by incubating the library with target molecules or target cells, so that the high affinity moieties can be captured, separated from those unbound moieties, and eluted from the target molecule or cells. In addition, counter selection might be performed to enhance the purity of the isolated targeting moiety. Amplification via PCR or cloning throguh transfected/infected cells will result in new libraries of targeting moieties enriched with higher affinity ones. The selection process may be repeated for several rounds, and the targeting moieties with the highest affinity to the target can be obtained for further functionalization of magnetic IO nanoparticles.

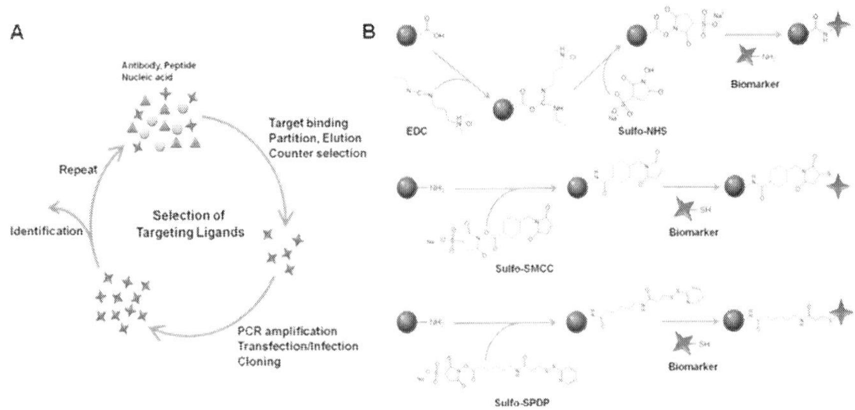

Fig. 2. (A) A schematic example of the selection process of targeting moieties. (B) Conjugation of IO nanoparticles with targeting ligands through maleimide reactions.

An active targeting approach in nanomedicine involves the direct conjugation of targeting ligands to the surface of nanoparticles rather than adsorption encapsulation. A variety of bioconjugation reactions have been developed by the incorporation of functional groups (e.g. carboxyl group, and amino group, thiol group) at the IO nanoparticle surface and in the targeting ligands. Besides affinity interactions, click chemistry, and streptavidin biotin reactions (Yang, Mao et al. 2009; Cutler, Zheng et al. 2010; Vigor, Kyrtatos et al. 2010), bioconjugation can be achieved by using linker molecules with carboxyl-, amine- or thiol-reactive groups, such as glutaraldehyde, 1-ethyl-3-(3-dimethylaminopropyl) carbodiimide hydrochloride (EDC), N-hydroxysuccinimide (NHS), succinimidyl-4-(N-maleimidomethyl)cyclohexane-1-carboxylate (SMCC), N-succinimidyl-3-(2-pyridyldithio)-propionate (SPDP), etc. (Lee, Huh et al. 2007; Lee, Li et al. 2008; Bi, Zhang et al. 2009; Yang, Mao et al. 2009; Yang, Peng et al. 2009; Hadjipanayis, Machaidze et al. 2010; Kumar, Yigit et al. 2010; Vigor, Kyrtatos et al. 2010; Yang, Park et al. 2010). For example, Yang et al. conjugated amphiphilic polymer-coated IO nanoparticles with amino-terminal fragment peptides via cross-linking of carboxyl groups to amino side groups through an EDC/NHS approach (Yang, Peng et al. 2009). The well developed bioconjugation methodologies advance the surface engineering of IO nanoparticles and expand the functionalities of IO nanoparticles.

4. Recent progress using IO nanoparticles for tumor imaging and therapy

With the emphasis on personalized medicine in future clinical oncology practices, the potential applications of biomarker-targeted imaging and drug delivery approaches are well recognized. Tumor-targeted IO nanoparticles that are highly sensitive imaging probes and effective carriers of therapeutic agents are the logical choice of a platform for future clinical development. Increasing evidence indicates that the selective delivery of nanoparticle therapeutic agents into a tumor mass can minimize toxicity to normal tissues and maximize bioavailability and cell killing effects of cytotoxic agents. This effect is mainly attributed to changes in tissue distribution and pharmacokinetics of drugs. Furthermore, IO nanoparticle-drugs can accumulate to reach high concentrations in certain solid tumors than free drugs via the enhanced permeability and retention effect (EPR). However, the EPR facilitates only a certain level of tumor targeting, while actively tumor-targeted IO nanoparticles may further increase the local concentration of drug or change the intracellular biodistribution within the tumor via receptor-mediated internalization.

4.1 Targeted IO nanoparticles for tumor imaging

Passive targeting of tumors with IO nanoparticles via the EPR effect plays an important role in the delivery of IO nanoparticles in vivo and can be used for tumor imaging. However, the biodistribution of such IO nanoparticles is non-specific, resulting in insufficient concentrations at the tumor site, and thus low sensitivity and specificity. The development of tumor-targeted IO nanoparticles that are highly sensitive and specific imaging probes may overcome such problems.

Various genetic alterations and cellular abnormalities have been found to be particularly distributed in tumors rather than in normal tissues. Such differences between normal and tumor cells provide a great opportunity for engineering tumor-targeted IO imaging probes. Antibodies, peptides and small molecules targeting related receptors on the surface of tumor cells can be conjugated to the surface of IO nanoparticles to enhance their imaging sensitivity and specificity. Many studies have reported using targeted IO nanoparticles for tumor imaging in vitro and in vivo, and such nanoparticles may have the potential to be used in the clinic in the near future.

Antibodies are widely used for engineering tumor targeted IO nanoparticles for *in vivo* tumor imaging due to their high specificity. The conjugation of antibodies to IO nanoparticles can maintain both the properties of the antibody and the magnetic particles. Monoclonal antibody-targeted IO nanoparticles have been well studied in vivo (Artemov, Mori et al. 2003; Serda, Adolphi et al. 2007; Kou, Wang et al. 2008; Chen, Cheng et al. 2009).

One well-known tumor target, the human epidermal growth factor receptor 2 (Her-2/*neu* receptor), has been found overexpressed in many different kinds of cancer such as breast, ovarian, and stomach cancer. Yang et al (Yang, Park et al. 2010) conjugated the HER2/neu antibody (Ab) to poly(amino acid)-coated IO nanoparticles (PAION), which have abundant amine groups on the surface. After conjungation, the diameter of PAION-Ab was 31.1 ± 7.8 nm, and the zeta-potential was negative (−12.93 ± 0.86 mV) due to the shield of amine groups by conjugated Her-2 antibodies. Bradford protein assay indicates that there are about 8 HER2/neu antibodies on each PAION. The T_2 relaxation times showed a significant difference between the PAION-Ab-treated (37.7 ms) and untreated cells (79.9 ms) in positive groups (SKBR-3 cells, overexpressing HER-2), while no significant difference was founded in T_2-weighted MR images of negative groups (H520 cells, HER-2 negative). The results demonstrated that HER2/*neu* antibody-conjugated PAION have specific targeting ability for HER2/*neu* receptors. Such HER2/*neu* antibody-conjugated PAION with high stability and sensitivity have potential to be used as an MR contrast agent for the detection of HER2/*neu* positive breast cancer cells. Herceptin, a well-known antibody against the HER2/*neu* receptor, which has been used in the clinic for many years, can also be conjugated to the IO nanoparticles for breast cancer imaging. Using such herceptin-IO nanoparticles, small tumors of only 50 mg in weight can be detected by MRI (Lee, Huh et al. 2007).

However, the relatively large size of intact antibodies limits their efficient conjugation because of steric effects. The specificity of antibody-conjugated IO nanoparticles may also decrease due to the interaction of antibody with Fc receptors on normal tissues. In addition, the expensive cost of intact antibodies further limits the application of antibody-targeted IO nanoparticles. Recently, more and more studies have reported engineering targeted IO nanoparticles using single chain antibodies (scFv) or peptides with small molecular weight and size. Compared with intact antibodies, there are many advantages of using scFv as tumor targeting ligands, 1) relatively small molecular weight and size; 2) no loss of antigen binding capacity; 3) no immune responses due to lack of Fc constant domain; 4) low cost and easily obtained.

The epidermal growth factor receptor (EGFR) signaling pathway is involved in the regulation of cell proliferation, survival, and differentiation, and it has been found overexpressed in many different kinds of cancer such as breast, ovarian, lung, head and neck cancer. By using a high-affinity single-chain anti-EGFR antibody (scFvB10, $K_D = 3.36 \times 10^{-9}$ M), Yang et al. has developed a EGFR-targeted amphiphilic triblock polymer coated IO nanoparticle for in vivo tumor imaging (Yang, Mao et al. 2009) (**Figure 3**). ScFvEGFR was conjugated to IO nanoparticles by crosslinking carboxyl groups to amino groups of the ScFvEGFR proteins mediated by ethyl-3-dimethyl amino propyl carbodiimide (EDAC). The in vitro results showed that the ScFvEGFR IO nanoparticles specifically bind to EGFR, which was demonstrated by Prussian blue staining and MRI (**Figure 4**). The EGFR-targeted or non-targeted IO nanoparticles were administrated via the tail vein to nude mice bearing orthotopical human pancreatic cancer xenograft. The results showed that the ScFvEGFR-IO nanoparticles could selectively accumulate within the pancreatic tumors, which was evidenced by a decrease in MRI signal in the tumor site and confirmed by histological examination of the pancreatic tissue, while non-targeted IO nanoparticles did not cause MRI signal changes in tumor.

A high affinity scFv reactive to carcinoembryonic antigen (CEA), sm3E, was covalently conjugated to superparamagnetic iron oxide nanoparticles (SPIONs), and the functionalized SPIONs could bind specifically to CEA while unmodified SPIONs did not show any binding ability. The ability of the targeted-SPIONs to specifically target and image CEA was further demonstrated by using the colorectal cancer cell line LS174T (CEA-expressing) and adherent melanoma cell line A375M (CEA negative). MR images showed 57% reduction in T_2 values compared with the 11% reduction induced by non-targeted SPIONs (Vigor, Kyrtatos et al. 2010).

Peptides that target specific receptors on the tumor cell surface can be used for engineering targeted IO nanoparticles for tumor imaging due to their small size and molecular weight. The urokinase plasminogen activator receptor (uPAR) is expressed in many different human cancers, and may play important roles in the tumor metastasis. The amino-terminal fragment (ATF) of urokinase plasminogen activator (uPA) can bind to uPAR on the cell surface, thus the ATF peptide is ideal for constructing uPAR-targeted IO nanoparticles for *in vivo* tumor imaging. Yang et al. purified the ATF peptide and conjugated it to amphiphilic polymer-coated IO nanoparticles (Yang, Mao et al. 2009). These uPAR-targeted IO nanoparticles showed selective accumulation at the tumor mass in orthotopical xenografted human pancreatic cancer model. More importantly, such uPAR-targeted IO nanoparticles could be internalized by both uPAR-expressing tumor cells and tumor-associated stromal cells, to further increase the amount and retention of the IO nanoparticles in a tumor mass, which increased the sensitivity of tumor detection by MRI. Pancreatic tumors as small as 1 mm^3 could be detected by a 3T clinical capable MRI scanner using the targeted IO nanoparticles. After labeling the ATF peptide with the near infrared (NIR) dye Cy5.5, the targeted IO nanoparticles enabled the detection of a 0.5 mm^3 intraperitoneal pancreatic cancer lesion by NIR optical imaging. Further study showed that NIR optical imaging detected tumor cell implants with only 1 × 10^4 tumor cells while MRI detected tumor cell grafts containing 1 × 10^5 labeled cells (**Figure 5**).

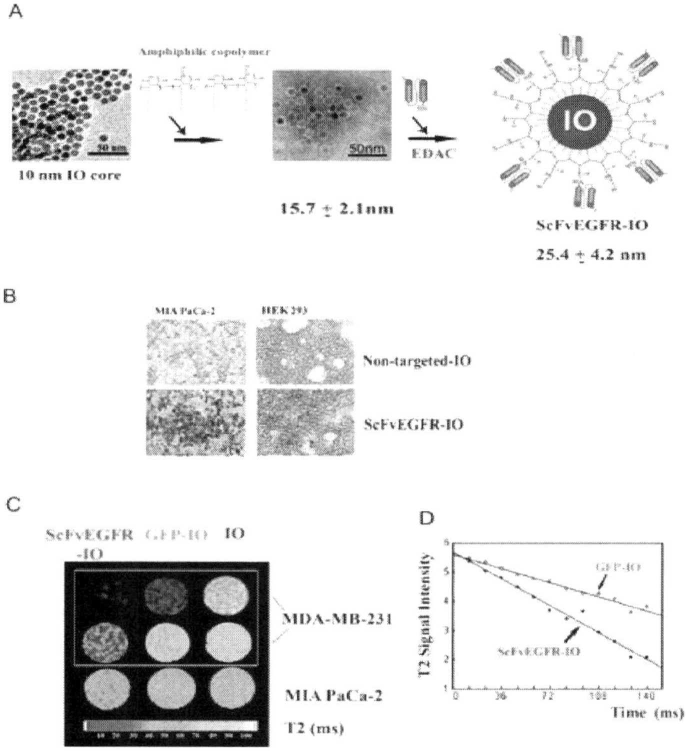

Fig. 3. ScFvEGFR-conjugated IO nanoparticles show high specificity to EGFR-overexpressing tumor cells and induce MRI signal changes in IO nanoparticle-bound tumor cells in vitro. A) ScFvEGFR-IO nanoparticle construct consists of uniform IO nanoparticles (10 nm core size) coated with amphiphilic copolymers modified with short PEG chains. ScFvEGFR proteins were conjugated to the IO nanoparticles mediated by EDAC. B) Prussian blue staining confirmed the specific binding of the ScFvEGFR-IO nanoparticles to tumor cells with EGFR overexpression . C) T_2 weighted MRI and T_2 relaxometry mapping showed significant decreases in MRI signals and T_2 relaxation times in the cells bound with ScFvEGFR-IO nanoparticles but not with GFP-IO nanoparticles or bare IO nanoparticles. MDA-MB-231 breast cancer cells and MIA PaCa-2 pancreatic cancer cells have different levels of EGFR expression and different levels of T_2 weighted contrast. A low T_2 value correlates with a higher iron concentration (red color), indicating higher level of specific binding of ScFvEGFR-IO nanoparticles to tumor cells. D) Multi-echo T_2 weighted fast spin echo imaging further confirmed the fastest T_2 value drop in MDA-MB-231 cells after incubation with ScFvEGFR-IO but not with control GFP-IO nanoparticles. Reproduced with permission from Yang, L., H. Mao, et al. (2009). "Single chain epidermal growth factor receptor antibody conjugated nanoparticles for in vivo tumor targeting and imaging." Small 5(2): 235-43.

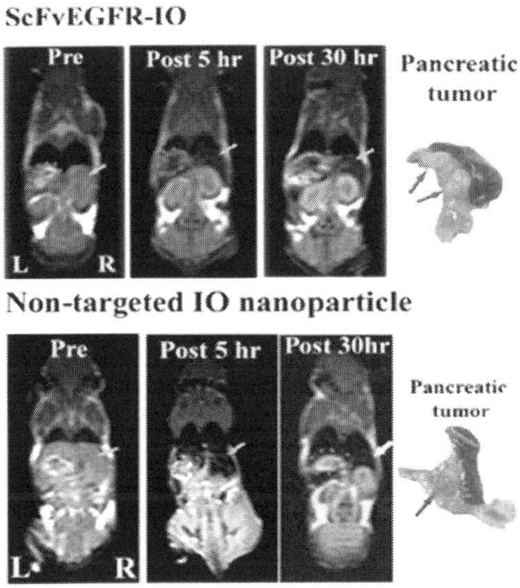

Fig. 4. Examination of target specificity of ScFvEGFR-IO nanoparticles by MRI using an orthotopic human pancreatic xenograft model, the areas of the pancreatic tumor were marked as pink dash-lined circle. Right is the picture of tumor and spleen tissues, showing sizes and locations of two intra-pancreatic tumor lesions (arrows) that correspond with the tumor images of MRI. Reproduced with permission from Yang, L., H. Mao, et al. (2009). "Single chain epidermal growth factor receptor antibody conjugated nanoparticles for in vivo tumor targeting and imaging." Small 5(2): 235-43.

The approach of using optically sensitive small dye molecules along with MRI-capable IO nanoparticles not only provides a potential multi-modal imaging capability for future application but also a way to validate and track the magnetic IO nanoparticles to investigate tumor targeting and biodistribution of nanoparticle constructs in animal models. Underglycosylated mucin-1 antigen (uMUC-1) is overexpressed in more than 50% of all human cancers and is located on the surface of tumor cells. The EPPT1 peptide, which is able to specifically bind to uMUC-1, has been synthesized and used by Moore et al. to fabricate uMUC-1-targeted superparamagnetic IO nanoparticles with dextran coating, their results showed that such targeted CLIO nanoparticles could induce a significant T2 signal reduction in uMUC-1-positive LS174T tumors compared with that of uMUC-1-negative U87 tumors in vivo (Moore, Medarova et al. 2004).

The luteinizing hormone releasing hormone (LHRH) (Chatzistamou, Schally et al. 2000) is a decapeptide, and more than half of human breast cancers express binding sites for receptors for LHRH. Leuschner et al synthesized LHRH-SPIO nanoparticles, and both in vitro and in vivo data showed that the IO nanoparticles selectively accumulated in both primary tumor cells and metastatic cells. The LHRH-conjugated SPIO nanoparticles may have potential to be used for detecting metastatic breast cancer cells *in vivo* in the future (Leuschner, Kumar et al. 2006).

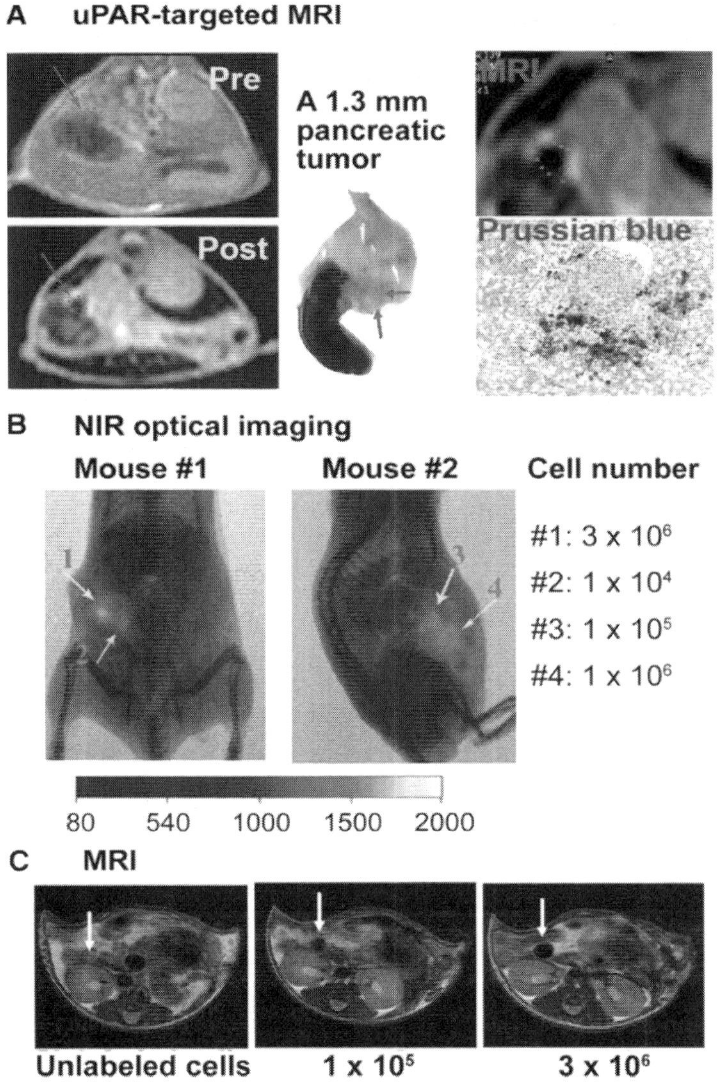

Fig. 5. Examination of sensitivity of in vivo tumor imaging. (A) uPAR-targeted MRI of an orthotopic pancreatic cancer. Tumor is marked as pink dotted circle. Prussian blue staining revealed the presence of IO nanoparticles in the tumor lesion with strong staining in tumor stromal areas. (B) NIR optical imaging and (C) MRI of injected labeled cells and nonlabeled cells in mouse pancreas. Reproduced with permission from Yang, L., H. Mao, et al. (2009). "Molecular imaging of pancreatic cancer in an animal model using targeted multifunctional nanoparticles." Gastroenterology 136(5): 1514-25.

In contrast, cost effective but high affinity small molecule targeting moities are not widely available or well tested. One exception is folic acid (FA), which targets the folate receptor, which is overexpressed on the surface of many human tumor cells and can thus be used as a target for tumor imaging. The vitamin FA has low molecular weight and has been widely studied as a targeting ligand. There are many advantages of using FA as a targeting ligand for synthesizing IO nanoparticles, 1) high binding affinity for its receptor ($K_d = 10^{-10}$ M), 2) low cost and easily obtained, 3) easy to be conjugated with the imaging agents, 4) lack of immunogenicity (Low, Henne et al. 2008). Sun et al constructed the FA-IO-nanoparticles, the *in vitro* experiments showed that FR-positive HeLa cells could uptake1.410 pg iron per cell after incubated with FR-targeted IO nanoparticles for 4 hrs, which was 12-fold higher than those cultured with non-targeted IO nanoparticles, and the increased internalization could be inhibited by increasing free FA concentration, and such targeting specificity of the FR-targeted IO nanoparticles could be further demonstrated by using FR-negative Human osteosarcoma MG-63 cells. The T_2-weighted MR phantom images of HeLa cells cultured with FR-targeted IO nanoparticles showed significantly lower T_2 values (23.5–14.2 ms) than those incubated with non-targeted IO nanoparticles (80.2–49.3 ms)(Sun, Sze et al. 2006). Another study also showed FA-targeted IO nanoparticles could selectively accumulate in human nasopharyngeal epidermoid carcinoma (KB) cells both in vitro and in vivo, which resulted in significant MRI signal changes (Chen, Gu et al. 2007).

Given the concerns regarding the delivery of fairly large nanoparticle constructs directly into the tumor, targeted imaging and drug delivery into the tumor vasculture, which is often associated with tumor angiogenesis, appears to be a feasible approach. Angiogenesis is essential for the development of tumors. As a marker of angiogenesis, the $\alpha_v\beta_3$ integrin locates on the surface of the tumor vessels and can be directly targeted via blood. The Arg-Gly-Asp (RGD) peptide, which can bind to the $\alpha_v\beta_3$ integrin receptor, has been well studied as a tumor vessel-targeted ligand. One study using RGD-USPIO nanoparticles for tumor vessel imaging showed that RGD-USPIO nanoparticles could target to the tumor vessels and resulted in a change in T_2 relaxation detected at the field strength of 1.5 T with a clinical MRI scanner, and the signal changes were correlated to the $\alpha_v\beta_3$ integrin expression level (Zhang, Jugold et al. 2007).

On the other hand, targeted delivery of biomarker-specific nanoparticle constructs to brain tumors needs to overcome the challenge of penatrating the intrinsic blood-brain barrier. Efforts have been made to identify the appropriate design of nanoparticle constructs for targeting brain tumors. It has been reported that matrix metalloproteinase-2 (MMP-2) is overexpressed in gliomas and other related cancers, and facilitates cancer invasion (Soroceanu, Gillespie et al. 1998; Deshane, Garner et al. 2003; Veiseh, Gabikian et al. 2007). The chlorotoxin (Cltx) is a small peptide (36-amino acid) which can recognize and bind to the MMP-2 endopeptidase, one study showed that Cltx-conjugated IO nanoparticles could be taken up in 9L glioma cells at significantly higher concentrations than that of their non-targeted counterpart, which further resulted in a significant difference in $R_2(1/T_2)$ relaxivity between Cltx-targeted IO nanoparticle- (5.20 $mm^{-1}s^{-1}$) and non-targeted IO nanoparticle- (0.22 $mm^{-1}s^{-1}$) treated tumor cells, and such R_2 change was also observed by MRI in vivo (Sun, Veiseh et al. 2008). One alternative and potential solution for overcoming the blood-brain barrier to deliver therapeutic IO nanoparticles is the use of conventional enhanced delivery, in which a magnetic IO nanoparticle suspension can be slowly infused into the tumor site via a minimally invasive procedure (Hadjipanayis, C. G., R. Machaidze, et al. (2010)).

There are still many issues that need to be addressed in the study of IO nanoparticles for tumor imaging, and which must be throughly investigated in future studies. These include: 1) the optimal coating of the IO nanoparticles, which may avoid non-specific binding to normal cells, prolong the blood circulation time, and make the IO nanoparticles more stable in physiological conditions; 2) quantification of the density of targeted ligand on the surface of IO nanoparticles, which may affect the binding and internalization of IO nanoparticles, as well as their in vivo biodistribution; 3) the long-term fate and toxicity of targeted IO nanoparticles in vivo. Until now, most tumor-targeted IO nanoparticles have only been applied in vitro or in small animal models for tumor imaging, and are not yet ready for clinical use. The development of tumor-targeted IO nanoparticles with high specificity and sensitivity in vivo for early stage detection of tumors, monitoring of tumor metastasis and response to therapy is greatly needed.

4.2 Tumor-targeted IO nanoparticles as selective drug delivery vehicles

The selective delivery of therapeutic agents into a tumor mass may enhance the antitumor efficacy while minimizing toxicity to normal tissues (Brigger, Dubernet et al. 2002; Maillard, Ameller et al. 2005; Shenoy, Little et al. 2005; Bae, Diezi et al. 2007; Gang, Park et al. 2007; Lee, Chang et al. 2007). While the delivery of small molecule drugs to the tumor is often limited by fast secretion, drug solubility and low intra-tumor accumulation, nanoparticle delivery vehicles can alter the pharmacokinetics and tissue distribution profile in favor of tumor specific accumulation. It is widely considered that nanoparticle-drugs can accumulate to higher concentrations in certain solid tumors than free drugs via the enhanced permeability and retention effect (EPR). In addition, actively tumor-targeted nanoparticles may further increase the local concentration of drug or change the intracellular biodistribution within the tumor via receptor-mediated internalization. With magnetic IO nanoparticles, the imaging capability allows for monitoring and potential quantification of the IO nanoparticle-drug complex in vivo with MRI.

Therapeutic entities, such as small molecular drugs, peptides, proteins and nucleic acids, can be incorporated in the IO nanoparticles through either loading on the surface layer or trapping within the nanoparticles themselves. When delivered to the target site, the loaded drugs are usually released by 1) diffusing; 2) vehicle rupture or dissolution; 3) endocystosis of the conjugations; 4) pH-sensitive dissociation, etc. Such delivery carriers have many advantages, including 1) water-soluble; 2) low toxic or nontoxic; 3) biocompatible and biodegradable; 4) long blood retention time; 5) capacity for further modification. Futhermore, these therapeutic IO conjugations enable the simultaneous estimation of tissue drug levels and monitoring of therapeutic response (Lanza, Winter et al. 2004; Atri 2006).

Conventional anti-cancer agents, such as doxorubicin, cisplatin, and methotrexate, have been conjugated with tumor-targeted IO nanoparticles to achieve effective delivery. Recently Yang et al (Yang, Grailer et al. 2010) developed folate receptor-targeted IO nanoparticles to deliver doxorubicin (DOX) to tumor cells. As shown in **Figure 6**, the hydrophillic IO nanoparticles were encapsulated in the multifunctional polymer vesicles in aqueous solution, the long hydrophilic PEG segments bearing the FA targeting ligand located in outer layers, while the short hydrophilic PEG segments bearing the acrylate groups located in inner layers. The anticancer drug (DOX) was conjugated onto the hydrophobic polyglutamate polymer segments via an acid-cleavable hydrazone bond, and could release at low pH value. The loading efficacy of DOX was about 14 wt %. The FA-conjugated SPIO/DOX-loaded vesicles demonstrated higher cellular uptake and cytotoxicity compared with FA-free vesicles due to folate receptor-mediated endocytosis.

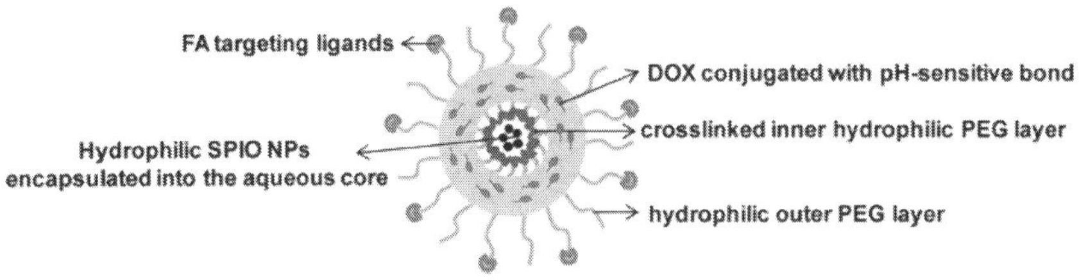

Fig. 6. Synthetic scheme of the amphiphilic triblock copolymers and the preparation process of the SPIO/DOX-loaded vesicles with cross-linked inner hydrophilic PEG layers. Reproduced with permission from Yang, X., J. J. Grailer, et al. (2010). "Multifunctional stable and pH-responsive polymer vesicles formed by heterofunctional triblock copolymer for targeted anticancer drug delivery and ultrasensitive MR imaging." ACS Nano 4(11): 6805-17.

Cisplatin (DDP) is one of the most widely used chemotherapy drugs in the treatment of cancers, including head and neck, testicular, bladder, ovarian, and non-small lung cancer. However, the major dose limiting toxicity of DDP is cumulative nephrotoxicity; severe and irreversible damage to the kidney will occur in about 1/3 of patients who receive DDP treatment. The selective delivery of DDP to tumor cells would significantly reduce drug toxicity, improving its therapeutic index. Recently, IO nanoparticles have been used as DDP carriers for targeted therapeutic applications. Sun's group (Cheng, Peng et al. 2009) reported DDP porous could be loaded into PEGylated hollow NPs (PHNPs) of Fe_3O_4 by using the nanoprecipitation method (**Figure 7**), which resulted in 25% loading efficacy. Herceptin was covalently attached to the amine-reactive groups on the Pt-PHNP surface, and such conjugation did not change the Herceptin activity. Results showed that DDP could release from the Her-Pt-PHNPs in the acidic endosomes or lysosomes after internalization by cells, and could significantly increase the cytotoxicity of DDP.

Methotrexate (MTX) can be used as both a targeting molecule for folate receptor (FR) and a therapeutic agent for cancer cells overexpressing FR on their surface. Its carboxyl end groups provide the opportunity to be conjugated on the IO nanoparticles with amine groups. Kohler et al. have demonstrated that the uptake of MTX-IO nanoparticles by FR-overexpressing cancer cells was significant higher than that of FR-negative control cells. This system showed high drug loading efficiency, about 418 MTX molecules could be loaded onto each IO nanoparticle with a core size of 10 nm diameter. Loaded MTX was only released inside the lysosomes at low pH condition after internalization by the targeted cells, and the drug delivery system could be monitored in vivo by MRI in real-time (Kohler, Sun et al. 2005).

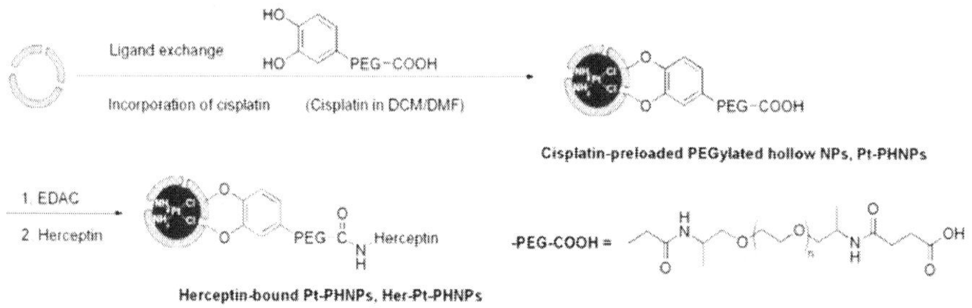

Fig. 7. Schematic illustration of simultaneous surfactant exchange and cisplatin loading into a PHNP and functionalization of this PHNP with Herceptin. Reproduced with permission from Cheng, K., S. Peng, et al. (2009). "Porous hollow Fe_3O_4 nanoparticles for targeted delivery and controlled release of cisplatin." J Am Chem Soc 131(30): 10637-44.

RNA interference (RNAi) has become a promising molecular therapeutic tool due to its high specificity. One of the big challenges for its in vivo application is that small interfering RNA (siRNA) cannot reach the target tissue at sufficient concentrations due to RNase degradation and inefficient translocation across the cell membrane. IO nanoparticles are expected to be applicable for delivering siRNA and monitoring the efficacy of therapy because of their unique characteristics as described above. It has been reported that BIRC5 could encode the antiapoptotic survivin proto-oncogene, and can be used as a good target for tumor therapy. The knockdown of BIRC5 by RNAi may mediate a therapeutic effect by inducing necrotic/apoptotic tumor cell death. Kumar et al (Kumar, Yigit et al. 2010) synthesized a novel tumor-targeted nanodrug (MN-EPPT-siBIRC5), which consists of 1) peptides (EPPT) that specifically target the antigen uMUC-1; 2) IO nanoparticles; 3) the NIR dye, Cy 5.5 and 4) siRNA that targets the tumor-specific antiapoptotic gene BIRC5 (**Figure 8**). Systemic delivery of MN-EPPT-siBIRC5 to nude mice bearing human breast adenocarcinoma tumors showed significant decrease of T_2 relaxation time of the tumor, which remained significantly lower than the preinjection values over time, suggesting that the concentration of nanodrug within the tumor tissue could be maintained. While this demonstrated that it is feasible to follow the accumulation and retention of drug-IO nanoparticles in vivo with MRI, the in vivo data also showed that MN-EPPT-siBIRC5 therapy can led to a 2-fold decrease in the tumor growth rate compared with the MN-EPPT-siSCR-treated group. The efficacy of MN-EPPT-siBIRC5 in the breast tumors was evaluated by H&E staining and TUNEL assay, which showed a 5-fold increase in the fraction of apoptotic nuclei in tumors in MN-EPPT-siBIRC5 treated mice via the MN-EPPT-siSCR group.

Tumor-targeted IO nanoparticles can also be used to "rescue" some anticancer drugs which show severe toxicity, low solubility or low antitumor efficacy in vivo. One example is the targeted delivery of noscapine, an orally available plant-derived anti-tussive alkaloid which shows antitumor activity by targeting tubulin, however, related preclinical studies did not exhibit significant inhibition of tumor growth even using high dosage (450 mg/kg), which may result from the shorter circulation time and lower drug uptake by tumor cells. Abdalla et al (Abdalla, Karna et al. 2010) have developed uPAR-targeted IO nanoparticles for selective delivery of noscapine to prostate cancer by conjugating the human ATF to the IO nanoparticles, and encapsulated about 80% of noscapine onto the uPAR-targeted nanoparticles via the interaction between the hydrophobic noscapine molecules and the hydrophobic segment of the amphiphilic polymer coating of nanoparticles. Their data showed the nanoparticles were uniformly sized and stable at physiological pH, while about 80% of drug molecules were efficiently released at pH 4 due to the onset of polymer degradation at lower pH, the breakage of hydrophobic interactions between polymer and drug molecules or hydrogen bonding. The hATF-Cy5.5-IO-Nos nanoparticles could significantly inhibit the proliferation of uPAR-positive human prostate carcinoma PC-3 cells compared with the nontargeted IO-Nos and free drug at the same concentration (10 μM). The uPAR-targeted NPs also delivered a significantly higher concentration of noscapine to the receptor positive cells, which led to a 6-fold enhancement in cell death compared to the free drug.

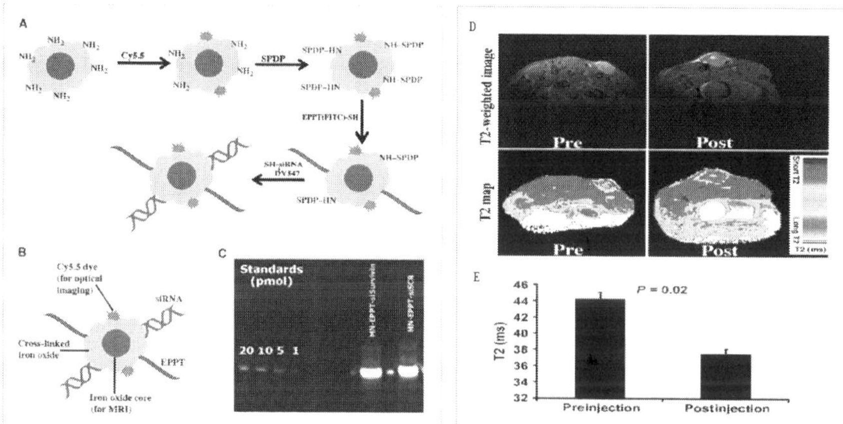

Fig. 8. A, flowchart of the synthesis. B, nanodrug characterization. The nanodrug consisted of dextran-coated MNs triple labeled with Cy5.5 dye, EPPT peptides, and synthetic siRNA duplexes. C, gel electrophoresis showing dissociation of siRNAs from the nanoparticles under reducing conditions. D, representative precontrast and postcontrast T_2-weighted images (top) and color-coded T_2 maps (bottom) of tumor-bearing mice injected i.v. with MN-EPPT-siBIRC5 (10 mg/kg iron). The tumors (outlined) were characteristically bright (T_2 long) before contrast. At 24 h after injection, there was a loss of signal intensity (T_2 shortening) associated with the tumors, indicative of nanodrug accumulation. E, quantitative analysis of tumor T_2 relaxation times. T_2 map analysis revealed a marked shortening of tumor T_2 relaxation times 24 h after nanodrug injection, indicating accumulation of MN-EPPT-siBIRC5.Reproduced with permission from Kumar, M., M. Yigit, et al. 2010 "Image-guided breast tumor therapy using a small interfering RNA nanodrug." Cancer Res 70(19): 7553-61.

Although much progress has been made in the development of tumor-targeted IO nanoparticles for the delivery of anticancer agents, there are still many obstacles to be overcome. First, the conjugation process during the synthesis of nano-drugs may induce a change in the chemical properties of the drugs or a loss in magnetization of the core magnetic material. Second, the drug loading efficiency is not high as expected for most nano-drugs. Third, controlling the drug release at the proper compartment within the tumor is still quite challenging, since most of the loaded drugs in nanoparticles release either prematurely or at a low rate from the nanoparticles. In this regard, novel strategies such as the development of magnetic IO nanoparticles for hyperthermia treatment and heating-induced drug release are under investigation and are expected to provide solutions for future clinical applications.

5. Conclusions and perspectives

Intensive investigations and the development of magnetic IO nanoparticles in the past decade have led to the much better understanding of the biological significances and potential biomedical applications of IO nanoparticles and a wide range of novel IO nanoparticle constructs designed for tumor targeted imaging and drug delivery. However, when constructing magnetic nanoparticles for tumor imaging and drug delivery, there are several goals that remain challenging to achieve, such as 1) specific accumulation in the tumor but minimal uptake in normal tissue and organs by selecting ideal tumor-targeted ligands; 2) modification of the surface and control of the size and charge of nanoparticles for adequate delivery; 3) regulation of blood circulation time; 4) stability of IO nanotherapeutics; 5) construction of smart tumor-targeted IO nanoparticles such that loaded drugs release only within tumor cells.

Recently, increasing concerns are focused on the safety of IO nanotherapeutic delivery systems. Although many animal studies have not shown visible toxicities, most of the available data come from mice with only a few studies conducted in rats, dogs and monkeys, and the sub-chronic and chronic toxicity studies for most IO nanoparticles have yet to be performed. Little is known about the long-term fate of IO nanoparticles and the pharmacokinetic/pharmacodynamic (PK/PD) changes in IO nanotherapeutics in vivo. The EPR effect constitutes only part of the drug targeting mechanism, and accumulating evidence has shown that tumor-targeted nanotherapeutics can internalize into tumor cells to a significantly higher concentration than their non-targeted counterparts. The majority of nanotherapeutic delivery systems are non-targeted, thus intensive studies using tumor-targeted nanoparticles as drug delivery carriers are needed.

6. Acknowledgment

This work was supported in part by grants from the National Institutes of Health (NIH), SPORE in Head & Neck Cancer (5P50CA128613-04), Center of Cancer Nanotechnology Excellence (CCNE, U54 CA119338-01), in vivo Cellular and Molecular Imaging Center (ICMIC, P50CA128301-01A10003) and Cancer Nanotechnology Platform Project (CCNP, 1U01CA151802-01 and 1U01CA151810-01).

7. References

Abdalla, M. O., P. Karna, et al. 2010 "Enhanced noscapine delivery using uPAR-targeted optical-MR imaging trackable nanoparticles for prostate cancer therapy." *J Control Release* 149(3): 314-22.

Agarwal, A., U. Gupta, et al. (2009). "Dextran conjugated dendritic nanoconstructs as potential vectors for anti-cancer agent." *Biomaterials* 30(21): 3588-3596.

Artemov, D., N. Mori, et al. (2003). "MR molecular imaging of the Her-2/neu receptor in breast cancer cells using targeted iron oxide nanoparticles." *Magn Reson Med* 49(3): 403-8.

Atri, M. (2006). "New technologies and directed agents for applications of cancer imaging." *J Clin Oncol* 24(20): 3299-308.

Bae, Y., T. A. Diezi, et al. (2007). "Mixed polymeric micelles for combination cancer chemotherapy through the concurrent delivery of multiple chemotherapeutic agents." *J Control Release* 122(3): 324-30.

Bi, F., J. Zhang, et al. (2009). "Chemical conjugation of urokinase to magnetic nanoparticles for targeted thrombolysis." *Biomaterials* 30(28): 5125-5130.

Brigger, I., C. Dubernet, et al. (2002). "Nanoparticles in cancer therapy and diagnosis." *Adv Drug Deliv Rev* 54(5): 631-51.

Chatzistamou, L., A. V. Schally, et al. (2000). "Effective treatment of metastatic MDA-MB-435 human estrogen-independent breast carcinomas with a targeted cytotoxic analogue of luteinizing hormone-releasing hormone AN-207." *Clin Cancer Res* 6(10): 4158-65.

Chen, H., Y. Gu, et al. (2007). "Characterization of pH- and temperature-sensitive hydrogel nanoparticles for controlled drug release." *PDA J Pharm Sci Technol* 61(4): 303-13.

Chen, H. W., L. Y. Wang, et al. (2010). "Reducing non-specific binding and uptake of nanoparticles and improving cell targeting with an antifouling PEO-b-P gamma MPS copolymer coating." *Biomaterials* 31(20): 5397-5407.

Chen, T. J., T. H. Cheng, et al. (2009). "Targeted Herceptin-dextran iron oxide nanoparticles for noninvasive imaging of HER2/neu receptors using MRI." *J Biol Inorg Chem* 14(2): 253-60.

Cheng, K., S. Peng, et al. (2009). "Porous hollow Fe(3)O(4) nanoparticles for targeted delivery and controlled release of cisplatin." *J Am Chem Soc* 131(30): 10637-44.

Cutler, J. I., D. Zheng, et al. (2010). "Polyvalent Oligonucleotide Iron Oxide Nanoparticle "Click" Conjugates." *Nano Letters* 10(4): 1477-1480.

Daou, T. J., G. Pourroy, et al. (2006). "Hydrothermal synthesis of monodisperse magnetite nanoparticles." *Chemistry of Materials* 18(18): 4399-4404.

Davis, M. E., Z. G. Chen, et al. (2008). "Nanoparticle therapeutics: an emerging treatment modality for cancer." *Nat Rev Drug Discov* 7(9): 771-82.

De Palma, R., S. Peeters, et al. (2007). "Silane ligand exchange to make hydrophobic superparamagnetic nanoparticles water-dispersible." *Chemistry of Materials* 19(7): 1821-1831.

Deshane, J., C. C. Garner, et al. (2003). "Chlorotoxin inhibits glioma cell invasion via matrix metalloproteinase-2." *J Biol Chem* 278(6): 4135-44.

Gang, J., S. B. Park, et al. (2007). "Magnetic poly epsilon-caprolactone nanoparticles containing Fe3O4 and gemcitabine enhance anti-tumor effect in pancreatic cancer xenograft mouse model." *J Drug Target* 15(6): 445-53.

Gu, B. H., J. Schmitt, et al. (1995). "Adsorption and desorption of different organic-matter fractions on iron-oxide." *Geochimica Et Cosmochimica Acta* 59(2): 219-229.

Gupta, A. K. and M. Gupta (2005). "Synthesis and surface engineering of iron oxide nanoparticles for biomedical applications." *Biomaterials* 26(18): 3995-4021.

Hadjipanayis, C. G., R. Machaidze, et al. (2010). "EGFRvIII antibody-conjugated iron oxide nanoparticles for magnetic resonance imaging-guided convection-enhanced delivery and targeted therapy of glioblastoma." *Cancer Research* 70(15): 6303-6312.

Hong, R. Y., B. Feng, et al. (2009). "Double-miniemulsion preparation of Fe3O4/poly(methyl methacrylate) magnetic latex." *Journal of Applied Polymer Science* 112(1): 89-98.

Hong, R. Y., B. Feng, et al. (2008). "Synthesis, characterization and MRI application of dextran-coated Fe3O4 magnetic nanoparticles." *Biochemical Engineering Journal* 42(3): 290-300.

Huang, J., L. H. Bu, et al. (2010). "Effects of Nanoparticle Size on Cellular Uptake and Liver MRI with Polyvinylpyrrolidone-Coated Iron Oxide Nanoparticles." *Acs Nano* 4(12): 7151-7160.

Huang, J., J. Xie, et al. (2010). "HSA coated MnO nanoparticles with prominent MRI contrast for tumor imaging." *Chemical Communications* 46(36): 6684-6686.

Hyeon, T., S. S. Lee, et al. (2001). "Synthesis of highly crystalline and monodisperse maghemite nanocrystallites without a size-selection process." *Journal of the American Chemical Society* 123(51): 12798-12801.

Kang, Y. S., S. Risbud, et al. (1996). "Synthesis and characterization of nanometer-size Fe3O4 and gamma-Fe2O3 particles." *Chemistry of Materials* 8(9): 2209-2211.

Kim, D. K., M. Mikhaylova, et al. (2003). "Starch-coated superparamagnetic nanoparticles as MR contrast agents." *Chemistry of Materials* 15(23): 4343-4351.

Kohler, N., C. Sun, et al. (2005). "Methotrexate-modified superparamagnetic nanoparticles and their intracellular uptake into human cancer cells." *Langmuir* 21(19): 8858-64.

Kou, G., S. Wang, et al. (2008). "Development of SM5-1-conjugated ultrasmall superparamagnetic iron oxide nanoparticles for hepatoma detection." *Biochem Biophys Res Commun* 374(2): 192-7.

Kumagai, M., Y. Imai, et al. (2007). "Iron hydroxide nanoparticles coated with poly(ethylene glycol)-poly(aspartic acid) block copolymer as novel magnetic resonance contrast agents for in vivo cancer imaging." *Colloids Surf B Biointerfaces* 56(1-2): 174-81.

Kumar, M., M. Yigit, et al. (2010). "Image-Guided Breast Tumor Therapy Using a Small Interfering RNA Nanodrug." *Cancer Research* 70(19): 7553-7561.

Lanza, G. M., P. Winter, et al. (2004). "Novel paramagnetic contrast agents for molecular imaging and targeted drug delivery." *Curr Pharm Biotechnol* 5(6): 495-507.

Lattuada, M. and T. A. Hatton (2007). "Functionalization of monodisperse magnetic nanoparticles." *Langmuir* 23(4): 2158-2168.

Laurent, S., S. Boutry, et al. (2009). "Iron oxide based MR contrast agents: from chemistry to cell labeling." *Current Medicinal Chemistry* 16(35): 4712-4727.

Laurent, S., D. Forge, et al. (2008). "Magnetic iron oxide nanoparticles: Synthesis, stabilization, vectorization, physicochemical characterizations, and biological applications." *Chemical Reviews* 108(6): 2064-2110.

Lee, H. Y., Z. Li, et al. (2008). "PET/MRI dual-modality tumor imaging using arginine-glycine-aspartic (RGD) - Conjugated radiolabeled iron oxide nanoparticles." *Journal of Nuclear Medicine* 49(8): 1371-1379.

Lee, J. H., Y. M. Huh, et al. (2007). "Artificially engineered magnetic nanoparticles for ultra-sensitive molecular imaging." *Nature Medicine* 13(1): 95-99.

Lee, J. H., M. V. Yigit, et al. (2010). "Molecular diagnostic and drug delivery agents based on aptamer-nanomaterial conjugates." *Advanced Drug Delivery Reviews* 62(6): 592-605.

Lee, S. W., D. H. Chang, et al. (2007). "Ionically fixed polymeric nanoparticles as a novel drug carrier." *Pharm Res* 24(8): 1508-16.

Lee, Y., J. Lee, et al. (2005). "Large-scale synthesis of uniform and crystalline magnetite nanoparticles using reverse micelles as nanoreactors under reflux conditions." *Advanced Functional Materials* 15(3): 503-509.

Leuschner, C., C. S. Kumar, et al. (2006). "LHRH-conjugated magnetic iron oxide nanoparticles for detection of breast cancer metastases." *Breast Cancer Res Treat* 99(2): 163-76.

Liang, X., X. Wang, et al. (2006). "Synthesis of nearly monodisperse iron oxide and oxyhydroxide nanocrystals." *Advanced Functional Materials* 16(14): 1805-1813.

Liu, X., B. Xu, et al. (2005). "[A method of showing thermal effect of iron oxide nanoparticles in alternating magnetic field]." *Ai Zheng* 24(9): 1148-50.

Low, P. S., W. A. Henne, et al. (2008). "Discovery and development of folic-Acid-based receptor targeting for imaging and therapy of cancer and inflammatory diseases." *Acc Chem Res* 41(1): 120-9.

Lutz, J. F., S. Stiller, et al. (2006). "One-pot synthesis of PEGylated ultrasmall iron-oxide nanoparticles and their in vivo evaluation as magnetic resonance imaging contrast agents." *Biomacromolecules* 7(11): 3132-3138.

Mahmoudi, M., A. Simchi, et al. (2008). "Optimal design and characterization of superparamagnetic iron oxide nanoparticles coated with polyvinyl alcohol for targeted delivery and imaging." *Journal of Physical Chemistry B* 112(46): 14470-14481.

Maillard, S., T. Ameller, et al. (2005). "Innovative drug delivery nanosystems improve the anti-tumor activity in vitro and in vivo of anti-estrogens in human breast cancer and multiple myeloma." *J Steroid Biochem Mol Biol* 94(1-3): 111-21.

Majumdar, D., X. H. Peng, et al. 2010 "The medicinal chemistry of theragnostics, multimodality imaging and applications of nanotechnology in cancer." *Curr Top Med Chem* 10(12): 1211-26.

Massart, R. (1981). "Preparation of aqueous magnetic liquids in alkaline and acidic media." *Ieee Transactions on Magnetics* 17(2): 1247-1248.

Moore, A., Z. Medarova, et al. (2004). "In vivo targeting of underglycosylated MUC-1 tumor antigen using a multimodal imaging probe." *Cancer Res* 64(5): 1821-7.

Muller, K., J. N. Skepper, et al. (2007). "Effect of ultrasmall superparamagnetic iron oxide nanoparticles (Ferumoxtran-10) on human monocyie-macrophages in vitro." *Biomaterials* 28(9): 1629-1642.

Namgung, R., K. Singha, et al. (2010). "Hybrid superparamagnetic iron oxide nanoparticle-branched polyethylenimine magnetoplexes for gene transfection of vascular endothelial cells." *Biomaterials* 31(14): 4204-4213.

Narain, R., M. Gonzales, et al. (2007). "Synthesis of monodisperse biotinylated p(NIPAAm)-coated iron oxide magnetic nanoparticles and their bioconjugation to streptavidin." *Langmuir* 23(11): 6299-6304.

Nath, S., C. Kaittanis, et al. (2009). "Synthesis, Magnetic Characterization, and Sensing Applications of Novel Dextran-Coated Iron Oxide Nanorods." *Chemistry of Materials* 21(8): 1761-1767.

Neuwelt, E. A., C. G. Varallyay, et al. (2007). "The potential of ferumoxytol nanoparticle magnetic resonance imaging, perfusion, and angiography in central nervous system malignancy: a pilot study." *Neurosurgery* 60(4): 601-11; discussion 611-2.

Park, J., K. J. An, et al. (2004). "Ultra-large-scale syntheses of monodisperse nanocrystals." *Nature Materials* 3(12): 891-895.

Park, J., E. Lee, et al. (2005). "One-nanometer-scale size-controlled synthesis of monodisperse magnetic iron oxide nanoparticles." *Angewandte Chemie-International Edition* 44(19): 2872-2877.

Peng, Z. G., K. Hidajat, et al. (2004). "Adsorption of bovine serum albumin on nanosized magnetic particles." *Journal of Colloid and Interface Science* 271(2): 277-283.

Santra, S., R. Tapec, et al. (2001). "Synthesis and characterization of silica-coated iron oxide nanoparticles in microemulsion: The effect of nonionic surfactants." *Langmuir* 17(10): 2900-2906.

Serda, R. E., N. L. Adolphi, et al. (2007). "Targeting and cellular trafficking of magnetic nanoparticles for prostate cancer imaging." *Mol Imaging* 6(4): 277-88.

Shenoy, D., S. Little, et al. (2005). "Poly(ethylene oxide)-modified poly(beta-amino ester) nanoparticles as a pH-sensitive system for tumor-targeted delivery of hydrophobic drugs: part 2. In vivo distribution and tumor localization studies." *Pharm Res* 22(12): 2107-14.

Sonvico, F., S. Mornet, et al. (2005). "Folate-conjugated iron oxide nanoparticles for solid tumor targeting as potential specific magnetic hyperthermia mediators: Synthesis, physicochemical characterization, and in vitro experiments." *Bioconjugate Chemistry* 16(5): 1181-1188.

Soroceanu, L., Y. Gillespie, et al. (1998). "Use of chlorotoxin for targeting of primary brain tumors." *Cancer Res* 58(21): 4871-9.

Sun, C., R. Sze, et al. (2006). "Folic acid-PEG conjugated superparamagnetic nanoparticles for targeted cellular uptake and detection by MRI." *J Biomed Mater Res A* 78(3): 550-7.

Sun, C., O. Veiseh, et al. (2008). "In vivo MRI detection of gliomas by chlorotoxin-conjugated superparamagnetic nanoprobes." *Small* 4(3): 372-9.

Sun, S. H. and H. Zeng (2002). "Size-controlled synthesis of magnetite nanoparticies." *Journal of the American Chemical Society* 124(28): 8204-8205.

Sun, S. H., H. Zeng, et al. (2004). "Monodisperse MFe2O4 (M = Fe, Co, Mn) nanoparticles." *Journal of the American Chemical Society* 126(1): 273-279.

Taniguchi, T., K. Nakagawa, et al. (2009). "Hydrothermal Growth of Fatty Acid Stabilized Iron Oxide Nanocrystals." *Journal of Physical Chemistry C* 113(3): 839-843.

Vayssieres, L., C. Chaneac, et al. (1998). "Size tailoring of magnetite particles formed by aqueous precipitation: An example of thermodynamic stability of nanometric oxide particles." *Journal of Colloid and Interface Science* 205(2): 205-212.

Veiseh, M., P. Gabikian, et al. (2007). "Tumor paint: a chlorotoxin:Cy5.5 bioconjugate for intraoperative visualization of cancer foci." *Cancer Res* 67(14): 6882-8.

Vigor, K. L., P. G. Kyrtatos, et al. (2010). "Nanoparticles functionalised with recombinant single chain Fv antibody fragments (scFv) for the magnetic resonance imaging of cancer cells." *Biomaterials* 31(6): 1307-1315.

Wan, J., W. Cai, et al. (2007). "Monodisperse water-soluble magnetite nanoparticles prepared by polyol process for high-performance magnetic resonance imaging." *Chemical Communications*(47): 5004-5006.

Wang, L., K. G. Neoh, et al. (2010). "Biodegradable magnetic-fluorescent magnetite/poly(DL-lactic acid-co-alpha,beta-malic acid) composite nanoparticles for stem cell labeling." *Biomaterials* 31(13): 3502-3511.

Xie, J., J. Huang, et al. (2009). "Iron Oxide Nanoparticle Platform for Biomedical Applications." *Current Medicinal Chemistry* 16(10): 1278-1294.

Xie, J., J. H. Wang, et al. (2010). "Human serum albumin coated iron oxide nanoparticles for efficient cell labeling." *Chemical Communications* 46(3): 433-435.

Yang, H. M., C. W. Park, et al (2010). "HER2/neu Antibody Conjugated Poly(amino acid)-Coated Iron Oxide Nanoparticles for Breast Cancer MR Imaging." Biomacromolecules. 11 (11): 2866–2872

Yang, L., H. Mao, et al. (2009). "Molecular imaging of pancreatic cancer in an animal model using targeted multifunctional nanoparticles." *Gastroenterology* 136(5): 1514-25 e2.

Yang, L., H. Mao, et al. (2009). "Single chain epidermal growth factor receptor antibody conjugated nanoparticles for in vivo tumor targeting and imaging." *Small* 5(2): 235-43.

Yang, L. L., X. H. Peng, et al. (2009). "Receptor-Targeted Nanoparticles for In vivo Imaging of Breast Cancer." *Clinical Cancer Research* 15(14): 4722-4732.

Yang, X., J. J. Grailer, et al. 2010 "Multifunctional stable and pH-responsive polymer vesicles formed by heterofunctional triblock copolymer for targeted anticancer drug delivery and ultrasensitive MR imaging." *ACS Nano* 4(11): 6805-17.

Zhang, C., M. Jugold, et al. (2007). "Specific targeting of tumor angiogenesis by RGD-conjugated ultrasmall superparamagnetic iron oxide particles using a clinical 1.5-T magnetic resonance scanner." *Cancer Res* 67(4): 1555-62.

Zhao, D. L., X. X. Wang, et al. (2009). "Preparation and inductive heating property of Fe3O4-chitosan composite nanoparticles in an AC magnetic field for localized hyperthermia." *Journal of Alloys and Compounds* 477(1-2): 739-743.

Zhou, Z. H., J. Wang, et al. (2001). "Synthesis of Fe3O4 nanoparticles from emulsions." *Journal of Materials Chemistry* 11(6): 1704-1709.

10

An Ancient Model Organism to Test *In Vivo* Novel Functional Nanocrystals

Claudia Tortiglione
Istituto di Cibernetica "E. Caianiello", National Research Council of Italy, Italy

1. Introduction

Scientific research largely depends on technological tools. If molecular biology allowed to manipulate the genome of complex organisms to investigate gene function, today nanotechnologies allow to synthesize objects at the same size scale as that of biological molecules, permitting the exploration of biological phenomena and dynamics at single molecule scale with unprecedented spatial precision and temporal resolution. Thanks to their superior physico-chemical and optoelectronic properties, colloidal semiconductor nanocrystals (NC), such as Quantum Dots (QD) and Quantum Rods (QR) have become attracting for investigators of different scientific fields. Their employment spans from electronics (tunable polarized lasers and organic-inorganic hybrid solar cells) (Hu et al., 2001; Huynh et al., 2002), to biology and medicine (biosensors, imaging and diagnostic contrast agents) (Alivisatos et al., 2005; Bruchez et al., 1998; Medintz et al., 2005). Recent advances in NC engineering, from synthesis to biofunctionalization, are being exploited to produce innovative nanodevices for drug delivery, gene silencing, hyperthermia treatments. However, their great potential to revolutionise basic and applied research founds its major concern in the lack of knowledge about their effects on biological systems, ranging from single cells to whole animals (Maynard et al., 2006). Nanocrystals size compares to that of biological molecules (nucleic acids, proteins, enzymes) and might interfere with the physiology/behaviour of the target living cell/animal, leading to unpredictable effects .

Among the factors to consider to predict the interaction of metal based nanocrystals with biological materials the core and the shell composition, the size and the surface charge of NC play crucial roles (Jiang et al., 2008). At the nanoscale, materials display properties profoundly different form their corresponding bulk chemicals, which may induce peculiar cellular responses, elicit several pathways of internalization, genetic networks, biochemical signalling cascades (Auffan et al., 2009; Choi et al., 2008; Demir E, 2010). The metal based core may adversely affect cell viability, unless properly shielded by surface coatings. Currently, increasing data addressing this important question relies on cell culture systems, and are focussed on the identification of the physicochemical parameters influencing the exposed cells (Hoshino and Yasuhara, 2004; Lewinski et al., 2008; Lovric et al., 2005b). Although cultured cells represent valid models to describe basic interactions with nanomaterials, they do not fulfil the *in vivo* response complexity.

It is a priority of the scientific community to evaluate the impact of novel nanostructrured materials *in vivo*, at level of whole animals (Fischer and Chan, 2007), and invertebrates represent valuable models for many reasons: they have a relatively short life span, with definite and reproducible staging for larval progression; the adult individual bodies are small and often transparent; the tests are quick, cost-effective and reproducible thanks to reliable standardized protocols, which makes them valuable systems for toxicity studies (Baun et al., 2008; Cattaneo, 2009).

In this chapter I will summarize some studies on the freshwater polyp *Hydra vulgaris*, a primitive organism at the base of metazoan evolution, to test NCs of different chemical composition, shell and surface coatings. The body structural complexity, simpler than vertebrates, with central nervous system and specialized organs, but much complex compared to cultured cells, makes *Hydra* comparable to a living tissue which cells and distant regions are physiologically connected. I will first generally describe the animal structural anatomy and physiology to allow non specialist readers to understand the mechanisms of tissue dynamics, reproduction, regeneration, on whose toxicity tests are relied. In the following sections I will describe the elicitation of different behaviours, internalization routes, toxicity effects, in response to different NCs, highlighting the advantages of using *Hydra* for fast, reliable assays of NC effect at whole animal level. Through the description of our studies using functionalized CdSe/ZnS QDs, unfunctionalized CdSe/CdS QRs, ultrasmall CdTe QDs, I will show that *Hydra*, up to now used mainly by a niche of biologists to study developmental and regeneration processes, have great potential to inspire scientists working in field of nanoscience, from chemists to toxicologists demanding new models to assess nanoparticle impact on human health and environment (Fischer and Chan, 2007), and to decipher the molecular basis of the bio-non bio interaction.

I would like to point out that all the data described in this chapter result from the interdisciplinary work with researchers in the field of nanomaterial science, which I sincerely thank. The continuous discussions and knowledge's exchanges between the different disciplines (chemistry, material science, biology, physiology), hided beyond each study, laid the foundations of an interdisciplinary platform for the smart design, testing and safe assessment of novel nanomaterials.

2. *Hydra vulgaris*: An ancient model system

Hydra belongs to the animal phylum Cnidaria that arose almost 600 million years ago (Lenhoff et al., 1968). Its body plan is very simple, consisting of a single oral-aboral axis with radial symmetry. The structures along the axis are a head, a body column and a foot to anchor to a substrate. The body has a bilayered structure, made of two unicellular sheets (ectoderm and endoderm) continuously dividing and migrating towards the animal oral and aboral extremities to be sloughed off. A third cell lineage, the interstitial stem cells lineage, is located in the interstices, among the epithelial cells of both layers (Fig. 1). These interstitial cells are multipotent stem cells that give rise to differentiated products: neurons, secretory cells, gametes, and nematocytes, phylum- specific mechano-sensory cells that resemble the bilaterian mechano-sensory cells in virtue of their cnidocil. Upon stimulation this cnidocil leads to the external discharge of an intracellular venom capsule (the nematocyst or cnidocyst), involved in the prey capture. Despite the simplicity of its nervous system, organized as a mesh-like network of neurons extending throughout the animal, the complexity of the mechanisms underlying neurotransmission resemble those of higher vertebrates, including both classical and peptidergic neurotransmitters (Pierobon et al., 2001; Pierobon et al., 2004). This makes *Hydra* an ideal system to study the behavioural response of a whole animal to an external stimuli, i.e. bioactive nanomaterials.

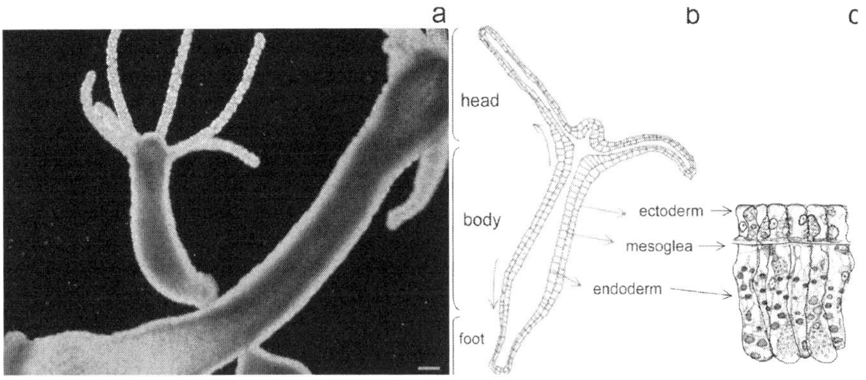

Fig. 1. Anatomical structure of *Hydra vulgaris*

Picture of living *Hydra*. a) The animal is shaped as a hollow tube with a head at the apical end, and a foot, or basal disc at the other. The head is in two parts, the hypostome (mouth) at the apex, and below that the tentacle zone from which a ring of six-eight tentacles emerges. The picture shows an adult animal with two buds emerging from the gastric region, facing two opposite parts. Scale bar 100 μm. b) Schematic representation of the bilayered structure of the animal: the body wall is composed of two self renewing cell layers, an outer ectoderm and an inner endoderm, separated by an extracellular matrix, the mesoglea. The arrows on the left side indicate the direction of tissue displacement. c) Along the animal body both ectoderm and endoderm layers are composed of epitheliomuscular cells, while interstitial stem cells and their intermediate and terminal derivatives (neurons, nematocytes and secretory cells) are interspersed among the two layers. Modified from (Tino, 2011).

Hydra polyps reproduce both sexually and asexually. Massive culturing is achieved thanks to fast mitotic reproduction, warranting a large number of identical clones (Loomis, 1956). The epithelial cells structuring the body continuously divide and contribute to the formation of new individuals, budding from the gastric region, and detaching from the mother in about 3 days (Figure 1A) (Galliot et al., 2006). Growth rate of *Hydra* tissue is normally regulated by a balance between epithelial cell cycle length, phagocytosis of ectodermal cell in "excess", and bud formation (Bosch and David, 1984). Environmental factors, such as the presence of pollutants or the feeding regime, can affect this balance. Thus, the population growth rate is an indirect measure of the *Hydra* tissue growth rate and cell viability.

Another peculiar feature of *Hydra* physiology is the remarkable capacity to regenerate amputated body parts. Polyps bisection at gastric or subhypostomal level in two parts generates stumps able to regenerate the missing parts (see Figure 2). Morphogenetic processes take place during the first 48 h post amputation (p.a.), followed by cell proliferation to restore adult size (Bode, 2003; Holstein et al., 2003). This highly controlled process relies on the spatio-temporal activation of specific genes and is object of wide investigations (Galliot and Ghila, 2010; Galliot et al., 2006). Moreover it can be adversely affected by the presence of organic and inorganic pollutants and specific assays have been developed to quantify this effect (Karntanut and Pascoe, 2000; Pollino and Holdway, 1999; Wilby, 1990).

Hydra is very sensitive to environmental toxicants and it has been used as biological indicator of water pollution. The responsiveness to different environmental stressors varies among different species, but it is always quantifiable by standardized protocols in terms of median lethal concentration and median lethal time (LC50 and LT50). For this reason short term (lethality) and long-term (sub-lethality) tests based on the evaluation of polyp morphology, reproductive activity and regeneration efficiency, can be used to test the potential toxicity/teratogenic effect of any kind of medium suspended compound.

Beside the effects detectable at macroscopic level, the availability of the genome sequence makes it possible to study the molecular mechanisms and gene pathways activated by the addition of external (chemical or physical) stressors. One of the main outcomes of the genomic sequencing projects of cnidarian species (corals, anemones, jellyfish and *Hydras*) (Chapman et al., 2010; Putnam et al., 2007) is the recognition that many genes, including those associated with diseases, are conserved in evolution from yeast to man (Steele et al., 2011). Remarkably, a surprisingly complexity was found in cnidarian genomes, in the range of higher vertebrates, while other invertebrates routinely used as model organisms, such as the fruit fly *Drosophila melanogaster* or the flatworm *Caernorabditis elegans*, have lost during speciation many genes belonging to the common eumetazoan primitive ancestor. In *Hydra*, the key pathways underlying development, regeneration and re-aggregation have been identified and their characterization showed the presence of almost complete gene repertoires: the canonical and non canonical Wnt pathways for maintaining and re-establishing apical organizer activity and for cellular evagination processes, respectively; the BMP/chordin pathway for axis patterning; the MAPK- CREB pathway for head regeneration; the FGF pathway for bud detachment, and the Notch pathway for differentiating some interstitial cell lineages (reviewed by Galliot, 2010; Galliot and Ghila, 2010).

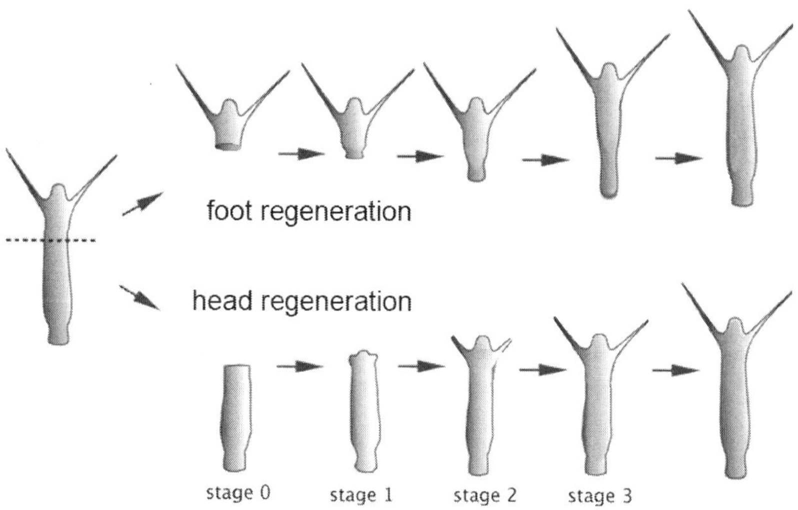

Fig. 2. The regeneration process in *Hydra vulgaris*

Hydra body column has a high capacity for regeneration of both the head and foot. Because of the tissue dynamics that take place in adult *Hydra*, the processes governing axial patterning are continuously active to maintain the form of the animal. Following amputation at mid-gastric level, the two polyp halves immediately initiate an asymmetric process at the wound site: the upper half undergoes foot regeneration in about two days, whereas the lower half initiates the head regeneration process, which is completed in three days. Biochemical, cellular and molecular analyses showed that these two regions immediately undergo different reorganization to become foot and head regenerating tips, respectively. Cell proliferation and differentiation during the late stages allow adult size to be restored.

3. *In vivo* interactions between semiconductor nanocrystals and *Hydra*

3.1 GSH functionalized QDs target specific cell types in *Hydra*

The tripeptide glutathione (g-L-glutamyl-L-cysteinylglycine, GSH) has been well-known to biochemists for generations. Both the reduced form (GSH) and its oxidized dimer (GSSG) have been implicated in a variety of molecular reactions throughout the animal kingdom. Although it is best known for its role as a free radical scavenger, GSH also performs a number of other functions in cell survival and metabolism, including amino acid transport, detoxification of xenobiotics, maintenance of protein redox state, neuromodulation, and neurotransmission. Almost 50 years ago, Loomis and Lenhoff suggested a role of GSH in signal transduction in *Hydra* (Loomis, 1955). A class of binding sites for GSH has been described (Bellis et al., 1994; Grosvenor et al., 1992), providing the basis for the behavioural response. However, up today, the GSH receptors have not been isolated. With the aim to identify in vivo GSH receptor/binding proteins we synthesized GSH functionalized fluorescent semiconductor quantum dots and analysed in vivo the elicitation of a behavioural response together with the localization of GSH targeted cells (Tortiglione et al., 2007). The choice of QD arose from the great advantages offered by these new nanotechnological probes over conventional ones which are revolutionising biology and medicine (Medintz et al., 2005). Colloidal semiconductor QD probes have unique photophysical properties, such as size-tuneable emission spectrum, narrow emission peak, broad absorption profile, and high brightness; they are much more stable to the permanent loss of fluorescence than conventional organic fluorophores (Michalet et al., 2005) becoming powerful investigation tools for multicolour, long-term, and high-sensitivity fluorescence imaging. QD functionalization with GSH was obtained by several reaction steps: core/shell CdSe/ZnS QDs were first water solubilized by the addition of an amphiphilic polymer coating (PC), then stabilized by Polyethylene Glycole (PEG) molecules, and finally covalently bound to GSH (Figure 3).

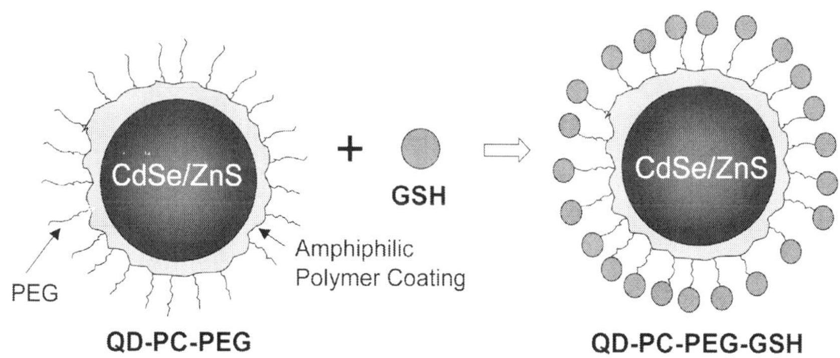

Fig. 3. Schematic representation of a GSH-QD conjugate.

Polymer-coated CdSe/ZnS core shell quantum dots were first conjugated to diamino-modified PEG molecules and then to GSH through amide bond formation. The resulting bioconjugated were extensively characterized to confirm the presence of the surface functionalizations (Tortiglione et al., 2007).

Both PEG-QDs and PEG-GSH-QDs were supplied to living polyps at different concentrations and then observed by fluorescence microscopy. A biological response consisting in mouth opening and QD entry into the gastric cavity was elicited by GSH-QDs. The elicitation of this behaviour, although slightly different from the classical feeding response (consisting of tentacle writhing and mouth opening) and occurring in a small percentage of animals (15%), was specific for GSH coated QDs, and indicated the bioactivity of the new GSH abduct. Fluorescent QD targeted cells were found within the inner endodermal cells, which internalized the QD upon mouth opening (see Figure 4) (Tortiglione et al., 2007).

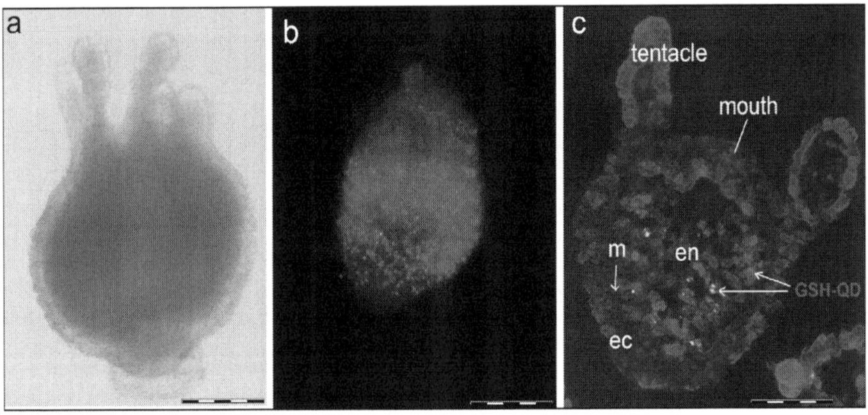

Fig. 4. *In vivo* fluorescence imaging of *Hydra* polyps treated with 300 nM GSH-QDs (emission max: 610 nm).
a) Bright field image of *Hydra* treated with GSH-QDs showing animal basic structure. The foot is on the lower part of the panel, while a crown of tentacles surrounds the mouth. b) Image taken 24 h after treatment: an intense fluorescence is distributed all along the gastric region. c) Cellular localization of QDs in *Hydra* cross sections. The whole *Hydra* was treated with 300 nM GSH-QDs for 24 h, fixed in 4% paraformaldehyde, and included for cryosectioning. Images were collected using an inverted microscope (Axiovert, 100, Zeiss) equipped with fluorescence filter sets (BP450-490/FT510/LP515). Endodermal cells(en) are separated from ectodermal cells (ec) by an extracellular matrix, the mesoglea (m), indicated by the arrow. Red fluorescence corresponds to GSH-QDs located specifically into endodermal cells. Scale bars: 500 μm in a, b; 200 μm in c

The fluorescence pattern and intensity lasted unaltered until the animals were fed again, after which the signal started to fade slowly and was diluted throughout the emerging buds (Figure 5).

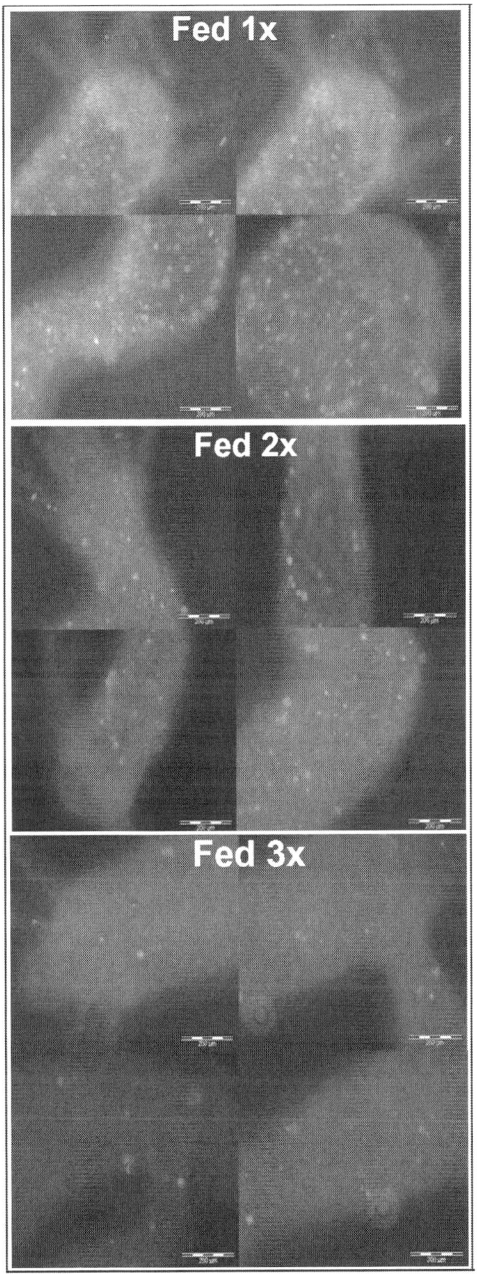

Fig. 5. Tracking QD fluorescence under normal feeding regime

GSH-QDs do not undergo degradation into the endodermal cells. They follow cell turnover and migration towards the animal ends and the developing bud. *Hydra* treated with GSH-QDs were fed on alternate days. After three feeding cycles GSH-QDs were found diluted among the endodermal cells, continuously diving. The orange fluorescent punctuated pattern decreases uniformly as new buds are formed on the mother (see lower panel, representing an adult with an emerging bud). Scale bars are 200 μm in all pictures.

The uptake of GSH-QDs was an active endocytotic process, as shown by its inhibition when performing the incubation at 4 °C. Tissue cryosection and dissociation of whole treated polyps into single cell suspensions confirmed the presence of QDs into cytoplasmic granular vesicles. In conclusion this first work showed that GSH-QDs alone can stimulate a response, although in a small percentage (15%) of the treated animals. Possible reasons for this low percentage could be a low concentration of the GSH molecules conjugated to the QD surface or the modified stereochemical conformation of the bound GSH molecules, which does not allow for correct interaction with the protein target. Although the bioactive GSH-QDs could target specific cells, as shown by the fluorescence of the endodermal layer, the nature of the GSH binding protein (as GSH receptor, GSH transporters...) remain to be determined. An important clue emerged from this study was the capability of PEG-QDs to be also internalized by endodermal cells, upong chemical induction of mouth opening. The uptake rate was lower compared to GSH-QDs, indicating different internalization routes and underlying mechanism for the two types of QDs. Considering the multiple roles played by glutathione in metabolic functions, and in particular in the nervous system of higher vertebrates, GSH functionalized nanocrystals prepared and tested in this work represent promising tools for a wide variety of investigations, such as the elucidation of the role played by GSH in neurotransmission and the identification of its putative receptor. Beside these considerations, the capability of PEG-QDs to be up taken by *Hydra* cells prompted us to investigate more in detail the mechanism of internalization of QDs, the role played by the surface ligand, the surface chemistry and charge, which underlies any bio-non -bio interaction.

3.2 Unfunctionalized Quantum Rods elicit a behavioural response in *Hydra vulgaris*

The capability of *Hydra* to internalize, upon chemical induction of mouth opening, PEG-QDs into endodermal cells suggested that also unfunctionalized nanocrystals can play active roles when interacting with living cells. Noteworthy attention should be paid to the chemical composition of surfactant-polymer-coated nanoparticles not only in determining their stability in aqueous media but also in investigating their interaction with cells and intracellular localization. With the aim to test the impact of a new kind of semiconductor nanocrystal on *Hydra* vulgaris, we demonstrated that specific behaviours might be induced by exposure of whole animals to unfunctionalized nanocrystals and that a careful investigation of the impact of the new material on living cells must be carried out before designing any nanodevice for biomedical purposes (Malvindi et al., 2008).

The nanocrystals under investigation were fluorescent CdSe/CdS quantum rods (from here named QRs). In addition to QD properties, such as bright photoluminescence (PL), narrow emission spectra, and broad UV excitation, QRs have larger absorption cross-sections, which might allow improvement to certain biological applications where extremely high brightness and photostability are required. QRs of length and diameter 35 ± 2 nm and 4.2 ± 0.4 nm, respectively, were synthesised according to a newly developed procedure (Carbone et al., 2007), and transferred to aqueous medium by using the same methodology described above for QDs (Pellegrino, 2004; Sperling, 2006; Williams, 1981). The resulting highly fluorescent PEG coated QRs (Figure 6) were challenged to living polyps, which were monitored over progressive incubation periods.

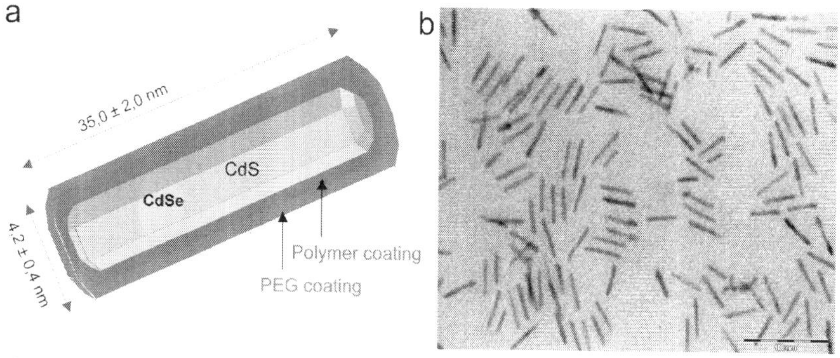

Fig. 6. A schematic representation of the CdSe/CdS rods used in this study

The scheme shows the asymmetrical shape derived from the synthesis procedure (Carbone et al, 2007). The method involves coinjecting Cd^{2+} and S^{2-} precursors and preformed spherical CdSe seeds into an environment of hot surfactants, well suited for the anisotropic growth of the second shell-material (CdS) on the first underlying core (CdSe). Resulting QRs are transferred from chloroform to water by wrapping them within an amphiphilic polymer shell (blue shell in the figure). To these polymer-coated QRs, polyethylene glycol (PEG) molecules (red shell) can be bound by using an EDC catalyzed cross linking scheme. The rod samples are an average of 35nm in length and 4 nm in diameter as confirmed by b) the TEM image of the corresponding sample (generously provided by Dr.A.Quarta, Italian Institute of Technology, Lecce, Italy)
Unlabelled cells were detectable by fluorescence microscopy, indicating that QRs were not uptaken by *Hydra* ectodermal cells. However, an unexpected animal behaviour was observed which consisted of an intense tentacle writhing, i.e. contractions and bending along the axial length of each tentacle, as shown in Figure 7.

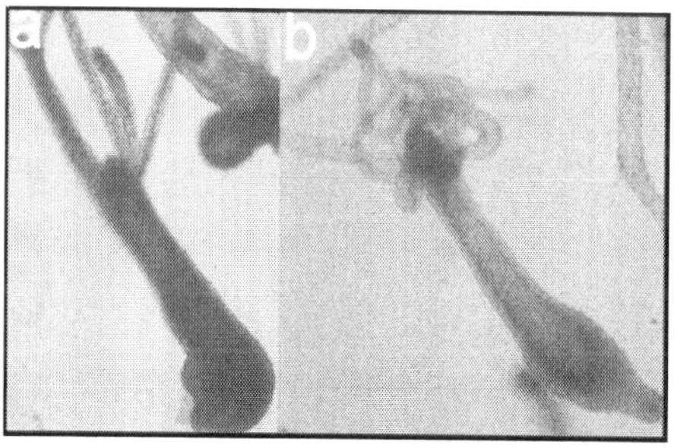

Fig. 7. Elicitation of tentacle writhing by QRs.

The test was initiated by adding CdSe/CdS core/shell QRs to each well containing six polyps and motor activity was monitored by continuous video recording using a Camedia-digital camera (Olympus) connected to a cold light Wild stereo microscope a) *Hydra* polyp in physiological condition show extended tentacles. b) Within seconds of addition of QRs to the culture medium the polyp's tentacle begin to writhe, bending toward the mouth. Contractions are not synchronous for all tentacles and lasted for an average of ten minutes (Malvindi et al., 2008).

The elicitation of this behaviour over an average period of ten minutes was dependent on the presence of calcium ions into *Hydra* medium, as shown by the inhibition of such activity by the calcium chelator EGTA. Interestingly, *Hydra* chemically depleted of neuronal cells were unresponsive to QRs, indicating that excitable cells are targeted by QRs. The mechanisms underlying neuron excitation are still under investigation, but the shape anisotropy has been shown involved in the elicitation of the activity, as nanocrystals of the identical chemical composition, but shaped as dots were ineffective. We suggested that CdSe/CdS QRs, regardless of surface chemical functionalization, may generate local electric fields associated with their permanent dipole moments that are intense enough to stimulate voltage dependent ion channels, thus eliciting an action potential resulting in motor activity. Results from a geometrical approximation (Malvindi et al., 2008) showed that a QR voltage potential of sufficient intensity to stimulate a voltage gated ion channel can be produced at nanometric separation distances, i.e. those lying between cell membranes and medium suspended QR, regardless of its orientation at the cell surface, thus it is theoretically possible for QRs to elicit neuronal activity. This hypothesis is currently under investigation in vertebrate model systems. In particular, we have preliminary data on the modulation of the electrophysiological properties of mammalian brain slices by QRs, (unpublished data) which indicate that QR response is not specific to our experimental model. Considering the challenges encountered in the design and synthesis of electrical nanodevices for neuronal stimulation (Pappas, 2007) we propose biocompatible, soluble QRs as a novel resource for neuronal devices, for diagnostic and therapeutic applications where non invasive probing and fine tuning of neuronal activity is required.

The peculiarities of our biological model system, such as the low-ionic-strength culture media and the presence of excitable cells directly facing the outer media, allowed us to highlight the neuronal stimulation by a nanometric inorganic particle, which might be difficult to study *in vivo* in a more complex whole organism. Avoiding the difficulties in investigating vertebrate brain behaviour *in vivo*, our cnidarian model organisms provided a simple, reliable, and fast system for screening nanoparticle activity *in vivo* on a functionally connected nerve net.

3.3 Unfunctionalized Quantum Rods reveals regulated portal of entry into *Hydra* cells

The complexity of the molecular interactions underlying the endocytosis suggests that a great evolutionary effort has been spent to regulate the cellular response to a variety of different environmental stimuli. In multicellular organisms the endocytic and secretory pathways evolved to control all aspects of cell physiology and intercellular communication (neurotransmission, immune response, development, hormone-mediated signal transduction). In this scenario, the emerging nanomaterials, variable in size (from 2 to 100 nm), chemical composition (gold, cadmium telluride, cadmium selenide, iron oxide) and physical properties (charge, spectral profile, colloidal stability, magnetism) represent a new class of compounds interacting with biological systems, which underlying mechanisms need to be carefully investigated. When studying the impact of CdSe/CdS QRs on *Hydra* (Malvindi et al., 2008), beside the detection of a specific behavioural response, an accurate microscopy analysis was performed in order to assess the putative internalization of the

QRs into *Hydra* cells. At neutral pH, QR uptake was never detectable at the concentrations (7nM) eliciting biological activity. By contrast, using the same concentration of CdSe/CdS QRs, but changing the pH of the *Hydra* medium toward mild acidic values (pH 4.5- 4), an intense fluorescence was observed (Tortiglione et al., 2009). The labelling pattern as soon as 30 minutes post incubation with QRs appeared like a uniform red fluorescence staining all around the animal (Figure 8a). In the following hours membrane bound nanocrystals appeared compacted within cytoplasmic granular structures, easily detectable as red spots at level of the tentacles first (Figure 8b), and then throughout the body (Figure 8c).

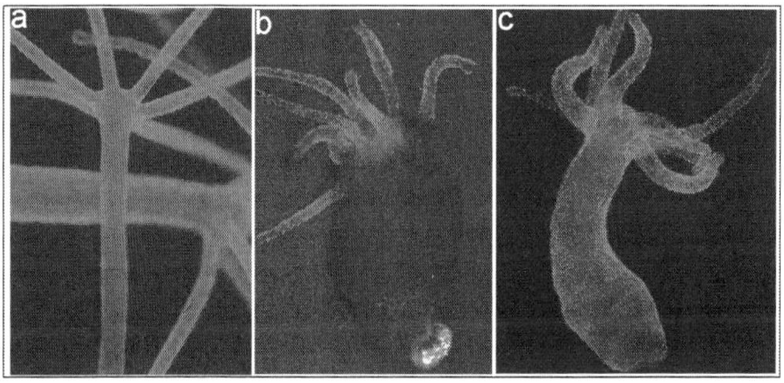

Fig. 8. *In vivo* fluorescence imaging of *Hydra vulgaris* exposed to QRs for different periods a) *In vivo* image of two *Hydra,* 30 minutes post incubation (p.i.): QR red fluorescence labels uniformly all body regions. A second *Hydra* is placed horizontally below b) *In vivo* image of a polyp 2h p.i. with QRs. A strong punctuated fluorescence labels the mouth, the tentacles and at a lower extent the animal body. c) Later on, in most of the animals, the punctuated fluorescence is evident also in body column.

Tissue cryosections made from treated animals allowed to detect not only the ectodermal localization of the internalized QRs, but also the dynamic of the labelled cells, at various time after incubation (Figure 9).

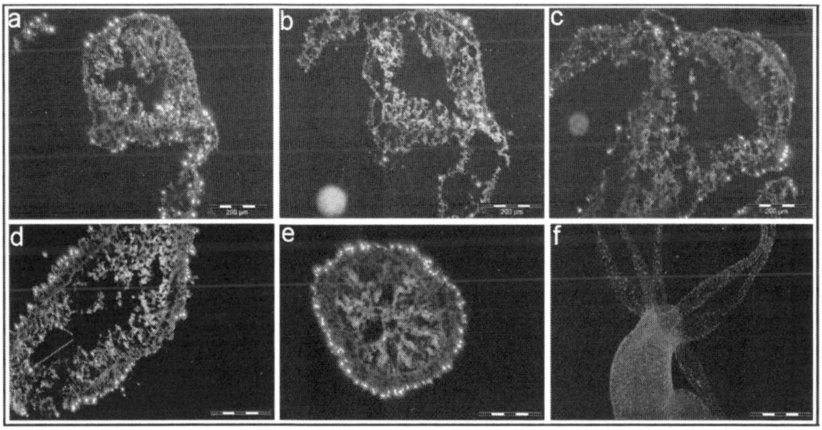

Fig. 9. Tissue localization of QRs in *Hydra* tissue sections.

Intact *Hydra* were treated with QRs at acidic pH for 4 h, and 24 h later fixed and processed for cryosectioning. The green colour is due to tissue autofluorescence, while the red staining indicate the QR presence. Serial longitudinal tissue cryosections obtained at level of the head (a, b and c) and body (d) show QRs located into the ectodermal cells, but also inside endodermal cells lining both the tentacles and gastric region. A transversal section (e) confirms the tissue distribution. The labelling pattern before sectioning is shown in (f). Scale bars: 200 μm (a-e), and 500 μm (f).

Remarkably, 24 h post treatment, fluorescent material appeared also into the endodermal cells lining the gastric cavity and the tentacles. At the tentacle base, the fluorescence draws a well defined strip along the tentacle length, shown by cross sections to be localised inside the endodermal cells and not in the tentacle lumen (Figure 9a, 9b, 9c). This cell dynamic, from ectoderm to endoderm, has never been described using conventional organic fluorophores and highlights the importance of using the innovative fluorophore to probe biological processes. The high photostability of the QRs allowed to study with unprecedented brightness and resolution endocytotic processes in *Hydra* and to track these phenomena over long periods. The same dynamic was observed also during regeneration of treated animals and it probably depends from autophagocytosis process occurring during head regeneration (Tortiglione et al., 2009). Beside these results, we determined the factors involved in the capability of *Hydra* to uptake QRs at acidic but not neutral pH and investigated the roles played by the nanocrystal surface at one side and by *Hydra* membranes at the other. QRs used in this study where stabilised by the addition of amino-PEG coating. Zeta potential measurement showed that at acidic pH QRs were positively charged, while at neutral pH their surface net charge was neutral or negative. Modifying the amounts of amino-PEG molecules present on QR surface we were able to tune the QR net charge and thus the up taking process. At acidic pH, the protonation of the PEG amino terminal groups (NH^{3+}) contributes to increase the positive charges while the protonation of the carboxyl groups of the amphiphilic polymer shell causes a reduction of the negative charges (COO^{2-}) at the nanoparticle surface and indeed the sum of the two effects results in a net positive surface of the QR (Figure 10). The different amounts of PEG molecules attached at the same QR surface account for the different behaviours displayed by diverse nanorod samples, independently from their size and shape. QRs presenting positive zeta potential bind to negatively charged membrane lipids, and stimulate endocytosis processes. A scheme of the QR protonation occurring at acidic pH is shown in Figure 10.

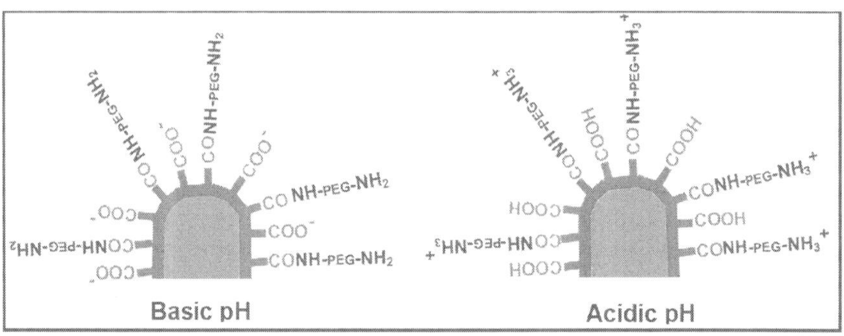

Fig. 10. Protonation/de-protonation state of the QRs.

A schematic view of the functional groups at the nanoparticle surface responsible for the switching of the surface charge. At basic pH, the carboxy groups are negatively charged and the amino groups are not protonated. At acidic pH, the carboxy and the amino groups are both protonated, which account for a positive zeta potential value measured. At neutral pH, the zeta potential measured in all cases is negative. The blue colour indicates the CdS/CdS core, while the amphiphilic polymer and PEG coatings are pink coloured. Modified from (Tortiglione et al., 2009).

We also investigated the biological factors involved in the internalization of QRs at acidic pH, and found the involvement of a peculiar protein displaying a pH dependent behaviour, named Annexin (ANX) (Moss and Morgan, 2004). ANXB12 is a *Hydra* protein belonging to the annexins superfamily, able to insert into lipidic membranes and to form ion channels at acidic but not neutral pH (Schlaepfer et al., 1992a; Schlaepfer et al., 1992b). As *Hydra* treatment with anti-ANX antibody prevented QR uptake, we suggest that ANX mediates the interaction with positively charged QRs, organizing membrane domains and uptake processes, probably throughout the specie-specific amino terminal domain. In presence of anti-ANX antibody, the endocytosis machinery is blocked, likely due to impairment of functional or structural important ANX extracellular domains.

In conclusion, the combined effect of nanorod positive surface charge and structural properties of cell membranes, at acidic pH, resulted in the active internalization of the fluorescent nanoparticles into specific cell types and according to a precise temporal dynamic. The availability of beautifully illuminated animals led to track fluorescent cells during developmental and regeneration processes, and to describe, beside known migration events, new cell dynamics and inter-epithelial/intercellular trafficking phenomena, which intriguing meaning lays the foundations for further investigations. Thus, we provide an example of how, probing cell and animal biology with nanosized compounds, we can uncover novel biological phenomena, aware of our capability of finely tuning and controlling this interaction for specific purposes.

The two examples of *Hydra*/QR interaction described in the two sections above show two biologically relevant responses induced by the same nanocrystal, determined in one case by the QR intrinsic shape dependent electrical properties, and in the other one by the QR positive surface charge. These studies show that presentation of chemical information at the same size scale as that of cell surface receptors may interfere with cellular processes, eliciting unexpected responses, such as the activation of a behavioural responses, or cell uptake, and that a simple experimental change, such as the pH of the medium used in the bioassay, may determinate dramatic difference in the evoked response. Thus, the interactions occurring at the interface bio-non bio are complex and depending on both players, which need to be fully characterized when designing nanodevices targeting biological systems.

3.4 Cadmium telluride QDs induce cytotoxic effects in *Hydra vulgaris*

The freedom to design and modify NCs to accomplish very specific tasks is currently being realized. However, their unique properties, not present in conventional bulk materials, such as enhanced magnetic, electrical and optical properties, have potential implications in NC toxicity, such as elemental composition, charge, shape, surface area and surface chemistry/derivatization. Several data of the inherent toxicity of some NCs are available and indicate that they can affect biological behaviour at the organ, tissue and cellular levels, and activate changes in the expression of stress-related or apoptotic genes (Choi et al., 2008; Rivera Gil et al., 2010). The great amount of data collected up to today regards different materials, biological systems, and are strictly dependent on the cell lines tested (Lewinski et al., 2008). This may be a result of interference with the chemical probes, differences in the innate response of particular cell types, as well as depending upon the different protocols used by different laboratories for the nanoparticle synthesis and characterization, giving rise to not identical nanomaterials. Therefore, for a single nanocrystal, the biological activities of NCs should be assessed by multiple cell-based assays and should more realistically rely on animal models (Fischer and Chan, 2007).

A primary source of QD toxicity results from cadmium residing in the QD core. Toxicity of uncoated core CdSe or CdTe-QD has been discussed in several reports and is associated, in part, with free cadmium present in the particle suspensions or released from the particle core intracellularly (Derfus, 2004; Kirchner et al., 2005; Lovric et al., 2005a). Free radical formation induced by the highly reactive QD core might also play crucial roles in the cellular toxicity. Encapsulation of the CdSe-QD with a ZnS shell or other capping materials has been shown to reduce toxicity, although much work remains to be completed in this field. However, to accurately assess safety of shell or capped particles, the degradation of the shell or capping material, along with its cytotoxicity must also be considered since several groups have found increased toxicity associated to capping materials such as mercaptoacetic acid and Topo-tri-n-octylphosphine oxide (TOPO) (Smith et al., 2008). Taken together, these reports suggest that the integrity of shell and capping materials, as well as toxicity, needs to also be more thoroughly assessed and that shell/capping materials must be assessed for different QD preparations.

Based on these considerations long term studies of effects on both cell viability and signal transduction are needed, and surely the animal studies are definitely required for proper assessment of QD toxicity. To date, rats have been used as model organisms for pharmacological studies, and only recently the use of invertebrates to test Cd based QDs is adding valuable informations in this field. For example, the freshwater macroinvertebrate, Daphnia magna, has been used to evaluate toxicity characteristics of CdSe/ZnSe in relation to surface coatings (Lee, 2009).

Cnidaria are sensitive to many environmental stressors and may become valuable indicators of exposure to disruptive chemicals and other stressors, such as nanomaterials. During animal evolution, an array of gene families and pathways (also known as "environmental genes") have evolved to face physical, chemical, and biological stressors. While the immune system responds to biotic stressors such as pathogens (Miller et al., 2007), another set of genes named "chemical defensome" (Goldstone, 2008), has been identified to sense, transform, and eliminate potentially toxic chemicals.

Hydra is sensitive to a range of pollutants and has been used to tests on water contamination by heavy metals (Holdway et al., 2001; Pascoe et al., 2003; Pollino and Holdway, 1999). Metal pollutants such as copper, cadmium and zinc have been tested against different *Hydra* species, and the relative toxicity based on the median lethal concentration (LC50) for all species was ranked from copper, the most toxic, to cadmium, with zinc least toxic (Karntanut and Pascoe, 2002; Karntanut and Pascoe, 2005). Drugs and pharmaceuticals targeted at mammalian receptors have also been shown to adversely affects *Hydra* (Pascoe et al., 2002), showing the feasibility to use this aquatic invertebrate to accurately assess the potential toxicological effect of any kind of molecule added to the animal culture medium.

In light of this knowledge we evaluated the possibility to use *Hydra* for nanotoxicology purposes. We addressed the toxicological effects of fluorescent CdTe QDs, presenting different chemical coatings on *Hydra* using several bioassays: 1) alteration of morphological traits, measurable as morphological median score values 2) alteration of reproductive capabilities, measurable as population growth rates 3) alteration of regeneration or pattern formation. These three phenomena are schematically drawn in Figure 11.

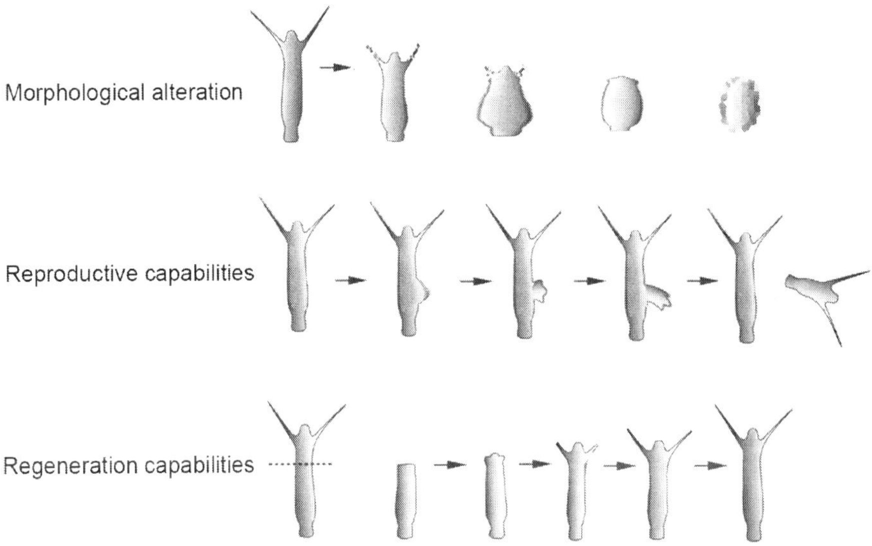

Fig. 11. Different developmental potentials available in the adult polyp.

The toxic effects of organic and inorganic pollutants, i.e, CdTe QDs, can be measured using *Hydra*, due to its unique developmental potentials. The toxicant under investigation can be added to the medium bathing living polyps and the effects on morphology, reproductive and regeneration capabilities can be quantified by standardised protocols. Upper panel: alteration of morphological traits can be measured by assigning numerical scores to progressive morphological changes (Wilby, 1988)(see below). Middle panel: upon regular feeding, the animals undergo asexual reproduction through budding: the number of buds produced by a single polyp over two weeks can be expressed as reproductive rate, which is altered in presence of toxicants. Lower panel: initially reported by A.Trembley (Trembley, 1744), Hydra polyps can regenerate any missing part after bisection of the body column performed at any level, and the presence of toxicants can irreversibly affect this capability.

CdTe nanocrystals are the most successful example of the colloidal quantum dots directly synthesized in aqueous solution. In Figure 12 a schematic representation of the synthesis of TGA-capped QDs is shown. The methodology was first described by Gao (Gao M, 1998) and it is routinely employed in many laboratories, although modifications have been further developed to increase photoluminescence, quantum yields, or for specific applications in various fields ranging from light harvesting and energy transfer to biotechnology (Gaponik and Rogach, 2010). The water-soluble CdTe QDs we analysed using *Hydra* were surface-capped with thioglycolic acid (TGA) or stabilized by glutathione (GSH), synthesized as described (Rogach and Lesnyak, 2007) and present a mean diameter of 3.1nm and 3.6nm, respectively .

In our previous studies using CdSe/ZnS QDs or CdSe/CdS QRs evident toxicity signs were not detected, even at the highest QD dose tested (300nM) (Tortiglione et al., 2007). In those cases, nanocrystal synthesis was accomplished by burying a CdSe inner core into a ZnS or CdS shell, then wrapping the metal core/shell by an amphiphilic polymer, further stabilised by conjugation to PEG molecules. The CdTe QDs are sized only a few nanometres and differ not only in chemical composition, but also in the synthetic route (directly in aqueous solution) employing different compounds (thioglycolic acid or glutathione...) as stabilising molecules. These differences drove our comparative toxicity studies using CdTe QDs and testing different concentrations and exposure times (Tino et al., 2011).

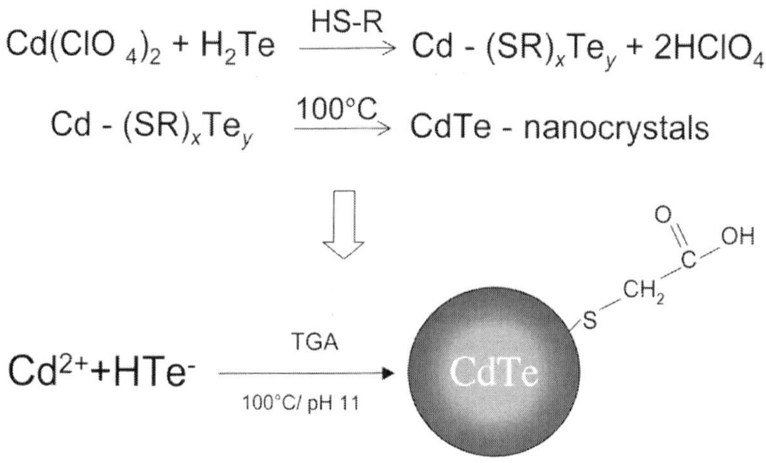

Fig. 12. Schematic representation of TGA capped QDs

The basics of the aqueous synthesis of thiol-capped CdTe NCs. In a typical standard synthesis, $Cd(ClO_4)$ salts are dissolved in water, and an appropriate amount of the thiol stabilizer is added under stirring, followed by adjusting the pH by dropwise addition of NaOH. Under stirring, H_2Te gas is then passed through the solution together with a slow nitrogen flow. CdTe NC precursors are formed at this stage; formation and growth of NCs proceed upon refluxing at 100°C under open-air conditions with a condenser attached (from (Rogach and Lesnyak, 2007).

When challenging living polyps to CdTe QDs, adverse effects on animal behaviour and morphology were immediately observed. In Figure 13 the pictures of polyps carrying progressive damages are shown. These different damages have been annotated using a scoring system ranging from 10 (healthy polyps) to zero (disintegrated animals) (Wilby, 1990), and already used for toxicological studies in *Hydra*. This system can be efficiently adopted to compare toxicity of diverse compounds or the sensitivity of different species to a given substance.

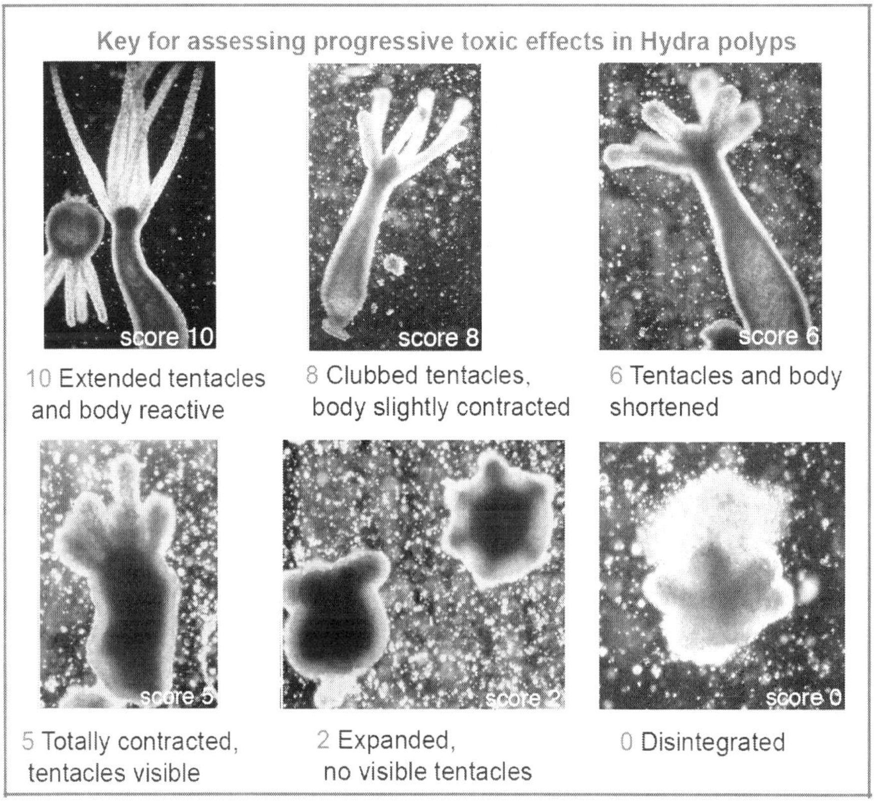

Fig. 13. Score system to assess toxic effects on *Hydra*

Examples of morphological alterations induced by treatment of living *Hydra* with CdTe QDs. Animals were incubated with TGA-QDs and observed by a stereomicroscope over a period of 72h. Images show progressive morphological changes scored from 10 down to 0, according to the scoring system previously developed (Wilby, 1988)

By fluorescence microscopy we observed intense staining in animals treated with the highest tested QD concentration (300nM), indicating QD uptake (Figure 14). At lower concentrations, the low fluorescent staining did not allow imaging.

Elemental analysis by Inductively Coupled Plasma Atomic Emission Spectrometer (ICP-AES) confirmed the internalization of the CdTeQDs (Ambrosone et al, unpublished).

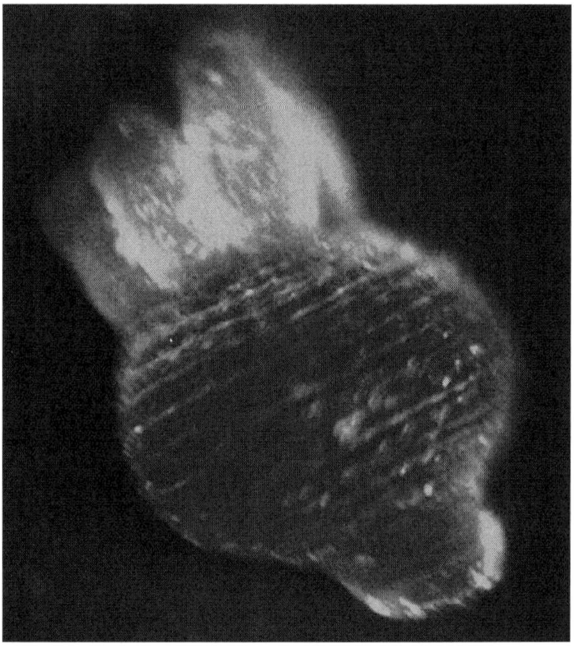

Fig. 14. *In vivo* fluorescence image of *Hydra* treated with 300nM TGA-QDs

Polyps were challenged with CdTe QDs and imaged after 2 hours of incubation. The polyp appears contracted, the tentacles clubbed, shortened. The fluorescence is uniform all along the animal (body and tentacles), drawing straight lines perpendicular to the main oral-aboral axis, and corresponding to membranes belonging to adjacent cells aligned during contraction. Granular structures are also present, indicating the initial uptake of QDs by ectodermal cells.

We performed acute toxicity tests (by exposing the animals for two hours to QDs and then monitoring the morphological scores), and chronic toxicity tests performing continuous incubation with the QDs (Ambrosone et al, unpublished). Under both acute and chronic treatment the median score values decreased with progressive exposure time, indicating toxic effect (see Figure 15A). After 72 hr of continuous incubation with 25nM QDs, all animals showed score value equal to zero, meaning that were all fully disintegrated. In Figure 15B, the distribution of the different scores among the treated animals is shown at each time point. Untreated animals showed always score 10 (blue bar, highlighted by the upper red arrow), while treatment with QDs causes a decrease in the score values, more pronounced for the higher QD concentration tested (25nM). In this latter case after 72 hr of continuous incubation all animals were fully disintegrated, as highlighted by the red arrows of Figure 15B.

The toxicity of CdTe QD to *Hydra* was further evaluated using a different method, based on mortality. The number of death animals was used for survival statistical analysis, and the Karber-Spearmann (Hamilton, 1977) method used to determinate the median lethal concentration and the median lethal scores, as shown in Figure 15C.

A

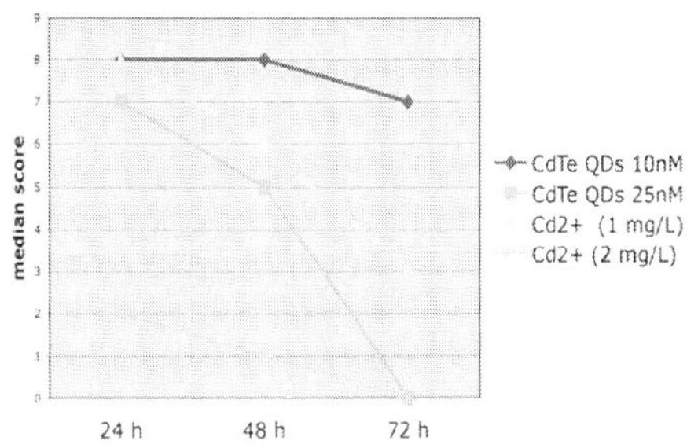

B

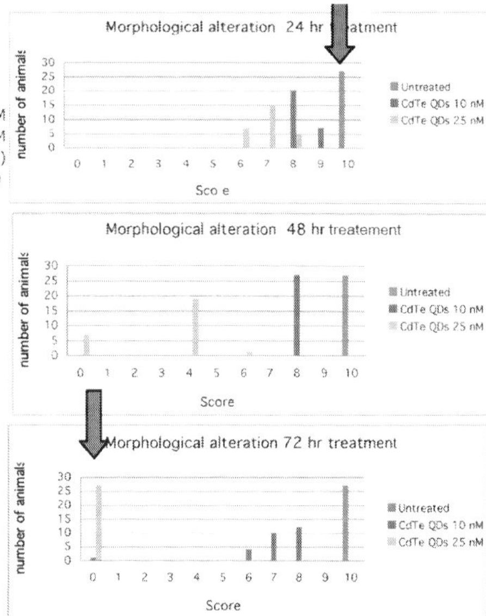

C

Time	LC50 (nM)
24 h	35.6
48 h	28.7
72 h	15.54

Conc.	LT50 (hr)
10nM	89.7
25nM	50.4

Fig. 15. Methods used to evaluate the toxicity of CdTe-QDs on *Hydra*

Two different methods can be used to assess the toxicity of a given compound on *Hydra*. The first method (used in A and B) is based on the evaluation of animal morphological traits, while the second one (C) is based on survival rates. In A the time response toxicity curves to equivalent TGA-QD concentrations are compared to the curves obtained by two different concentrations of Cd salts. 25 *Hydra* were treated with the indicated compound and morphological scores were monitored over 24, 48 and 72hr. In B the number of the animals presenting different scores are reported for each time point in the three graphs (24, 48, 72hr). The red arrows highlights that the score values decreasing from ten (untreated animals) to zero obtained with 25nM concentration, after 72hr of incubation. In C the median lethal time and median lethal concentration were calculated using the Sperman-Karber method.

In this way sub-lethal doses were determined and used for assessing the potential long-term toxic effects induced by CdTe QDs on *Hydra* reproductive capabilities (Ambrosone et al., 2011; Tino et al., 2011). Growth rate of *Hydra* tissue is regulated by the epithelial cell cycle, which normal length (about 3 days) is controlled by environmental conditions, i.e., the feeding regime (Bosch and David, 1984). Thus, for a given feeding condition, the growth rate is an indirect measure of the *Hydra* tissue growth and cell viability. The number of individuals generated by an adult polyps over two-three weeks can be used to calculate the growth rates constant (k), which is the slope of the regression line using the standard equation of logarithmic growth: $\ln (n/n^{\circ}) = kt$ (where n is the number of individuals at the time t, and n° is the number of the founder polyps). Representative growth rate curves determined for QD treated and untreated animals are shown in the graph of Figure 15, and indicate k values lower for QD treated animals compared to control. These differences were found significant by statistical analysis of repeated experiments (Ambrosone et al, unpublished).

Regeneration efficiencies were also estimated bisecting the animals and allowing regeneration in presence of QDs. During the first 48-72hr post amputation a great percentage of animals treated with the highest QD concentration were unable to regenerate a head and were found as stumps without tentacles (stage 0).
Moreover, about 30% of the bisected animals died, demonstrating the high QD toxicity (see Figure 16, upper panel).

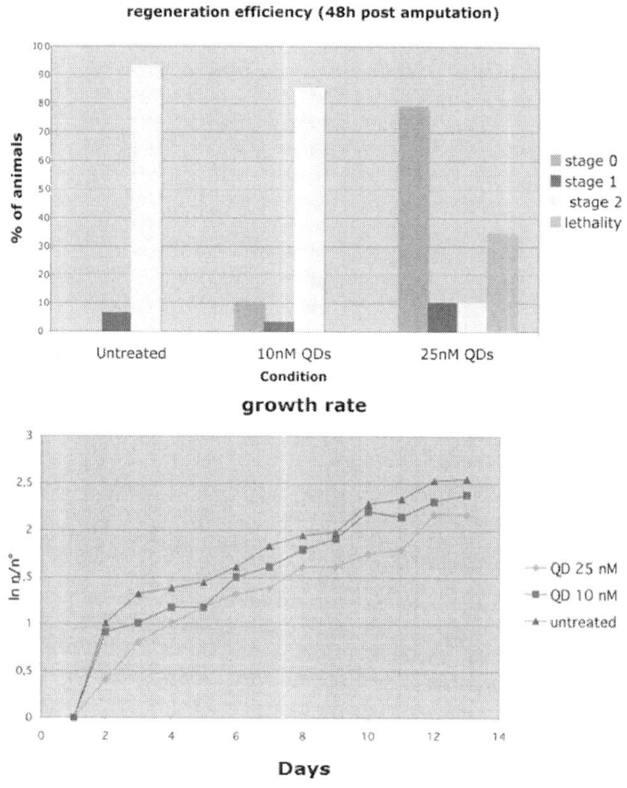

Fig. 16. Impact of CdTe QDs on regeneration efficiency and growth rates

Upper panel: representative histogram showing the impact of QDs on *Hydra* head regeneration. The regeneration stages are classified as in Fig.2. Basically, stage zero indicate the complete inhibition of regeneration (zero tentacles); stage 1, indicates heads with aberrant tentacles (one or two), while stage 2 indicates normal regeneration (tentacles from four to six at this time). The lowest QD concentration tested, 10nM, does not impair head regeneration, while the 25nM dose inhibits the whole process, and furthermore, causes lethality. Lower panel: influence of the QD treatment on *Hydra* population growth rate. Population growth test started with a population of four full-grown *Hydra*, incubated 24h with the indicated dose of QD, washed out and monitored every day for bud detachment. The logarithmic growth rate constant (k) is the slope of the regression line using the standard equation of logarithmic growth: ln (n/n0) = kt. In this representative graph the regression line is not drawn. Polyps treated with the highest QD concentration were impaired in the reproductive capabilities, as shown by the altered ratio n/n° along the monitored period (Ambrosone et al, unpublished).

We also compared the effects of thioglycolic acid capped QDs (TGA-QDs) and glutathione capped QDs (GSH-QDs), by using the same approaches and observed that although both nanocrystals were toxic, the most severe effects were induced by TGA capped QDs (Tino et al., 2011). This confirms the importance of the nanocrystal surface chemistry in the interaction with living cells.

The availability of a *Hydra* whole genome sequence allowed us to study the nanoparticle-induced cellular changes at three levels: non-genomic, genomic and epigenetic. The genes selectively involved in the apoptosis or in the necrosis process, as diverse as the Hymyc transcription factor, Caspase 3, Superoxide dismutase, Hsp70 have been analysed by quantitative real time PCR, and compared to the expression of animals treated with free cadmium salts (Ambrosone et al, unpublished). Aside from genotoxic effects, as nanoparticles could cause more subtle changes to living cells, such as long-term effects on gene expression, after the QD signal has been removed, epigenetic effects are being addressed. At the current stage of investigation, the elucidation of the possible molecular pathways activated by CdTe QDs appears rather complex, and it may concern universal stress response genes, Cd specific response genes or novel unidentified signalling cascades, initiated by the QDs at the cell surface.

In conclusion, by using different approaches, from *in vivo* evaluation of morphological traits to the impact on growth rate and regeneration, to the molecular analysis of the genes potentially involved in the QD response, we determined animal behaviours and toxicological effects played by CdTe QDs, and proposed *Hydra* as a valuable model for nanotoxicology studies.

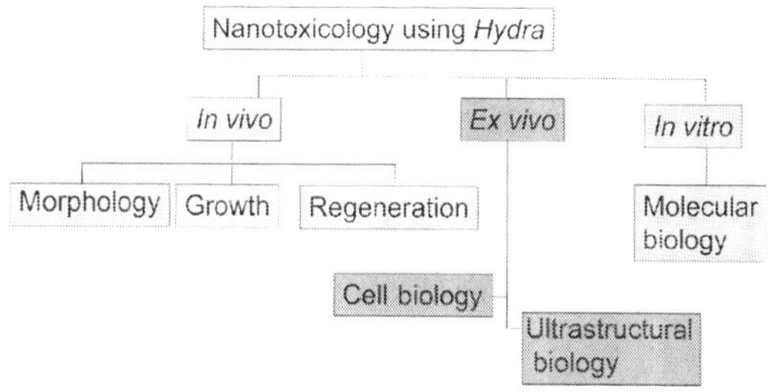

Fig. 17. Methodological approaches for nanotoxicology using *Hydra* as model system

The impact of nanoparticles on a living organism can be assessed by using the freshwater polyp *Hydra*. This system allows to evaluate *in vivo*, *ex vivo* and *in vitro* the responses of a whole animal to short or long exposures of any organic and inorganic compound, unless unstable in *Hydra* culture medium.

4. *Hydra* as a widely applicable tool for high-throughput screens of nanoparticles biocompatibility and (eco)toxicity

The use of simple model organisms to dissect complex biological processes has permitted biology to advance at an impressive pace, and the knowledge generated by integrating genetic and biochemical studies has allowed scientists to begin to understand the molecular basis of complex diseases such as cancer and diabetes. Several pharmaceutical companies developed research programs that use simple organisms to identify and validate drug targets. Since the production of newer engineered nanomaterials and their applications has exponentially increased, high-throughput screens (HTS) are required to evaluate their impact on human and environmental health. In the above sections I gave some examples demonstrating the use of *Hydra* as valuable model system for the dissection of biological processes evoked by metal based nanocrystals. Because of the small size, short generation time, high fecundity and cost effective maintenance, it can also be used for HTS of nanoparticle biocompatibility, environmental and animal impact. Standard microtiter plates can be used for whole animal assays to assess toxicity and identify the underlying mechanisms by simply changing multiple experimental conditions in adjacent wells, such as medium composition, pH, presence of specific inhibitors/competitors/agonists, and the trials can all be run in parallel, in large scale enabling statistical treatment of the data.

In addition, the new genomic resources open the way to the molecular toxicology field. Several gene families that defend against chemical stressors have been identified in other cnidarians and include oxidases, various conjugating enzymes, ATP-dependent efflux transporters, oxidative detoxification proteins, as well as various transcription factors (Goldstone, 2008; Goldstone et al., 2006). The modulation of their expression in *Hydra* exposed to the new class of stressors, i.e. nanomaterials, may easily help to dissect the mechanisms underlying nanoparticle toxicity, and to identify those shared by other stressors and those unique to the nanomaterial under investigation.

Considering the key role played by cnidarians in freshwater, estuarine and reefs environments, the obtained results would be of invaluable importance for ecotoxicological studies as well. As nanoparticles may enter natural waters through sewage effluent and landfill leakages and present unknown risk to aquatic species, invertebrate testing may be used not only to advance the level of knowledge in nanoecotoxicology, but also for investigating behaviour and bioavailability of engineered nanoparticles in the aquatic environments.

5. Conclusion

Since the first publication on *Hydra* challenged with functional QDs (Tortiglione et al., 2007), the scientific community caught the advantages offered by this simple model to address nanotechnological issues, and many groups involved in the synthesis of nanomaterials demanded to test their synthetic products on *Hydra*. A picture of living polyps exposed to different nanoparticles is shown in Figure 18. We are currently investigating for each material the cell and molecular bases of interaction with *Hydra*, from the internalization route relying on the chemistry surface properties, to the molecular machinery activated by these nanosized objects. These results would be of valuable help when designing nanodevices to be interfaced with eukaryotic living cells. Once established the rules governing such interactions we will move toward the functionalization of the nanoparticles, combing the new size dependent physical properties to the specificity of the bioactive conjugated moiety to achieve targeted functioning.

Despite the initial studies limited to fluorescent semiconductor nanocrystals (QDs and QRs) for imaging purposes, the wide arrays of physical properties offered by nanoparticles of different materials supplies a corresponding wide repertoire of new tools to probe biological phenomena. Superparamagnetic nanoparticles (Fe_xO_y) could be employed for local heat generation (magnetic hyperthermia) under an alternating magnetic field, and thus exploited for selective cell destruction. Up to date, magnetic hyperthermia has been studied for cancer treatment but not applied to basic research, i.e. to obtain loss of function by cell ablation. Similarly, the property of some nanomaterials to strongly absorb NIR irradiation for conversion into thermal energy has been tested for phototherapy in cellular models, but not as universal tool for cell/animal biology. Nowadays nanotechnology allow to revisit traditional methodologies and extract yet unobserved or inaccessible information *in vitro* or *in vivo*. Only the cross-talk between different disciplines (biologists /chemists/physics) can bridge separate expertises, develop innovative tools and successfully apply them to modern research.

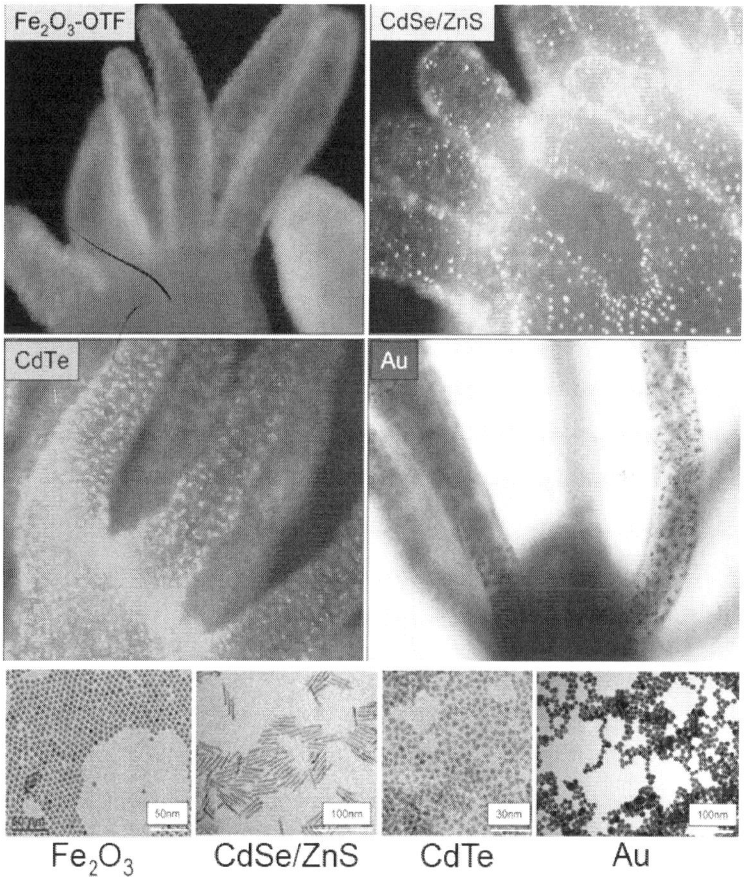

Fig. 18. Labelling *Hydra* with nanocrystals

In vivo imaging of polyps incubated with different nanocrystals, whose interaction with *Hydra* in terms of biocompatibility and toxicology is currently in progress. Upper left panel: picture of a living *Hydra* incubated with bifunctional conjugates (Fe_2O_3-OTF) based on the linkage of inorganic Fe_2O_3 nanoparticles to organic oligothiophene fluorophores (OTFs). Nanoparticle core diameter: 8nm; emission λmax= 605nm (Quarta et al., 2008). The presence of the fluorophore allows to track nanoparticle cell uptake, while the magnetic properties can be exploited for magnetic separation of the labelled cells. Upper right panel: *Hydra* labelled with fluorescent rod shaped nanocrystals, PEG coated CdSe/ZnS QRs. Nanoparticle diameter: 3,5nm, lenght 34nm; emission λmax= 592 nm. These two type of nanocrystals were a precious gift from Dr. Teresa Pellegrino (Italian Institute of Technology, Genova, Italy). Lower left panel: CdTe QD amino stabilised, by cysteamine, (emission λmax= 510nm, diameter: 2.6nm) were added to the medium bathing living *Hydras* and imaged after 4 hr. These nanocrystals were a generous gift from Dr. Andrey Rogach, City University of Hong Kong, Hong Kong, SAR. Lower right panel: *Hydra* treated with PEG coated gold nanoparticles (diameter: 14nm) These nanocrystals were surface modified to introduce positive charges on the surface (de la Fuente et al, unpublished) and are internalized at high rate by *Hydra* ectodermal cells. These nanocrystals were supplied by Dr. Jesus de la Fuente, University of Zaragoza, Spain. At the bottom representative TEM images of the samples above described were generously supplied by the corresponding providers.

6. Acknowledgment

I sincerely thank all the co-authors of the papers on *Hydra*/nanoparticles that I mentioned in this chapter, and those that are in preparation. As I stated earlier, these interdisciplinary works were made possible by the tight collaboration between different groups and expertises, and a great effort stands beyond each one. In particular, I thank Dr. Teresa Pellegrino (Italian Institute of Technology, Genova, Italy), as with her precious collaboration in material synthesis the whole research line was launched; dr.Angela Tino, (Institute of Cybernetics, National research Council of Italy) for daily discussions and data analysis; and people from my lab which shared challenges and enthusiasm for this work.
This work is supported by the NanoSci-ERA net project NANOTRUCK (2009-2012).

7. References

Alivisatos, A.P., Gu, W. and Larabell, C. (2005) Quantum dots as cellular probes. *Annu Rev Biomed Eng*, 7, 55-76.

Ambrosone, A., Marchesano, V., Mattera, L., Tino, A., Tortiglione, C. (2011) Bridging the fields of nanoscience and toxicology: nanoparticle impact on biological models. In Parak, W.J., Yamamoto, K., Osinski, M. (ed.), *Colloidal Quantum Dots/Nanocrystals for Biomedical Applications VI*. SPIE, Bellingham, WA, Washington, USA, Vol. 7909.

Auffan, M., Rose, J., Bottero, J.Y., Lowry, G.V., Jolivet, J.P. and Wiesner, M.R. (2009) Towards a definition of inorganic nanoparticles from an environmental, health and safety perspective. *Nat Nanotechnol*, 4, 634-641.

Baun, A., Hartmann, N.B., Grieger, K. and Kusk, K.O. (2008) Ecotoxicity of engineered nanoparticles to aquatic invertebrates: a brief review and recommendations for future toxicity testing. *Ecotoxicology*, 17, 387-395.

Bellis, S.L., Laux, D.C. and Rhoads, D.E. (1994) Affinity purification of Hydra glutathione binding proteins. *FEBS Lett*, 354, 320-324.

Bode, H.R. (2003) Head regeneration in Hydra. *Dev Dyn*, 226, 225-236.

Bosch, T.C. and David, C.N. (1984) Growth regulation in Hydra: relationship between epithelial cell cycle length and growth rate. *Dev Biol*, 104, 161-171.

Bruchez, M., Moronne, M., Gin, P., Weiss, S. and Alivisatos, A.P. (1998) Semiconductor nanocrystals as fluorescent biological labels. *Science*, 281, 2013-2016.

Carbone, L., Nobile, C., De Giorgi, M., Sala, F.D., Morello, G., Pompa, P., Hytch, M., Snoeck, E., Fiore, A., Franchini, I.R., Nadasan, M., Silvestre, A.F., Chiodo, L., Kudera, S., Cingolani, R., Krahne, R. and Manna, L. (2007) Synthesis and micrometer-scale assembly of colloidal CdSe/CdS nanorods prepared by a seeded growth approach. *Nano Lett*, 7, 2942-2950.

Cattaneo, A.G.G., R; Chiriva-Internati, M; Bernardini, G (2009) Ecotoxicology of nanomaterials: the role of invertebrate testing. *ISJ - Invertebrate Survival Journal,*, 6, 78-97.

Chapman, J.A., Kirkness, E.F., Simakov, O., Hampson, S.E., Mitros, T., Weinmaier, T., Rattei, T., Balasubramanian, P.G., Borman, J., Busam, D., Disbennett, K., Pfannkoch, C., Sumin, N., Sutton, G.G., Viswanathan, L.D., Walenz, B., Goodstein, D.M., Hellsten, U., Kawashima, T., Prochnik, S.E., Putnam, N.H., Shu, S., Blumberg, B., Dana, C.E., Gee, L., Kibler, D.F., Law, L., Lindgens, D., Martinez, D.E., Peng, J., Wigge, P.A., Bertulat, B., Guder, C., Nakamura, Y., Ozbek, S., Watanabe, H., Khalturin, K., Hemmrich, G., Franke, A., Augustin, R., Fraune, S., Hayakawa, E., Hayakawa, S., Hirose, M., Hwang, J.S., Ikeo, K., Nishimiya-Fujisawa, C., Ogura, A., Takahashi, T., Steinmetz, P.R., Zhang, X., Aufschnaiter, R., Eder, M.K., Gorny, A.K., Salvenmoser, W., Heimberg, A.M., Wheeler, B.M., Peterson, K.J., Bottger, A., Tischler, P., Wolf, A., Gojobori, T., Remington, K.A., Strausberg, R.L., Venter, J.C., Technau, U., Hobmayer, B., Bosch, T.C., Holstein, T.W., Fujisawa, T., Bode, H.R., David, C.N., Rokhsar, D.S. and Steele, R.E. (2010) The dynamic genome of Hydra. *Nature*, 464, 592-596.

Choi, A.O., Brown, S.E., Szyf, M. and Maysinger, D. (2008) Quantum dot-induced epigenetic and genotoxic changes in human breast cancer cells. *J Mol Med*, 86, 291-302.

Demir E, V.G., Kaya B, Creus A, Marcos R. (2010) Genotoxic analysis of silver nanoparticles in Drosophila. *Nanotoxicology*, in press, 1-8.

Derfus, A.C., WCW; Bhatia, SN. (2004) Probing the Cytotoxicity of Semiconductor Quantum Dots. *Nano Letters*, 4, 11-18.

Fischer, H.C. and Chan, W.C. (2007) Nanotoxicity: the growing need for in vivo study. *Curr Opin Biotechnol*, 18, 565-571.

Galliot, B., Chera, S. (2010) The Hydra model: disclosing an apoptosis-driven generator of Wnt-based regeneration. *Trends Cell Biol*, 20, 514-523.

Galliot, B. and Ghila, L. (2010) Cell plasticity in homeostasis and regeneration. *Mol Reprod Dev*, 77, 837-855.

Galliot, B., Miljkovic-Licina, M., de Rosa, R. and Chera, S. (2006) Hydra, a niche for cell and developmental plasticity. *Semin Cell Dev Biol*, 17, 492-502.

Gao M, K.S., Mvhwald H, Rogach AL, Kornovski A, Eyhmiller A, Weller Horst. (1998) Strongly photoluminescent CdTe nanocrystals by proper surface modification. *J Phys Chem Biol*, 102, 8360–8363.

Gaponik, N. and Rogach, A.L. (2010) Thiol-capped CdTe nanocrystals: progress and perspectives of the related research fields. *Phys Chem Chem Phys*, 12, 8685-8693.

Goldstone, J.V. (2008) Environmental sensing and response genes in cnidaria: the chemical defensome in the sea anemone Nematostella vectensis. *Cell Biol Toxicol*, 24, 483-502.

Goldstone, J.V., Hamdoun, A., Cole, B.J., Howard-Ashby, M., Nebert, D.W., Scally, M., Dean, M., Epel, D., Hahn, M.E. and Stegeman, J.J. (2006) The chemical defensome: environmental sensing and response genes in the Strongylocentrotus purpuratus genome. *Dev Biol*, 300, 366-384.

Grosvenor, W., Bellis, S.L., Kass-Simon, G. and Rhoads, D.E. (1992) Chemoreception in hydra: specific binding of glutathione to a membrane fraction. *Biochim Biophys Acta*, 1117, 120-125.

Hamilton, M.A., Russo, R.C., Thurston, R.V. (1977) Trimmed Spearman-Karber Method for Estimating Median Lethal Concentrations in Toxicity Bioassays. *Environmental Science & Technology*, 11, 714-719.

Holdway, D.A., Lok, K. and Semaan, M. (2001) The acute and chronic toxicity of cadmium and zinc to two hydra species. *Environ Toxicol*, 16, 557-565.

Holstein, T.W., Hobmayer, E. and Technau, U. (2003) Cnidarians: an evolutionarily conserved model system for regeneration? *Dev Dyn*, 226, 257-267.

Hoshino, A., Fujioka, K., Oku, T., Suga, M., Sasaki, Y.F., Ohta, T., and Yasuhara, M., Suzuki, K., and Yamamoto, K. . (2004) Physicochemical properties and cellular toxicity of nanocrystal quantum dots depend on their surface modification. *Nano Lett.*, 4, 2163-2169.

Hu, J., Li, L., Yang, W., Manna, L., Wang, L. and Alivisatos, A.P. (2001) Linearly polarized emission from colloidal semiconductor quantum rods. *Science*, 292, 2060-2063.

Huynh, W.U., Dittmer, J.J. and Alivisatos, A.P. (2002) Hybrid nanorod-polymer solar cells. *Science*, 295, 2425-2427.

Jiang, W., Kim, B.Y., Rutka, J.T. and Chan, W.C. (2008) Nanoparticle-mediated cellular response is size-dependent. *Nat Nanotechnol*, 3, 145-150.

Karntanut, W. and Pascoe, D. (2000) A comparison of methods for measuring acute toxicity to Hydra vulgaris. *Chemosphere*, 41, 1543-1548.

Karntanut, W. and Pascoe, D. (2002) The toxicity of copper, cadmium and zinc to four different Hydra (Cnidaria: Hydrozoa). *Chemosphere*, 47, 1059-1064.

Karntanut, W. and Pascoe, D. (2005) Effects of removing symbiotic green algae on the response of Hydra viridissima (Pallas 1776) to metals. *Ecotoxicol Environ Saf*, 60, 301-305.

Kirchner, C., Liedl, T., Kudera, S., Pellegrino, T., Munoz Javier, A., Gaub, H.E., Stolzle, S., Fertig, N. and Parak, W.J. (2005) Cytotoxicity of colloidal CdSe and CdSe/ZnS nanoparticles. *Nano Lett*, 5, 331-338.

Lee, J.J., K.; Kim, J.; Park, K.; Lim, K.H.; Yoon, T.H.; Choi, K. (2009) Acute Toxicity of Two CdSe/ZnSe Quantum Dots with Different Surface Coating in Daphnia magna Under Various Light Conditions. *Environmental Toxicology*, 25.

Lenhoff, H.M., Muscatine, L. and Davis, L.V. (1968) Coelenterate biology: experimental research. *Science*, 160, 1141-1146.

Lewinski, N., Colvin, V. and Drezek, R. (2008) Cytotoxicity of nanoparticles. *Small*, 4, 26-49.

Loomis, W.F. (1955) Glutathione control of the specific feeding reactions of Hydra. *Ann. N. Y. Acad. Sci*, 62, 208-209.

Loomis, W.F., and Lenhoff, H. M. (1956) Growth and sexual differentiation of Hydra in mass culture. . *J. Exp. Zool.* , 132, 555-574.

Lovric, J., Bazzi, H.S., Cuie, Y., Fortin, G.R., Winnik, F.M. and Maysinger, D. (2005a) Differences in subcellular distribution and toxicity of green and red emitting CdTe quantum dots. *J Mol Med*, 83, 377-385.

Lovric, J., Cho, S.J., Winnik, F.M. and Maysinger, D. (2005b) Unmodified cadmium telluride quantum dots induce reactive oxygen species formation leading to multiple organelle damage and cell death. *Chem Biol*, 12, 1227-1234.

Malvindi, M.A., Carbone, L., Quarta, A., Tino, A., Manna, L., Pellegrino, T. and Tortiglione, C. (2008) Rod-shaped nanocrystals elicit neuronal activity in vivo. *Small*, 4, 1747-1755.

Maynard, A.D., Aitken, R.J., Butz, T., Colvin, V., Donaldson, K., Oberdorster, G., Philbert, M.A., Ryan, J., Seaton, A., Stone, V., Tinkle, S.S., Tran, L., Walker, N.J. and Warheit, D.B. (2006) Safe handling of nanotechnology. *Nature*, 444, 267-269.

Medintz, I.L., Uyeda, H.T., Goldman, E.R. and Mattoussi, H. (2005) Quantum dot bioconjugates for imaging, labelling and sensing. *Nat Mater*, 4, 435-446.

Michalet, X., Pinaud, F.F., Bentolila, L.A., Tsay, J.M., Doose, S., Li, J.J., Sundaresan, G., Wu, A.M., Gambhir, S.S. and Weiss, S. (2005) Quantum dots for live cells, in vivo imaging, and diagnostics. *Science*, 307, 538-544.

Miller, D.J., Hemmrich, G., Ball, E.E., Hayward, D.C., Khalturin, K., Funayama, N., Agata, K. and Bosch, T.C. (2007) The innate immune repertoire in cnidaria--ancestral complexity and stochastic gene loss. *Genome Biol*, 8, R59.

Moss, S.E. and Morgan, R.O. (2004) The annexins. *Genome Biol*, 5, 219.

Pappas, T.C., Wickramanyake, W.M., Jan, E., Motamedi, M., Brodwick, M., Kotov, N.A. (2007) Nanoscale engineering of a cellular interface with semiconductor nanoparticle films for photoelectric stimulation of neurons. *Nano Lett*, 7, 513-519.

Pascoe, D., Carroll, K., Karntanut, W. and Watts, M.M. (2002) Toxicity of 17alpha-ethinylestradiol and bisphenol A to the freshwater Cnidarian Hydra vulgaris. *Arch Environ Contam Toxicol*, 43, 56-63.

Pascoe, D., Karntanut, W. and Muller, C.T. (2003) Do pharmaceuticals affect freshwater invertebrates? A study with the cnidarian Hydra vulgaris. *Chemosphere*, 51, 521-528.

Pellegrino, T., Manna, L., Kudera, S., Liedl, T., Koktysh, D., Rogach, A., Keller, S., Radler, J., Natile, G., Parak, WJ. (2004) Hydrophobic nanocrystals coated with an amphiphilic polymer shell: A general route to water soluble nanocrystals. *Nano Lett.* , 4, 703-707.

Pierobon, P., Minei, R., Porcu, P., Sogliano, C., Tino, A., Marino, G., Biggio, G. and Concas, A. (2001) Putative glycine receptors in Hydra: a biochemical and behavioural study. *Eur J Neurosci*, 14, 1659-1666.

Pierobon, P., Sogliano, C., Minei, R., Tino, A., Porcu, P., Marino, G., Tortiglione, C. and Concas, A. (2004) Putative NMDA receptors in Hydra: a biochemical and functional study. *Eur J Neurosci*, 20, 2598-2604.

Pollino, C.A. and Holdway, D.A. (1999) Potential of two hydra species as standard toxicity test animals. *Ecotoxicol Environ Saf*, 43, 309-316.

Putnam, N.H., Srivastava, M., Hellsten, U., Dirks, B., Chapman, J., Salamov, A., Terry, A., Shapiro, H., Lindquist, E., Kapitonov, V.V., Jurka, J., Genikhovich, G., Grigoriev, I.V., Lucas, S.M., Steele, R.E., Finnerty, J.R., Technau, U., Martindale, M.Q. and Rokhsar, D.S. (2007) Sea anemone genome reveals ancestral eumetazoan gene repertoire and genomic organization. *Science*, 317, 86-94.

Quarta, A., Di Corato, R., Manna, L., Argentiere, S., Cingolani, R., Barbarella, G. and Pellegrino, T. (2008) Multifunctional nanostructures based on inorganic nanoparticles and oligothiophenes and their exploitation for cellular studies. *J Am Chem Soc*, 130, 10545-10555.

Rivera Gil, P., Oberdorster, G., Elder, A., Puntes, V. and Parak, W.J. (2010) Correlating physico-chemical with toxicological properties of nanoparticles: the present and the future. *ACS Nano*, 4, 5527-5531.

Rogach, A.L.F., T.; Klar, T. A.; Feldmann, J.; Gaponik, N.; and Lesnyak, V.S., A.; Eychmuller, A.; Rakovich, Y. P.; Donegan, J. F. (2007) Aqueous Synthesis of Thiol-Capped CdTe Nanocrystals: State-of-the-Art. *J Phys Chem C*, 111, 14628-14637.

Schlaepfer, D.D., Bode, H.R. and Haigler, H.T. (1992a) Distinct cellular expression pattern of annexins in Hydra vulgaris. *J Cell Biol*, 118, 911-928.

Schlaepfer, D.D., Fisher, D.A., Brandt, M.E., Bode, H.R., Jones, J.M. and Haigler, H.T. (1992b) Identification of a novel annexin in Hydra vulgaris. Characterization, cDNA cloning, and protein kinase C phosphorylation of annexin XII. *J Biol Chem*, 267, 9529-9539.

Smith, A.M., Duan, H., Mohs, A.M. and Nie, S. (2008) Bioconjugated quantum dots for in vivo molecular and cellular imaging. *Adv Drug Deliv Rev*, 60, 1226-1240.

Sperling, R.A., Pellegrino, T., Li, J.K., Chang, W.H. & Parak, W.J. . (2006) Electrophoretic separation of nanoparticles with a discrete number of functional groups. *Adv. Funct. Mater.*, 16, 943-948.

Steele, R.E., David, C.N. and Technau, U. (2011) A genomic view of 500 million years of cnidarian evolution. *Trends Genet*, 27, 7-13.

Tino, A., Ambrosone, A., Mattera, L., Marchesano, V., Susha, A., Rogach, A., Tortiglione, C. (2011) A new in vivo model system to assess the toxicity of semiconductor nanocrystals. *International Journal of Biomaterials*. Volume 2011, Article ID 792854, 8 pages, doi:10.1155/2011/792854

Tortiglione, C., Quarta, A., Malvindi, M.A., Tino, A. and Pellegrino, T. (2009) Fluorescent nanocrystals reveal regulated portals of entry into and between the cells of Hydra. *PLoS One*, 4, e7698.

Tortiglione, C., Quarta, A., Tino, A., Manna, L., Cingolani, R. and Pellegrino, T. (2007) Synthesis and biological assay of GSH functionalized fluorescent quantum dots for staining Hydra vulgaris. *Bioconjug Chem*, 18, 829-835.

Trembley, A. (1744) *Memoires PourServira l'Histoire d'un Genre de Polypes d'EauDouce, a Bras en Forme deCornes.*

Wilby, O., Tesh JM. (1990) The Hydra assay as an early screen for teratogenic potential. *Toxicol in vitro*, 4, 582-583.

Wilby, O.K. (1988) The Hydra regeneration assay. *Proceedings of workshop organised by Association Francaise de Teratologie,*, 108–124.

Williams, A.I., I.T. . (1981) Carbodiimide chemistry: recent advances. *Chem. Rev*, 81, 589-636.

11

Nanocrystalline Thin Ceramic Films Synthesised by Pulsed Laser Deposition and Magnetron Sputtering on Metal Substrates for Medical Applications

Adele Carradò[1], Hervé Pelletier[2,3] and Thierry Roland[3]
[1]*Institut de Physique et Chimie des Matériaux de Strasbourg, UMR 7504 UDS-CNRS,*
[2]*Institut Charles Sadron, CNRS UPR 22, Strasbourg*
[3]*Institut National des Sciences Appliquées, Strasbourg*
France

1. Introduction

A suitable design of an implant material is aimed to provide an essential functionality, durability and biological response. Functionality and durability depend on the bulk properties of the material, whereas biological response is governed by the surface chemistry, surface topography, surface roughness, surface charge, surface energy, and wettability (Oshida et al., 2010). The implants biocompatibility has been shown to depend on relationship with biomaterials, tissue, and host factors, being associated with both surface and bulk properties.

Research area of thin and nano-structured films for functional surfaces interests to enhance the surface properties of materials. Thin films are an important and integral part of advanced material, conferring new and improved functionalities to the devices. Also processing of thin coatings with reproducible properties is a major issue in life-time of implanted biomaterial.

Currently in the implantology, hydroxyapatite (HA), alumina (Al_2O_3) and titanium nitride (TiN) have been widely chosen as thin biofilms to be coated on metal implants such as titanium materials and surgical 316L stainless steel.

HA coatings on titanium implants have been proposed as a solution for combining the mechanical properties of the metals with the bioactive character of the ceramics, leading to a better integration of the entire implant with the newly remodelled bone. HA has drawn worldwide attention as an important substitute material in orthopaedics and dentistry because of its chemical and biological nature similar to that of bone tissue (~70%) (de Groot, 1983; Kohn & Ducheyne, 1992; LeGeros & LeGeros, 1993; Elliot, 1994), its biocompatibility, bioactivity and osteoconductivity (Hench, 1991).

Al_2O_3 for its excellent wear resistance (Husmann et al., 1998) high chemical inertness under physiological conditions and TiN for its chemical stability are also commonly used as biomaterials (Staia et al.,1995). This last one interlayer plays a role as a diffusion barrier and it exhibits excellent mechanical properties and chemical stability (Iliescu et al., 2004).

Titanium materials (commercially pure titanium ASTM Grades 1 through 4 or Ti-based alloys) are considered to be the most biologically compatible materials to vital tissue (Oshida et al., 2010). Their more recent applications are in maxillofacial, oral and cardiovascular-surgery, as well as in orthopaedics indicating a superiority of titanium materials compared to stainless steel, Co-Cr-Mo alloys (Kasemo, 1983). However, they have no bioactivity as bone-substitute implant materials. These results in mechanical bonding rather than direct chemical bonding between the titanium implant material and the host bone tissue (Long & Rack, 1998). According to various in-vitro and in-vivo tests, HA implant coatings have shown an improved bone apposition as compared to uncoated implants in the first several weeks after operation (Tisdel et al., 1994).

Surgical AISI 316L stainless steel is widely used in orthopaedic implantology, although biological complications may result from its insufficient mechanical and tribological properties (Bordji et al., 1996). 316L contains enough chromium to confer corrosion resistance by passivity. Nevertheless the passive layer is not enough stable and because of poor corrosion resistance of 316L stainless steel under high stressed and oxygen-depleted regions, it is suitable to use it in temporary implant devices or coated with bioinert films.

Nowadays there are numerous thin film deposition techniques; most common are molecular beam epitaxy, plasma spray (PS), dipping, electro-codeposition, sol-gel-derived coating, magnetron sputtering (MS) and pulsed laser deposition (PLD) methods that have been developing rapidly during the last decades. Between them, MS and PLD are very powerful process, which are employed successfully in biomedical, functional and protective films. MS and PLD processes allow the control of the interface layer between the substrate material and the thin film, which in turn can be used to substantially improve the film adhesion to substrate. They are useful method for making thin films of functional biomaterials. A considerable amount of researches has been devoted to develop techniques for coating HA on titanium (Long & Rack, 1998) such as plasma spraying (Yang, 1995; Weng et al.,1995), dipping (Li et al., 1996), electro-codeposition (Dasarathy et al., 1996), PLD (Cotell, 1994), sputtering (Yang et al., 2005) and sol-gel-derived coating (Carradò & Viart, 2010).

Moreover, PLD (Pelletier et al., 2011) and MS (Carradò et al., 2010) can make thin TiN coatings, favourable for high fatigue resistance. In addition, TiN films should have good mechanical properties, i.e. a very strong adherence to the substrate, and hardness, Young modulus, stiffness and mechanical wear similar to those specific to human bone. Also a large variety of deposition techniques like PS (Liu et al. 2003), PLD (Carradò et al., 2008), MS (Trinh et al., 2008; Carradò et al., 2008), dipping and spinning (Babaluo et al., 2004) and sol-gel (G. Ruhi et al., 2008) have been approached for obtaining these oxides (Al_2O_3).

We reported some example of bioinert alumina, titanium nitride and bioactive hydroxyapatite coated on titanium and stainless steel substrates and we investigated the micro-structural and mechanical characteristics of these bioceramic coatings on their substrates. Among the different methods to obtain ceramic coatings that we have chosen PLD and MS due to their versatility and controllability, the aptitude to synthesize and deposit uniform films, with an accurate control of the stoichiometry and crystallinity. Various microscopic observations and mechanical characterisations by nanoindentation and scratch tests were used in order to connect the mechanical response to the microstructure of the coatings. Our studies revealed that the pulsed-laser deposition and magnetron sputtering technique appear as extremely versatile technologies in biomedical applications.

2. Ceramic thin films for biomedical

Many commercial replacement materials now have been developed as biomaterial for thin films, including metal, natural and synthetic polymers, corals and its derivatives and synthetic ceramics. These last ones can be divided roughly into three main types governed by the tissue response. In broad terms:

1. bioinert (alumina, titanium nitride, titanium dioxide, zirconia) materials have no or negligible tissue response;
2. bioresorbable (tricalcium phosphate (TCP), $Ca_3(PO_4)_2$) materials degradable and absorbed by the body;
3. bioactive materials (hydroxyapatite (HA), $Ca_{10}(PO_4)_6(OH)_2$), bioactive glasses (CaO-SiO_2-P_2O_5-Na_2O), and glass ceramics), encourage bonding to surrounding tissue with, for example, new bone growth being stimulated, or porous for tissue in growth (HA coating, and bioglass coating on metallic materials) (Hench, 1991; Cao & Hench, 1996; Hench, 1998).

2.1 Bioactive ceramic films

Hydroxyapatite (HA) forms a real bond with the surrounding bone tissue when implanted. Even so, due to the poor mechanical properties of bulk HA ceramic, it cannot be used as implant devices to replace large bony defects or for load-bearing application as was described by Hench (Hench & Wilson, 1993). Koch (Koch et al., 1990) presented HA has low mechanical strength, but very good osteointegration and biocompatibility. The use of HA coatings on titanium alloys leads to a structure that has good mechanical strength and good osteointegration properties at the surface (Lacefield, 1998). It has also been demonstrated that the bond between HA and bone is better than the bond between titanium and bone (Radin & Ducheine, 1992; Filiaggi et al., 1993).

2.2 Bioinert ceramic films

Alumina (Al_2O_3) is a highly inert material (Chiba et al., 2003) and resistant to most corrosive environments, including the highly dynamic environment that is the human body. Under physiological conditions, it is also extremely unreactive and is classed as nearly inert, eliciting little if any response from surrounding tissues and remaining essentially unchanged after many years of service. Due to its ability to be polished to a high surface finish and its excellent wear resistance, Al_2O_3 is often used for wear surfaces in joint and hip replacement prostheses (Hatton et al., 2002). Nevertheless, the body recognizes it as a foreign material and does attempt to isolate it by forming a layer of non adherent fibrous tissue around the implant where possible.

Titanium nitride (TiN) is known for its high surface hardness and mechanical strength. It was also reported that the dissolution of Ti ions is very low (Tamura et al., 2002). TiN coatings are often employ for improving the tribological performance in industrial applications due to its mechanical (Leng et al., 2001) and chemical properties including high hardness, low wear coefficient (Holmberg & Matthews, 1994). It is biologically inert and tolerated by living tissues (Kao et al., 2002). Moreover, the TiN interlayer produces improvement of HA film mechanical performances, by increasing its bond strength and adherence (Nelea et al., 2002; Ducheyne et al., 1993).

3. Deposition techniques

3.1 Magnetron sputtering (MS)

Magnetron sputtering (MS) is a very powerful technique which is used in a wide range of applications due to its excellent control over thickness and uniformity, excellent adherence of the films and its versatility in automatization (Wasa et al. 2003).

A strong potential difference is applied in a gas, generally of argon, with possibly reactive gases (O_2, N_2, etc.). It causes the ionization of the gas atoms and the creation of plasma. These ions are accelerated by the potential difference and strike the target surface. Target atoms are then ejected by mechanical action and condense on the substrate. Target electrons are also ejected and enter in collision with gas atoms, which causes their ionization and allows the maintenance of plasma (Fig. 1). Two types of power supply can be used: alternate radio frequency (RF) or direct current (DC). RF is used to deposit insulators, indeed in DC one uses a stronger tension to compensate for the resistivity of the target.

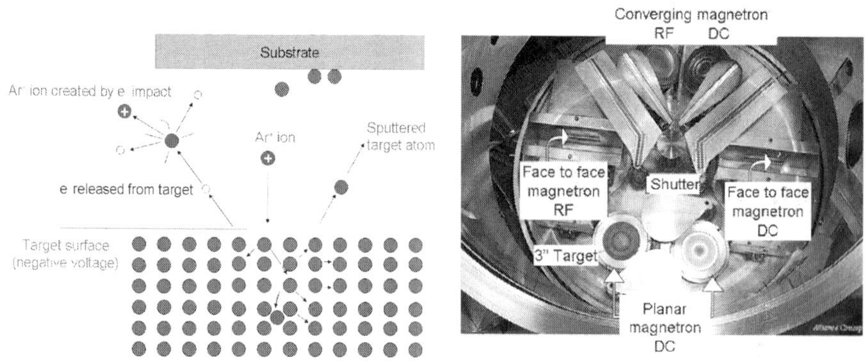

Fig. 1. Schematic principle of magnetron sputtering (MS) and picture of MS apparatus

3.2 Pulsed Laser Deposition (PLD)

Pulsed laser deposition (PLD) is for many reasons a versatile technique. Since with this method the energy source is located outside the chamber, the use of ultrahigh vacuum as well as ambient gas is possible (Krebs et al., 2003) (Fig. 2). Combined with a stoichiometry transfer between target and substrate this allows depositing all kinds of different materials (e.g. oxides, nitrides, carbides, semiconductors, metals and even polymers) can be grown with high deposition rates. The preparation in inert gas atmosphere makes it even possible to tune the properties (stress, texture, reactivity, magnetic properties...) by varying the kinetic energy of the deposited particles. All this makes PLD an alternative deposition technique for the growth of high-quality thin films (Fernandez-Pradas et al., 1998; Jelínek et al., 1995; Mayor et al., 1998; Fernández-Pradas et al., 2002; Arias et al., 1997).

Because of its capability to restore complex stoichiometry and to produce crystalline and adherent films, PLD stands for a challenge to plasma spraying that for the moment is the only commercially available technique for HA coatings deposition used in bone implantology (Zeng & Lacefield, 2000; Chen et al., 1997; Feng et al., 2000). However, it is generally accepted nowadays that plasma spraying produces porous films with poor crystallinity, exhibiting a low adherence to the metallic substrate (Carradó, 2010). PLD is an alternative method to coat metal substrates with HA in order to improve both the chemical homogeneity and the mechanical properties of calcium phosphate coatings (Nelea et al., 2006). PLD has successfully produced HA coatings with various compositions and crystallinity (Arias et al., 2002). Moreover, PLD can synthesize thin HA coatings, adequate for high fatigue resistance.

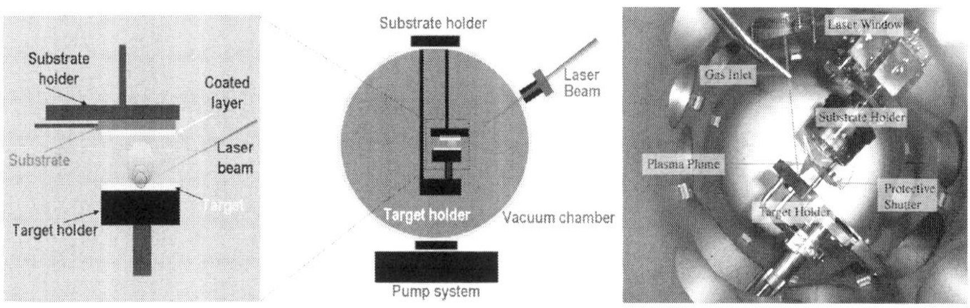

Fig. 2. Schematic principle of Pulsed laser deposition (PLD)

4. Experimental details

4.1 Bioinert Al_2O_3 interlayer

Al_2O_3 was deposed on stainless steel (grade 304L, Table 1) substrate– square pieces (1×1×10 mm^3). Al_2O_3 was applied as an inert interlayer to improve the adhesion of bio-ceramic films to the metallic substrate. The surgical stainless steel substrate was mechanically polished and then cleaned with methylene chloride and methanol. A dynamical pressure of O_2 was stabilized inside the PLD chamber and maintained during the whole deposition cycle. During the deposition, the stainless steel substrate was kept at 200 °C.

Prior deposition the substrates of stainless steel were mirror-polished and then cleaned ultrasonically in CH_2Cl_2 and CH_3OH. The studied alumina coatings were deposited onto these substrates by PLD and MS.

	Alloy composition [wt%]							
	C max	Si max	Mn max	S max	Cr	Ni	N	Cu
316 L	0.03	1.0	2.0	0.03	17.5/19.5	8.0/10.0	0.045	≤0.11

Table 1. Chemical composition in wt of surgical 304L stainless steel

Magnetron sputtered samples were prepared at low substrate temperature (200 °C) by reactive (O_2) direct current sputtering on a planar magnetron. The deposition parameters are summarized in Table 2. Before deposition, the surface of the substrates was cleaned by a 30 minutes plasma etching.

PLD coatings were produced using an excimer laser KrF* emitting at λ= 248 nm, by 20 ns pulses at 10 Hz and a sintered alumina target. As for MS samples, the substrates were maintained at 200 °C during the deposition time. Prior to the deposition, the pressure in the chamber was 5×10^{-6} Pa. Table 3 sums up the deposition parameters.

Sample	MS
Target	Al
Substrate temperature [°C]	200
Dynamical pressure [Pa]	0.4 with Ar 15 sccm and O_2 8 sccm
I_{DC} [mA]	600
P [W]	180
Deposition time [h]	17.5
Coating thickness [μm]	1.0

Table 2. Experimental conditions for MS Al_2O_3 coatings

Samples	PLD 4	PLD 5	PLD 6
Fluency [J/cm^2]	1.5		
Dynamical pressure [Pa]	6×10^{-5}	5 Pa with O_2 10 sccm	1 Pa with O_2 10 sccm
Deposition time (hours)		4.5	
Coating thickness (μm)	1.2	0.6	1.2
Pulse duration (ns)		20	
Pulse repetition rate (Hz)		10	
Number of pulses	150,000	150,000	180,000
Substrate temperature (°C)		200	
Ra (μm)	0.01	0.03	0.04

Table 3. Experimental conditions for Pulsed Laser Deposition Al_2O_3 coatings

The coatings surface morphology was investigated using a field emission microscope JEOL JSM-6700F. The chemical analysis of the thin films was investigated using an energy dispersive X-ray analyzer (Oxford Instruments). The crystal structure of the films was studied with a Selected Area Electron Diffraction (SAED) of Transmission Electron Microscopy (TEM) with a Topcom EM 002B microscope equipped with a small dose sensitive camera and a Si/Li detector.

4.2 Bioactive hydroxyapatite coatings: experimental details

An UV KrF* laser source (λ = 248 nm, τ = 10 ns), placed outside the irradiation chamber, was used. The laser radiation was focused with a an anti-reflection coated MgF_2 cylindrical lens with a focal length of 30 cm and was incident at 45° onto the target surface. The targets were mounted in a special holder which was rotated and/or translated during the application of the multi-pulse laser irradiation in order to avoid piercing and to continuously submit a fresh zone to laser exposure. A multi structure of the type HA/Ti/ was grown on a titanium substrate. A multi-target carousel was used to facilitate the target exchange, in order to avoid exposition of growing films to open air. Commercial titanium (Ti grade 4), and 99.98% pure HA targets have been subsequently used.

Two Ti Grade 4 substrates (Ø = 15 mm, thickness = 2 mm) were prepared with a final polishing by silicon carbide sandpaper (1200#) and finally treated chemically. The chemical etching consisted in a pre-treatment by specimen immersion in 1 M sodium hydroxide and 0.5 M hydrogen peroxide at 75 °C for 10 minutes for cleaning and decontaminating the titanium surface from embedded particles and machining impurities. After 10 minutes of treatment in 0.2 M oxalic acid at 85°C to produce a microporous surface and a final immersion in nitric acid for final passivation was done. The Ti interlayer was interposed between the initial titanium substrate and the HA film, to minimize interface stresses. Finally, one sample was kept as it was (HA-2, Table 4) and the second was treated for 6 hours in an atmosphere enriched in water vapours (HA-1, see Table 4) in order to improve the HA crystallinity status and to restore the loss of OH groups from the HA molecule. The deposition conditions are collected in Table 4.

	Target	Temperature [°C]	Pression [Torr]	Pulses	Water vapours treatment
HA-1	Ti	RT	10^{-6}	40000	
	HA	400	10^{-6}	500	
	HA	400	0.35 H_2O	30000	*
HA-2	Ti	RT	10^{-6}	40000	
	HA	400	10^{-6}	500	
	HA	400	0.35 H_2O	30000	without treatment

Table 4. Experimental conditions of HA films with and without water vapours

5. Structural and microstructural characterisation

Preliminary X-ray diffraction was performed for detecting the crystalline phases of the coatings. Only the characteristic peak pattern of austenitic Fe corresponding of 33-0397 JCPDS was displayed. Consequently the alumina coatings seem to be amorphous. Nonetheless, in case of MS Al_2O_3 films grown at 200 °C, selected area electron diffraction (SAED) reveals a fine crystallization in the γ-Al_2O_3 phase (Fig. 3b). The SAED pattern corresponds to the tetragonal γ-Al_2O_3 polycrystalline structure, with reticular parameters a = b = 0.57 nm and c = 0.79 nm. The MS film deposited shows the characteristic 311, 400, 511, 440 and 444 rings of polycrystalline aluminium oxide and the continuity of the rings in the first selected area diffraction indicates the presence of randomly oriented grains of very fine dimension (Fig. 3a). Whereas, as clearly shown in PLD Al_2O_3 films at 200 °C (Fig. 3c) samples is generally amorphous with a reduced number of small grain (Carradò et al., 2008). Laser deposited coatings have a smooth surface (Fig. 4a), with alumina particulates deposited on the film or embedded into the film. These particulates generally are either spherical, with a diameter between several hundreds of nanometers and one micrometer, or discoidal, with a diameter usually exceeding one micrometer (Fig. 4b,c). MS samples exhibit a smooth surface which follows closely the topography of the substrate. Spherical alumina particulates with approximately 100 nm diameter lay on top of the alumina film. They are generally agglomerated in structures resembling coral (Fig. 4d).

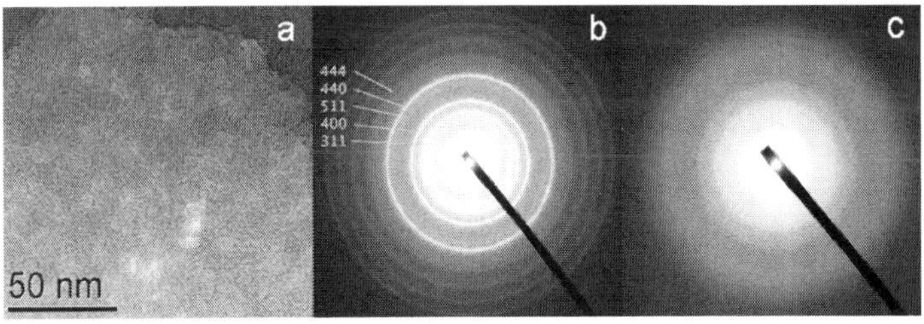

Fig. 3. High-resolution TEM (HRTEM) plan-view image or Bright field of MS film (a) and SAED patterns of MS2 (b) and of PLD5 (c)

These structures are spread on areas up to 60 μm diameter. EDS measurements demonstrate that the coatings have a chemical composition close to stoichiometric Al_2O_3 (Al: 34%, O: 66%, for MS coatings, and Al: 38%, O: 62%, for PLD coatings).

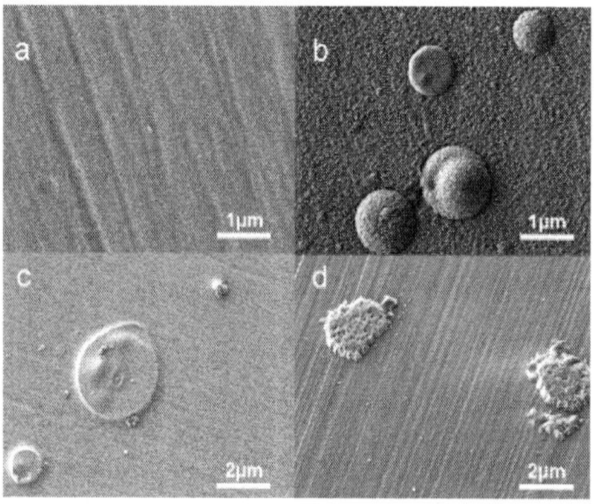

Fig. 4. (a-c) Typical SEM micrographs of an Al_2O_3 film consisting evidencing a smooth film with embedded droplets. (a) PLD4 sample, without O_2; (b) PLD 5 working pressure of 5 Pa, with O_2 10 sccm. The scale bar is 1 μm (c) PLD 6 coatings deposed with working pressure of 1 Pa, with O_2 10 sccm. (d) MS coatings deposed with working pressure of 0.4 with Ar 15 sccm and O_2 8 sccm

In Fig. 5 some typical SEM micrographs of the PLD HA film are given. The surface is compact and well-crystallized and exhibits an irregular morphology principally due to the chemical etching of the substrate. Some grain-like particles and droplets were observed on the surface of the film, characteristic to PLD coatings (Cottel, 1994). The morphology of the droplets suggests that they might be a result of target splashing in liquid phase (Fig. 5b, insert), since the droplet diameter is much smaller than the particle size of the powder used to prepare the HA target. SAED-TEM image (insert in Fig. 6) reveals a polycrystalline structure of the ceramic film, consisting of nanometric crystalline HA domains. The desired formation of a graded layer of about 20–25 nm thickness can be clearly observed. Atomic plane of grains are visible in some regions, demonstrating the polycrystalline structure of the HA layer.

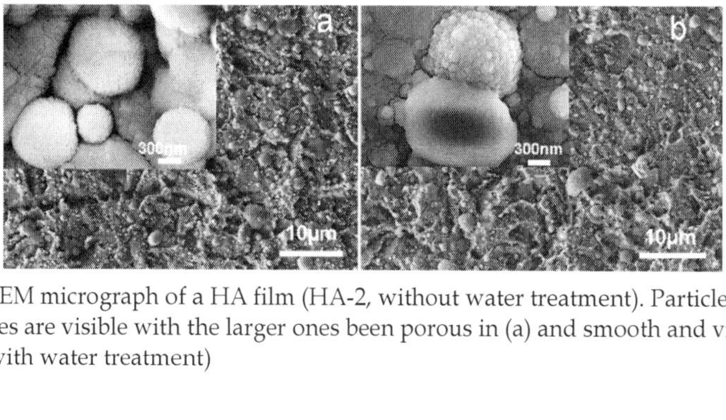

Fig. 5. (a) SEM micrograph of a HA film (HA-2, without water treatment). Particles of various sizes are visible with the larger ones been porous in (a) and smooth and vitreous in (b, HA-1, with water treatment)

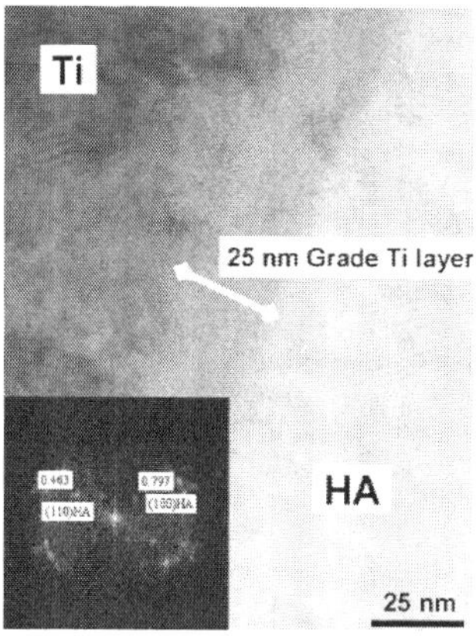

Fig. 6. HRTEM image of the HA/Ti interface. The presence of the graded layer is evidenced

6. Mechanical and tribological characterization

As described before, bioceramics such as Al_2O_3 and HA are currently used as biomaterials for many biomedical applications partly because of their ability to form a real bond with the surrounding tissue when implanted (Cao et al, 1996). However, usually the main weakness of this material lies in their poor mechanical strength that makes them unsuitable for loads bearing applications.

Our study is focused on understanding the mechanical characteristics and the tribological behaviour of a bioinert Al_2O_3 and a bioactive HA according to their micro-structural features processed by MS or PLD under several deposition conditions. The micro hardness, *H*, and elastic modulus, *E*, of the layers were measured using a nanoindentation system and a nano scratch experiments were employed to understand their wear mechanisms.

The literature devoted to mechanical properties of bioceramics is not sufficiently exhaustive and this section intends to give some clarifications.

6.1 Nanoindentation

The mechanical properties of the Al_2O_3 and HA bioceramics coated by MS or PLD were analysed by nanoindentation technique using a Nanoindenter XP developed by MTS Systems Corporation. In this technique, a diamond tip (Berkovich indenter) was drawn into the surface under very fine depth and load control. The reaction force (P) was measured as a function of the penetration depth (h), both during penetration (loading phase) and during removal (unloading phase), with high load and displacement resolutions (50 nN and 0.04 nm respectively). *H* and *E* were deduced from the recorded load-displacement curve using the Oliver and Pharr procedure (Oliver et al. 1992). The force required to indent for a particular applied load (and its corresponding penetration depth) gives a measure of the hardness of the material, while the response of the material during removal indicates the apparent elastic modulus. Due to the low thicknesses of the coatings (500 to 1200 nm), the indentation tests were performed at shallow indentation depth to avoid or limit the effect of the substrate. Moreover, to follow the evolution of *H* and *E* values (in accordance to the indentation depth during loading phase) several partial unloading phases were introduced in order to estimate the different contact stiffnesses. Consequently, the substrate effect on nanoindentation measurements was deduced. Prior to test, the Berkovich triangular pyramid was calibrated using the fused-silica samples following the Oliver and Pharr procedure (Oliver et al., 1992).

Fig. 7 illustrates the experimental load-displacement curves obtained from the different bilayer Al_2O_3/304L systems (samples MS and PLD 5) whereas Fig. 8 shows the evolution of *H* and *E*, estimated on the 304L substrate as a function of the applied load (P) and the corresponding penetration depth (h).

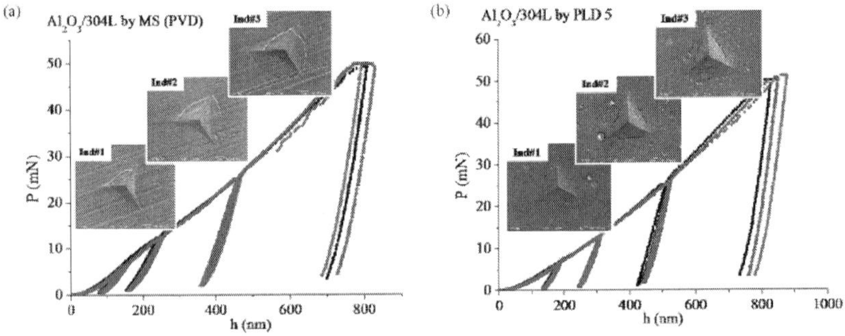

Fig. 7. Load-displacement curves obtained on Al_2O_3/304L systems processed by (a) MS and (b) PLD 5

To obtain the *H* of a coated film, the indentation depth should be about ten times smaller than the film thickness, in case of a harder film deposited on a soft substrate (Buckle, 1973). Nevertheless, it mainly depends on (i) the mechanical properties of the film and of the substrate (ratios H_f/H_s and E_f/E_s), (ii) the indenter shape and (iii) the interface adhesion (Sun, 1995). Basically, the substrate effect on the determination of the H_f and E_f by nanoindentation is directly related to the expansion of the elastically and plastically deformed volume underneath the indenter during the loading phase. This critical depth normalized by the film thickness (h_c/t) may vary between 0.05 and 0.2. The evolution of the composite hardness with indentation depth was predicted by various methods and models.

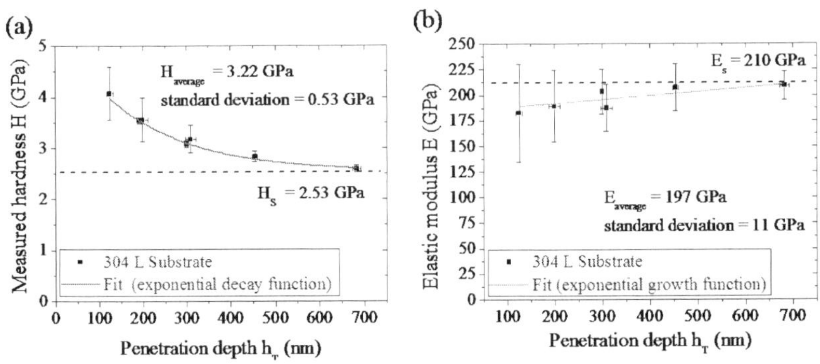

Fig. 8. (a) Hardness and (b) elastic modulus as function of penetration depth determined from the 304L substrate without coating

In our study, due to the deposition of a hard film on a softer substrate, the analytical expression of Eq. 1 (Korsunsky, 1998) was used to extract the true H_f and E_f for the MS and PLD Al_2O_3 films:

$$H_{mes} = H_s + \frac{H_f - H_s}{1 + k\left(\frac{h_c}{t}\right)^2} \quad (1)$$

where k is a fitting parameter. Here again, the contact depth is determined according to the Oliver and Pharr procedure (Oliver, 1992).

Fig. 9 shows the evolutions of the composite hardness as a function of the indentation contact depth normalized to the coating thicknesses of the samples PLD 4, PLD 5 and PLD 6 and it can be seen that the previous equation can successfully described the shape of these curves.

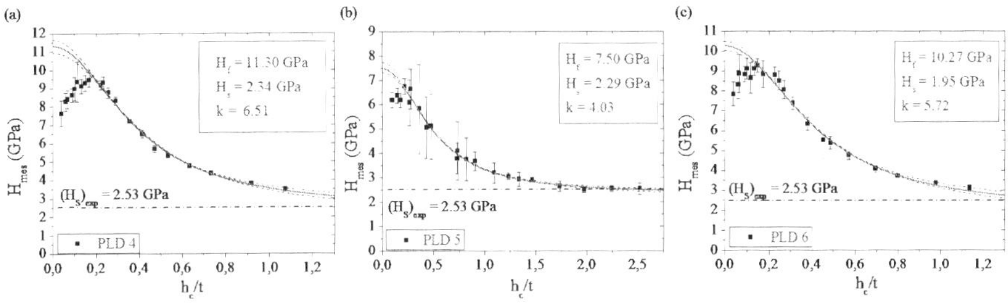

Fig. 9. Evolution of the harness according to the ratio (h_c/t) for the sample (a) PLD 4, (b) PLD 5 and (c) PLD 6

Using the same fitting equation (Eq. 1) the hardness of the MS sample was measured. Figure 10 shows MS sample hardness measured values compared to PLD 4. The values of H_f, H_s and E_f are reported in Table 5. To determine the elastic modulus E_f of a film deposited on a substrate, a model should also be used to account for the substrate effect (Saha and Nix, 2002). But, in a first approach, the average of elastic modulus is obtained by the plateau region of the curves (see Fig. 10 and Fig. 11). From these curves, an average value of E_f was obtained and reported in Table 5, assuming a Poisson coefficient of $\upsilon = 0.3$ and $\upsilon = 0.25$ for the 304L substrate and for the coatings respectively.

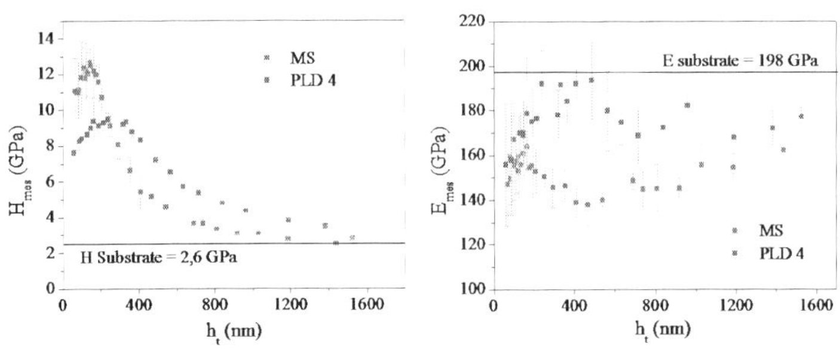

Fig. 10. Hardness and elastic modulus evolutions as function of the penetration depth (h_t) of MS and PLD 4 samples

Sample	H_f [GPa]	H_s [GPa]	E_f [GPa]
MS	12.10 ± 1.23	2.60 ± 0.30	158 ± 13
PLD 4	11.29 ± 0.35	2.34 ± 0.30	180 ± 15
PLD 5	7.50 ± 0.25	2.29 ± 0.10	150 ± 20
PLD 6	10.27 ± 0.25	1.95 ± 0.30	178 ± 13

Table 5. Mechanical properties of Al_2O_3 films determined by nanoindentation (using Eq. 1)

Fig. 9 illustrates a small difference between the experimental data and the fitting curves that could be explained by fracture phenomenon around the tip, defined by the physical meaning of the k parameter. In fact, SEM observations of the residual imprints (Fig. 12) show the formation of cracks in the contact zone for MS and PLD 5 layers. These cracks are related to the local microstructure and are predominately present on sample processed by MS and PLD5. They indicated the fragility of Al_2O_3 films compared to other ones which seem more ductile. Furthermore, it could also be linked to the smaller thickness of the Al_2O_3 coating in case of PLD 5 (0.5 μm) compared to PLD 4 and PLD 6 (1.2 μm).

It appears clearly that nanoindentation was relevant to extract the mechanical properties of the bioceramics films combined with microstructural observations showing the fragility aspects of the MS and PLD 5 films. For all samples, H_f and E_f values were in good agreements with those found by Ahn (Ahn, 2000) or Knapp (Knapp, 1996) for Al_2O_3 deposited by Radio Frequency sputtering or pulsed laser deposition respectively.

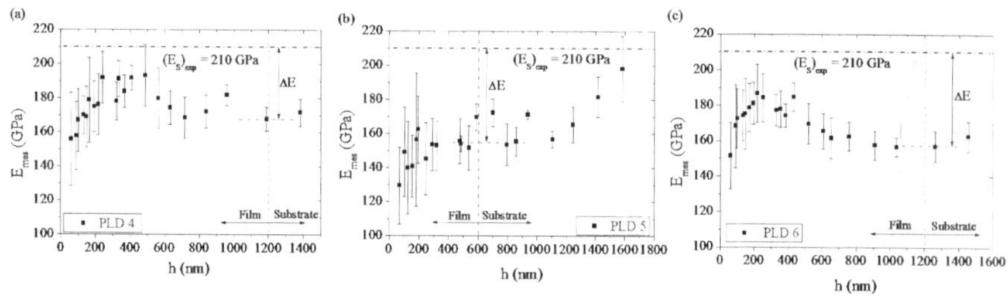

Fig. 11. Evolution of the elastic modulus for composite systems PLD 4, PLD 5 and PLD6

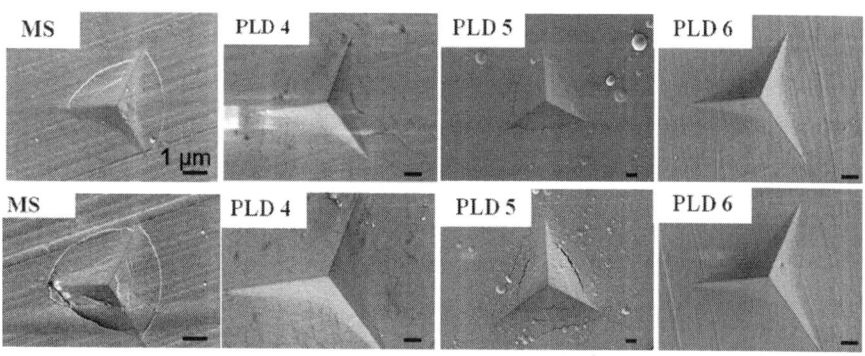

Fig. 12. SEM observations of the residual imprints for indentation test performed at h_T = 0.5 μm (first line of images) and h_T = 1 μm (second range of images)

Nanoindentation experiments on bioactive hydroxyapatite layer (HA-1 and HA-2) PLD coated on massive Ti substrate were carried out and treated as described in this section. Due to the high porous and heterogeneous HA morphology (Fig. 5) a high scattering data was shown. Indeed, at low load, the scattering is related to the surface roughness and the surface morphology. Using a linear approximation, it was further possible to estimate the *H* and *E* values at the penetration depth of 100 nm that corresponds to several percent of the film thickness and thus to the intrinsic values of the mechanical properties of the tested HA coatings. Table 6 summarizes the obtained results.

Sample	H [GPa]	E [GPa]
HA-1	2.5 ± 0.5	80 ± 20
HA-2	1.7 ± 0.5	65 ± 20

Table 6. Experimental values of H and E for HA coatings determined by nanoindentation

The values of nanohardness and elastic modulus experimentally determined in this study are in good agreements with the literature (Nieh, 2001; Deg, 2009). Most of them reported values of E and H determined by nanoindentation technique with a Berkovich indenter for plasma sprayed HA coatings on Ti ranging from 83 to 123 GPa and 4 to 5 GPa, respectively (Zhang, 2001).

6.2 Nanoscratch

In recent years, scratch testing has become a more popular and meaningful way to address coating damage and seems able to overcome the deficiencies found in other more subjective test methods. It involves the translation of an indenter of a specified geometry subjected to a constant or progressive normal load across a surface for a finite length at either constant or increasing speed. At a certain critical load the coating may start to fail. The beginning of the scratch can be taken as truly representative of the resistance of the investigated materials towards penetration of the indenter before scratching. The critical loads can be confirmed and correlated with observations from optical microscope. Fig. 13 schematically describes the scratch tester.

The scratch testers measure the applied normal force, the tangential (friction) force and the penetration and the residual depth (Rd). These parameters provide the mechanical signature of the coating system. Using this general protocol, it becomes possible to effectively replicate the damage mechanisms and observe the complex mechanical effects that occur due to scratches on the surface of the coating.

A typical scratch experiment is performed in three stages: an original profile, a scratch segment and a residual profile (Fig. 13). The actual penetration depth (h_T) of the indenter and the sample surface are estimated by comparing the indenter displacement normal to the surface during scratching with the altitude of the original surface, at each position along the scratch length.

The original surface morphology is obtained by profiling the surface under a very small load at a location where the scratch is to be performed. Figure 13 defines the different steps of a classical scratch procedure. Roughness and slope of the surface are taken into account in the calculation of the indenter penetration.

The parameter commonly used to define the scratch resistance of the material, when fracture is involved, is the *critical load*. This parameter is the load at which the material first

fractures. LC1 and LC2 are the *critical load* values which correspond, respectively, to failure and detachment of the coating. The fracture events can be visible on both the microscope view and the penetration curves.
All scratch experiments were performed with a spherical indenter with a tip radius R = 5 µm and at a constant sliding velocity of V_{tip} = 10 µm s^{-1}. The parameters used for these experiments are reported in Table 7.

Scratch	Starting load [mN]	Maximum load [mN]	Loading rate [mN/s]	Scratch length L_R [µm]
#1	1	16	0.3	500
#2	10	25	0.3	500
#3	20	40	0.4	500
#4	40	80	0.4	1000

Table 7. Scratch parameters

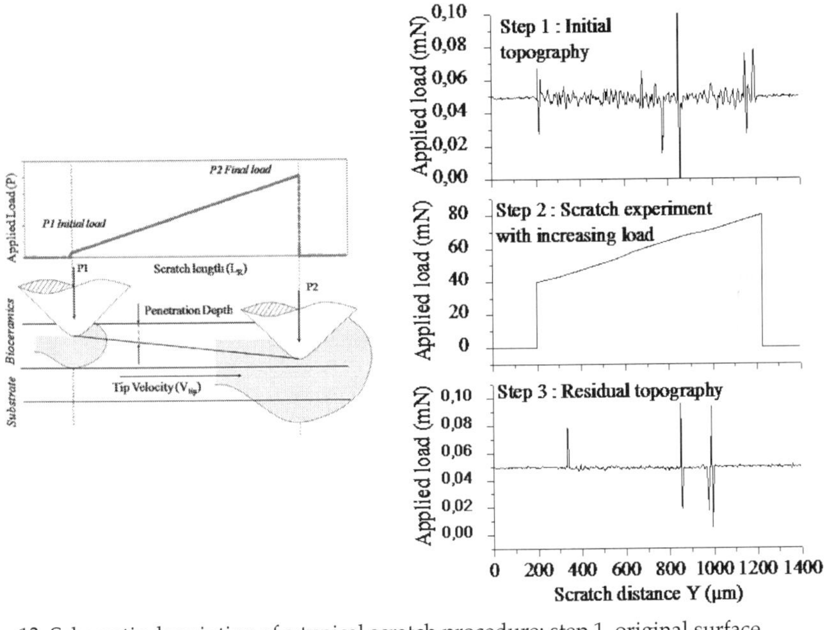

Fig. 13. Schematic description of a typical scratch procedure: step 1, original surface morphology, step 2, penetration depth during scratch, step 3, residual depth of the scratch groove.

Scratch experiments are known to be a more qualitative method compared to nanoindenation, and it is especially applied to compare the tribological response to friction of the tested surface during the same experimental procedure. In particular, scratch testing is widely used to determine the critical parameters for failure, such as the critical load which can be clearly seen when discontinuities appear on the different curves h_T versus F_N or F_T versus F_N. A further parameter of importance for tribological behaviour of films is the friction coefficient, defined as the ratio F_T/F_N.

In our study, residual scratch tracks were observed by SEM and compared to the experimental load-displacement curves during scratch to get access to the tribological properties of the deposited bioceramics in function of the used processes of elaboration (MS or PLD).

As observed for MS and PLD 5 samples, the failure and then detachment of the Al_2O_3 coating result in a abrupt changes in load-displacement curves, shown in Fig. 14(a-b), that show that critical load were reached. This is characteristic of an important release of an elastic energy during the propagation of cracks into Al_2O_3 films and then in the interface between the film and the underlying substrate, yielding to delamination. By contrast for the PLD 6 sample (Fig. 14c), no change in the h_T versus F_N curves is observed, proving that no ductile-brittle transition occurs for the tested normal load range. Same trend was observed for the PLD 4 sample but not presented here.

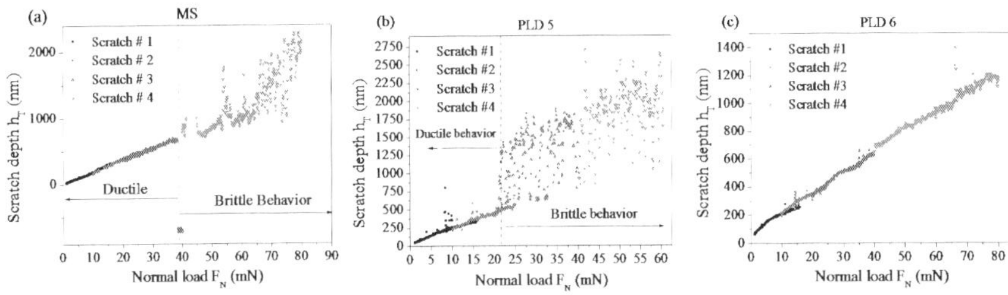

Fig. 14. Penetration depth as a function of the applied load during scratch measurements numbered 1 to 4 for (a) MS and (b-c) PLD 5 and PLD 6 samples.

SEM observations (Fig. 15), showing the scratch morphologies, clearly indicate that the initiation of failure occurs at the beginning of the scratch experiments for sample PLD 5 where partial cone track is initiated at the trailing edge of the spherical indenter, rapidly followed by delamination process of the Al_2O_3.

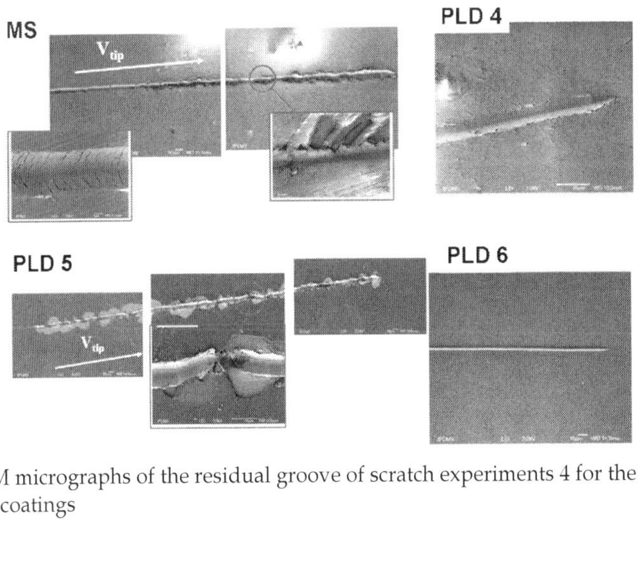

Fig. 15. SEM micrographs of the residual groove of scratch experiments 4 for the MS and PLD Al_2O_3 coatings

For MS sample, failure events can be seen with cracks perpendicular to the scratch direction that appear on the bottom of the groove. These cracks are essentially due to the tensile stress at the trailing edge of the contact during friction. Furthermore, others cracks are visible on both sides of the scratch (Fig. 15). In contrast, PLD 4 and PLD 6 samples show no evidence of failure and a rather ductile behavior as seems to indicate the allure of the load-displacement curves for these samples (Fig. 14).
As mentioned with nanohardness measurements, the mechanical properties of PLD 6 are higher. It is important to note that the harder film (PLD 6) appears to be tougher than the softer (PLD 5), as determined by nanoindentation experiments exposed in the above section. However, failure processes are dependent on the deposition routes through residual stresses generated at the interface between film and substrate and also on the adhesion energy which can explain that MS sample (which shows the higher hardness compared to any PLD samples) is subject to cracking under nanoscratch. We can, however, notice that in comparison to PLD 5, these failure events appear with some delay and for a higher load.
Using the same tribological experimental conditions scratch tests were performed on the HA samples. Some results are given in Fig. 16 with increasing load from 0.75 to 15 mN (realized in three steps) at the sliding speed of 10 μm·s^{-1} (length scratch was 500 μm).
The HA tribological behaviour is opposed to one of Al_2O_3 layer. It is due to the surface morphology of this last one which is a dense, homogeneous and with weak roughness. Opposite tribological performance of the PLD HA on Ti substrate is conditioned by its topography presenting a high roughness due to the presence of droplets of different diameters and nanoaggregates. This can de described by the high level of oscillations in the penetration curves. The HA-1 and HA-2 analysis of curves cannot clearly show a distinct mechanical behaviour within the tested range of load.

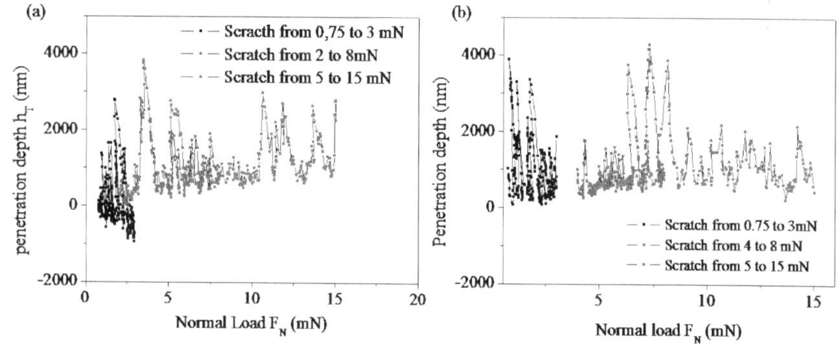

Fig. 16. Resistance to Penetration curves determined by scratch experiments on (a) HA-1 and (b) HA-2

7. Conclusions

Morphological, structural, nanoscratch and nanoindentation studies were performed to evaluate the composition, crystallinity status and mechanical properties of Al_2O_3/304L and HA/Ti structures synthesized by PLD and MS. We compared the characteristics of the substrates and their coatings deposited in different conditions. Alumina nanostructured films had a smooth surface, with few alumina particulates deposited on. They were stoichiometric, partially crystallized with an amorphous matrix. The obtained values of hardness and elastic modulus of the studied films are in good agreements with those found in literature. Different mechanical behaviours were observed in relation to different parameter of deposition (with or without working pressure in O_2). By nanohardness and wear measurements, the mechanical properties of PLD 6 are higher. The harder PLD 6 film appears to be tougher than the softer films MS and PLD 5, as determined by nanoscratch experiments and validate by tribological tests. We also compared the characteristics of the HA synthesized with (HA-1) and without (HA-2) a post-deposition heat treatment in water vapour showing a well-crystallized, polycrystalline structure and an irregular HA morphology due to the chemical etching of the substrate and the presence of some HA particles and droplets, characteristic to PLD coatings.

Tribological behaviour of HA samples is mainly conditioned by the surface morphology as detected by the numerous oscillations on the scratch penetration curves. During scratching, the plastic strain is the leading deformation mechanism without failure event, at least in the tested load range.

These studies reveal that the pulsed-laser deposition and magnetron sputtering techniques appears extremely versatile technology and good candidates in tribological applications.

8. Acknowledgements

The authors wish to thank Prof I.N. Mihailescu and Dr. Sorin Grigorescu for performing PLD HA INFLPR of Bucharest in Romania; Mr. Jacques Faerber (IPCMS) for SEM characterizations; Mr. Guy Schmerber for preparing the MS alumina samples (IPCMS) and Mr. Gilles Versini (IPCMS) for the elaboration of PLD alumina samples. We acknowledge the financial support of Egide–Centre français pour l'accueil et les échanges internationaux by the PAI Brancusi (08867SD) and PAI IMHOTEP (12444SH) projects.

9. References

Ahn H. and Kwon D. (2000), Micromechanical estimation of composite hardness using nanoindentation technique for thin film coated system *Materials Science and Enigineering A* vol 285 p. 172 - 179, ISSN 09215093.

Arias J.L., Mayor M.B., Garcia-Sanz F.J., Pou J., Leon B., Perez-Amor M. & Knowles J.C. (1997). Structural analysis of calcium phosphate coatings produced by pulsed laser deposition at different water-vapour pressures. *Journal of Materials Science: Materials in Medicine*, Vol. 8, No 12, pp. 873-876, ISSN 0957-4530.

Arias J.L., Mayor M.B., Pou J., León B. & Pérez-Amor M. (2002). Transport of ablated material through a water vapor atmosphere in pulsed laser deposition of hydroxylapatite. *Applied Surface Science*, Vol. 186, No 1-4, 28 January 2002, pp. 448-452, ISSN 0169-4332.

Babaluo A. A., Kokabi M., Manteghian M., Sarraf-Mamoory R. (2004). A modified model for alumina membranes formed by gel-casting followed by dip-coating. *Journal of the European Ceramic Society*, Vol. 24, No 15-16, pp. 3779-3787, ISSN 0955-2219.

Bordji G., Jouzeau J-Y., Mainard D., Payan E., Delagoutte J-P. & Netter P. (1996). Evaluation of the effect of three surface treatments on the biocompatibility of 316L stainless steel using human differentiated cells. *Biomaterials*, Vol. 17, No 9, pp. 491-500, ISSN 0142-9612.

Buckle H., Applications to other material properties, in: J.W. Westbrook, H. Conrad (Eds.) *The science of hardness testing and its research Applications*, ASM, Metals Park, OH, 1973 p. 453 - 491.

Cao W. & Hench L. L., (1996). Bioactive ceramics. *Ceramics International* Vol. 22, pp. 493–507, ISSN 0272-8842.

Carradò A., Pelletier H., Fabre A., Barrallier L. & Mihailescu I.N. (2008). A perspective of pulsed laser deposition in surface engineering: alumina coatings and substrates. *Key Engineering Materials*, Vol. 384, pp. 185-212, ISBN0-87849-372-7.

Carradò A., Schmerber G. & Pelletier H. (2010), Structural and mechanical investigations of magnetron sputtering TiO2/Ti/TiN multilayer films on Si(100) substrate. *Journal of Coatings Technology and Research*, Vol. 7, No 6, pp. 821-829, ISSN 1547-0091.

Carradò A. & Viart N., (2010). Nanocrystalline spin coated sol-gel hydroxyapatite thin films on Ti substrate: towards potential applications for implants. *Solid State Science*, Vol. 12, No. 7, pp. 1047-1050, ISSN 1293-2558.

Carradò A., (2010). Structural, Microstructural, and Residual Stress Investigations of Plasma-Sprayed Hydroxyapatite on Ti-6Al-4V. *ACS Applied Materials & Interfaces*, Vol. 2, No. 2, pp. 561–565, ISSN 1944-8252.

Carradò A., Taha M. A. & El Mahallawy N. A., (2010), Nanocrystalline γ-Al_2O_3 thin film deposited by magnetron sputtering (MS) at low temperature. *Journal of Coatings Technology and Research*, Vol. 7, No 4, pp. 515-519, ISSN 1547-0091.

Chen J., Tong W., Cao Y., Feng J. & Zhang X. (1997). Effect of atmosphere on phase transformation in plasma-sprayed hydroxyapatite coatings during heat treatment. *Journal of Biomedical Materials Research*, Vol. 34, No. 1, pp. 15–20. ISSN 1549-3296

Chiba A., Kimura S., Raghukandan K. & Morizono Y., (2003). Effect of alumina addition on hydroxyapatite biocomposites fabricated by underwater-shock compaction. *Materials Science and Engineering A*, Vol. 350, No 1-2, pp. 179-183. ISSN 0921-5093.

Cotell C.M., Pulsed laser deposition of biocompatible thin films, in: D.B. Chrisey, G.K. Hubler (Eds.), Pulsed Laser Deposition of Thin Films, Wiley, New York, (1994).

Dasarathy H., Riley C., Coble H.D., Lacefield W.R. & Maybee G. (1996). Hydroxyapatite/metal composite coatings formed by electrocodeposition. *Journal of Biomedical Materials Research*, Vol. 31, No. 1, pp. 81–89. ISSN 1549-3296

de Groot K., Bioceramics of Calcium Phosphate. CRC Press, Boca Raton, FL, (1983).

Ducheyne P., Radin S. & King L., (1993). The effect of calcium phosphate ceramic composition and structure on in vitro behavior. I. Dissolution. *Journal of Biomedical Materials Research*, Vol. 27, No.1, pp. 25–34. ISSN 1549-3296.

Elliot J.C., Structure and Chemistry of the Apatites and Others Orthophosphates, Elsevier, Amsterdam, (1994).

Filiaggi M.J., Pilliar R.M., Coombs N.A. (1993). Post-plasma-spraying heat treatment of the HA coating/Ti-6Al-4V implant system. *Journal of Biomedical Materials Research*, Vol. 27, No. 2, pp. 191–198, ISSN 1549-3296.

Feng C.F., Khor K.A., Liu E.J. & Cheang P., (1999). Phase transformations in plasma sprayed hydroxyapatite coatings. *Scripta Materialia*, Vol. 42, No; 1, pp. 103-109, ISSN 1359-6462.

Fernandez-Pradas J.M., Sardin G., Cleries L., Serra P., Ferrater C. & Morenza J.L.. (1998). Deposition of hydroxyapatite thin films by excimer laser ablation. *Thin Solid Films Vol.* 317, No 1-2, pp. 393-396 , ISSN 0040-6090.

Fernández-Pradas J.M., García- Cuenca M.V., Clèries L., Sardin G. & Morenza J.L. (2002). Influence of the interface layer on the adhesion of pulsed laser deposited hydroxyapatite coatings on titanium alloy. *Applied Surface Science,* Vol. 195, No. 1-4, pp. 31-37, ISSN 0169-4332.

Hatton A., Nevelos J. E., Nevelos A. A., Banks R. E., Fisher J. & Ingham E. (2002). Alumina-alumina artificial hip joints. Part I: a histological analysis and characterisation of wear debris by laser capture microdissection of tissues retrieved at revision. *Biomaterials*, Vol. 23, No 16, pp. 3429-3440, ISSN 0142-9612.

Hench L. L. (1991). Bioceramics: from concept to clinic. *Journal of the American Ceramic Society,* Vol. 74 pp. 1487–1510, ISSN 0002-7820.

Hench L.L. & Wilson J., (1993). Introduction. In: L.L. Hench , J. Wilson, Editors, An introduction to bioceramics, Advanced series in ceramics vol. 1, World Scientific, Singapore 1993; pp. 1-24.

Hench L. L. (1998). Bioceramics. *Journal of the American Ceramic Society,* Vol. 81, No. 7, pp. 1705–1728, ISSN 0002-7820.

Holmberg K. & Matthews A. Coatings-tribology. Amsterdam: Elsevier; 1994.

Husmann A., Gottmann J., Klotzbücher T. & Kreutz E.W. (1998). Pulsed laser deposition of ceramic thin films using different laser sources. *Surface and Coatings Technology,* Vol. 100-101, pp. 411-414, ISSN 0257-8972.

Iliescu M., Nelea V., Werckmann J. & Mihailescu I. N. (2004). Transmission electron microscopy investigation of pulsed-laser deposited hydroxylapatite thin films prepared by tripod and focused ion beam techniques. *Surface and Coatings Technology,* Vol. 187, No 1, pp. 131-140, ISSN 0257-8972.

Jelínek M., Olsan V., Jastrabík L., Studnicka V., Hnatowicz V., Kvítek J., Havránek V., Dostálova T., Zergioti I., Petrakis A., Hontzopoulos E. & Fotakis C., (1995). Effect of processing parameters on the properties of hydroxylapatite films grown by pulsed laser deposition. *Thin Solid Films,* Vol. 257, No 1, 15 February 1995, pp. 125-129, ISSN 0040-6090.

Kao C.-T., Ding S.-J., Chen Y.-C. & Huang T.-H. (2002). The anticorrosion ability of titanium nitride (TiN) plating on an orthodontic metal bracket and its biocompatibility. *Journal of Biomedical Materials Research,* Vol. 63, No. 6, pp. 786–792. ISSN 1549-3296.

Kasemo, B. (1983); Biocompatibility of titanium implants surface science aspects. *Journal of Prosthetic Dentistry.* Vol. 49, pp. 832-837. ISSN 0022-3913.

Knapp J.A., Follstaedt D.M., Myers S.M. (1996), precipitate hardened aluminium alloys formed using pulse laser deposition, *Journal of Applied Phyics* Vol. 79, Issue 2 p. 1116- 1122. ISSN 00218979.

Koch B., Wolke J.G.C. & de Groot K., (1990). X-ray diffraction studies on plasma-sprayed calcium phosphate-coated implants. *Journal of Biomedical Materials Research* Vol. 24, pp. 655–667. ISSN 1549-3296.

Kohn D.H., Ducheyne P. Materials for bone and joint replacement. In: Williams DF, editor. Medical and dental materials. Materials science and technology (a comprehensive treatment), Vol. 14. RW Cahn, P Haasen, EJ Kramer, collection editors. Weinheim:

Korsunsky A.M., McGurk M.R., Bull S.J., Page T.F., on the hardness of coated systems, *Surface and Coatings Technology*, 99 (1998) pp.171–183. ISSN 02578972.

Krebs H.-U., Störmer M., Faupel J., Süske E., Scharf T., Fuhse C., Seibt N., Kijewski H., Nelke D., Panchenko E. & Buback M. (2003). Pulsed laser deposition (PLD) - a versatile thin film technique. *Advances in Solid State Physics*, Vol. 43, pp. 505-517. ISSN 1438-4329.

Lacefield W.R. (1998). Current status of ceramic coatings for dental implants. *Implant Dentistry* Vol. 7, No 4, pp. 315–322, ISSN 1056-6163.

Legeros R.Z. & Legeros J.P., (1993). Dense hydroxyapatite. In: L.L. Hench & J. Wilson, Editors, An introduction to bioceramics. Advanced series in ceramics Vol. 1, pp. 139 World Scientific, Singapore.

Leng Y. X., Yang P., Chen J. Y., Sun H., Wang J., Wang G. J., Huang N., Tian X. B. & Chu P. K. (2001). Fabrication of Ti–O/Ti–N duplex coatings on biomedical titanium alloys by metal plasma immersion ion implantation and reactive plasma nitriding/oxidation. *Surface and Coatings Technology*, Vol. 138, No 2-3, pp. 296-300, ISSN 0257-8972.

Li T.T., Lee J.H., Kobaysi T. & Aoki H. (1996). Hydroxyapatite coating by dipping method, and bone bonding strength. *Journal of Materials Science: Materials in Medicine*, Vol. 7, No 6, pp. 355-357, ISSN 0957-4530.

Liu Y., Fischer T.E. & Dent A., (2003). Comparison of HVOF and plasma-sprayed alumina/titania coatings—microstructure, mechanical properties and abrasion behaviour. *Surface and Coatings Technology*, Vol. 167, No 1, pp. 68-76, ISSN 0257-8972.

Long M. & Rack H.J. (1998). Titanium alloys in total joint replacement—a materials science perspective. *Biomaterials* Vol. 19, No. 18, p. 1621- 1639, ISSN 0142-9612.

Mayor B., Arias J., Chiussi S., García F., Pou J., León B. & Pérez-Amor M. (1998). Calcium phosphate coatings grown at different substrate temperatures by pulsed ArF-laser deposition. *Thin Solid Films*, Vol. 317, No 1-2, pp. 363–366, ISSN 0040-6090.

Nelea V., Pelletier H., Muller D., Broll N., Mille P., Ristoscu C. & Mihailescu I.N. (2002). Mechanical properties improvement of pulsed laser-deposited hydroxyapatite thin films by high energy ion-beam implantation. *Applied Surface Science*, Vol. 186, No. 1-4, pp. 483-489, ISSN 0169-4332.

Nelea V., Jelinek M. & Mihailescu I. N., (2006). Biomaterials: new issues and breakthroughs for biomedical applications in: R. Eason (Ed.) Pulsed Laser Deposition of thin films: applications-lead growth of functional materials", Wiley & Sons, New York.

Nieh T.G, Jankowski A.F, Koike J. (2001), Processing and characterization of hydroxyapatite coatings on titanium produced by magnetron sputtering, *Journal of Materials Research* Vol 16, pp 3238 -3245, ISSN 08842914.

Oshida Y., Tuna E.B., Aktören O. & Gençay K. (2010). Dental Implant Systems. *International Journal of Molecular Science*, Vol. 11, No 4, pp. 1580-1678, ISSN 1422-0067.

Oliver W.C., Pharr G.M. (1992), Measurement of hardness and elastic modulus by instrumented indentation, *Journal of Materials Research* Vol. 7, issue 4, pp1564-1583.

Pelletier H., Carradò A., Faerber J. & Mihailescu I. N., (2011). Microstructure and mechanical characteristics of hydroxyapatite coatings on Ti/TiN/Si substrates synthesized by pulsed laser deposition. *Applied Physics A: Materials Science & Processing*, 2011, Vol. 102, No. 3, pp. 629-640, ISSN 1432-0630.

Radin S.R. & Ducheine P. (1992). Plasma spraying induced changes of calcium phosphate ceramic characteristics and the effect in vitro stability. *Journal of Materials Science: Materials in Medicine*, Vol. 3, No 1, pp. 33-42, ISSN 0957-4530.

Ruhi G., Modi O.P., Sinha A.S.K.& Singh I.B. (2008). Effect of sintering temperatures on corrosion and wear properties of sol-gel alumina coatings on surface pre-treated mild steel. *Corrosion Science*, Vol. 50, No 3, pp. 639-649. ISSN 0010-938X.

Saha R. and Nix W.D. (2002), Effect of the substrate on the determination of thin film mechanical properties by nanoindentation, *Acta Materialia*, Vol 50, No 11, pp. 23 - 38, ISSN 1359-6454.

Staia M.H., Levis B., Cawley J. & Hendson T., (1995). Chemical vapour deposition of TiN on stainless steel. *Surface and Coatings Technology*, Vol. 76-77, No 1, pp. 231-236, ISSN 0257-8972.

Sun Y., Bell T., Zheng S. (1995) Finite element analysis of the critical ratio of coating thickness to indentation depth for coating property measurements by nanoindentation, *Thin Solid Films*, Vol. 258, No 1, pp. 198-204, ISSN 00406090

Tamura, Y., Yokoyama, A., Watari, F. & Kawasaki, T. (2002). Surface properties and biocompatibility of nitrided titanium for abrasion resistant implant materials. *Dental Material Journal*, Vol. 21, pp. 355–372. ISSN 02874547.

Tisdel C. L., Golberg V. M, Parr J. A., Bensuan J. S., Staikoff L. S. & Stevenson S. (1994). The influence of a hydroxyapatite and tricalcium-phosphate coating on bone growth into titanium fiber-metal implants. *Journal of Bone & Joint Surgery (US Volume)*,Vol. 76, No 2, pp. 159–171. ISSN 00219355.

Trinh D.H., Kubart T., Nyberg T., Ottosson M., Hultman L. & Högberg H. (2008). Direct current magnetron sputtering deposition of nanocomposite alumina – zirconia thin films. *Thin Solid Films, Vol.* 516, No 23, pp. 8352-8358, ISSN 0040-6090.

Wasa K., Kitabatake M., Adachi H., Thin Film Materials Technology: Sputtering of Compound Materials, Noyes Publications, 2003.

Weng J., Liu X.G., Li X.D. & Zhang X.D., (1995). Intrinsic factors of apatite influencing its amorphization during plasma-spray coating. *Biomaterials*, Vol. 16, No. 1, 1995, pp. 39-44, ISSN 0142-9612

Yang C.Y., Wang B.C., Chang E. & Wu J.D. (1995). The influences of plasma spraying parameters on the characteristics of hydroxyapatite coatings: a quantitative study. *Journal of Materials Science: Materials in Medicine*, Vol. 6, pp. 249–257, ISSN 0957-4530.

Yang Y., Kim K-H & Ong J. L. (2005). A review on calcium phosphate coatings produced using a sputtering process—an alternative to plasma spraying. *Biomaterials,* Vol. 26, No. 3, pp. 327-337, ISSN 0142-9612.

Zhang C., Leng Y., Chen J. (2001), amorphous and recristallisation during plasma spraying of hydroxyapatite, *Biomaterials,* Vol. 22, No 11, pp. 1357 -1363.

Zeng H. & Lacefield W.R. (2000). XPS, EDX and FTIR analysis of pulsed laser deposited calcium phosphate bioceramic coatings: the effects of various process parameters. *Biomaterials,* Vol. 21, No 1, pp. 23-30, ISSN 0142-9612.

12

Micro-Nano Technologies for Cell Manipulation and Subcellular Monitoring

M.J. Lopez-Martinez[1,2] and E.M. Campo[1,3]
[1]*IMB-CNM CSIC*
[2]*University of Groningen,*
[3]*University of Pennsylvania,*
[1]*Spain*
[2]*Netherlands*
[3]*US*

1. Introduction

Currently, mechanistic and biological phenomena within the cellular level are not well understood (Bao & Suresh, 2003) and the evolution of those during disease or treatment is also unclear. Cells are complex structures with nuclei and organelles, whose dimensions require the development of micro and nanotechnologies for effective manipulation and monitoring. Indeed, sizes of nuclei vary from 3 to 7 μm for differentiated cells. In embryos, nuclei are not surrounded by a membrane although the genetic material is mostly compounded in a 9μm diameter region. Other organelles, with specific functions in eukaryotic cells like mithocondria, can have smaller sizes (1 μm). In addition, histologists know that important parameters such as pH or Ca/Na/K concentration can greatly vary locally within the cytoplasmic region. Recently, Weibel (Weibel et al., 2007) argued the need for microbiology to evolve into a quantitative field. The argument predicted the development of microsystem tools to enable individual cell manipulation, growth, and the study of **subcellular organization**, while mechanisms of differentiation and communication between cells would be unveiled. Indeed, current research efforts aim at investigating the genetic, biochemical, and behavioural differences among cells. On-going development of microstructures to quantitatively study parameters within single cells will lead to a thorough understanding of subcellular activity, including pathogenesis with an unprecedented level of detail. In addition, these efforts will pave the way for highly-effective, cell-tailored, drug delivery. The problems are of course how to effectively manipulate cells, how to position a sensor at specific locations within the cell, and even how to penetrate the different organelles, as depicted in Figure 1. This chapter will review current concerns on cell manipulation and recent developments in micro and nanofabrication technologies aiming at the increased functionality of cellular tools.

2. Microfabrication technologies for cellular handling

A first step in the study of cells inevitably starts by designing tools and protocols for cell handling, as the manipulation of the uttermost external membranes in life cells are likely to introduce perturbations in the system that could ultimately impact either the sub-cellular or intercellular processes to be elucidated. Pipettes are typically pulled and thinned by pullers, cut to the appropriate inner diameter by microforging techniques, and polished. Human fertility scientists identified earlier (Huang et al., 1996) the difficulties around tool preparation, and the importance of appropriate cell handling during in vitro fertilization (IVF) procedures. Following this line of thought, and in view of the traditional manufacturing approach currently active in the trade, technologists have pondered whether cell handling is hindered by rudimentary-manufactured manipulators (Campo et al., 2009 a and b).

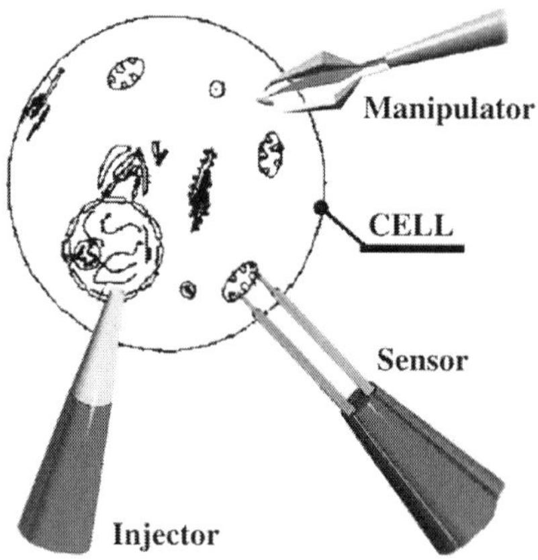

Fig. 1. Schematic describing functionalities of intracellular manipulator.
After Kometani et al., 2005b[1].

Conventional pipettes consist of borosilicate glass capillaries that are subsequently thinned, cut, and polished to achieve appropriate tip geometries with adequate dimensions. Figure 2 shows commercially available glass capillaries whose difference in geometry has been controlled by a puller with a combination of axial tension and thermal treatment (Sutter Instruments, 2008). In recent years, cell microinjection has become a crucial procedure in cell and reproductive biology. Microinjection of cells is routinely used in various biotechnological and biomedical applications such as reproductive cloning of animals by nuclear transfer (Kishigami et al., 2006), production of transgenic animals by DNA injection into embryos (Ittner and Götz 2007) or in vitro fertilization of oocytes by intracytoplasmic sperm injection (ICSI) (Palermo et al. 1992; Yoshida and Perry 2007). Higher cell survival rates have been reported to result from minimized microinjection damage when high quality pipettes are used. With common-practice microinjection methods, 5-25% of mouse oocytes lyse during ICSI (Lacham-Kaplan & Trounson, 1995) and 20-30% of mouse embryos lyse after pronuclear microinjection of DNA (Nagy et al. 2002). With all, experimental evidence suggests that crucial conventional pipette manufacturing procedures involve tedious artisanal methods that are prone to failure (Yaul et al., 2008; Ostadi et al., 2009).

---

[1] Reprinted from *Nuclear Instruments and Methods in Physics Research Section B: Beam Interactions with Materials and Atoms*, Vol. 232, No. 1-4, Kometani, R.,Hoshino, T., Kanda, K., Haruyama, Y., Kaito, T., Fujita, J., Ishida, M., Ochiai, Y., & Matsui, S. , Three-dimensional high-performance nano-tools fabricated using focused-ion-beam chemical-vapor-deposition, pp. (362-366), 2005, with permission from Elsevier

Despite the absence of a thorough bio-mechanistic explanation to pipette-cell interaction, trial and error-based initiatives have accumulated a wealth of specifications applicable to tools and piercing techniques in different scenarios. Figure 2 shows electron microscopy images of pre-processed pipettes (top) and optical microscopy images of conventionally processed pipettes to different geometries. In particular, for most applications involving oocytes and embryos, injection pipettes must be bevelled and often spiked at the tip (Yaul et al. 2008; Nagy et al. 2002). Bevelled spiked tips (as those shown in Figure 3) favour penetration through a thick zona pellucida and an elastic plasma membrane.

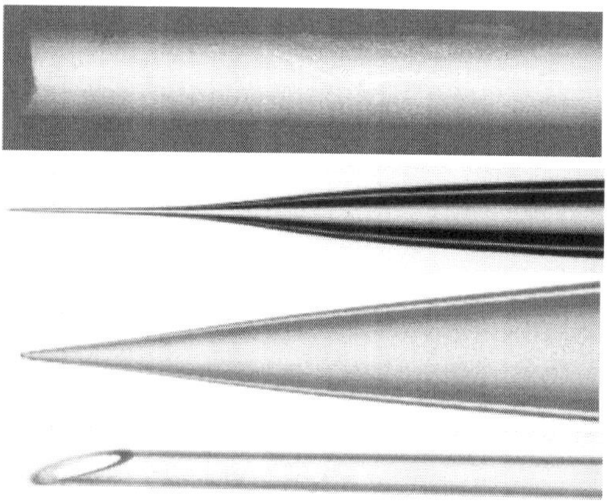

Fig. 2. Electron and optical microscopy images of pre-processed (top) and conventionally processed capillaries.

The different geometries achieved by forging and polishing techniques have some versatility to accommodate for different piercing scenarios. Microinjection protocols for sperm injection, particularly those used for injecting mouse oocytes, occasionally need flat-end micropipettes to first "core" through the zona pellucida and then through the oolemma using minute vibrations from a piezo device. Pipettes used with a piezo drill require a clean 90-degree break at the tip (amenable to be produced by a microforge) and a bevel or spike at the tip is not needed to assist perforation. The inner diameter of these pipettes must be carefully controlled for the pipette to be most effective. The pulled pipette is usually cut on a microforge to the appropriate diameter (Sutter Instruments, 2008). Figure 3 shows SEM images of tips from glass pipettes, revealing rough edges in pre-processed pipettes and polished edge in a conventionally-used pipette in human ICSI; where smooth edges and a bevelled tip with a spike assist during perforation.

Indeed, edge finish is an important factor in pipette quality. Abrasion, acid and fire polishing are common techniques to remove morphological irregularities from pipette edges. In a recent study, Yaul and coworkers (Yaul et al., 2008) investigated the impact of different gas chemistries during fire-polishing of IVF pipettes. Typically in IVF industry, glass micro tools are drawn from hollow glass capillaries of 1 mm diameter (Yaul et al., 2008). These thinned capillaries are cut manually to a length of 100 mm from hollow glass rods resulting in sharp and chipped edges, similar to those shown in Figure 3 (left). Resulting sharp and uneven edges are known to easily pick up debris, rendering them ineffective for IVF treatments. Yaul's experiments involved analysis of fire polishing process using candle, butane, propane, 2350 butane propane, and oxyacetylene gas flames to find the appropriate gas chemistry, the optimum distance of the capillary relative to the flame, and the optimum heating and cooling times as the tip morphology is modified by the glass phase transition. The results show that the temperature range in 2350 butane propane gas (between 925–1,015°C) is optimum for fire polishing of borosilicate glass capillaries, as the softening point of borosilicate glass is 820°C and the working temperature lies between 1,000 to 1,252°C.

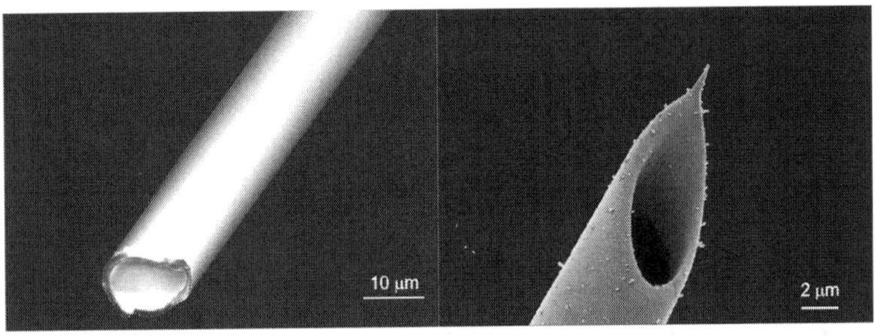

Fig. 3. Electron microscopy images of unpolished glass pipette (left) and commercially-polished (Humagen, Virginia) pipette (right).

The uneven pattern in heat radiance from a non-punctual heating source was also tentatively addressed by exposing capillaries to the top, middle, and bottom section of the flame, as shown in Figure 4. Inspection of edge roughness was conducted by optical microscopy and discussion was only provided in a qualitative manner.

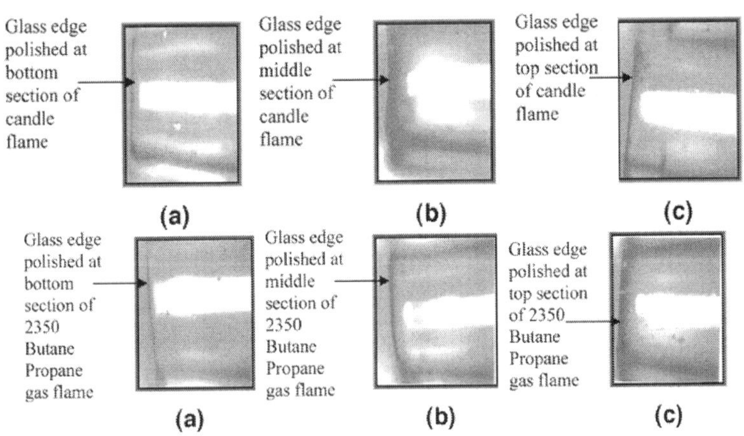

Fig. 4. Optical microscopy images showing the effects of pipette exposure to candle flame (above) and to 2350 Butane Propane (below) at different sections in the candle flame. (after Yaul et al., 2008)[2]

[2] With kind permission from Springer Science+Business Media: *Biomedical Microdevices*, Evaluating the process of polishing borosilicate glass capillaries used for fabrication of in - vitro fertilization (iVF) micro-pipettes, Vol. 10, No. 1, (2008), pp. (123-128), Yaul, M., Bhatti, R., & Lawrence, S. Figures 8 and 9.

Reportedly, fire-polished capillaries were tested in IVF clinics in the UK, with great acceptance over pipettes with non-fired polished edges. Although fire polishing seems to have an impact on pipette performance, there is still a lack of quantitative measure of both thermal parameters (for automation) and effects of this treatment on edge roughness.

At this time, it is unclear what levels of roughness are acceptable for adequate cell handling. A number of questions arise as the importance of the edge surface to be atomically flat for cell handling or even for organelle perforation. Incidentally, Malboubi and coworkers (Malboubi et al., 2009) unequivocally correlated pipette surface roughness (in the order of nanometers) with giga-seal formation in patch clamping, providing semi-quantitative evidence of improved roughness based on the resolution provided by electron microscopy images. Commonly used characterization techniques to measure roughness in microelectronics, such as atomic force microscopy (AFM) are amenable to be deployed in the context of tools for the biological sciences. This is possibly the most sensible step looking forward in the process to understand edge roughness and its consequences on cellular manipulation.

To this effect, a number of efforts to introduce current microtechnologies into the context of pipette processing (Kometani et al., 2005-2008; Malboubi et al., 2009; Campo et al., 2010a) and piercing techniques (Ergenc & Olgac, 2007) have appeared in the literature. In particular, the use of focus ion beams and electron microscopy may have opened a new avenue to the generation of improved or even, altogether new, tools in the biomedical sciences. In the next sub-sections we will review the functionalities of focus ion beams and the incipient efforts to apply those to the life sciences.

2.1 Micro-nano fabrication using focus ion beam technologies

In the last few decades, technological advancements in computing capacity, vacuum pumps, and differential vaccumm columns among others have had a large impact on electron and ion microscopy. Scanning electron microscopes (SEMs) can now operate in dry vacuum or wet mode, possibilitating imaging of hydrated specimens in their native environment. To the myriad of developments, it is worth emphasizing the revolutionary contribution of dual focus ion beam systems (FIBs), where the usual single electron gun in SEM is now complemented with a gallium ion gun. The complementary gun keeps a coincidental point with the electron gun, and their intersecting angle depends on the manufacturer. In addition, the systems are usually complemented with in situ gas sources. The action of a focus beam of gallium ions is schematically depicted in Figures 5 and 6.

Gallium ions are larger and heavier than electrons. When accelarated, they (brown spheres in Figure 5) impinge on a surface and their interaction with the outmost atoms on the substrate will result in atomic ionization and breaking of chemical bonds. As a result, outer atoms in the substrate are sputtered away, as seen in the grey spheres in Figure 5. The availiability of gas injectors in the FIB chamber can actually assist the atom ejection process by first adsorbing, and then chemically etching the targeted surface (blue spheres in Figure 5). The use of gases can acelarate milling in large regions and facilitate etching through deep trenches. In addition, gallium ions are likely to be unintentionally implanted during etching. Unintentional gallium ion implantation could have deleterious effects over the applicability of biomedical tools, as will be discussed later.

The other-less known- functionality adscribed to FIB is the gas-assisted deposition of metals and insulators, as seen in Figure 6. In this scheme, the combined action of gallium ions (brown spheres) and gas molecules (blue and green sphere-coplexes) emerging from the in

situ sources, results in the adsorption of gas molecules to the substrate, which leads to a thermally-driven gas molecule disocciation. Finally, the unwanted dissociated species are sputtered. Similarly to milling, implantation of both gallium ions and dissociated species are likely to occur during deposition.
The reader is directed to the monograph on Focus Ion Beams by Lucille Giannuzzi and Fred Stevie (Giannuzzi & Stevie, 2005) for a thorough and rigorous description of the technique.

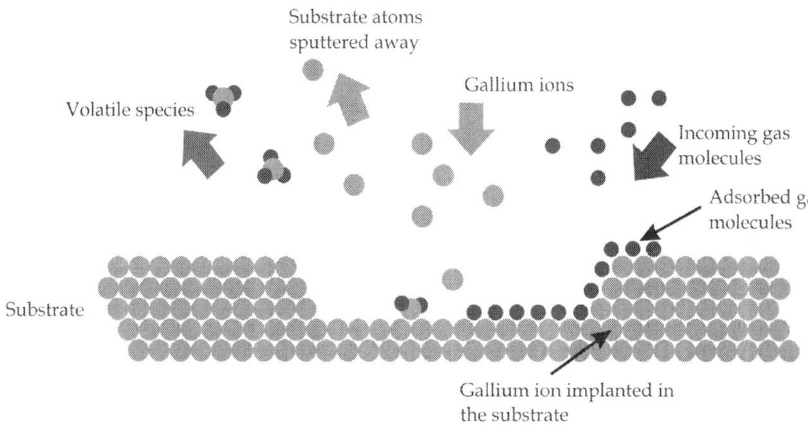

Fig. 5. Schematic describing atomic processes during ion beam-promoted sputtering.

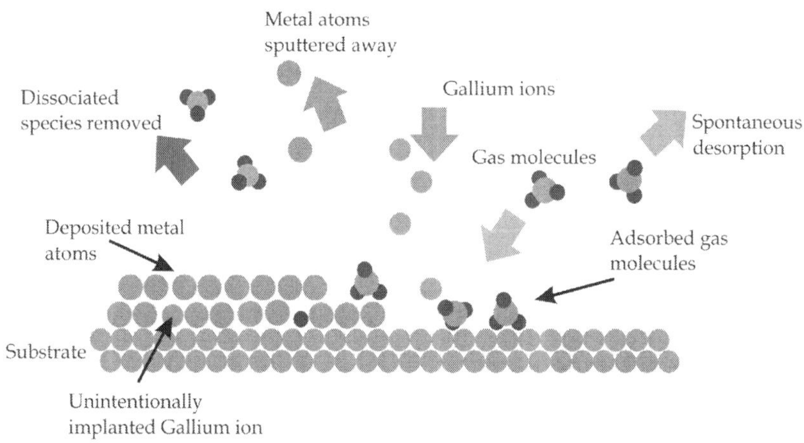

Fig. 6. Schematic describing atomic porcesses during ion-beam assistend gass deposition.

2.2 FIB micro-nano fabrication for customized pipettes

Fabrication of microinjection pipettes and micromanipulators with finely-controlled piercing angles, nanometer polishing, and versatile tip geometries is the next step to improve cell manipulation efficiency. Microsystem-based technologies hold the promise to mass-manufacture such highly functional tools with highly customized tips. This high customization is likely to have an impact on both current and future cell handling and cell probing. In particular, FIB micromachining has been receiving some attention lately in this application context. Indeed, FIB is rapidly becoming useful in diverse environments, serving multiple applications. Some of which differ greatly from the initial aims of FIB towards, for example, identification of failure mode analysis in the semiconductor industry or the thinning of lamellas (Gianuzzi and Stevie, 2005) for transmission electron microscopy inspection in materials science.

The pervasive nature of FIB capabilities, combined with the increasing cross-talk between the physical and the life sciences have been conducive to the pursuit of FIB as means of pipette customization. Some of the first evidence in this effort came from Kometani and coworkers, who retrofitted conventional glass pipettes (glass capillaries) by building nanostructured nozzles (Kometani et al., 2005a). The process is depicted in Figure 7 (Kometani et al., 2005b), where a conventional pipette is subjected to pulling (for thinning purposes), gold coating (to minimize electrical charing during electron and ion beam bomdardment), and FIB customization by chemical vapor deposition (CVD) and further milling.

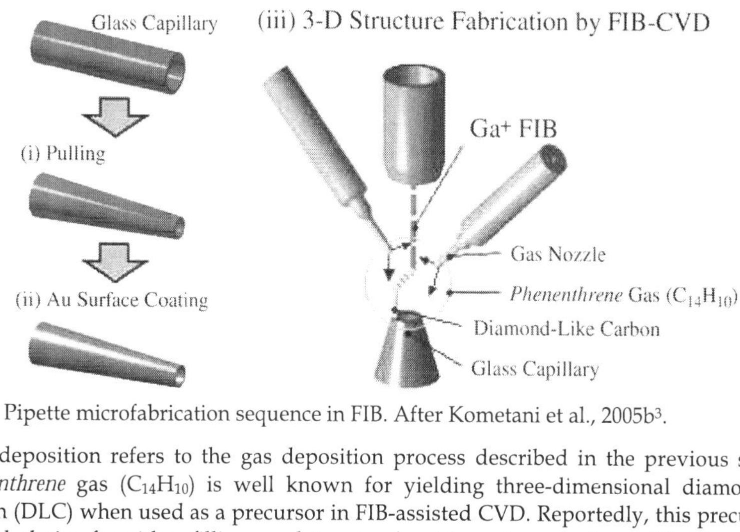

Fig. 7. Pipette microfabrication sequence in FIB. After Kometani et al., 2005b[3].

CVD deposition refers to the gas deposition process described in the previous section. *Phenanthrene* gas ($C_{14}H_{10}$) is well known for yielding three-dimensional diamond-like carbon (DLC) when used as a precursor in FIB-assisted CVD. Reportedly, this precursor is a good choice for either filling predetermined voids or for growing a fill tube directly above a fill hole (Biener et al. 2005). Other precursor gases are readily available on conventional commercial FIBs, such as tungstene (W) and silicon oxide (SiO_2), opening up the materials space to applications with conductivity and structural requirements (Kometani et al., 2007).

[3] Reprinted from *Nuclear Instruments and Methods in Physics Research Section B: Beam Interactions with Materials and Atoms*, Vol. 232, No. 1-4, Kometani, R.,Hoshino, T., Kanda, K., Haruyama, Y., Kaito, T., Fujita, J., Ishida, M., Ochiai, Y., & Matsui, S. , Three-dimensional high-performance nano-tools fabricated using focused-ion-beam chemical-vapor-deposition, pp. (362-366), 2005, with permission from Elsevier

In this scheme, nozzle structures were first fabricated on silicon substrates (Kometani et al., 2003). Irradiation of selected areas in the surface under a constant *phenanthrene* gas flow was performed following a scanning sequence dictated by a function generator. This function generator specified the pathway of the ion beam which determines the local DLC deposition, as depicted in Figure 6, with nanometric presicion. The pathway is not only being dictated on the x-y plane perpendicular to the tip by the usual lateral scanning action of beams. It also suffers modification on the vertical z axis, parallel to the pippette axis, presumably by varying the focal depth of the ion beam. The convolution of both lateral scanning and vertical height variation, would produce a helix trayectory, as shown in the schematic of Figure 8 top, which summarizes the synthesis of nozzle structures by DLC deposition. Nozzle fabrication is followed by spot milling of the inner channel, and tip customization by sectioning at specific angles.
Figure 8 (middle row) shows the progression of nozzle building with final inner and outer channels of 150 nm and 1580 nm at tip and base, respectively. The post-fabrication cross-section images (as seen in the last images in middle and bottom row) suggests even deposition and absence of voids, although the DLC surface has probably been unintentionally polished during FIB cross-sectioning. Further discussion would be needed to clarify the structural quality of as-grown DLC in these architectures.

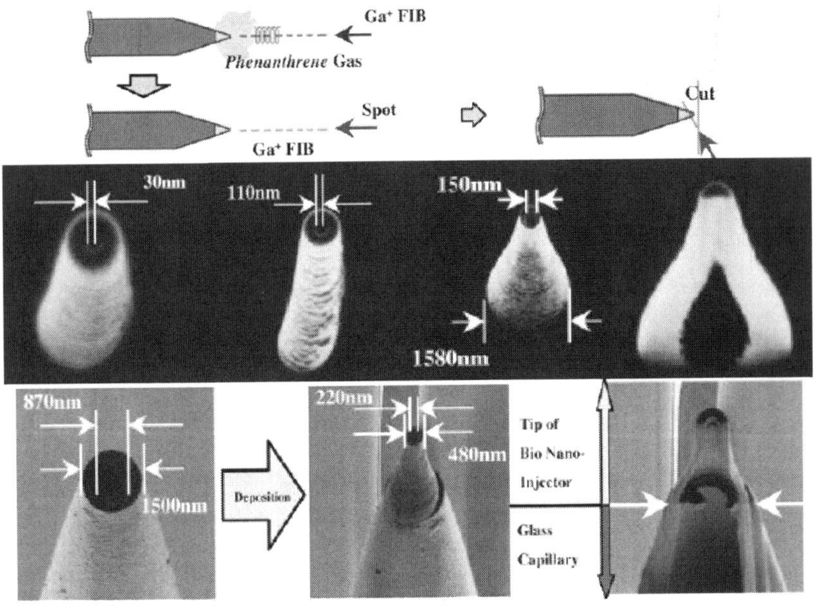

Fig. 8. FIB sequence for pipette micromanufacturing through vapor deposited DLC. After Kometani et al., 2003[4].

[4] This material is the reproduction from . *Japanese Journal of Applied Physics*, Vol. 42, No. 6B, (February 2003), pp. 4107-4110, Nozzle-Nanostructure Fabrication on Glass Capillary by Focused-Ion-Beam Chemical Vapor Deposition and Etching, 2003, Kometani, R., Morita T., Watanabe, K., Kanda K., Haruyama, Y., Kaito, T., Fujita, J., Ishida, M., Ochiai, Y., & Matsui, S.

Similarly, nozzle architectures can be implemented on pipette surfaces (Kometani et al., 2003). Again, by combining etching and deposition FIB capabilities, a final nozzle of 220 nm tip inner diameter can be tightly sculpted on the edges of a commercial glass pipette, as seen in Figure 8 (bottom row). In this process, an initial polishing of the edges takes place to subsequently facilitate a smooth deposition. The function generator designed for sculpting this nozzle tapered a cone-like shell, from 1500 nm to 480 nm outer diameters and from 870 nm to 220 nm inner diameters. A cross-section view of the structure shows the sharp interface between glass and DLC. Although values of interface strength were not reported along with fabrication methodology, this approach could be sound for cellular handling.

We have mentioned earlier how the versatility of FIB milling and deposition is not only due to the high position ability of the ion beam itself, but also to the high programmability of the scanning lenses (magnetic fields). Coupled with design software, sophisticated 3-dimensional patterns can be sculpted at pipette edges, as seen in Figure 9 (Kometani et al., 2005a, and 2006). Nanonets could be sculptured at the edges of pipettes (Kometani, 2005b) (not shown), offering a singular approach to collecting 2μm polystyrene spheres submerged in an aqueous environment.

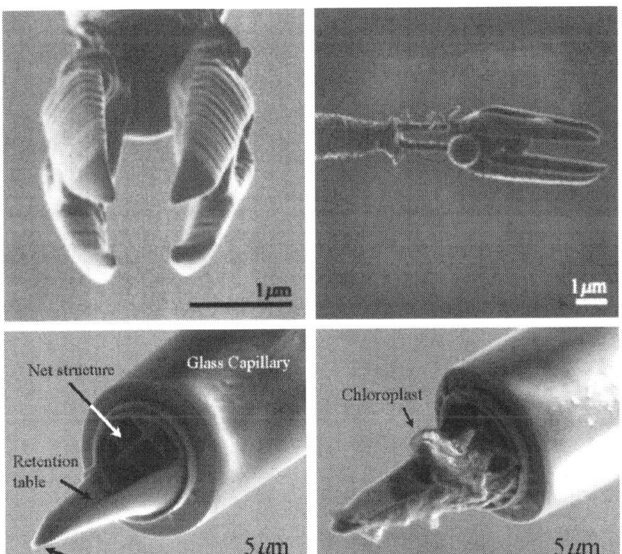

Fig. 9. SEM images of nozzle architectures, after Kometani et al., 2005a[5], and 2006[6].

[5] Reprinted with permission from *Journal of Vacuum Science & Technology B: Microelectronics and Nanometer Structures*, Vol. 23, No. 1, pp. (298-301), Performance of nanomanipulator fabricated on glass capillary by focused-ion-beam chemical vapor deposition, Kometani, R., Hoshino, T., Kondo, K., Kanda, K., Haruyama, Y., Kaito, T., Fujita, J., Ishida, M., Ochiai Y., & Matsui, S. (2005) American Vacuum Society.

[6] Reprinted from *Microelectronic Engineering*, Vol. 83, No. 4-9, , Kometani, R., Funabiki, R., Hoshino, T., Kanda, K., Haruyama, Y., Kaito, T., Fujita, J., Ochiai, Y., & Matsui, S., Cell wall cutting tool and nano-net fabrication by FIB-CVD for subcellular operations and analysis, pp. (1642-1645), (2006), with permission from Elsevier

The nanonet design serves as a proof of concept conducive to manipulation and analysis of subcellular organelles. Design possibilities go beyond passive components and an electrostatically-active manipulator has also been demonstrated, as shown in Figure 9 (top) by a 4-finger nanomanipulator, clampling 1μm-diameter latex microspheres. The scenario to selectively capture subcellular organelles of a specific size in a cell of choice was explored by constructing a multi-component tool. The multicomponent tool consisted of a cell wall-cutting needle and a nano-net of a pre-defined mesh size (Figure 9 bottom). Chloroplasts in an Egeria densa leaf were selectively captured by size-filtration in a nanonet. Filtration was activated by the naturally-occurring capillary suction at the tip of the pipette (Kometani 2006). Indeed, the filtering tool was manipulated to approach a specific cell (Kometani 2006), and the needle was inserted into the cell wall with the assistance of an external micromanipulator. Filtering of smaller organelles took place, leaving chloroplasts in the cell cutting component, also acting as a surgical scoop. Reportedly, this process was completed in 7 s, and the filtered chloroplasts from the cell of interest are shown in Figure 9 (bottom right).

The wealth of examples provided by Kometani and co-workers has paved the way for a radical approach to pipette design and manufacturing, opening a whole new perspective in procedures for biological handling at the cellular and subcellular level. Following the initial stages of proof of concept, a few questions arise regarding reliability; such as the mechanical properties of the ensemble. As-deposited FIB DLC shows a large Young's modulus (600 GPa-Kometani 2003 and references therein), yielding a stiffness comparable to other ceramics such as SiC and WC. In addition, the nanomanipulators did survive tests involving microsphere manipulation and chloroplast filtration. However, a more detailed analysis of mechanical durability of these structures in the relevant context applications is necesary.

Albeit, questions regarding toxicity and biocompatibility need urgent attention (Campo et al., 2011). It is worth emphasizing that gallium ions are likely to be implanted during both milling and deposision in FIB. Further studies are needed to address the impact of ion implantated tools on cellular activity. The next section will describe the work by Campo and co-workers who milled conventional glass pipettes at specific angles (Campo et al., 2010a) by FIB, yielding extremely polished edges with high precision. Tests during mouse embryo piercing, correlated increased penetration rates with decreased pipette angle. In addition, optimum embryo development after manipulation revealed little impact of residual implanted gallium ions, suggesting biocompatibility. It was also observed that milled pipettes maintain structural integrity after repeated piercing. Micromachining of glass pipettes by FIB could be amenable to mass production, presenting a promising avenue for future, increasingly demanding, cell handling.

2.3 FIB microfabrication for cell handling: Piercing and biocompatibility

Recapitulating, prior sections have described how manufacturing embryo injection pipettes is a delicate task. Typically conducted manually, trial-and-error pulling and heating control the inner and outer diameters as well as the length of the taper (Nagy et al., 2002). In FIB, areas can be milled selectively by gallium ions, as discussed earlier. In this section, we will describe how careful choice of time and current in the ion beam allows for high-quality polishing, providing qualitatively smooth, regular tapers. The high spatial selectivity in FIB has been effectively used to design sharp pipette tips, creating highly customized capillaries (Campo et al., 2010a). In this context, customization involved controlled bevelled angles as well as regular taper finishes. In an attempt to address the usability of FIB-customized pipettes in an impactful application context and also to partially address biocompatibility, mouse oocytes and embryos were used in piercing tests. Mouse embryos pose an ideal test bench for initial assessment of biocompatibility since small perturbations at the initial developmental stages are likely to impact embryonic development.

Important technological advances have taken place on oocyte and embryo microinjection recently. Oocyte and embryo microinjection can be performed with flat-ended pipettes which are easier to fabricate but often require piezoelectric-driven drilling to mechanically advance the pipette tip through the zona pellucida and plasma membrane (Yoshida & Perry, 2007). Piezo-driven drilling has been key to the success of experimental procedures involving microinjection of mouse oocytes in processes such as ICSI. The high elasticity of mouse oocyte plasma membrane complicates manual perforation without rupture using conventional bevelled and spiked pipettes, systematically requiring piezo-drilling. Although not strictly necessary, piezo-driven drilling greatly simplifies mouse embryo piercing. In this scheme, a small amount of mercury is typically loaded in the micropipette to minimize lateral vibrations, preventing cell damage (Ediz & Olgac, 2005). However, the additional cost of piezo-drills and, more importantly, toxicity issues arising from the use of mercury, have limited the use of piezo-assisted microinjection to just a few species (Yoshida & Perry, 2007; Ergenc et al., 2008).

Following this line of research and given the increasing need to improve current cell piercing (Ergenc & Olgac, 2007) and pipette quality (Yaul et al. 2008; Ostadi et al. 2009), Campo and coworkers (Campo et al., 2010) have sharpened conventional glass capillaries by FIB and tested them in mouse embryos. For the first time, the effect of sub-nanometer pipette polishing on zona pellucida and plasma membrane piercing is investigated. In addition, in vitro development of injected embryos was monitored, providing an early assessment on damage and toxicity from FIB-processed pipettes. A total of three capillaries were sharpened at 30, 20, and 15° (capillaries number 1,2, and 3, respectively), with profiles shown in Figure 10. The resulting edges were smooth after successive polishing. The insert in Figure 10a (previously shown in Figure 3 right) shows a commercial glass pipette used in human ICSI (Humagen, Virginia) featuring a sharp spike that, according to commercial specifications, has an angle between 25 and 30°. This angle is similar to those of pipettes number 1 and 2. Table 1 lists the different capillaries describing the final angular features.

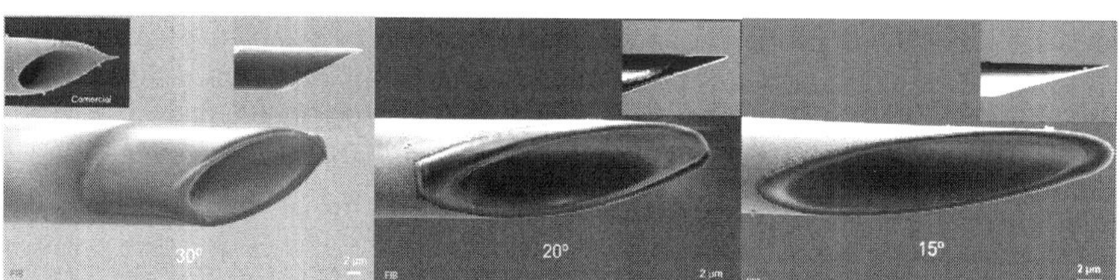

Fig. 10. SEM images of pipettes (left) 1, (centre) 2 , and (right) 3, sharpened at 30°, 20°, and 15°, respectively and showing beveled cut. Insert in (a) top left shows a commercial ICSI pipette. Inserts in (a), (b), and (c) top right show side-views of the milled pipettes.[7]

[7] With kind permission from Springer Science+Business Media: *Biomedical Microdevices*, Focus Ion Beam Micromachined Glass Pipettes for Cell Microinjection., Vol. 12, No.2, 2010, pp. (311-316), Campo, E.M., Lopez-Martinez, M. J., Fernández, E., Barrios, L., Ibáñez, E., Nogués, C., Esteve, J., & Plaza, J.A.

Capillaries number 1, 2, and 3 were used to pierce zona pellucida and plasma membrane of mouse embryos at the one cell stage (Figure 11). When successful, once inside the perivitelline space, the sharp tip was positioned to deform the plasma membrane and pierce it, penetrating within the cytoplasm. This process was conducted with a micromanipulator; applying pressure manually, in the absence of piezo-drilling.
A total of 20 embryos were used to test the injection efficiency of each pipette and the results are summarized in Table 1. Successful penetration of both the zona pellucida and the plasma membrane was achieved with all pipettes tested, with varying efficiencies and rates of embryo lysis. Pipette number 1 went through the zona pellucida in 60% of the tested embryos, leaving 40% unperforated. Further plasma membrane penetration was achieved with a 45% success rate, applying high pressures that resulted in extensive embryo deformation, possibly promoting lysis. All of the tested embryos were perforated with pipette number 2, totaling 75% penetration rate of both the zona pellucida and the plasma membrane. Pipette number 2 failed to perforate the plasma membrane in only 25% of the tested embryos. Finally, zona pellucida and plasma membrane penetration was achieved in 100% of the embryos punctured with pipette number 3.

Pipette number	Beveled angle [°] of micropipette	Number of embryos used	Penetration of ZP and PM (%)*	Penetration of ZP only (%)**	Lysis (%)[b]
1	30	20	9 (45)[a]	3 (15)[a]	3 (33.3)[a]
2	20	20	15 (75)[a]	5 (25)[a]	7 (46.7)[a]
3	15	20	20 (100)[b]	-	6 (30)[a]

* ZP: zona pellucida; PM: plasma membrane
** Number (percentage) of embryos that lysed after successful penetration of both ZP andPM
a-b Values with different superscripts within the same column differ significantly ($p < 0.05$).

Table 1. Injection efficiency and rates of lysis in mouse embryos penetrated with capillaries beveled at different angles.[8]

Lysis was observed only in embryos in which both the zona pellucida and the plasma membrane penetration was successful. Rates of embryo lysis were 33%, 46.7%, and 30% for capillaries number 1, 2, and 3, respectively. Pipettes were structurally sound, as no chips or fractures developed after piercing multiple embryos. Embryos that survived micromanipulation with pipette number 3 (n=14) were kept in culture for 96 h, and their development was assessed every 24 h, as seen in Table 2. These will be referred to as micromanipulated embryos throughout this discussion. An additional collection of embryos that were cultured in parallel with the micromanipulated embryos but without going through micromanipulation was used for comparison. We will refer to these as control embryos (n=23). In vitro embryo development results are summarized in Table 2. Control and micromanipulated embryos cleaved at similar rates (86.9% and 92.8%, respectively) and developed to the blastocyst stage (see Figure 12) also at similar rates (82.6% and 78.6%, respectively).

[8] With kind permission from Springer Science+Business Media: *Biomedical Microdevices,* Focus Ion Beam Micromachined Glass Pipettes for Cell Microinjection., Vol. 12, No.2, 2010, pp. (311–316), Campo, E.M., Lopez-Martinez, M. J., Fernández, E., Barrios, L., Ibáñez, E., Nogués, C., Esteve, J., & Plaza, J.A

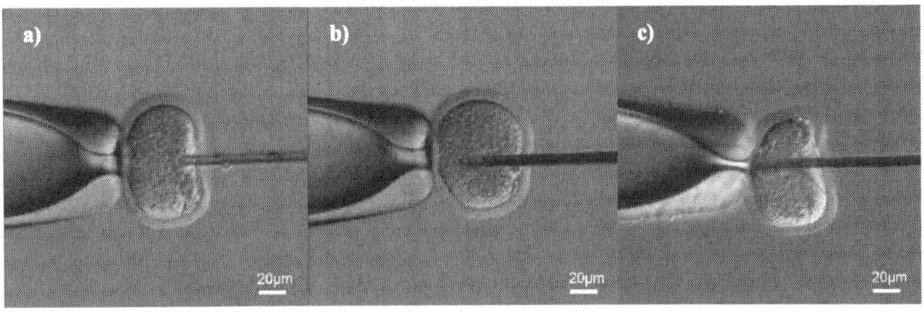

Fig. 11. Optical images of injection with pipettes number (a) 1 (b) 2, and (c) 3. The images were acquired at different stages in the piercing process. The observed embryo deformation is not indicative of the penetration depth prior to piercing.[9]

Group of embryos	Number of embryos	Embryos (%) developed to			
		2-cell	4-cell	Monula	Blastocyst
Micromanipulated	14	13 (92.8)	13 (92.8)	13 (92.8)	11(78.6)
Control	23	20 (86.9)	20 (86.9)	20 (86.9)	19 (82.6)

Table 2. In vitro development of mouse embryos successfully penetrated with pipette number 3.[10]

Summarizing, only pipette number 3 could penetrate the zona pellucida and the plasma membrane with 100% success and avoid lysis with 70% success. Piercing with pipettes 1 and 2 resulted in a more difficult plasma membrane penetration, as summarized in Table 1. Penetration rates increase with a decreased pipette angle. However, some lysis was unavoidable for all three pipettes. The correlation between sharpness and lysis is unclear, as sharper tips do not appear to minimize damage during piercing or decrease lysis. The finish in the pipette surely has an impact both in the piercing effect and in embryo development. Indeed, roughness and chipped edges in pipette tips are thought to be responsible for introducing contaminants into the oocyte, therefore inhibiting fertilization (Yaul et al., 2008). Some additional work has also been done assessing the effect of FIB- taper finish on penetration and damage (Campo et al., 2009b), although only in a qualitative fashion. These results show that capillary number 3 with 15°-sharp, smooth, finished tips by FIB could penetrate the zona pellucida and the plasma membrane efficiently, in good agreement with classic piezo-assisted drilling (Nagy et al., 2002).

[9] With kind permission from Springer Science+Business Media: *Biomedical Microdevices,* Focus Ion Beam Micromachined Glass Pipettes for Cell Microinjection., Vol. 12, No.2, 2010, pp. (311–316), Campo, E.M., Lopez-Martinez, M. J., Fernández, E., Barrios, L., Ibáñez, E., Nogués, C., Esteve, J., & Plaza, J.A.

[10] With kind permission from Springer Science+Business Media: *Biomedical Microdevices,* Focus Ion Beam Micromachined Glass Pipettes for Cell Microinjection., Vol. 12, No.2, 2010, pp. (311–316), Campo, E.M., Lopez-Martinez, M. J., Fernández, E., Barrios, L., Ibáñez, E., Nogués, C., Esteve, J., & Plaza, J.A.

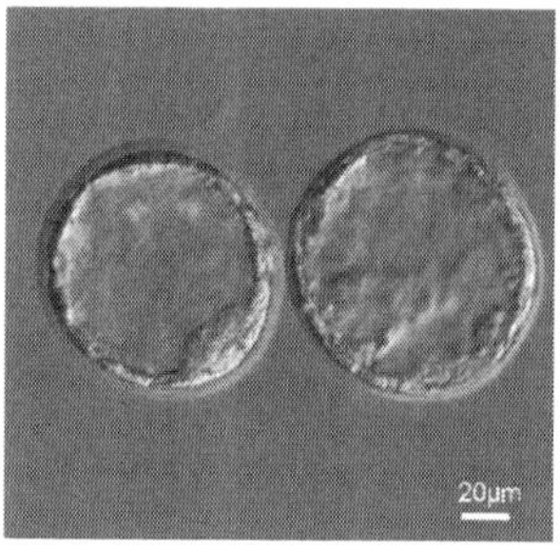

Fig. 12. Optical images of previously injected embryos showing development to the blastocyst stage.[11]

Survival rates during the in-vitro development of embryos previously manipulated with pipette number 3 were similar to survival rates of control, non-manipulated embryos (Table 2). All 14 embryos pierced with pipette number 3 were monitored for in-vitro development, noting the survival rates at the two-cell, four-cell, morula, and blastocyst stages. Most micromanipulated embryos successfully developed to the two- and four-cell stages as well as at morula. The survival rate at all these stages was constant at 93%. Similarly, control embryos maintained a constant 87% survival rate at the same intervals. Only one of the 14 micromanipulated embryos remained arrested at the one-cell stage. This phenomenon was also observed in control embryos, suggesting that causes inhibiting division might be unrelated to micromanipulation factors.

Gallium ions (unintentionally implanted during pipette milling) did not appear to affect development of mouse embryos to the blastocyst stage. While more detailed analyses are needed to fully address biocompatibility, these preliminary results are encouraging and could ultimately lead to improved piercing and survival rates during cell handling.

3. Sub-cellular monitoring, drug-delivery and manipulation

The prior section reviewed recent developments in technologies aiming at improving the funtionalities of celllular tools (mostly manipulators and injectors) and addressing the quality of finishes in injection pipettes. In the spirit of completeness, in this section we will describe in a cursory manner, some of the current landscape for subcellular technology.

3.1 Monitoring and drug-delivery by sub-cellular smart particles

The idea of targeting specific areas within the cell for detailed study is not new. Dyed biocompatible polymeric nanoparticles have been used for apoptosis imaging (Kim et al., 2006), and morphology of intracellular polymeric systems have been studied to address bio-compatibility along with their suitability as imaging markers and as drug delivery carriers (Nishiyama, 2007). Carrier morphology studies suggest that particles of specific sizes are

---

[11] With kind permission from Springer Science+Business Media: *Biomedical Microdevices,* Focus Ion Beam Micromachined Glass Pipettes for Cell Microinjection., Vol. 12, No.2, 2010, pp. (311-316), Campo, E.M., Lopez-Martinez, M. J., Fernández, E., Barrios, L., Ibáñez, E., Nogués, C., Esteve, J., & Plaza, J.A.

required to prevent deleterious interaction with cell organelles. On those lines, vehicle morphology studies concluded that phagocitic cells responded differently to micelles (assemblies of hydrophobic/hydrophilic block-copolymers) of different sizes (Geng et al., 2007). Walter et al. examined polymeric spheres that were phagocited for drug delivery (Walter et al., 2001) and Akin et al. (Akin et al., 2007) used microbots (nanoparticles attached to bacteria) to deliver therapeutic cargo to specific sites within a cell. Microbots delivered nanoparticles of polystyrene carrying therapeutic cargo and DNA into cells by taking advantage of invasive properties of bacteria. Recently, Kataoka's group (Mirakami et al., 2011) has sucessfully delivered chemotherapeutic drugs to the nuclear area of cancerous cells using micelles carriers. The specific delivery to the nuclear region is believed to have played a role in inhibiting the development of drug-resistance tumors.

Within the subcellular domain, different approaches have aimed at manufacturing devices to interact with organelles. Some groups have contemplated the possibility of constructing micro total analysis stystems (μTAS) suitable for biological applications (Voldman et al., 1999), where the mechanisms to extract information out of the cellular entity are challenging. However, few attempts have been made to address viability and functionality of standard microtechnology processed systems. Recently, our group has reported silicon microparticles embedded in live cells, suggesting an outstanding compatibility between conventional microtechnology devices and live systems down to the cellular level (Fernandez-Rosas et al., 2009; Gomez-Martinez et al., 2010). In terms of sensing, initial functionality mechanisms have identified apoptosis. These revolutionary findings constitute a paramount paradigm shift on cellular metrology, histology, and drug delivery; which are likely to have a profound impact in future research lines.

3.2 Manipulation by biomimetics

Another approach to sub-cellular exploration is inspired by nature. Indeed, understanding, mimicking, and adapting cellular and molecular mechanisms of biological motors in vitro has been forecast to produce a revolution in molecular manufacturing (Dinu et al., 2007, and Iyer et al., 2004). Biomolecular motors are biological machines that convert several forms of energy into mechanical energy. During a special session at Nanotech 2004 in Boston, MA, DARPA commissioned-overview by Iyer argued that functions carried out within a cell by biomolecular motors could be similar to man-made motors (i.e. load carrying or rotational movement). Researchers have already pondered about ways to transport designated cargo, such as vesicles, RNA or viruses to predetermined locations within the cell (Hess et al., 2008). Professor Hess during his keynote lecture at SPIE Photonics West (January 2008) also proposed biomolecular motors as imaging and sensing devices. Biomolecular motors such as the motor protein kinesin have been suggested as efficient tractor trailers within the cell. Efficiency of these systems could generate useful tools (conveyor belts and forklifts) as nanoscale bio-manufacturing tools. Kinesin moves along a track and is responsible for transporting cellular cargo such as organelles and signaling molecules. However, a detailed explanation of this walking mechanism is still missing (Iyer et al., 2004), currently inhibiting spatial and temporal control of kinesin molecular motors.

3.3 Monitoring and manipulation by FIB and microfluidics

Trends to intracellular manipulation also revolve around scaling down conventional pipettes. This trend is facilitated by microfluidics. Microsystem technologies have produced in the last decade an array of microfluidic devices (Verpoorte & De Rooig, 2003) that could

potentially probe the subcellular domain. By combining our prior experience learned in FIB glass pipettes (Campo et al. 2010a) with microfluidics (Lopez-Martinez et al. 2008 and 2009), micropipettes have been milled and tested in live embrios (Campo et al., 2009a and b). In this approach, micropipettes dimensions are comparable to some organelles and the sharp tips are likely to induce less damage on external cell walls. Details on the bottom-up microfabrication squeme can be found elsewhere (Lopez-Martinez et al., 2009). Similar experiments to those with glass pipettes (described in Section 2.3) revealed that silicon oxide (SiO_2) FIB-sharp nozzles successfully pierced mouse oocytes and embryos, without prejudice to the embryo and without producing structural damage to the nozzle.
Lack of structural damage is an important concern in FIB-modified structures as puncture devices reside on mechanical strength. Ideally, micronozzles will be sturdy enough to perforate zona pellucida and membrane without curving the tip of the micropipette or causing any other structural damage such as cracking or fragmentation. The tested micropipettes mantained their structural alumina layer, which provided sturdier structures. Figure 13 shows the structural layer (darker filler) surrounded by the silicon oxide channel. The tips did not show signs of mecanical failure during puncturing, as seen in Figure 14, or after repeated puncturing. Success from this initial assessment on mechanical strength and sucessful piercing has led to further work on hollow, fully microfluidic-functional micropipettes (*Lopez-Martinez & Campo-under preparation*). In addition, a study to assess viability and the adequate angular range for embryo piercing is underway. A better understanding of this procedure could eventually lead to commercial production and set pattern in cell handling.

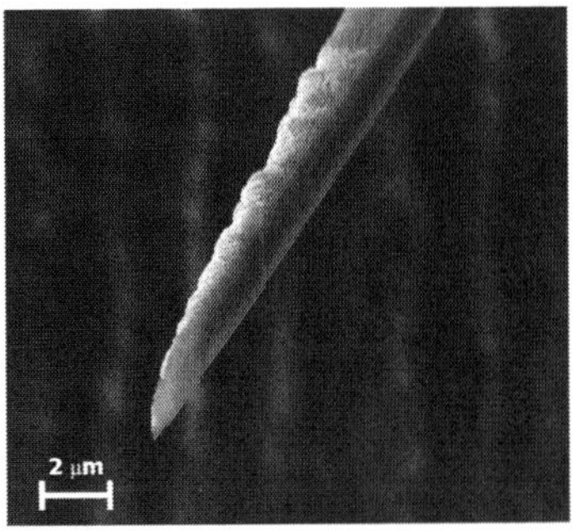

Fig. 13. SEM image of a 2 µm-wide silicon oxide nozzles FIB-sharpened at 5° (after Lopez-Martinez et al. 2009).[12]

Scaling down further to nanofluidics has also been achieved by ingenious building of carbon nanopipettes on conventional glass pipettes (Schrlau et al., 2008). Compared to conventional glass pipettes, these structures have suggested enhanced performance for intracellular delivery and cell physiology due to their smaller size, breakage and clogging resistance. Carbon nanopippettes have been reportedly used for concurrent injection and electrophysiology.

[12] Reproduced with permission from IOP: *Journal of Micromechanics and Microengineering*, Versatile micropipette technology based on Deep Reactive ion Etching and anodic bonding for biological applications, . (2009), Vol. 19, No. 10, pp. 105013, Lopez-Martinez, M.J. , Campo, E. M., Caballero, D., Fernandez, E., Errachid, A., Esteve, J., & Plaza, J.A

3.4 Smart materials in the sub-cellular domain

Materials science also has an important role in the development of cellular tools. Indeed, development of biocompatible smart materials with novel functionalities could provide the needed non-incremental advancement for sub-cellular monitoring and manipulation. Historically, there is a large presence of polymers in biomedicine. In fact, liquid crystal elastomers have been proposed as artificial muscles under the heating action of infrared lasers (Shenoy et al., 2002 and Ikeda et al., 2007), and an early proof-of-concept observed liquid crystal elastomers "swimming away" from the actuating light (Camacho-Lopez et al., 2004). This rudimentary motor was submerged in water and the source was an Ar+ ion laser (514 nm). Despite their potentially large application space, photoactuating materials have not been used in the broader context of biological systems (Campo et al., 2010b), posing an unique research opportunity for innovative functionalities.

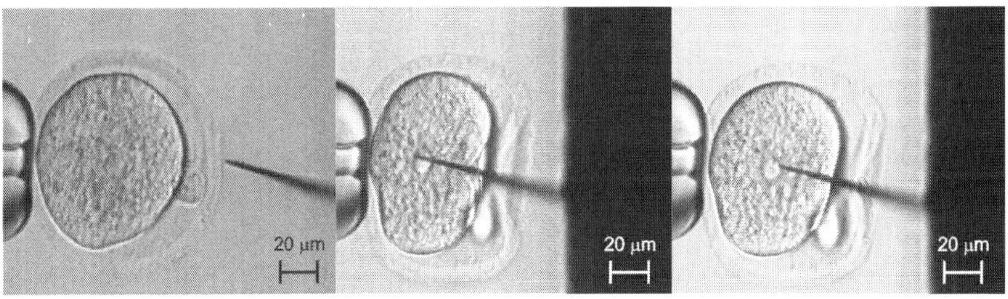

Fig. 14. Optical images of piercing test progress, (left) microdispenser nozzle outside a embryo, (centre) nozzle trying to penetrate embryo and (right) nozzle inside the embryo. (After Lopez-Martinez et al., 2009)[13]

4. Conclusions and future directions

An engineering analysis of the currently restrictive designs, finishes, and probing methods of glass pipettes and micromanipulators, suggests that those suffer from limited functionality and often damage cells; ultimately resulting in lysis. With all, the physical parameters that identify a high-quality pipette for a specific application need of a more quantitative description. In particular, the finishes of a pipette seem to be lacking a quantitative measure that could be provided by commonly-used characterization techniques in microsystem technologies, such as atomic force microscopy.

There seems to be plenty of leeway in advancing the state of the art in pipette design, manufacturing and piercing techniques. The great flexibility posed by microsystem technologies in the context of microfluidic devices and micromanufacturing with ion beams, present an unique opportunity in the biomedical sciences. In this scheme, tools for cell handling and monitoring can be tailored to specific tasks with unprecedented level of detail. Indeed, the possibility of affordable custom-made tools opens the door to improved sucess rates in common cellular procedures such as cell piercing. Highly-customized tools can also be designed to accomplish subcellular manipulation that would be, otherwise, unattainable

[13] Reproduced with permission from IOP: *Journal of Micromechanics and Microengineering,* Versatile micropipette technology based on Deep Reactive ion Etching and anodic bonding for biological applications, . (2009), Vol. 19, No. 10, pp. 105013, Lopez-Martinez, M.J. , Campo, E. M., Caballero, D., Fernandez, E., Errachid, A., Esteve, J., & Plaza, J.A

with the limitted functionalities of conventional pipettes. The use of ion beams for surface finishes can possibly alivieate some of the tedious work often involved in finishing capilaries. Ion beam polishing could also contribute to the characterization of roughness and finishes in a quantitative manner. In fact, ion beam milling is a useful tool to reverse engineer the morphology of pipettes altogether by sequential polishing and further image reconstruction (Ostadi et al., 2009). These tomographic capabilities could prove useful in quality control assessment of current and upcomming cellular tools.

Kometani et al. have provided a wealth of examples in highly customized micromanipulators, pending application in relevant cellular and subcellular scenarios. Future experiments should aim at inseminating mouse oocytes with FIB-polished glass pipettes, as initial tests by Campo et al. merely addressed piercing feasibility, i.e. mechanical sturdiness, sharpness, and early indication of biocompatibility. However, the real application scenario has not yet been demonstrated since no injection tests have been performed to show functionality. Similarly, FIB-sharpened microfluidic-pipettes are pending injection testing. In addition, microfulidic-pipettes manufacturing is ameanable to exploring materials other than silicon oxide, that could be of interest to complementary applications such as electrophysiology. Similarly to glass pipettes, microfluidic pipettes could be fitted with additional components, either by bottom-up or top-down microtechnologies. Resulting structures from the addition of sensors and actuators with different functionalities need to be tested in adequate scnearios and further assess biocompatibility.

We have discussed in detail how FIB with the assistance of gallium ions and carbon deposition, has gone well beyond proof of concept in terms of innovative design and micromanufacturing. Future directions in the microtechnology applications to the life sciences are likely to build upon FIB capabilities and also explore upcomming ion-bem microscopies. Looking forward, building upon FIB capabilities could be explored in the materials space, as well as in the functionality space of ion beam-produced tools. On the materials front, most FIB manufacturing for cellular tools has exploited the structural robustness of DLC. However, a number of chemistries are available in commercial FIB, with increasingly purified sources (Botman et al., 2009). Deposition of gold (Au), paladium (Pd), and platinum (Pt) could be specially interesting for devices requiring electrical conduction, such as those used in electrophysiology. Tipically, higher purity nanostructures are deposited by ion beam than by electron beam-assited deposition (Utke, 2008). However, further work will need to assess the effects of source purity on chemistry and mechanical characteristics of ion beam-deposited structures.

Amongst emergent novel micromachining and micromanufacturing technologies ameanable to contributing to cellular tools, Helium Ion Microscopy (HIM) is possibly the most relevant. Seminal papers describe this novel microscopy that serves both as a characterization (Scipioni et al., 2009) and a manufacturing tool (Postek et al., 2007, Maas et al., 2010) in micro-nano systems. With the use of hellium (He) ions and, smilarly to FIB, highly customizable milling capabilities, HIM could have a possitive impact on the pending biocompatibility assessment. Adequate biocompatibility studies are needed to assess ion dose implantation on tools and devices and the effects at the subcellular and cellular levels, as well as in vivo. These will be critical parameters that could hinder the implementation of ion-beam technologies in the life sciences. In all likelihood, these strategies will need to be developed by multidisciplinary teams. In fact, assembly of highly multidisciplinary teams, encompassing bio-medical scientists and microsytem technologists, are surely needed to fully explore the possibilities of impactful task-specific tools in the context of subcellular manipulation.

It is also crucial to develop a mechanistic understanding of how design, manufacturing, and piercing techniques affect cellular structures. Indeed, the impact of pipette parameters on handling is unclear, as mechanisms responsible for different failure modes during conventional piezo-assisted piercing only recently have been subject of investigation (Ediz et al., 2005). Mechanistic studies would establish a much-needed correlation between the (quantifiable) physical parameters of pipettes and piercing techniques with cellular response in the context of elasticity theory and biology. In terms of operator training and quantification of the exerted force, the advent of haptics in the context of robotics could provide quantification of cell injection force and also to improve success statistics in piercing and other operational procedures. There is already enough evidence suggesting that the combination of haptic and visual feedback improves handling (Pillaresetti et al., 2007). Further development of these technologies will, most likely, make them available to the bio-medical community at large. Novel piercing technologies have also appeared in the recent literature, such as Ross-Drill, promoting a rotational approach to cell piercing, rather than tangential (tipical of piezo-assited drilling) and claiming decreased training effort for operators. The possibility of combining Ross-Drill with FIB-polished pipettes has already been sugested (Campo et al., 2010a).

SPECIALTY	APPLICATION	CITATION
CELL INJECTION	ROTATIONAL OSCILLATION-DRILL	ERGENC, EDIZ & OLGAC
CELL INJECTION	MICROMANUFACTURING OF CUSTOMIZED TIPS IN GLASS CAPILARIES AND MICROFLUIDIC PLATFORMS	CAMPO & PLAZA
CELL INJECTION	3-D STUDY OF GLASS PIPETTE GEOMETRY BY MICROMACHINING TECHNIQUES	OSTADI & OLGAC
CELL MICROINJECTION	USE OF CARBON NANOTUBES FOR ELECTROPHYISIOLOGY AND NANOFLUIDIC INJECTION	SCHRLAU&BAU
CELLULAR/ SUBCELLULAR HANDLING	MICROMANUFACTURING OF CUSTOMIZED MANIPULATORS IN GLASS CAPILARIES	KOMETANI& MATSUI
SUBCELLULAR MONITORING	MICROMANUFACTURIG OF CUSTOMIZED SENSORS AND ACTUATORS IN GLASS CAPILARIES	KOMETANI& MATSUI
SUBCELLULAR DRUG DELIVERY	POLYMERIC MICELLE CARRIERS	GENG & DISCHER
SUBCELLULAR DRUG DELIVERY	BACTERIA-MEDIATED DRUG DELIVERY	AKIN&BASHIR
SUBCELLULAR DNA DELIVERY	POLYMER MICROSPHERES	WALTER & MERKLE
SUBCELLULAR MONITORING AND DELIVERY*	PROOF OF CONCEPT: BIOCOM-PATIBLE INSERTION OF MICROCHIPS ON CELLS	FERNANDEZ-ROSAS, GOMEZ-MARTINEZ & PLAZA
SMART MATERIALS**	PROOF OF CONCEPT: LCE PHOTO-PROPELLED IN AN AQUOUS ENVIRONMENT	CAMACHO-LOPEZ, PALFFY-MUHORAY & SHELLEY
MECHANICAL ACTUATORS*	PROOF OF CONCEPT: BIMORPH THERMAL NANO- ACTUATORS BY FIB	CHANG & LIN
HAPTIC TECHNOLOGY IN CELLULAR HANDLING	HAPTIC FEED-BACK IN COMBINATION WIH VISUAL INSPECTION DURING CELL PIERCING	PILLARISETTI & DESAI

*This is a promising approach in subcellular monitoring and delivery.

* *This approach has not been applied to cellular or subcellular environments.

Table 3. List of highlighted technologies according to specialty, detailing specific application and citation included in the references in Section 6.

Future directions in micro-nanotechnologies applied to the life sciences are likely to build upon the approaches described in this chapter, which have been summarized in Table 3. Beyond piercing, technological developments such as cell-embedded silicon microparticles are likely to develop into micro-chips in the near future; posing a new paradigm shift in sub-cellular probing. In addition, novel actuation capabilities have been temptatively explored by Kometani's group producing an electrostatic-operated micromanipulator. Further, Chang et al., (Chang, 2009) have recently discussed a bimorph thermal actuator that combined thermal conductivity of FIB-depostied tungsten (W) with structural rigidity of DLC. This work is innovative as it introduces smart materials in microtechnology manufacturing in the production of cellular tools. On-going efforts to incorporate electro and photoactuators in the biomedical arena as artificial muscles are likely to expand to the subcellular domain and potential application contexts will be suggested, further paving the way for the incorporation of nano-opto-mechanical-systems (NOMS) in main stream research (www.noms-project.eu).

5. Acknowledgments

The authors gratefully acknowledge mentorship from Jose A. Plaza and Jaume Esteve at IMB-CNM CSIC and the cooperation of Elizabeth Fernandez-Rosas, (who conducted the cell biology experiments), Leonard Barrios, Elena Ibanez y Carmen Nogues from the Biology Department at the Universitat Autonoma de Barcelona. We are also indebted to Dr. Núria Sancho Oltra from the Department of Chemical and Biomolecular Engineering at the University of Pennsylvania for useful discussions. This work was partially supported by the Spanish government under Juan de la Cierva Fellowship, MINAHE 2 (TEC2005-07996-C02-01) and MINAHE 3 (TEC2008-06883-C03-01) projects and by the European Union FP7 under contract NMP 228916.

6. References

Akin, D., Sturgis, J., Ragheb, K., Sherman, D., Burkholder, K., Robinson, J.P., Bhunia, A.K., Mohammed, S., & Bashir, R. (2007). Bacteria-mediated delivery of nanoparticles and cargo into cells nature. Nature Nanotechnology, Vol. 2 (April 2007), pp. (441 - 449), ISSN: 1748-3387

Bao, G., & Suresh, S. (2003). Cell and molecular mechanics of biological materials. Nature materials, Vol. 2 (November 2003), No. 11, pp. (715-725), ISSN : 1476-1122

Biener, J., Mirkarimi, P.B., Tringe, J.W., Baker, S.L., Wang, Y.M., Kucheyev, S.O., Teslich, N.E., Wu, K.J., Hamza, A.V., Wild, C., Woerner, E., Koidl, P., Bruehne, K., & Fecht, H.-J. (2006). Diamond Ablators for Inertial Confinement Fusion. *Fusion Science & Technology*, Vol. 49, No. 4, pp. (737-742), ISSN: 1536-1055

Biggers, J.D., McGinnis, L.K., & Raffin, M. (2000). Amino Acids and Preimplantation Development of the Mouse in Protein-Free Potassium Simplex Optimized Medium. *Biology of Reproduction*, Vol. 63, No. 1, (July 2000), pp. (281-293), ISSN: 0006-3363

Botman, A., Mulders, J. J. L., & Hagen C.W. (2009) Creating pure nanostructures from electron-beam-induced deposition using purification techniques: a technology perspective *Nanotechnology*, Vol. 20, pp(372001 (17pp), ISSN: 1748-3387

Camacho-Lopez, M., Finkelman, H., Palffy-Muhorray, P., & Shelley, M (2004) Fast liquid-crystal elastomer swims into the dark. *Nature Materials,* Vol. 3 (May 2004), pp. (307-310), ISSN: 1476-4660

Campo, E.M., Lopez-Martinez, M.J., Fernandez, E., Ibanez, E., Barros, L., Nogues, C., Esteve, J., & Plaza, J.A. (2009). Sharpened transparent micronozzles fabrication for cell membrane piercing. *Proceedings of SPIE, the International Society for Optical Engineering.* ISBN 978-0-8194-7450-6, San Jose, California, United States, January 2009

Campo, E.M., Lopez-Martinez, M. J., Fernández, E., Esteve, J., & Plaza, J.A. (2009). Implementation of Ion-Beam techniques in microsystems manufacturing: Opportunities in cell biology. *Proceedings of SPIE, the International Society for Optical Engineering, Scanning Microscopy.* ISSN 0277-786X , Monterey, May 2009

Campo, E.M., Lopez-Martinez, M. J., Fernández, E., Barrios, L., Ibáñez, E., Nogués, C., Esteve, J., & Plaza, J.A. (2010). Focus Ion Beam Micromachined Glass Pipettes for Cell Microinjection. *Biomedical Microdevices,* Vol. 12, No.2, (April 2010), pp. (311–316), ISSN 1572-8781 .

Campo, E.M., Campanella, H., Huang, Y.Y., Zinoviev, K., Torras, N., Tamargo, C., Yates, D., Rotkina, L., Eteve, J., & Terentjev, E.M. (2010). Electron Microscopy of Polymer-Carbon Nanotube Composites. *Proceedings of SPIE, the International Society for Optical Engineering, Scanning Microscopy.* ISBN: 978-0-8194-8217-4 , Monterey, May 2010

E.M. Campo, B. Mamojka, D. Wenn, I. Ramos, J. Esteve, and E.M. Terentjev, "*Education and dissemination strategies in photoactuation,*", in preparation, SPIE NanoScience + Engineering August 2011

Chang, J., Min, B.K., Kim, J. & Lin, L. (2009) Bimorph nano actuators synthesized by focused ion beam chemical vapor deposition, *Microelectronic Engineering* 86, pp.(2364–2368), ISSN: 0167-9317

Dinu, C.Z., Chrisey, D.B., Diez, S., & Howard, J. (2007). Cellular Motors for Molecular Manufacturing. *The Anatomical Record,* Vol. 290, No. 10, (Setember 2007), pp. (1203-1212), ISSN: 1932-8494

Ediz, K., & Olgac, N. (2005). Effect of Mercury Column on the Microdynamics of the Piezo-Driven Pipettes. *Journal of Biomechanical Engineering-Transactions of the ASME,* Vol. 127, No. 3, (June 2005), pp. (531-535), ISSN: 0148-0731

Ergenc, A., & Olgac, N. (2007). New technology for cellular piercing: rotationally oscillating μ-injector, description and validation tests. *Biomedical Microdevices,* Vol. 9, No. 6, (December 2007), pp. (885-891), ISSN: 1387-2176

Fernandez-Rosas, E., Gomez, R., Ibañez, E., Barrios, L., Duch, M., Esteve, J., Nogues, C., & Plaza, J.A. (2009) Intracellular Polysilicon Barcodes for Cell Tracking. *Small,* Vol. 5, No. 21, (November 2), pp. (2433–2439), ISSN: 1613-6829

Geng, Y., Dalhaimer, P., Cai, S., Tsai, R., Tewari, M., Minko, T., & Discher, D.E. (2007). Shape effects of filaments versus spherical particles in flow and drug delivery. *Nature Nanotechnology,* Vol. 2, (April 2007), pp. (249-255), ISSN: 1748-3387

Giannuzzi, A., & Stevie, F. A. (2005). *Introduction to Focused Ion Beams: Instrumentation, Theory, Techniques and Practice* (1st edition), NY: Springer, ISBN 978-0-387-23116-7 North Carolina State University (Eds.)

Gomez-Martinez, R., Vázquez P., Duch, M., Muriano, A., Pinacho, D., Sanvicens, N., Sánchez-Baeza, F., Boya, P., de la Rosa, E., J, Esteve, J., Suárez, T., & Plaza, J.A. (2010). Intracellular silicon chips in living cells. *Small*, Vol. 6, No. 4, (February 2010) pp. (499-502), ISSN: 1613-6829

Hess, H., Fischer, T., Agarwal, A., Katira, P., Finger, I., Mobley, E., Tucker, R., Kerssemakers, J., & Diez, S. (2008). Biomolecular motors challenge imaging and enable sensing. *Progress in biomedical optics and imaging, Proceedings of SPIE, Nanoscale imaging, sensing, and actuation for biomedical applications V*, ISSN: 1605-7422, San Jose, January 2008

Hoshino, T., Kawamori, M., Suzuki, T., Matsui, S., & Mabuchi, K. (2004). Three dimensional and multimaterial microfabrication using focused-ion-beam chemical-vapor deposition and its application to processing nerve electrodes. *Journal of Vacuum Science & Technology B*, Vol. 22, No. 6, (November 2004) pp. (3158-3162), ISSN: 1071-1023

Huang, T.,Kimura, Y., &Yanagimachi, R. (1996). The use of piezo micromanipulation for intracytoplasmic sperm injection of human oocytes. *Journal of Assisted Reproduction and genetics*, Vol. 13, No. 4, pp.(320-328), ISSN: *1573-7330*

Ikeda, T., Mamiya, J., & Yu, Y. (2007). Photomechanics of Liquid-Crystalline Elastomers and Other Polymers. *Angewandte Chemie International Edition*, Vol. 46, No.4 (January 2007), pp. (506 - 528), ISSN: 1521-3773

Ittner, L., & Götz, J. (2007). Pronuclear injection for the production of transgenic mice. *Nature protocols*, Vol 2, No. 5, (April 2007), pp. (1206-1215), ISSN: 1754-2189

Iyer, S., Romanowicz, B., & Laudon, M. (2004). Biomoleculars motors. *Proceedings Nanotech, the Nanotechnology Conference and Trade Show*, Boston, March 2004

Kim, K., Lee, M., Park, H., Kim, J., Kim, S., Chung, H., Choi, K., Kim, I., Seong, B.L., & Kwon, I.C. (2006). Cell-Permeable and Biocompatible Polymeric Nanoparticles for Apoptosis Imaging. *Journal of the American Chemical Society*, Vol. 128, No. 11, (March 2006), pp. (3490-3491), ISSN: 0002-7863

Kishigami, S., Hikichi, T., Van Thuan, N., Ohta, H., Wakayama, S., Bui, H.T., Mizutani, E., & Wakayama, T. (2006). Normal specification of the extraembryonic lineage after somatic nuclear transfer. *FEBS Letters*, Vol. 580, No. 7, (March 2006), pp. (1801-1806), ISSN 0014-5793

Kometani, R., Morita T., Watanabe, K., Kanda K., Haruyama, Y., Kaito, T., Fujita, J., Ishida, M., Ochiai, Y., & Matsui, S. (2003). Nozzle-Nanostructure Fabrication on Glass Capillary by Focused-Ion-Beam Chemical Vapor Deposition and Etching. *Japanese Journal of Applied Physics*, Vol. 42, No. 6B, (February 2003), pp. 4107-4110, ISSN: 0021-4922

Kometani, R., Hoshino, T., Kondo, K., Kanda, K., Haruyama, Y., Kaito, T., Fujita, J., Ishida, M., Ochiai Y., & Matsui, S. (2005). Performance of nanomanipulator fabricated on glass capillary by focused-ion-beam chemical vapor deposition. *Journal of Vacuum Science & Technology B: Microelectronics and Nanometer Structures*, Vol. 23, No. 1, (January/February 2005), pp. (298-301), ISSN 0734-211X

Kometani, R.,Hoshino, T., Kanda, K., Haruyama, Y., Kaito, T., Fujita, J., Ishida, M., Ochiai, Y., & Matsui, S. (2005). Three-dimensional high-performance nano-tools fabricated using focused-ion-beam chemical-vapor-deposition. *Nuclear Instruments and Methods in Physics Research Section B: Beam Interactions with Materials and Atoms*, Vol. 232, No. 1-4, (May 2005), pp. (362-366), ISSN 0168-583X

Kometani, R., Hoshino, T., Kondo, K., Kanda, K., Haruyama, Y., Kaito, T., Fujita, J., Ishida, M., Ochiai, Y., & Matsui, S. (2005). Fabrication of nanomanipulator with SiO_2/DLC heterostructure by focused-ion-beam chemical vapor deposition. *Japanese journal of applied physics*, Vol. 44, No. 7B, (July 2005), pp. 5727–5731, ISSN 0021-4922

Kometani, R., Funabiki, R., Hoshino, T., Kanda, K., Haruyama, Y., Kaito, T., Fujita, J., Ochiai, Y., & Matsui, S. (2006). Cell wall cutting tool and nano-net fabrication by FIB-CVD for subcellular operations and analysis, *Microelectronic Engineering*, Vol. 83, No. 4-9, pp. (1642-1645), ISSN: 0167-9317

Kometani, R., Koike, H., Kanda, K., Haruyama, Y., Kaito, T., & Matsui, S. (2007). Evaluation of a Bio Nano-Sensing Probe Fabricated by Focused-Ion-Beam Chemical Vapor Deposition for Single Organelle Analyses. Japanese Journal of Applied Physics, Vol. 46, No. , (December 2007), pp. (7963-7965), ISSN 0021-4922

Lacham-Kaplan, O., & Trounson, A. (1995). Intracytoplasmic sperm injection in mice: increased fertilization and development to term after induction of the acrosome reaction. *Human Reproduction*, Vol. 10, No. 10, (October 1995), pp. (2642-2649), ISSN 0268-1161

Lopez-Martinez, M. J., Caballero, D., Campo, E. M., Perez-Castillejos, R., Errachid, A., Esteve, J., & Plaza, J. A. (2008). FIB assisted technology in sub-picolitre micro-dispenser fabrication. *Journal of Micromechanics and Microengineering*, Vol. 18, No. 7, (July 2008), 075021, ISSN 1361-6439

Lopez-Martinez, M.J. , Campo, E. M., Caballero, D., Fernandez, E., Errachid, A., Esteve, J., & Plaza, J.A. (2009). Versatile micropipette technology based on Deep Reactive ion Etching and anodic bonding for biological applications. *Journal of Micromechanics and Microengineering*, Vol. 19, No. 10 (October 2009), 105013, ISSN 1361-6439

Maas, D., van Veldhoven, E., Chen, P., Sidorkin, V., Salemink, H., van der Grift, E, & Alkemade, P. (2010). Nanofabrication with a Helium Ion Microscope. *Proceedings of SPIE, the International Society for Optical Engineering, Scanning Microscopy*. Vol. 7638, ISSN 0277-786X , Monterey, May 2009

Malboubi, M., Ostadi, H., Wang, S., Gu, Y., & Jiang, K. (2009). The Effect of Pipette Tip Roughness on Giga-seal Formation. *Proceedings of the World Congress on Engineering 2009 Vol II WCE 2009*, ISBN: 978-988-18210-1-0 London, U.K. July, 2009

Morita, T., Kometani, R., Watanabe, K., Kanda, K., Haruyama, Y., Hoshino, T., Kondo, K., Kaito, T., Ichihashi, T., Fujita, J., Ishida, M., Ochiai, Y., Tajima, T., & Matsui, S. (2003). Free-space-wiring fabrication in nano-space by focused-ion-beam chemical vapor deposition. *Journal of Vacuum Science & Technology B*, Vol. 21, No. 6, (November 2003), pp. (2737-2741), ISSN: 1071-1023

Mirakami, M., Cabral, H., Matsumoto, Y., Wu, S., 3 Kano, M.R., Yamori, T. , Nishiyama, N., Kataoka, K. (2011) Improving Drug Potency and Efficacy by Nanocarrier-Mediated Subcellular Targeting. Science of Translational Medicine 3, 64ra2 , ISSN: 1946-6242

Nagy, A. , Gertsenstein, M., Vintersten, K., & Behringer, R. (2002) *Manipulating the Mouse Embryo: A laboratory Manual*, 3rd ed, Cold Spring Harbor Laboratoy Press, ISBN 978-087969591-0, New York

Nishiyama, N. (2007). Nanocarriers shape up for long life. *Nature Nanotechnology*, Vol. 2 (April 2007), pp. 203-204, ISSN: 1748-3387

Ostadi, H., Malboubi, M., Prewett, P.D., & Jiang, K. (2009). *Microelectronic Engineering.* 3D reconstruction of a micro pipette tip, Vol. 86, No. 4-6, (April-June 2009), pp. (868-870), ISSN: 0167-9317

Palermo, G. , Joris, H., Camus, M., Devroey, P., & Van Steirteghem, A. C. (1992). Pregnancies after intracytoplasmic injection of single spermatozoon into an oocyte. *Lancet,* Vol. 4, No. 340, (July 1992), pp. 8810-8817, ISSN 0140-6736

Pillarisetti, A., Pekarev, M., Brooks, A.D., & Desai, J.P. (2007) "Evaluating the Effect of Force Feedback in Cell Injection," *IEEE Transactions on Automation Science and Engineering,* vol. 4(3), pp. (322-331), ISSN: 1545-5955

Postek, M., Vladár, A.E., Kramar,J., Stern, L.A., Notte, J., & McVey, S. (2007) "The helium ion microscope: a new tool for nanomanufacturing", . *Proceedings of SPIE, the International Society for Optical Engineering, Instrumentation Metrology and Standards for nanomanufacturing,* Vol. 6648 (2007)

Schrlau, M., Brailoiu, E., Patel, S., Gogotsi, Y., Dun. J., & Bau, H.H. (2008). Carbon nanopipettes characterize calcium release pathways in breast cancer cells. *Nanotechnology,* Vol. 19, No. 32, (July 2008), 325102, ISSN 1361-6528

Scipioni, L., Sanford, C., Notte, J., Thompson, B.,& McVey, S. (2009). Understanding imaging modes in the helium ion microscope. *Journal of Vacuum Science and Technology B,* Vol. 76, No. 6 (November-December 2009), pp. (3250-3255), ISSN 1520-8567

Shenoy, D.K., Thomsen III, D.L., Srinivasanb, A., Kellerc, P., & Ratna, B.R. (2002). Carbon coated liquid crystal elastomer film for artificial muscle applications. *Sensors and Actuators A: Physical,* Vol. 96, No. 2-3, (February 2002), pp. (184-188), ISSN: 0924-424

Sutter Instruments. (2008). P-97 Pipette cookbook (Rev. D). Retrieved from www.sutter.com

Utke, I., Hoffmann, P., Melngailis, J. (2008). Gas-assisted focused electron beam and ion beam processing and fabrication. *J. Vac. Sci. Technol. B* 26, pp.(1197-1272), ISSN ISSN 0734-211X

Verpoorte, E., & De Rooig, N.F. (2003). Microfluidics meets MEMS. *Proceedings of the IEEE,* Vol. 91, No. 6 (June 2003), pp. (930 - 953), ISSN: 0018-9219

Voldman, J., Gray, M.L.,& Schmidt, M.A. (1999) Microfabrication in Biology and Medicine. *Annual Review of Biomedical Engineering,* Vol. 01, (August 1999), pp. (401–425), *ISSN*:1523-9829

Walter, E., Dreher, D., Kok, M., Thiele, L., Kiama, S.G., Gehr, P., & Merkle, H.P. (2001). Hydrophilic poly(DL-lactide-co-glycolide) microspheres for the delivery of DNA to human-derived macrophages and dendritic cells. *Journal of Controlled Release,* Vol. 76, No.1-2, (Setember 2001), pp. (149–168), ISSN: 0168-3659

Weibel, D.B., DiLuzio, W.R., & Whitesides, G.M. (2007). Microfabrication meets microbiology. *Nature Reviews Microbiology,* Vol. 5, No. 3, (March 2007), pp. (209-218), ISSN: 1740-1526

Yaul, M., Bhatti, R., & Lawrence, S. (2008) Evaluating the process of polishing borosilicate glass capillaries used for fabrication of in - vitro fertilization (iVF) micro-pipettes. *Biomedical Microdevices,* Vol. 10, No. 1, (February 2008), pp. (123-128), ISSN: 1387-2176

Yoshida, N., & Perry, A. C. F. (2007). Piezo-actuated mouse intracytoplasmic sperm injection (ICSI). *Nature Protocols,* Vol. 2, No. 2, (March 2007) pp. (296-304), ISSN: 1754-2189

13

Nanoparticles in Biomedical Applications and Their Safety Concerns

Jonghoon Choi[1] and Nam Sun Wang[2]
[1]*Department of Chemical Engineering, Massachusetts Institute of Technology, Cambridge, MA,*
[2]*Department of Chemical and Biomolecular Engineering, University of Maryland, College Park, MD, USA*

1. Introduction

In this chapter, we will discuss the fate of nanoparticles when they are introduced into a system. Recent advances in synthesis and functionalization of nanoparticles have brought a significant increase in their biomedical applications, including imaging of cell and tissues, drug delivery, sensing of target molecules, etc. For example, iron oxide nanoparticles (Feridex) have been clinically administered as a contrast agent in magnetic resonance imaging (MRI).

Their superb magnetic properties provide a significant contrast of tissues and cells where particles were administered. The use of Feridex as a MRI contrast agent enables a facile diagnosis of cancers in diverse organs in their early stages of development. As the range of different nanoparticles and their biomedical applications continue to expand, safety concerns over their use have been growing as well, leading to an increasing number of research on their *in vivo* toxicity, hazards, and biodistributions.

While the number of studies assessing *in vivo* safety of nanoparticles has been increasing, a lack of understanding persists on the mechanisms of adverse effects and the distribution pathways. It is a challenge to correlate reports on one type of particles to reports on other types due to their intrinsic differences in the physical properties (particle size, shape, etc.) and chemical properties (surface chemistry, hydrophobicity, etc.), methods of preparation, and their biological targets (cells, tissues, organs, animals).

Discrepancies in experimental conditions among different studies is currently bewildering the field, and there exists a critical need to arrive at a consensus on a gold standard of toxicity measure for probing *in vivo* fate of nanoparticles. This chapter summarizes recent studies on *in vivo* nanoparticle safety and biodistribution of nanoparticles in different organs. An emphasis is placed on a systematic categorization of reported findings from *in vivo* studies over particle types, sizes, shapes, surface functionalization, animal models, types of organs, toxicity assays, and distribution of particles in different organs.

Based on our analysis of data and summary, we outline agreements and disagreements between studies on the fate of nanoparticles *in vivo* and we arrive at general conclusions on the current state and future direction of *in vivo* research on nanoparticle safety.

2. Nanoparticles in biomedical applications

Particles in nanosize have significantly different characteristics from particles not in nanoscale. Since these nanoparticle properties are often in many applications, they have been applied in a wide variety of medical research. (Bystrzejewski, Cudzilo et al. 2007; Yu 2008; Nune, Gunda et al. 2009; Yaghini, Seifalian et al. 2009)

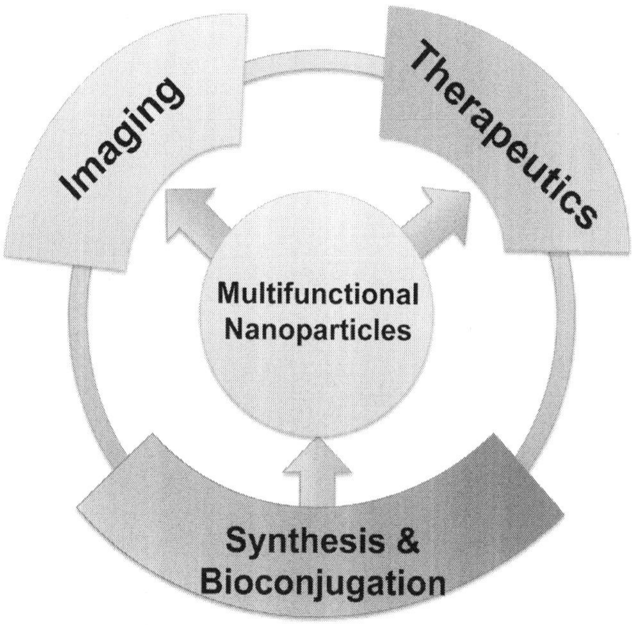

Fig. 1. Multifunctional nanoparticles in bioimaging and medicine. Developed synthesis and bioconjugation strategies for multifunctional nanoparticles helps enabling applications of multifunctional nanoparticles in *in vivo* imaging and therapy.

In this chapter, nanoparticles of different kinds will be reviewed for their applications in biomedical imaging and therapeutics. Popular nanoparticles in biomolecular and biomedical imaging include fluorescent particles for optical imaging, such as quantum dots, gold nanoparticles and magnetic particles for MRI. Nanoparticle derives therapeutics includes heat ablation of target tumours, or delivery of drugs. Figure 1 summarizes the attributes of multifunctional nanoparticles that have attracted the field of bioimaging and medicine. Multiple modalities of these particles enable the accurate, less-invasive diagnosis and therapeutic approaches.

2.1 Imaging

Nanoparticles in imaging applications have been increasingly developed in last 20 years. Because of the superior photo stability, narrow range of emission, broad excitation wavelength, multiple possibilities of modification, quantum dots have gathered much attention from engineering and scientists who are interested in bio markers, sensors or drug targeting. (Willard and Van Orden 2003; Qi and Gao 2008; Ghaderi, Ramesh et al. 2010; Han, Cui et al. 2010; Li, Wang et al. 2010) Commercially available binary quantum dots from Qdot have been successfully applied for above purposes during the last 10 years and reported in a vast number of literatures. Small size comparable to biomolecules (antibody, RNA, virus, etc.), high quantum yields and high magnetism are few representative advantages of nanoparticles that makes them to be a next generation imaging tools for *in vivo* imaging applications.

2.1.1 Nanoparticles for optical imaging

The most widely used nanoparticles in optical imaging are semiconductor nanocrystals, known as quantum dots. Their size dependent optical properties are unique in their applications to the efficient labelling of biomolecules and tissues where the traditional fluorescent labels have been hardly accessible to because of the size restrictions. In contrast, the size and shape of fluorescent nanoparticlces can be rather easily controllable during their synthesis. Semiconductor quantum dots are about 100 times brighter, have narrow emission spectra and broader excitation than traditional organic dye molecules. Since the quantum dots share the similar excitation wavelength and the emission is size tunable, multiple color imaging with single excitation.

Recent developments of conjugating particle surface with biomolecules allowed cell targeting using quantum dots. (Hoshino, Hanaki et al. 2004; Jaiswal, Goldman et al. 2004) Targeting of cells with quantum dots, however, often faces the issues in their accessibility of internalization. Larger size particles will affect protein trafficking and the viability of the cells.

Whether fluorescent nanoparticles are uptaken into the cell or not is critical decision maker in application of them for *in vivo* imaging. The number of nanoparticles in the cell cytoplasm should be to enough to enlighten the cell in the deep tissue. Although there have been efforts to enhance the fluorescent signal in the deep tissue by using a two-photon microscope or upconversion nanoparticles, it is still important to have enough number of nanoparticles per cell to be able to clearly visualize the target. A difficulty here is, the increased number of nanoparticles will increase toxicity of them to the cells. Therefore, the development of fluorescent nanoparticles for *in vivo* imaging is still an open challenge.

In vivo imaging of the target cells by fluorescent nanoparticles are often achieved by first labeling cells with particles then injecting them in the target. Loading of nanoparticles into human cancer cells in vitro has been shown successfully (Sage 2004; Li, Wang et al. 2006; Xing, Smith et al. 2006) and their *in vivo* application in mice model (Kim, Jin et al. 2006; DeNardo, DeNardo et al. 2007; Goldberg, Xing et al. 2011) was evaluated as well. It showed the division of human cancer cells and their reforming of tumour tracked by fluorescence. In imaging of lymphatic or cardiovascular systems, fluorescent nanoparticles have shown their potentials. Sentinel lymph systems in small animals were imaged by using a near infrared emitting quantum dots. (Parungo, Colson et al. 2005; Soltesz, Kim et al. 2006; Frangioni, Kim et al. 2007) Trafficking of quantum dots in those lymphatic systems was rather investigated by other groups as well. Lymph node imaging is beneficial to the surgeons for them to locate the exact position of the target.

Another example of *in vivo* imaging application using fluorescent nanoparticles is imaging of cardiovascular systems. Sensitivity and stability of fluorophore is always been a challenge in cardiovascular imaging. Coronary vasculature of a rat heart has been imaged with near IR emitting nanoparticles with high sensitivity. (Morgan, English et al. 2005)

Early detection of cancerous cells is the topic of interest for applications of quantum dots. Multiplexing of quantum dots for the better targeting and sensitivity has been a candidate for this purpose. Surface receptors are available on cancer cells that can be targeted by the multiplxed nanoparticles. Antibody coated quantum dots that are specific to the surface markers on cancer cells were demonstrated to label them in mice. Currently, targeting tumours are based on such an approach that functionalizing quantum dots with molecules specific to the target.

Since *in vivo* imaging requires high quantum efficiency of quantum dots to penetrate deep tissue and organs, its bioconjugation strategy should also be compatible to keep the initial brightness. In that regards, near IR emitting quantum dots are believed to be the optimal candidates for *in vivo* optical imaging. Infrared has the long wavelength that it can penetrate the deep tissues relatively better than other visible lights. It will also minimize the possible false positive signal by autofluorescence from the background since near IR is not relatively absorbed well by water or hemoglobin in the system.

Gold nanoparticles have been the popular choice for near IR emitting nano fluorophores since it is relative biocompatible and easy to synthesize. (Lee, Cha et al. 2008; Shang, Yin et al. 2009) The surface plasmon resonance is dependent on the size of the nanoparticles that it moves towards red with increasing particle size. Other types of gold nanomaterials such as gold nanorods and gold nanoshells were also popularly used in bioimaging because of its tunable surface plasmon bands and controllable position of the resonance by varying the synthesis conditions.

Several imaging methodologies were developed to be able to use gold nanoparticles and their derivatives in bioimaging. Optical Coherence Tomography (OCT) uses the scattering function of gold nanoshells for *in vivo* imaging. (Agrawal, Huang et al. 2006; Adler, Huang et al. 2008; Skrabalak, Chen et al. 2008) The accumulation of gold nanoshells at the tumour increases scattering at that location that provides the contrast. Another imaging tool for gold nanomaterials is using photoacoustic imaging. The photoacustic imaging adapts a pulse of near IR that causes thermal expansion nearby and sound wave detectable at the surface. Distinctive sound wave generated by gold nanoparticles can be separated from background signal by surrounding tissues and organs.

Another approach of adapting gold nanomaterials for *in vivo* imaging is using a two-photon fluorescence spectroscopy. Since gold nanomaterials possess the strong surface plasmon resonance, it can increase occurrence rate of two-photon excitation and relaxation of energy through fluorescence.

Lastly, Raman spectroscopy can be used for enhanced Raman effect at the surface of gold nanomaterials. Location of gold nanoparticles in animal model was demonstrated by using a Raman effect of reporter dye on the gold surface of particles. (Christiansen, Becker et al. 2007; Lu, Singh et al. 2010)

Although quantum dots are useful as a tagging material, they also have several disadvantages. First and the most serious demerits of binary quantum dot is that it is toxic to cells. Most popular components of binary quantum dots are cadmium / serenide which are deleterious to cells. Because of the intrinsic toxicity of binary quantum dot, very thick surface coating is required. The final size of quantum dot is almost twice as thick as the initial core size and hinders the applications of quantum dots in a cell. Another drawback of binary quantum dot is its blinking behavior when a single binary quantum dot is observed with confocal fluorescent microscope. (Durisic, Bachir et al. 2007; Lee and Osborne 2009; Peterson and Nesbitt 2009) Its blinking behavior hinders the tracking of quantum dot targeted bio molecule in a bio system.

Because of drawbacks of binary quantum dots, silicon nanocrystal has been studied to overcome the demerits of commercially available quantum dots and be used as a substituting fluorophore with traditional organic dyes. Silicon nanocrystals' superiorities as a fluorophore are summarized in Table 1. Silicon is basically non-toxic to cells so that it does not require a thick surface coating to prevent exposure of core to the environment. Therefore, its average size remains close to its core size.

	Silicon Nanocrystal	Binary Quantum dot	Organic dye
Average Size	1~4 nm (in dimeter)	10~20 nm (in diameter)	0.5~10 nm
Quantum Yield	< 60 %	>50 %	>90 %
Photostability	> 6 month	No data	1 day
Blinking	No data	Micro second	No data

Table 1. Comparison of characteristic properties of Silicon nanocrystal with binary quantum dots and traditional organic dyes.

2.1.2 Magnetic nanoparticles

Recently, various non-invasive imaging methods have been developed by labeling stem cells using nanoparticles such as magnetic nanocrystals, quantum dots, and carbon nanotubes. Among these, magnetic nanocrystals provide the excellent probe for the magnetic resonance imaging (MRI), which is widely used imaging modality to present a high spatial resolution and great anatomical detail.

In the last decade, superparamagnetic iron oxide (SPIO) nanoparticle has become the gold standard for MRI cell tracking, and has even entered clinical use. However, in many cases, SPIO-labeled cells producing hypointensities on T_2/T_2^*-weighted MR images, cannot be distinguished from other hypointense regions such as blood clots or scar tissues in some experimental disease models. Moreover, the susceptibility artifact or "blooming effect" resulting from the high susceptibility of the SPIO may distort the background images.

Gd complex based contrast agents can be good alternative MRI contrasts to generate the unambiguous positive contrast (hyper-intensity) and developed. Even if they produce positive contrast and increase the visibility of cells in low signal tissue, they have short residence time and can't pass through the cell membrane easily. Therefore, there have been developed some of Gd ion based nanopaticulate contrast agents to overcome these disadvantages of the complex agents. (Ananta, Godin et al. 2010)

MnO nanoparticles have also been recently explored as a new T_1 MRI contrast agent and fine anatomical features of the mouse brain were successfully obtained. These MnO nanoparticles were also used to demonstrate feasibility of cell labeling and *in vivo* MRI tracking. (Baek, Park et al. 2010) However, under existing MnO based nanoparticle systems, the contrast is weak and the duration of signal is short for the long time *in vivo* MRI tracking.

Therefore, it is required the further development of the MnO based contrast agent with high relaxivities and improved cellular uptake to stem cells which is more difficult to label due to the lack of substantial phgocytic capacity. (Kim, Momin et al. 2011)

2.2 Multifunctional nanoparticles in therapy

Multifunctional nanoparticles are in the process of being evaluated as new tools for therapy in biomedical research. In the United States 15 out of every 100,000 persons are diagnosed with brain cancer every year.

The most common type of adult brain tumor is malignant glioma with median survival rate of 10-12 month. Due to the complexity of the brain, the most practical treatment remained surgical removal of the tumor that frequently results in reoccurrence of the disease.

A new type of nanoparticles is suggested that it cannot only be used for imaging but also can be used as a therapeutic agent. These new nanoparticles can be activated either by using radiofrequency (RF) pulses or infrared light to release the drug.

2.2.1 Hyperthermia

In order to implement hyperthermia treatment, magnetic nanoparticles can be introduced in the body through magnetic delivery systems (high gradient magnetic fields) or local injection to the affected area. (Corchero and Villaverde 2009)

MRI utilizes RF pulses to generate coherent magnetization from the magnetic moments of water molecules in the sample that can then be detected. Since RF energy can also be converted into heat (e.g. similar to using a microwave to boil water) if the MRI agents can absorb RF energy efficiently, then a localized heating is possible during MR image collection. This idea of RF induced hyperthermia, or in other words, RF ablation has been studied in cancer research since the 1950's.

Certain parameters should be evaluated before deciding the contrast agent for the best hyperthermia applications. The best candidate nanoparticles are selected following these categories; specific absorption rate, size, biocompatibility.

Tumor treatment by hyperthermia has limitations, however, that the most of nanoparticles do not have high specific absorption rate. At least 10% of tumor weight should be absorbed in order to be effective to heat-ablate tumors through hyperthermia.

Treatment of malignant tumors at any site in the body is expected to be possible if agents that convert RF energy into heat can be delivered to the malignant cells. However, RF ablation suffers from the disadvantage that it is an invasive method that often requires insertion of electrodes into the body to deliver RF to the tumor sites.

Superparamagnetic iron oxide nanoparticles of a correctly determined size are appropriate for *in vivo* hyperthermia applications, as they have no net magnetization without the external magnetic field. No net magnetization without the external magnetic field would eliminate the possible particle aggregation in the system. Aggregated particles often experience non-specific engulfment by reticular endothelial system that will significantly reduce the contrast.

Plasmonic photothermal therapy is another new technology to treat tumor by using nanoparticles. (Chen, Frey et al. 2010) Plasmonic photothermal therapy is based on the surface plasmon resonance effect in nanoparticles when the light activates them. Most common example of this therapy is using gold nanoshells that we discussed before to achieve localised, irreversible thermal ablation of the tumor.

In future direction of the research, the MRI will be used passively to visualize the tumor and actively to eradicate it. Multifunctional nanoparticles have a tremendous potential for RF activated heating and triggering since they possess magnetic properties to generate MRI contrast, have the ability to absorb remote RF energy, and can deliver/release anti-cancer drugs in a controlled manner.

2.2.2 Photodynamic therapy

Singlet oxygen ($^1O_2$), as a part of reactive oxygen species (ROS) is useful tool to destruct cancer cells at the local site when singlet oxygen is concentrated. Photodynamic therapy is a new technology to treat tumor based on nanoparticle generated ROS at the tumor site. (Takahashi, Nagao et al. 2002; Oberdanner, Plaetzer et al. 2005) Photosensitizers, such as nanoparticles, can produce ROS when they are activated with the appropriate wavelength of excitation light. Nanoparticles as photosensitizers must be in close proximity to the tumor cells that they are usually administered at the tumor site directly. Photodynamic therapy is desirable in that it is relatively non-invasive and low toxicity. The major technical barrier, however, of this therapy is its difficulty in systemic introduction of photosensitizer to the tumor site and local irradiation to activate them. Tumors that have disseminated throughout the whole body may not be adequate for this therapy since the current technology is not available to irradiate the whole body. In addition, UV light is the wavelength of choice for the most of traditional photosensitizers that cannot efficiently penetrate into deep tissue.

Therefore, the new class of nanoparticles called up-converting nanocrystals was introduced to alleviate these issues. (Vetrone, Naccache et al. 2010) Up-converting nanoparticles are excited by near infrared light that can efficiently penetrate tissues deeper than UV-VIS light, which allows for the non-invasive application of the method. Functionalized surface on up-converting nanoparticles can direct particles to the specific tumor site that will concentrate ROS production.

There are still few disadvantages of up-converting nanoparticles that their size is intrinsically large. The size of them is usually around 100 nm that may not be appropriate for *in vivo* imaging. Furthermore, ROS are produced at the surface shell of up-converting nanoparticles that its efficiency may be degraded while diffusing out to the surrounding environment.

3. Toxicity

Production and exposure of nanoparticles less than 100 nm in diameter may pose unknown risks since the responses of biological systems to novel materials of this size have not been adequately studied.

The high surface area to volume ratio makes nanoparticles particularly good catalysts and such particles readily adhere to biological molecules. The size and surface charge of nanoparticles enable them to access places where larger particles may be blocked, including passage through cellular membranes. However, the wider application of semiconductor quantum dots as biological probes has been held back by their inherent chemical toxicity, which necessitates encapsulating them in a robust inert shell that increases the diameter of the probe.

Although there are studies (Zhu, Oberdorster et al. 2006; Rogers, Franklin et al. 2007; Teeguarden, Hinderliter et al. 2007; Warheit, Hoke et al. 2007; Clift, Rothen-Rutishauser et al. 2008; Prow, Bhutto et al. 2008; Simon-Deckers, Gouget et al. 2008; Zhu, Zhu et al. 2008; Crosera, Bovenzi et al. 2009; Kramer, Bell et al. 2009; Marquis, Love et al. 2009; Monteiro-Riviere, Inman et al. 2009; Simeonova and Erdely 2009; Warheit, Reed et al. 2009; DeVoll 2010; Li, Muralikrishnan et al. 2010; Maurer-Jones, Lin et al. 2010; Samberg, Oldenburg et al. 2010; Yang, Liu et al. 2010; Zhu, Chang et al. 2010) on both known and unknown hazards of several kinds of nanoparticles, many questions remain unanswered. Furthermore, there are few systematic studies dealing with both cytotoxicity and inflammatory responses of cells treated with nanoparticles.

How will a biological system react when exposed to nanoparticles? What is the fate of the nanoparticles once they are presented to a population of cells? If the nanoparticles enter into the cell, what effects do they exert internally? These questions must be answered in order to ensure safety to the patient if nanoparticles are incorporated in biomedical applications.

In this chapter, we will discuss nanoparticles as for any diagnostic or medicinal tool and point out that nanoparticles can only be applicable to *in vivo* applications on humans when they pass the assessment for their toxicity. To the fact that the number of different nanomaterials synthesized and potentially targeted for *in vivo* applications is much more than the number of toxicity assessment for them, these investigations are only at the very early stage.

Noticeable conclusions from those studies have been already distress the field and public to strengthen the extended investigation requirement before pursuing any further research. Recent reviews on the toxicity assessment of nanoparticles keep pointing out that the experimental conditions, preparations of nanoparticles and protocols the investigators use all affect the results. These discrepancies between studies even for the same kind of nanoparticle result from the complexity of the investigated systems and potential interference of nanomaterials to the assay techniques.

3.1 Nanoparticle toxicity assessment in *in vitro* assays

Growing public concern regarding the unknown toxicological effects of nanoparticles has spawned cooperative efforts by government agencies and academia to closely investigate these issues.

In vitro assay	Assay mechanism	Detection	Tested nanoparticles	Pros	Cons
MTT (or MTS)	Dead cells cannot reduce MTT (MTS).	Absorption	Quantum dots, gold nanoparticles	Widely used, relatively simple, low cost	Metabolic activity can be affected by multiplexed effects
Calcein AM	Dead cells cannot cleave the acetomethoxy group of calcein AM	Fluorescence	Gold nanoshells	Widely used fluorescence assay, relatively simple, low cost	Fluorescent nanoparticles interfere with calcein dyes.
Protease activity assays (e.g., CytoTox-Glo)	Substrates bind to dead cells' proteases in the media to produce a fluorescence signal.	ELISA/fluorescence colorimeter	Fullerene, carbon black, quantum dots	Cytotoxicity can be probed based on the activity of various proteases	Expensive; fluorescent nanoparticles in the cell interfere with the signal.
Blood contact properties (e.g., hemolysis)	Hemoglobin released from cells is oxidized and quantified by its absorbance	ELISA/ absorption colorimeter	PAMAM dendrimers, TiO_2 nanoparticles	Widely used, relatively simple, low cost	No established positive control for nanomaterials; possible interference
Macrophage functions (cytokine induction)	Nitric oxides, various cytokines (e.g., interleukins, TNF-alpha) are induced	ELISA/absorption/fluorescence colorimeter	Si nanoparticles	Widely used fluorescence assay, relatively simple, low cost	Fluorescent nanoparticles interfere with detection dyes

Table 2. Summary of popular cytotoxicity and inflammatory response assays used for nanoparticles

Nanoparticles may not be filtered by the body's defense mechanisms because of their small size, which suggests that they may cause inflammatory and/or toxic responses. The reported cytotoxicity and immune response studies on nanoparticles have been based mainly on *in vitro* assays such as cell viability tests, cytokine release analyses and cell

function degradation analyses upon the exposure of a bulk culture of cells to nanoparticles (see available assays: http://ncl.cancer.gov/working_assay-cascade.asp).
However, no validated standard or protocol has yet been established to test biological responses to nanoparticles. Table 2 lists a representative selection of cytotoxicity and inflammatory response assays used to test biological responses to nanoparticles.

3.1.1 Nanotoxicity: Complex system to investigate

The number of reports on assessment of the nanoparticle toxicity has been growing with the number of biomedical research associated with them. It is noticeable that the reports are not consistent in terms of particles' toxicity results. Some reports on popular nanoparticles such as cadmium selenide, iron oxide, gold and silica nanoparticles all have non-consistent conclusions about their toxicity to the biological system. These inconsistent conclusions result from the fact that there is currently no standard protocol for the assessment of the toxicity of nanomaterials. Variation of experiment parameters as well as interference of nanoparticles to the measuring instruments is prime reasons that make it impossible to compare the results between different studies.

3.1.2 Cytotoxicity

The cytotoxicity of a nanomaterial is influenced by the following parameters: cell line, culture conditions for *in vitro* studies, how to introduce particles in *in vivo* studies, nanoparticle concentration, size and duration of exposure. No standard protocol is available at the current stage in terms of setting those parameters relatively be consistent. It is challenging, furthermore, to decide whether the reported range of particle concentration is physiologically relevant to the *in vivo* system.
The cell line to test *in vitro* is a critical factor determining the degree of cytotoxicity of nanomaterials. In one study, nanoparticle uptake rate and resulted cytotoxicity was compared in the same cell line but prepared by following different protocols. It was found that the cytotoxicity could be varied among the cell lines depending on how they were prepared.
Another factor for observed discrepancies between the results of toxicity assays is different testing methods applied on the same nanomaterial.
In most of the *in vitro* cytotoxicity studies, cell death is investigated using colorimetric assays such as shift of absorption or emission of markers. For example, Trypan blue dye exclusion assay provides information of cell death by showing dye staining on cells that were ruptured. Potential issue here is that nanoparticles applied are usually strongly emit or absorb light. Nanoparticles absorb or emit light may give false positive signal.
Cytotoxicity assays commonly used are to measure the effect of test compound that can rather quickly diffuse into the target cell that they can be assayed within the time frame when the dye still can be effective. Therefore, cytotoxicity assays are rarely run for over few days. Another potential issue here is that nanoparticles are less mobile than the most chemical compounds resulting that they will require longer duration of assays. This would require the modification of the cytotoxicity protocols that should be used for nanoparticles and nanomaterials.
Physical and chemical characterizations of nanoparticles are critically important for cytotoxicity assays. For size analysis, either dynamic light scattering (DLS) or transmission electron microscopy (TEM) is the method of choice for the most of nanoparticles. The nanoparticles that are well dispersed in water would not show a significant aggregation or morphological variations in TEM images.

However, it is often pointed out in many studies that there are some discrepancies in mean particle size between that measured by TEM or by DLS. (Teeguarden, Hinderliter et al. 2007; Warheit, Hoke et al. 2007; Marquis, Love et al. 2009; Monteiro-Riviere, Inman et al. 2009; Vippola, Falck et al. 2009) These discrepancies may be due to differences in both preparation and the inherent limitations of nanoparticle sizing methods, and emphasize the necessity to apply multiple techniques for determining particle sizes in polydisperse batches. While TEM can serve as a tool to capture the size of each individual particle, it is limited in that it can only measure particles after they have been suspended and then dried, it requires measurements of many different particle regions to appropriately represent the entire particle batch, and complex geometries of particles or agglomerates may make characterization difficult. The solvent used to disperse the particles prior to drying for TEM analysis may also affect the measurements.

While dynamic light scattering is performed in solutions, the suspending media and how the particle sample was mixed (i.e. sonication intensity and exposure time) and pre-filtered can significantly affect the particle hydrodynamic size analysis. Moreover, particle agglomeration and time-dependent sedimentation of large (i.e. > 100 nm) and dense silver particles may affect the DLS measurement reliability even during the short measurement time period (2-5 min).

DLS measurements of highly polydispersed particle solutions are also dependent on the main analysis parameter. In an intensity-based DLS analysis of a polydisperse particle sample, smaller particles are under-represented due to weaker light scattering and particle shape effects. For this reason, a number-based DLS analysis would be more appropriate to highlight the most abundant particle size population so that one could make limited comparisons between the different particles, especially when the particles are not pre-filtered and the effect of media on nanoparticle size, agglomeration, and polydispersity are significant.

In general, all of the aqueous particles demonstrate an increase in particle size and/or agglomeration, either by DLS measurement or visually, when mixed with DPBS media due to reaction with chloride ions and the presumable formation of poorly soluble silver chloride.

Surface chemistry of nanoparticles is also another important factor that will affect cytotoxicity of nanoparticles. Citrate is the conjugate base of citric acid, which is a popular reducing agent used in silver and gold production, and provides a negatively charged surface moiety that stabilizes nanoparticle colloids through Columbic repulsion. The citrate-stabilized nanoparticles suspended in water acquired a significant negative charge and acidified the aqueous solution.

However, in comparing the nano-sized particles, it was found that particles share the similar pH and zeta potentials when they are diluted in PBS solution regardless of the degree of citrate coating on each particle. Furthermore, no significant differences in cytotoxicity levels between the nano-sized particles argues in favor of particle size as a stronger determinant of toxicity rather than initial surface chemical properties. This also emphasizes the potential importance of plasma proteins in altering the surface properties of nanoparticles by coating them and affecting their biocompatibility.

3.2 Nanoparticle toxicity analysis toward its *in vivo* applications

In general, the smaller the nanoparticle is the greater the toxicity. This is due in part to the fact that small nanoparticles are more readily uptaken into the cell or even near the nucleus. Larger nanoparticles may therefore be less cytotoxic simply because their cellular uptake is limited at that same concentration.

In order to consider and predict possible nanoparticles toxicity in *in vivo* applications, few things should be carefully examined.

First of all, *in vitro* studies for cytotoxicity should carefully be used to extrapolate expected results in *in vivo* studies. Nanoparticles in *in vivo* system would experience much more complicated perturbations because of a wide variety of proteins and small biomolecules present around them. Because of these neighboring biomolecules, nanoparticles can be degraded, engulfed by phagocytic cells, or traveled away from the target site by lymphatic system. Assay responses obtained from well-controlled environment such as in culturing plate may not always present the same results obtained in *in vivo* environment. Therefore, it will be inadequate to draw any conclusions from the *in vitro* assay for nanoparticle responses in *in vivo* system until following experiments at least in animal model is performed.

Second of all, limitations of current assays performed for cytotoxicity or inflammatory responses of cells to the nanomaterials should be carefully recognized and further endeavors to advance technologies for better assaying nanoparticles should be invested. Studies of *in vitro* cytotoxicity and the inflammatory response to nanoparticles have adopted conventional assays developed for chemical toxins or microparticles. These reports provide little insight into how individual cells react when exposed to nanoparticles. Also, the analysis of these assay results is prone to error because cells can behave differently depending on the assays employed.

The limitations of current cytotoxicity and immune response assays for the assessment of nanoparticles can be summarized as follows. First, cells cannot be recovered after the single assay readout; thus the possibilities for time-dependent monitoring of changes in a cell's activity are limited. Second, the assays' readings are averaged over all the cells present. Therefore, a single cell's responses to the nanoparticles cannot be individually recorded from the assay. Third, nanoparticles inside a cell may interfere with the fluorescence signal produced by the dye used in the assay. Additionally, nanoparticles may interact with and/or bind to dyes, altering their absorption and/or fluorescence. Nanoparticles can also adsorb to proteins and other biomolecules in the cell culture medium, which can interfere with the particles' normal interactions with cells. Furthermore, nanoparticles can bind to cytokines released from the cells; this may artificially reduce an assay's positive signal. Flow cytometry is a commonly used method in biological response assays, but the technique requires that cells be detached from the cell culture plate, which may alter the cells' mortality. Finally, multiplexed analyses of nanoparticles in the same well with single cells have not been performed. Because of these limitations, there is an emergent need to develop a solid assay that overcomes the above-mentioned problems with conventional assays and is able to evaluate biological responses to nanoparticles in a multiplexed, high-throughput manner.

Cutting-edge single-cell assay techniques have been developed for assessing cytotoxic and inflammatory responses to nanoparticles in a multiplexed manner. The multiplexed analysis strategy will be used in safety studies of various nanoparticles. Time-dependent analysis of a single cell's responses to nanoparticles may elucidate the mechanism of toxicity for nano-sized particles. Such single-cell analyses will be used in concert with conventional bulk assays. The approaches discussed will benefit nanotoxicological studies and help the broader nanotechnology community by providing proof of concept for an efficient analytical tool with which to investigate the safety of nanoparticles at the single-cell level in a high-throughput and multiplexed fashion.

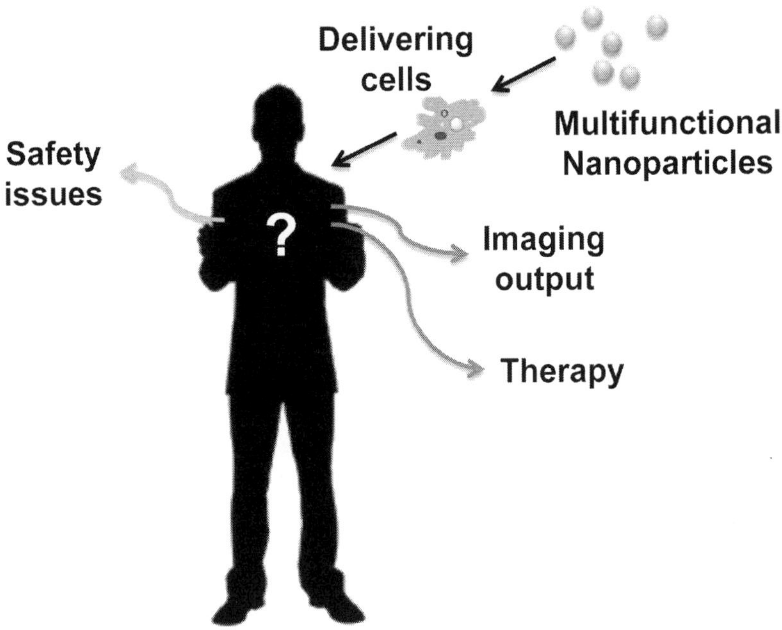

Fig. 2. Safety concerns about nanoparticles in *in vivo* applications grows and it is still a "black box" that has not been clearly shown its potential hazards.

4. Conclusion

The toxicity of nanoparticle is critically important topic for researchers both in material science and biomedical fields. Toxicity assessment so far has been informative but it could not catch up the development of technology especially in biological application of nanoparticlces as covered in earlier sections in this chapter. Even in *in vitro* assays, assay results were often challenged by their inconsistencies. For *in vivo* application it is even more important to have well defined, consistent assay protocol and techniques so that one can try to discover the key to the unknown, "black box" of particle toxicity *in vivo* (Figure 2). The immediate need in this regard will be the standardization of assessment protocols for nanoparticle toxicity. Government, academics and worldwide cooperation are desirable to facilitate this process for standardization of assays. *In vitro* findings should be carefully integrated to the *in vivo* behavior of nanoparticles since it is fairly different environment that nanoparticles will experience. For *in vivo* applications, therefore, extra care should be taken in prediction of potential toxicity of nanoparticles before their actual implementation.

5. Acknowledgment

JC acknowledges Professor J. Christopher Love at MIT and Dr. Peter L. Goering at FDA for useful discussion on the subject.

6. References

Adler, D. C., S. W. Huang, et al. (2008). "Photothermal detection of gold nanoparticles using phase-sensitive optical coherence tomography." *Opt Express* 16(7): 4376-4393.

Agrawal, A., S. Huang, et al. (2006). "Quantitative evaluation of optical coherence tomography signal enhancement with gold nanoshells." *J Biomed Opt* 11(4): 041121.

Ananta, J. S., B. Godin, et al. (2010). "Geometrical confinement of gadolinium-based contrast agents in nanoporous particles enhances T1 contrast." *Nat Nanotechnol* 5(11): 815-821.

Baek, M. J., J. Y. Park, et al. (2010). "Water-soluble MnO nanocolloid for a molecular T1 MR imaging: a facile one-pot synthesis, in vivo T1 MR images, and account for relaxivities." *ACS Appl Mater Interfaces* 2(10): 2949-2955.

Bystrzejewski, M., S. Cudzilo, et al. (2007). "Carbon encapsulated magnetic nanoparticles for biomedical applications: thermal stability studies." *Biomol Eng* 24(5): 555-558.

Chen, Y. S., W. Frey, et al. (2010). "Enhanced thermal stability of silica-coated gold nanorods for photoacoustic imaging and image-guided therapy." *Opt Express* 18(9): 8867-8878.

Christiansen, S. H., M. Becker, et al. (2007). "Signal enhancement in nano-Raman spectroscopy by gold caps on silicon nanowires obtained by vapour-liquid-solid growth." *Nanotechnology* 18(3): 035503.

Clift, M. J., B. Rothen-Rutishauser, et al. (2008). "The impact of different nanoparticle surface chemistry and size on uptake and toxicity in a murine macrophage cell line." *Toxicol Appl Pharmacol* 232(3): 418-427.

Corchero, J. L. and A. Villaverde (2009). "Biomedical applications of distally controlled magnetic nanoparticles." *Trends Biotechnol* 27(8): 468-476.

Crosera, M., M. Bovenzi, et al. (2009). "Nanoparticle dermal absorption and toxicity: a review of the literature." *Int Arch Occup Environ Health* 82(9): 1043-1055.

DeNardo, S. J., G. L. DeNardo, et al. (2007). "Thermal dosimetry predictive of efficacy of 111In-ChL6 nanoparticle AMF--induced thermoablative therapy for human breast cancer in mice." *J Nucl Med* 48(3): 437-444.

DeVoll, J. R. (2010). "Nanoparticle toxicity." *Aviat Space Environ Med* 81(2): 152-153.

Durisic, N., A. I. Bachir, et al. (2007). "Detection and correction of blinking bias in image correlation transport measurements of quantum dot tagged macromolecules." *Biophys J* 93(4): 1338-1346.

Frangioni, J. V., S. W. Kim, et al. (2007). "Sentinel lymph node mapping with type-II quantum dots." *Methods Mol Biol* 374: 147-159.

Ghaderi, S., B. Ramesh, et al. (2010). "Fluorescence nanoparticles "quantum dots" as drug delivery system and their toxicity: a review." *J Drug Target*.

Goldberg, M. S., D. Xing, et al. (2011). "Nanoparticle-mediated delivery of siRNA targeting Parp1 extends survival of mice bearing tumors derived from Brca1-deficient ovarian cancer cells." *Proc Natl Acad Sci U S A* 108(2): 745-750.

Han, C., Z. Cui, et al. (2010). "Urea-type ligand-modified CdSe quantum dots as a fluorescence "turn-on" sensor for CO3(2-) anions." *Photochem Photobiol Sci* 9(9): 1269-1273.

Hoshino, A., K. Hanaki, et al. (2004). "Applications of T-lymphoma labeled with fluorescent quantum dots to cell tracing markers in mouse body." *Biochem Biophys Res Commun* 314(1): 46-53.

Jaiswal, J. K., E. R. Goldman, et al. (2004). "Use of quantum dots for live cell imaging." *Nat Methods* 1(1): 73-78.

Kim, T., E. Momin, et al. (2011). "Mesoporous silica-coated hollow manganese oxide nanoparticles as positive t(1) contrast agents for labeling and MRI tracking of adipose-derived mesenchymal stem cells." *J Am Chem Soc* 133(9): 2955-2961.

Kim, T. H., H. Jin, et al. (2006). "Mannosylated chitosan nanoparticle-based cytokine gene therapy suppressed cancer growth in BALB/c mice bearing CT-26 carcinoma cells." *Mol Cancer Ther* 5(7): 1723-1732.

Kramer, J., R. Bell, et al. (2009). "Silver nanoparticle toxicity and biocides: need for chemical speciation." *Integr Environ Assess Manag* 5(4): 720-722.

Lee, S., E. J. Cha, et al. (2008). "A near-infrared-fluorescence-quenched gold-nanoparticle imaging probe for in vivo drug screening and protease activity determination." *Angew Chem Int Ed Engl* 47(15): 2804-2807.

Lee, S. F. and M. A. Osborne (2009). "Brightening, blinking, bluing and bleaching in the life of a quantum dot: friend or foe?" *Chemphyschem* 10(13): 2174-2191.

Li, J. J., S. Muralikrishnan, et al. (2010). "Nanoparticle-induced pulmonary toxicity." *Exp Biol Med (Maywood)* 235(9): 1025-1033.

Li, Z., K. Wang, et al. (2006). "Immunofluorescent labeling of cancer cells with quantum dots synthesized in aqueous solution." *Anal Biochem* 354(2): 169-174.

Li, Z., Y. Wang, et al. (2010). "Rapid and sensitive detection of protein biomarker using a portable fluorescence biosensor based on quantum dots and a lateral flow test strip." *Anal Chem* 82(16): 7008-7014.

Lu, W., A. K. Singh, et al. (2010). "Gold nano-popcorn-based targeted diagnosis, nanotherapy treatment, and in situ monitoring of photothermal therapy response of prostate cancer cells using surface-enhanced Raman spectroscopy." *J Am Chem Soc* 132(51): 18103-18114.

Marquis, B. J., S. A. Love, et al. (2009). "Analytical methods to assess nanoparticle toxicity." *Analyst* 134(3): 425-439.

Maurer-Jones, M. A., Y. S. Lin, et al. (2010). "Functional assessment of metal oxide nanoparticle toxicity in immune cells." *ACS Nano* 4(6): 3363-3373.

Monteiro-Riviere, N. A., A. O. Inman, et al. (2009). "Limitations and relative utility of screening assays to assess engineered nanoparticle toxicity in a human cell line." *Toxicol Appl Pharmacol* 234(2): 222-235.

Morgan, N. Y., S. English, et al. (2005). "Real time in vivo non-invasive optical imaging using near-infrared fluorescent quantum dots." *Acad Radiol* 12(3): 313-323.

Nune, S. K., P. Gunda, et al. (2009). "Nanoparticles for biomedical imaging." *Expert Opin Drug Deliv* 6(11): 1175-1194.

Oberdanner, C. B., K. Plaetzer, et al. (2005). "Photodynamic treatment with fractionated light decreases production of reactive oxygen species and cytotoxicity in vitro via regeneration of glutathione." *Photochem Photobiol* 81(3): 609-613.

Parungo, C. P., Y. L. Colson, et al. (2005). "Sentinel lymph node mapping of the pleural space." *Chest* 127(5): 1799-1804.

Peterson, J. J. and D. J. Nesbitt (2009). "Modified power law behavior in quantum dot blinking: a novel role for biexcitons and auger ionization." *Nano Lett* 9(1): 338-345.

Prow, T. W., I. Bhutto, et al. (2008). "Ocular nanoparticle toxicity and transfection of the retina and retinal pigment epithelium." *Nanomedicine* 4(4): 340-349.

Qi, L. and X. Gao (2008). "Emerging application of quantum dots for drug delivery and therapy." *Expert Opin Drug Deliv* 5(3): 263-267.

Rogers, N. J., N. M. Franklin, et al. (2007). "The importance of physical and chemical characterization in nanoparticle toxicity studies." *Integr Environ Assess Manag* 3(2): 303-304.

Sage, L. (2004). "Finding cancer cells with quantum dots." *Anal Chem* 76(23): 453A.

Samberg, M. E., S. J. Oldenburg, et al. (2010). "Evaluation of silver nanoparticle toxicity in skin in vivo and keratinocytes in vitro." *Environ Health Perspect* 118(3): 407-413.

Shang, L., J. Yin, et al. (2009). "Gold nanoparticle-based near-infrared fluorescent detection of biological thiols in human plasma." *Biosens Bioelectron* 25(2): 269-274.

Simeonova, P. P. and A. Erdely (2009). "Engineered nanoparticle respiratory exposure and potential risks for cardiovascular toxicity: predictive tests and biomarkers." *Inhal Toxicol* 21 Suppl 1: 68-73.

Simon-Deckers, A., B. Gouget, et al. (2008). "In vitro investigation of oxide nanoparticle and carbon nanotube toxicity and intracellular accumulation in A549 human pneumocytes." *Toxicology* 253(1-3): 137-146.

Skrabalak, S. E., J. Chen, et al. (2008). "Gold nanocages: synthesis, properties, and applications." *Acc Chem Res* 41(12): 1587-1595.

Soltesz, E. G., S. Kim, et al. (2006). "Sentinel lymph node mapping of the gastrointestinal tract by using invisible light." *Ann Surg Oncol* 13(3): 386-396.

Takahashi, M., T. Nagao, et al. (2002). "Roles of reactive oxygen species in monocyte activation induced by photochemical reactions during photodynamic therapy." *Front Med Biol Eng* 11(4): 279-294.

Teeguarden, J. G., P. M. Hinderliter, et al. (2007). "Particokinetics in vitro: dosimetry considerations for in vitro nanoparticle toxicity assessments." *Toxicol Sci* 95(2): 300-312.

Vetrone, F., R. Naccache, et al. (2010). "Luminescence resonance energy transfer from an upconverting nanoparticle to a fluorescent phycobiliprotein." *Nanoscale* 2(7): 1185-1189.

Vippola, M., G. C. Falck, et al. (2009). "Preparation of nanoparticle dispersions for in-vitro toxicity testing." *Hum Exp Toxicol* 28(6-7): 377-385.

Warheit, D. B., R. A. Hoke, et al. (2007). "Development of a base set of toxicity tests using ultrafine TiO2 particles as a component of nanoparticle risk management." *Toxicol Lett* 171(3): 99-110.

Warheit, D. B., K. L. Reed, et al. (2009). "A role for nanoparticle surface reactivity in facilitating pulmonary toxicity and development of a base set of hazard assays as a component of nanoparticle risk management." *Inhal Toxicol* 21 Suppl 1: 61-67.

Willard, D. M. and A. Van Orden (2003). "Quantum dots: Resonant energy-transfer sensor." *Nat Mater* 2(9): 575-576.

Xing, Y., A. M. Smith, et al. (2006). "Molecular profiling of single cancer cells and clinical tissue specimens with semiconductor quantum dots." *Int J Nanomedicine* 1(4): 473-481.

Yaghini, E., A. M. Seifalian, et al. (2009). "Quantum dots and their potential biomedical applications in photosensitization for photodynamic therapy." *Nanomedicine (Lond)* 4(3): 353-363.

Yang, Z., Z. W. Liu, et al. (2010). "A review of nanoparticle functionality and toxicity on the central nervous system." *J R Soc Interface* 7 Suppl 4: S411-422.

Yu, W. W. (2008). "Semiconductor quantum dots: synthesis and water-solubilization for biomedical applications." *Expert Opin Biol Ther* 8(10): 1571-1581.

Zhu, S., E. Oberdorster, et al. (2006). "Toxicity of an engineered nanoparticle (fullerene, C60) in two aquatic species, Daphnia and fathead minnow." *Mar Environ Res* 62 Suppl: S5-9.

Zhu, X., Y. Chang, et al. (2010). "Toxicity and bioaccumulation of TiO2 nanoparticle aggregates in Daphnia magna." *Chemosphere* 78(3): 209-215.

Zhu, X., L. Zhu, et al. (2008). "Comparative toxicity of several metal oxide nanoparticle aqueous suspensions to Zebrafish (Danio rerio) early developmental stage." *J Environ Sci Health A Tox Hazard Subst Environ Eng* 43(3): 278-284.

14

Male Circumcision: An Appraisal of Current Instrumentation

Brian J. Morris[1] and Chris Eley[2]

[1]*School of Medical Sciences, The University of Sydney, Sydney,*
[2]*Editor, www.circlist.com, London,*
[1]*Australia*
[2]*United Kingdom*

1. Introduction

The topic of male circumcision (MC) is of considerable current interest, largely because of widespread publicity generated by research findings attesting to its ability to prevent HIV infection during heterosexual intercourse. In addition, its long-recognized ability to protect against other sexually transmitted infections (STIs) has also been well publicized in recent times, especially now that support has been provided by large randomized controlled trials (RCTs).

While MC can be performed at any age, the ease with which circumcision can be performed in infancy makes this time of life preferable to intervention later in childhood or in adulthood. As well as the issue of safety, convenience, simplicity and consequent cost reductions, circumcision in infancy provides greater net benefits over the lifetime of the individual.

It provides immediate 10-fold protection against urinary tract infections and thus kidney damage in baby boys, and greater protection against penile cancer than circumcision later in life, virtually eliminating the risk of this disease with its high morbidity and mortality (Morris, 2007; Morris, 2010; Tobian *et al.*, 2010; Morris *et al.*, 2011). Another benefit is prevention of phimosis, a common cause of sexual problems in adolescent boys and men, and a major risk factor for penile cancer. It also lowers to risk of inflammatory skin conditions such as balanoposthitis. Circumcised men have superior hygiene (O'Farrell *et al.*, 2005) and half the prevalence of thrush (Richters *et al.*, 2006). As far as protection against STIs is concerned, the most notable is human papillomavirus (HPV), the pathogen not only responsible for most cervical cancers in women, but also a proportion of penile cancers in men (Morris et al., 2011). MC also reduces the incidence of ulcerative STIs, including syphilis, chancroid, *Trichomonas vaginalis*, and herpes simplex virus type 2 (HSV-2) (Weiss *et al.*, 2006; Morris & Castellsague, 2010; Tobian et al., 2010). Circumcised men have lower genital ulcer disease as a result of this and the reduction in penile injury arising from tearing of the foreskin and frenulum during sexual activity (Bailey & Mehta, 2009). MC reduces sexual problems with age and diabetes (Morris, 2007; Morris, 2010; Tobian et al., 2010; Morris et al., 2011), and has no adverse effect on sexual function, sensation or acceptability (Morris, 2007; Tobian et al., 2010), if anything the reverse (Krieger *et al.*, 2008). MC provides a public health benefit to women by lowering their risk of various STIs, including high-risk HPV types that cause cervical cancer, HSV-2,

Chlamydia trachomatis that can cause pelvic inflammatory disease, ectopic pregnancy and infertility, as well reducing the risk of bacterial vaginosis (Morris, 2007; Morris, 2010; Tobian et al., 2010; Morris et al., 2011; Wawer *et al.*, 2011).

If one tallies up all of the conditions listed above, 1 in 3 uncircumcised men will require medical attention from a condition stemming from their uncircumcised state (Morris, 2007). Moreover, such an analysis shows that the benefits exceed the risks by over 100 to 1, and far more if one factors in the severity of the consequences, including mortality and morbidity, that can occur in uncircumcised males and their sexual partners in adulthood.

MC is, without doubt, a multi-benefit procedure. Yet many analyses of its benefits make the mistake of addressing its effect with respect to just one medical condition. For a true assessment of its value it is necessary to carry out a summation of all the benefits, quoting the total inclusive of spin-offs every time.

Because of the current focus on efficient and effective MC in regions of the world where HIV prevalence is high, in the present chapter we will begin by summarizing the HIV findings. In the context of biomedical engineering, we will then examine the devices that have been devised for the surgical procedure itself. The intention of these devices has been to help reduce risk to delicate penile structures during surgery and also to ensure a favourable cosmetic outcome of the circumcision procedure.

2. Male circumcision for HIV prevention

In 2007 MC was endorsed by the World Health Organization (WHO) and the Joint United Nations Programme on HIV/AIDS (World Health Organisation and UNAIDS, 2007a) as being an important, proven strategy for prevention of heterosexually-transmitted HIV in high prevalence settings. Such advice was the culmination of 20 years of research that led to the findings of three large randomized controlled trials in different parts of sub-Saharan Africa (Auvert *et al.*, 2005; Bailey *et al.*, 2007; Gray *et al.*, 2007). After rigorous examination of the data, the Cochrane committee concluded that "inclusion of male circumcision into current HIV prevention guidelines is warranted" and that "No further trials are required" (Siegfried *et al.*, 2009; Siegfried *et al.*, 2010). A recent analysis of data from 18 sub-Saharan African countries found the protective effect after adjustment for number of lifetime sexual partners and socio-demographic variables was 5-fold (Gebremedhin, 2010). As a result, large-scale MC programmes are being rolled out across sub-Saharan Africa in societies where traditional circumcision has not in recent times been the norm.

Therefore, whilst the long-term goal should be one of circumcising in infancy, the immediate need in settings where life-threatening HIV prevalence is high is to circumcise uninfected heterosexually-active adult and adolescent males.

Critics of this approach cite the "ABC" policy (**A**bstinance, **B**ehaviour, **C**ondoms) (Coates *et al.*, 2008) as being sufficient. While condoms are 80–90% effective if always used properly (Halperin *et al.*, 2004), including during foreplay, the reality is that for a host of reasons such as passion over-riding common sense, dislike for condoms, reckless behaviour often fuelled by inebriation, and/or not having a condom available, many people either do not use them consistently or at all (Donovan & Ross, 2000; Szabo & Short, 2000; Caballero-Hoyos & Villasenor-Sierra, 2001; Ferrante *et al.*, 2005; Jadack *et al.*, 2006; Kang *et al.*, 2006; Sanchez *et al.*, 2006; Yahya-Malima *et al.*, 2007; Munro *et al.*, 2008; Wawer *et al.*, 2009). This research included RCTs in which men were given counselling and free condoms (Wawer et al., 2009). A review of 10 studies from Africa found that overall there was no association between condom use and reduced HIV infection, with two studies actually showing a positive association between use of a condom and HIV infection (Slaymaker, 2004; Lopman *et al.*, 2008). Part of the reason, however, is that condom use is likely to be higher when one person knows they are HIV-positive and does not want to infect their partner. Circumcision can thus be regarded as providing backup protection. It is much like seatbelts and airbags used in combination to reduce the road toll (Cooper *et al.*, 2010). Buckling up the seatbelt has to be done, whereas the airbag is always there. Imperfect though it is, once circumcised a male enjoys a guaranteed degree of protection for life. The widespread acceptance of MC as an important HIV prevention measure has led to a new "ABC" now being advocated: **A**ntivirals, **B**arriers and **C**ircumcision. Not instead of the original ABC, but additionally. This clearly recognizes that MC is part of a package of prevention measures.

An as-treated meta-analysis of the initial findings from the three RCTs found that the protective effect was 65% (Weiss *et al.*, 2008). This was identical to the summary risk ratio for the 15 observational studies that adjusted for potential confounders. Follow-up analyses have indicated an increase in the 60% protective effect seen in the Kenyan trial to 65% at 3.5 years (Bailey *et al.*, 2008) and 4.5 years (Bailey *et al.*, 2010) In the Ugandan trial by 5 years the protective effect had increased to 73% (Kong *et al.*, 2011). Such a level of protection is similar to that afforded by influenza vaccines (Fiore *et al.*, 2007; Kelly *et al.*, 2009). Even higher protection (80%) was found in the analysis of data from 18 sub-Saharan African countries (Gebremedhin, 2010).

The high protective effect of MC should not detract from the need to adopt the other ABC measures as well.

MC also reduces HIV infection in women by 20-46% (Baeten *et al.*, 2009; Weiss *et al.*, 2009; Baeten *et al.*, 2010; Hallett *et al.*, 2010). Economic analyses have estimated enormous savings in lives and cost by adoption of widespread MC in high risk settings (Williams *et al.*, 2006) and has the potential to abate the epidemic over the next 10-20 years (Gray *et al.*, 2008). Even in low prevalence settings such as the USA, infant MC was shown to be cost-saving for HIV prevention (Sansom *et al.*, 2010).

Several different partial remedies can act cumulatively, each contributing not just towards a reduction in infection rates but also towards the ultimate public health goal of herd immunity. It is here, rather than in the realms of individual healthcare, that the true value of MC lies. Not surprisingly, MC is now regarded as a "surgical vaccine" (Morris, 2007; Schoen, 2007b; Ben *et al.*, 2009). It provides a behaviour-independent secure foundation upon which other forms of protection can build.

As a prelude to the discussion of MC technique and the various devices for achieving foreskin removal, it is important to emphasize the biological evidence that has now accumulated that indicates the vulnerability of the inner lining of the foreskin to infection of the man by HIV.

During an erection the foreskin can either retract fully or only partially. Either way, during intercourse the thin, mucosal inner surface of the foreskin is exposed to the partner's body fluids (Szabo & Short, 2000). The foreskin then traps the infectious inoculum when the penis becomes flaccid again (Cameron *et al.*, 1989). The mucosal inner lining is only lightly keratinized (Patterson *et al.*, 2002; McCoombe & Short, 2006; Ganor *et al.*, 2010) and is rich in Langerhans cells (Patterson et al., 2002). Dendrites from these project to just under the surface (McCoombe & Short, 2006). The higher susceptibility of the inner lining to infection by live, tagged HIV has been demonstrated in cultured tissue (Patterson et al., 2002). Internalization of HIV involves the presence on Langerhans cells of the c-type lectin,

Langerin, that can bind HIV and internalize it (Turville *et al.*, 2002). The Langerin is then involved in its transport to regional lymph nodes (Turville *et al.*, 2002). In the inner (but not the outer) foreskin, tumor necrosis factor-α can activate Langerhan's cells; stimulatory cytokines then cause an influx of CD4+ T-cells into the epithelial layer (Fahrbach *et al.*, 2010). The higher permeability of the inner foreskin is associated with increased interaction of HIV target cells with external factors, such as HIV. HIV can, moreover, infect T-cells independently of Langerhans cells (Boggiano & Littman, 2007). HIV's success in establishing a systemic infection might nevertheless depend on its early interaction with Langerhans cells (Boggiano & Littman, 2007; Hladik *et al.*, 2007). At low viral levels Langerin is able to clear HIV, shunting it to intracellular granules for degradation, but this mechanism becomes overwhelmed at higher viral loads (de Witte *et al.*, 2007; Schwartz, 2007). By confocal imaging microscopy and mRNA quantification, the demonstration of abundant and superficially present potential HIV target cells (CD3+ and CD4+ T-cells, Langerhans cells, macrophages and submucosal dendritic cells) has provided anatomical support for the protective effect of circumcision (Hirbod *et al.*, 2010). There was no difference between positive and negative HSV-2 serostatus.

In 2010 it was found that HIV infected cells, but not free HIV, form viral synapses with apical foreskin keratinocytes, followed by rapid internalization by Langerhans cells, whose projections (dendrites) weave up between the keritanocytes in the inner foreskin, the infection occurring within 1 hour (Ganor & Bomsel, 2010; Ganor et al., 2010). The Langerhans cells then formed conjugates with T-cells thereby transferring the HIV. The thick keratin layers in the outer foreskin prevent infection (Ganor & Bomsel, 2010).

Ulcerative disease and tearing are more common in uncircumcised men, adding to the risk of HIV entry (Alanis & Lucidi, 2004). A large 2-year RCT found significantly lower penile coital injuries amongst men in the circumcised arm of the trial, adjusted odds ratio being 0.71 for soreness, 0.52 for scratches/abrasions/cuts, and 0.62 for bleeding (Mehta *et al.*, 2010). HSV-2 infection increases HIV risk in men and women by 3-fold (Freeman *et al.*, 2006). Men with a higher foreskin surface area appear more likely to be infected with HIV (Kigozi *et al.*, 2009b). Inflammation of the epithelium of the foreskin is another factor that can increase infection risk and has been noted in 4.2% of men with neither HIV nor HSV-2, 7.8% of men with HSV-2 only, 19% of men with just HIV, and 32% of men with both (Johnson *et al.*, 2009). For stromal inflammation, the figures were 14%, 30%, 33% and 61%. Both epithelial and stromal inflammation were more common in men with accumulations of smegma. Even in the absence of visible lesions the mucosal tissue can show histological signs of inflammation (Hirbod et al., 2010). Wetness under the foreskin is an indicator of poor hygiene and is associated with a 40% increase in risk of HIV infection (O'Farrell *et al.*, 2006). A wet penis may enhance attachment of infectious virions for longer, reduce healing after trauma, or may lead to balanitis under the foreskin and consequent micro-ulcerations (O'Farrell et al., 2006).

In high HIV prevalence settings, MC has been shown to be cost-effective for prevention of this virus (Williams et al., 2006; Uthman *et al.*, 2011). In sub-Saharan Africa the cost of MC is always lower than the cost of anti-retroviral treatment; by how much depends on the method of circumcision used. Prevention is of enhanced importance here, because no outright cure currently exists for HIV infection.

As mentioned earlier, even in settings in which HIV prevalence is low – such as the USA – calculations by the Centers for Disease Control and Prevention (CDC) have indicated that circumcision of infants would be cost-saving for HIV prevention (Sansom et al., 2010). The CDC has been giving favourable consideration, based on the wide-ranging benefits, to encouraging infant MC in the USA (Smith *et al.*, 2010). Earlier analyses, based on just some of the benefits, were favourable (Schoen *et al.*, 2006). These did not consider the benefits to women such as reduction in cervical cancer and various STIs besides oncogenic HPV (Morris *et al.*, 2006).

The ongoing penetration of HIV into the heterosexual community and rise in the number and proportion of new diagnoses from heterosexually-acquired infection in previously low HIV prevalence settings has led to calls for MC to be encouraged strongly in infancy (Cooper et al., 2010).

3. Rates of circumcision

Worldwide 30-32% of males are circumcised (World Health Organization, 2008b). Most are a consequence of Muslim tradition that mandates MC. Religion dictates MC at day 8 for Jewish infants. In much of sub-Saharan Africa and other parts of the world such as indigenous peoples of Australia and the Pacific islands, MC is performed as part of coming of age ceremonies for boys. In the 1800s MC became popular in Britain and countries with an Anglo-Celtic heritage such as the USA and Australia. While a decline took place in the UK starting in the 1930s and in Australia and New Zealand in the 1970s, rates in the USA have remained high amongst Anglo-Celtic whites and Afro-American blacks (Xu *et al.*, 2007). Hospital discharge data that suggest a decline do not take into account earlier discharge from maternity wards shifting the procedure from hospitals (where circumcisions are recorded in official statistics) to doctor's offices (where they are not), and the fact that not all hospitals record infant MC after delivery. The campaigning by MC opponents that led to withdrawal of Medicaid funding for MC in 17 states has had an adverse effect on the ability of the poor to access MC services for their children (Leibowitz *et al.*, 2009; Morris *et al.*, 2009). In a 2008 report, hospital discharge data in Maryland found 75.3% of 96,457 male infants were circumcised after birth and survey data from 4,273 mothers showed a rate of 82.3% (Cheng *et al.*, 2008). Rate was higher in white and Afro-American blacks and lower amongst Hispanic and Asian infants. The continued influx of migrants, mostly Hispanic, in whom MC is culturally foreign, has been a major factor in the declining prevalence of MC in the US population as a whole. Subsequent generations are, however, more likely to adopt local US customs by having their baby boys circumcised. In Australia a reversal of the downward trend has become evident, no doubt fuelled by widespread news media publicity of the many benefits, especially in HIV prevention.

4. Circumcision style: Terminology

Excision of the foreskin can adopt various styles. These can be divided into what is referred to commonly as either a "high'" or a "low" style (Fig. 1).

There is no published evidence as to whether one style or the other offers greater protection from HIV. The RCTs of MC for HIV prevention used either the forceps-guided method (which is "moderately high and loose": http://www.circlist.com/instrstechs/forcepsguide.html) (Auvert et al., 2005; Bailey et al., 2007) or the sleeve technique (which is "high" and either "tight" or "loose": http://www.circlist.com/ instrstechs/doublecirc.html) (Gray et al., 2007). Proponents of the "low" style argue that the antigen receptor cells responsible for admitting HIV to the uncircumcised male are concentrated in the frenulum and inner foreskin, implying that this tissue should be removed completely in order to obtain maximum benefit from the circumcision. Opponents consider that post-circumcision changes in residual mucosal tissue (changes that are loosely termed "keratinization") render its removal unnecessary. The authors'

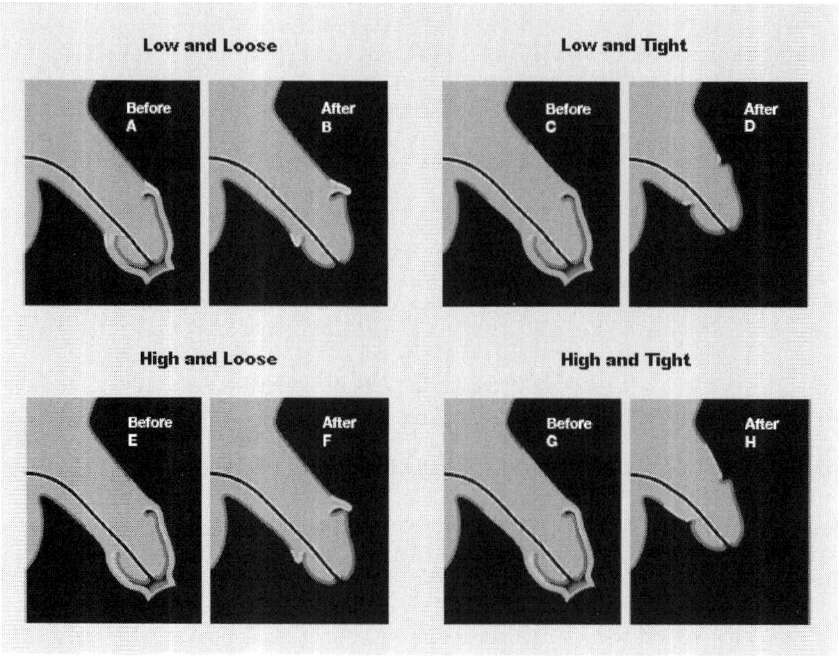

Fig. 1. Depiction of flaccid penis before and after circumcision showing what gets removed for extremes of style; in each case the tissue to be removed is shown in orange. (A) before and (B) after for the "low and loose" style: Almost all the inner foreskin has been removed along with an equal amount of outer foreskin. No tension has been placed in the shaft skin, with the result that the flaccid penis droops and the sulcus is not held fully open. Thus, despite circumcision, it remains possible for smegma to accumulate. (C) before and (D) after for the "low and tight" style: The maximum possible amount of inner foreskin has been removed along with the whole of the outer foreskin *plus* a considerable portion of shaft skin. This has placed the residual shaft skin under tension, with the result that the flaccid penis appears to be short and semi-erect. The sulcus is held fully open; therefore it is not possible for smegma to accumulate. (E) before and (F) after for the "high and loose" style: Much of the of inner foreskin has been retained, folded back on itself to face outwards and assume the role of shaft skin. The outer foreskin has been removed along with some shaft skin, but not enough to place the residue under tension. Thus the flaccid penis still droops as it did before circumcision. The sulcus is not held fully open; therefore it is still possible for smegma to accumulate. (G) before and (H) after for the "high and tight" style: Much of the inner foreskin has been retained, folded back on itself to face outwards and assume the role of shaft skin. The outer foreskin has been removed, as has a considerable amount of shaft skin. This has placed the residual shaft skin under tension, with the result that the flaccid penis appears to be short and semi-erect. The sulcus is held fully open; therefore it is not possible for smegma to accumulate. Diagrams from: http://www.circlist.com/styles/page1.html#terminology

view is that, unless or until proof positive emerges to the effect that a "high" style confers as great a degree of prophylaxis as a "low" style, the Precautionary Principle should be applied and circumcisions should be done in the "low" style.
Traditional circumcisions done using "tug-&-chop" methods (Fig. 2) already provide us with ample examples of residual inner foreskin. There appears to be scope for a population study here, comparing HIV infection rates amongst groups with "high" and "low" styles of circumcision.

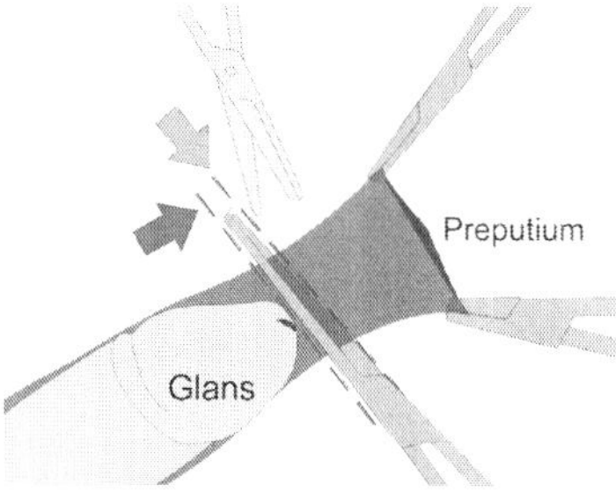

Fig. 2. The "tug-and-chop" method of circumcision.

Another somewhat contentious style issue is the matter of tightness. Often, tightness is considered to be nothing more than a cosmetic matter. However, theoretical models of STI transmission tend to suggest that benefit is gained from the sulcus being dry. This implies that circumcisions should be sufficiently tight to hold the sulcus open, such that no moisture will accumulate there.
The third style issue to be resolved relates to removal or retention of the frenulum. As well as having high concentrations of antigen receptor cells targeted by HIV, the highly vascular frenulum is particularly susceptible to tearing or other damage during intercourse, as well as being a frequent site of lesions produced by other STIs (Szabo & Short, 2000). Persistent debate relates to resulting changes in sexual sensitivity; anecdotal evidence from those who have had their frenulum surgically removed suggest that no loss of sensitivity occurs. It is also worthy of note that the frenulum can be lost as a result of tearing; such loss does not appear to give rise to complaint about effects long-term.
In the light of all of the above, there appears to be a good cause not just to circumcise but to circumcise in a particular way. It seems appropriate for the surgery to specifically target certain classes of cells for removal, at the same time achieving a result that holds the sulcus open so that it remains dry and clean, unable to harbour a viral payload either in smegma or in residues of erogenously triggered body fluids.

5. Methods of circumcision

We will now present information on current approaches to circumcision, mostly stemming from experience in developed nation settings, the USA in particular. We will start with infants and then move on to adults and older boys. We will end with speculation about what is needed for low-resource settings in terms of devising novel devices.
There is no standard circumcision procedure and the issue of standards has been a rallying call for years. At the Western Section American Urological meeting in 2007 Dr Sam Kunin,

who practices in Los Angeles, compared and contrasted clamps and discussed what he considered should be the minimal standards for circumcision (Kunin, 2007a).
The postnatal period provides an ideal window of opportunity for circumcision (Schoen, 2007a). The newborn, having recently experienced the considerable trauma of birth, has elevated levels of normal stress-resistance hormones. Neonates heal quickly, are resilient, and use of local anaesthesia means little or no pain. Since the inner and outer foreskin layers readily adhere to each other afterwards, sutures are rarely needed in this age group.

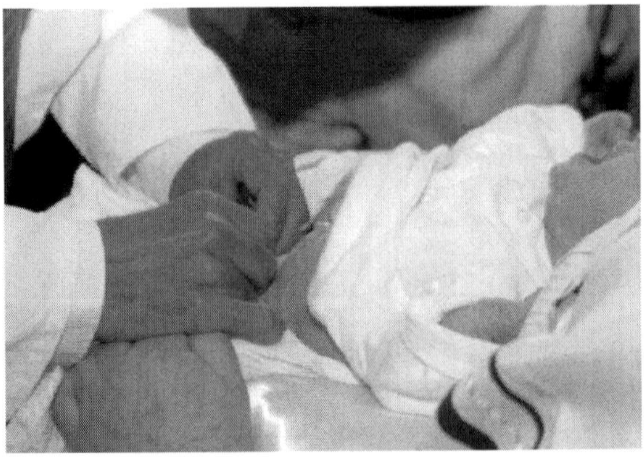

Fig. 3. Photo of a baby boy having a circumcision.

There is no evidence of any long-term psychological harm arising from circumcision. The risk of damage to the penis is extremely rare and avoidable by using a competent, experienced doctor. Unfortunately, because it is such a simple, low-risk procedure, it had once been the practice to assign this job to junior medical staff, with occasional devastating results. Anecdotes of such rare events from the past should be viewed in perspective. Parents or patients nevertheless need to have some re-assurance about the competence of the operator. Also the teaching of circumcision to medical students and practitioners needs to be given greater attention because it is performed so commonly and needs to be done well. Models to teach interns and others have, moreover, been produced (Erikson, 1999; Cohen, 2002).

6. Traditional circumcision of infants

Surgical methods often use a procedure that protects the penis during excision of the foreskin.
Safe implementation of the Jewish tradition of circumcision on the eighth day of life led to the development of what is termed the "Traditional Jewish Shield". At one time made from silver (a material chosen for its natural aseptic qualities), the identical method is now to be found in conjunction with single-use disposable equipment. The objective of the device is to prevent accidental injury to the glans.
The traditional Jewish equipment typifies the "Tug-&-Chop" method. Similar shielding can equally be achieved with forceps or a haemostat, whereupon it becomes known as the forceps-guided technique. Cutting can be done with scissors, a scalpel or an electrocautery device. In all instances the mucosal skin that is stretched between the sulcus and the distal

face of the shield remains intact. Given the current state of knowledge, such a style of circumcision must be regarded as sub-optimal.

Wholly freehand circumcisions did occur, but at theoretically greater risk of injury to the glans.

None of the traditional devices automatically result in removal of the frenulum. If that is required, it must be done as a separate procedure.

7. Medical circumcision of infants and very young boys

In the 1930s in the United States, the search for a means of bloodless circumcision of infants began. Yellen set out the principles involved (Yellen, 1935), but it fell to others (Goldstein, 1939; Ross, 1939; Bronstein, 1955; Kariher & Smith, 1955) to produce workable devices to implement the concept. Numerous patent applications for circumcision instruments were filed during this period, especially in the United States as can be seen by referring to the US Patent and Trademark Office database (USPTO), but few of the inventions passed into mass production and routine use. Meantime, in Europe, a similar but apparently unpatented device known as the Winkelmann Clamp was gaining favour (untraced in the European Patent Office database).

Such devices can be divided into two categories: Those that rely on ischaemic necrosis and those that do not. Ischaemic necrosis involves the deliberate killing-off of tissue by strangulation of its blood supply for a period of days, as in the Ross Ring and the Plastibell® (the trade name given to Kariher and Smith's device). The other devices first crush the blood vessels, typically for a period of some minutes, and then provide protection for the glans when the foreskin is severed. Conventional wound healing follows. In infants, the crushing action is sufficient to seal the wound such that sutures are not normally needed.

In consequence of the design fundamentals of the Gomco (**GO**ldstein **M**edical **CO**mpany) clamp (the trade name given to Goldstein's device) and the Winkelmann Clamp, these two clamps have the potential to remove almost all inner foreskin. The inner, "bell" component reaches beneath the prepuce in a way that places the cut near to the coronal rim of the glans. In consequence, as regards HIV prophylaxis, the resulting style of a circumcision done with these clamps is preferable to any "Tug-&-Chop" method.

In the USA the most commonly used devices are the Gomco clamp (67%), the Mogen clamp (10%) and the Plastibell (19%) (Stang & Snellman, 1998). Pictures of these appear later and can also be found in references: (Langer & Coplen, 1998; Alanis & Lucidi, 2004). The latter article in particular discusses the procedure, as well as contraindications. A technique that uses the Plastibell as a template for paediatric circumcision has been developed (Peterson *et al.*, 2001). Rather than waiting for the bell to slough off days later, sutures are made at the time and the bell is removed. A similar "adult circumcision template" was later created for use in men, with good results (Decastro *et al.*, 2010).

The various devices serve to protect the penis when excising the prepuce. The type of clamp used affects the time taken for the procedure, being on average 81 seconds for the Mogen clamp and 209 seconds for the Gomco clamp (Kurtis *et al.*, 1999). In a head-to-head trial of length of procedure the Mogen took 12 minutes, compared with 20 minutes for the Plastibell (Taeusch *et al.*, 2002). The latter time is far greater than others generally achieve (see 8.2.4 below). Although simpler to use and more pain-free than the other two (Kurtis et al., 1999; Kaufman *et al.*, 2002; Taeusch et al., 2002), the Mogen clamp removes less foreskin. The Gomco is the oldest and is the most refined instrument (Wan, 2002). Its use is widespread, a study in Togo confirming its superiority to grips-only circumcision (Gnassingbé *et al.*, 2010).

Since some of these more elaborate methods can take up to 30 minutes to perform they therefore expose the baby to a greater period of discomfort. In contrast, a circumcision can be completed in 15-30 seconds by a competent practitioner using methods that are part of traditional cultures.

Interestingly, strict sterile conditions were reported not to be necessary to prevent infection in ritual neonatal circumcision in Israel (Naimer & Trattner, 2000).

Rather than tightly strapping the baby down, swaddling and a pacifier has been suggested (Herschel *et al.*, 1998; Howard *et al.*, 1998; Howard *et al.*, 1999). A special padded, "physiological" restraint chair has moreover been devised and shown to reduce distress scores by more than 50% (Stang *et al.*, 1997). Exposure to a familiar odour (the mother's milk or vanilla) reduces distress after common painful procedures in newborns (Goubet *et al.*, 2003; Rattaz *et al.*, 2005; Goubet *et al.*, 2007).

Dr Tom Wiswell and other experts strongly advocate the neonatal period as being the best time to perform circumcision, pointing out that the child will not need sutures (owing to the thinness of the foreskin (Schoen, 2005)) nor general anaesthesia, or additional hospitalization (Wiswell & Geschke, 1989; Wiswell & Hachey, 1993; Wiswell, 1995; Wiswell, 1997; Wiswell, 2000). Wiswell pointed out (personal email communication in Apr 2009) that "starting in the 1970s there was a movement away from delivery room circumcisions at minutes of life until several hours to several days of life. This was mainly because of the recognition of the transition period to extrauterine life that babies go through. 'Stresses' can have an adverse effect on this process, particularly on the heart and lungs. In an otherwise healthy infant, though, there is no need to delay until 2 weeks of age."

All circumcisions should involve adequate anaesthesia, using either EMLA cream, dorsal penile nerve block, penile ring block, or a combination of these prior to the operation (http://www.circinfo.net/anesthesia.html). Without an anaesthetic the child experiences pain, during the procedure and for a maximum of 12-24 hours afterwards. That the baby could remember for a *short* time was suggested by a greater responsiveness to subsequent injection for routine immunization (Taddio *et al.*, 1997). The child does not, however, have any long-term memory of having had a circumcision performed and there are no other long-term adverse effects (Fergusson *et al.*, 2008). Local anaesthesia is therefore advocated.

Whatever the method, post-operative care, as advised by the doctor, must be undertaken, usually by the parents. Cosmetic results have met with unanimous parental acceptance (Duncan *et al.*, 2004).

Healing is rapid in infancy (Schoen, 2005), complication rate is very low (0.2%-0.6%) (Wiswell & Geschke, 1989; Cilento *et al.*, 1999; Christakis *et al.*, 2000; Ben Chaim *et al.*, 2005), and cost is much lower than when performed later in life (Schoen et al., 2006).

For males with haemophilia, special pre-operative treatment is required (Balkan *et al.*, 2010; Yilmaz *et al.*, 2010). A satisfactory outcome can be achieved with a specialized cost-effective device (Karaman *et al.*, 2004; Sewefy, 2004). Just as for healthy individuals (see below), cyanoacrylate tissue adhesives (Glubran and Glubran 2) have been found to be effective for circumcision of haemophilia patients (Haghpanah *et al.*, 2011).

8. Circumcision of adults and boys post-infancy

8.1 Freehand methods

Circumcision is more traumatic, disruptive and expensive for men and older boys than it is for infants (Schoen, 2007a). For those aged 4 months to 15 years some authorities advocate a general anaesthetic. Others strongly disagree, saying that since a general anaesthetic carries a small risk, a local anaesthetic, often with a mild sedative, is what should be used for all children (Schoen, 2007a).

Unlike infant circumcisions, sutures/stitches or wound staples are usually needed for men and older children, although use of synthetic tissue adhesives such as 2-octyl-cyanoacrylate (Dermabond) (Cheng & Saing, 1997; Subramaniam & Jacobsen, 2004; Ozkan *et al.*, 2005; Elmore *et al.*, 2007; Elemen *et al.*, 2010; Lane *et al.*, 2010; D'Arcy & Jaffry, 2011) have proven to be effective alternatives. These are safe, easy to use, reduce operating time, lower postoperative pain and give a better cosmetic appearance (Ozkan et al., 2005; Elmore et al., 2007).

Excellent cosmetic results were reported for all of 346 patients aged 14 to 38 months using electro-surgery, which presents a bloodless operative field (Peters & Kass, 1997). Metal of any kind (such as the Gomco clamp that is used commonly in infant MC) has to of course be avoided in this procedure.

Laser surgery is gaining popularity, but requires both specialized equipment and training. The method has its own associated shields (Chekmarev, 1989; Zhenyuan, 1989; Gao & Ni, 1999).

Gentle tissue dissection with simultaneous haemostasis has been achieved using an ultrasound dissection scalpel for circumcision (Fette *et al.*, 2000).

A randomized trial found that a bipolar diathermy scissors circumcision technique led to less blood loss (0.2 versus 2.1 ml), shorter operating time (11 versus 19 min) and lower early and late postoperative morbidity as compared with a standard freehand scalpel procedure (Méndez-Gallart *et al.*, 2009). Bipolar scissors also appear to offer a method of bloodless removal of the frenulum prior to application of any one of a number of circumcision clamps for the remainder of the procedure.

Unless combined with other surgery, circumcision later obviously requires a separate (occasionally overnight) visit to hospital. Healing is slower than in newborns and the rate of complications is greater, but still low: 1-4% (Auvert et al., 2005; Cathcart *et al.*, 2006; Bailey et al., 2007; Gray et al., 2007; Krieger *et al.*, 2007). Most common is postoperative bleeding (0.4-0.8%), infection (0.2-0.4%), wound disruptions (0.3%), problems with appearance (0.6%), damage to the penis (0.3%), insufficient skin removed (0.3%), delayed wound healing (0.1%), delayed healing (0.2%), swelling at the incision site or haematoma (0.1-0.6%) or need to return to the theatre (0.5%). An average of 3.8% adverse events has been seen for the first 1-100 circumcisions a clinician does (Krieger et al., 2007). For the next 100 this decreases to 2.1% and by the time they have done 200-400 it drops to less than 1%. Beyond 400 it is 0.7%. The incidence of penile adhesions after a circumcision decreases with age, but at any age they often resolve spontaneously (Ponsky *et al.*, 2000). Pain sometimes can last for days afterwards and those older than 1 to 2 years may remember.

Cost is also much greater than for neonatal circumcision. Cost can be reduced by having the surgery performed on an outpatient basis.

A local anaesthetic is all that is needed for MC, so reducing anaesthetists' charges which can be quite high for a general anaesthetic. The WHO has produced a manual for circumcision of men under local anaesthesia (World Health Organisation, 2006). Various methods can be used for local anaesthesia, including dorsal penile nerve block and ring block. Recently, a no-needle jet of 0.1 ml 2% lidocaine solution sprayed at high pressure directly on to the penile skin circumferentially around the proximal third of the penis has proven to be quick and effective, and has obvious appeal (Peng *et al.*, 2010a).

Conventional surgery under general anaesthetic normally uses the sleeve-resection technique, described in a series of diagrams with technical details by Elder (2007). This method takes longer and for this reason many surgeons will insist on using a general anaesthetic. By its nature sleeve resection removes mainly shaft skin, not foreskin, so having potential implications for HIV infection. An alternative is the Dissection Method. These two methods are often confused. Illustrated by Mousa (Mousa, 2007), the Dissection Method separates inner and outer foreskin in a manner similar to a very loose "tug and chop" circumcision, but then proceeds to excise most of the inner and all of the outer foreskin along with some shaft skin. The amount of shaft skin removed depends on the tightness required; inner foreskin is left only as necessary to provide an anchorage for sutures reconnecting the shaft skin to the sulcus.

Interestingly, genital surgery in women often involves a course of topical estrogen in advance in order to increase thickening, cornification and keratinization of the vaginal epithelium (Short, 2006). This helps surgical outcome and has led to the suggestion that similar pre-treatment be carried out prior to circumcision in men.

Pain from conventional surgery can last for up to a week or longer afterwards, during which time absence from work may be required. Some men, however, report no pain, just minor discomfort from the stitches. A large RCT found that at the 3-day post-circumcision follow-up, 48% reported no pain, 52% very mild pain, and none moderate or severe pain (Bailey et al., 2007). By 8 days, 89% had no pain and 11% mild pain. Vasectomy in men circumcised previously as adults (and who can thus attest to the difference) is said to be much more painful.

8.2 Instruments developed over earlier years

The following devices were in common use for male circumcision prior to the start of the HIV epidemic. The patent information quoted relates to the country of residence of the inventor(s). In many instances other patents exist, especially in the USA, the European Union and, since its formation in 1967, the records of the World Intellectual Property Organisation (WIPO).

8.2.1 Traditional Jewish shield

Inventor: Unknown
Primary patent: None: historic
Patent priority date: Not applicable
Patient age range: Full-term neonate to adult
Category: Tug-&-Chop shield

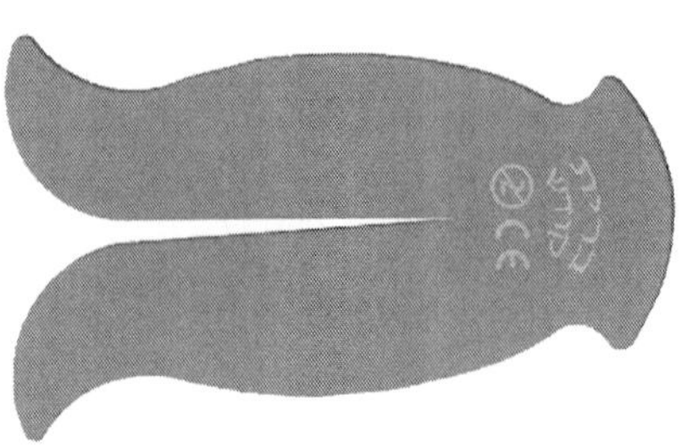

Fig. 4. The traditional Jewish shield.

Procedure: The foreskin is pulled forward and the shield slipped over it. The excess prepuce is then excised by running a scalpel or similar knife across the distal face of the device.

8.2.2 Gomco Clamp

Inventor:	Goldstein, A.A.
Primary patent:	United States Design Patent USD119180 (no Utility Patent has been traced)
Patent priority date:	16 Mar 1939
Patient age range:	Full-term neonate to adult
Category:	Bell clamp / scalpel guide

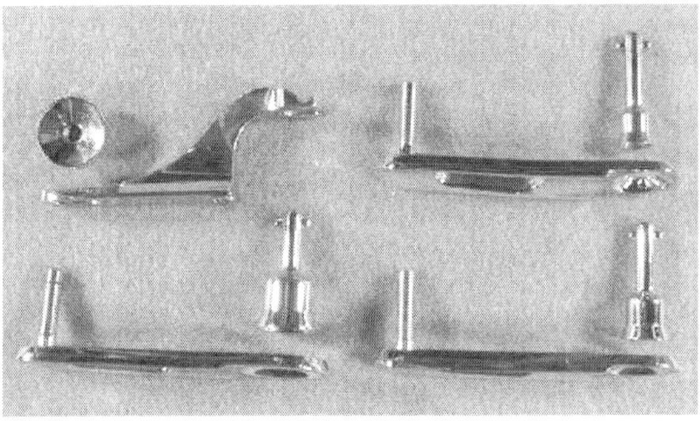

Fig. 5. The Gomco Clamp showing components, in a range of sizes, that are assembled during the procedure described in the text.

Procedure: First of all, a dorsal slit is made in the foreskin and the foreskin is separated from the glans. The bell of the Gomco clamp is then placed over the glans, and the foreskin is pulled over the bell. The base of the Gomco clamp is placed over the bell, and the Gomco clamp's arm is fitted. After the surgeon confirms correct fitting and placement (and the amount of foreskin to be excised), the nut on the Gomco clamp is tightened, causing the clamping of nerves and blood flow to the foreskin. The Gomco clamp is left in place for about 5 minutes to allow clotting of blood to occur, then the foreskin is dissected off using a scalpel. The Gomco's base and bell are then removed, and the penis is bandaged. It is a fairly bloodless circumcision technique. The circumcision is relatively quick compared to the Plastibell. It was the most popular method for circumcisions between 1950 and 1980 and is still common today, especially in the USA. A training video of a neonatal Gomco circumcision using dorsal penile nerve block and a sucrose pacifier, conducted by Dr Richard Green, Stanford University School of Medicine, is available at http://newborns.stanford.edu/Gomco.html

Dr Sam Kunin, an experienced urological surgeon in Los Angeles, has developed a clever, and very effective, method in which local anaesthetic is injected into the distal foreskin (Kunin, 2007b). Doing so separates the inner and outer foreskin therefore allowing the inner layer to be pulled against the bell of the Gomco clamp, and results in a maximum amount of inner layer being removed (http://www.samkuninmd.com). He points out that the inner lining is the area most prone to adhesions, irritations, yeast and bacterial infections, particularly in diabetics.

Gomco clamps exist in sizes from neonatal to adult. Suturing is required post-infancy.

8.2.3 Winkelmann Clamp

Inventor:	Provisionally attributed to the German urological surgeon Karl Winkelmann (1863-1925).
Primary patent:	None traced
Patent priority date:	None traced
Patient age range:	Infant to mid-puberty, according to manufacturer.
Category:	Bell clamp / scalpel guide

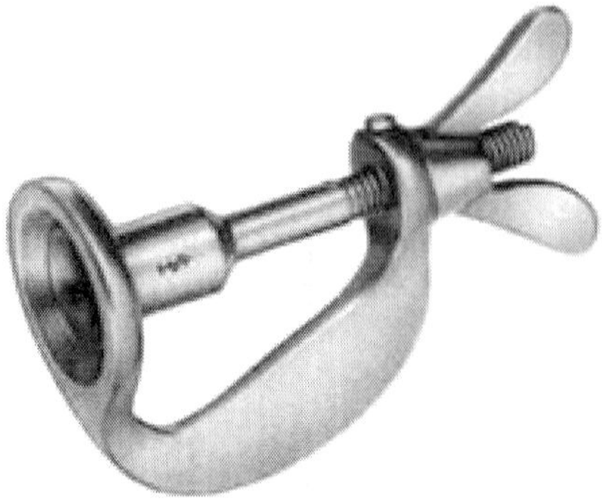

Fig. 6. The Winkelmann Clamp.

Procedure: Nominally the same as the Gomco clamp described above. Despite its ready availability, the Winkelmann Clamp appears not to have been trialled in connection with the search for devices suitable for campaigns of mass circumcision.

8.2.4 Plastibell

Inventors:	Kariher, D.H. and Smith, T.W.
Primary patent:	US3056407
Patent priority date:	18 May 1955
Patient age range:	Full-term neonate to onset of puberty
Category:	Ischaemic necrosis device using string ligature

Procedure: The Plastibell is a clear plastic ring with handle and has a deep groove running circumferentially. The adhesions between glans and foreskin are divided with a haemostat (artery forceps) or similar probe. Then the foreskin is cut longitudinally starting at the distal end dorsally to allow it to be retracted so that the glans (the head of penis) is exposed (Elder, 2007). The appropriately sized device is chosen and applied to the exposed glans. The ring is then covered over by the foreskin. A ligature is tied firmly around the foreskin, crushing the skin against the groove in the Plastibell. Then the excess skin protruding beyond the ring is trimmed off, something that is possible using surgical scissors rather than a scalpel. Finally, the handle is broken off. The entire procedure takes 5 to 10 minutes, depending on the experience and skill of the operator. The compression against the underlying plastic shield causes the foreskin tissue to necrotize. The ring falls off in 3 to 7 days leaving a circumferential wound that will heal over the following week. Typically, the glans will appear red or yellow until it has cornified (Gee & Ansell, 1976; Holman *et al.*, 1995).

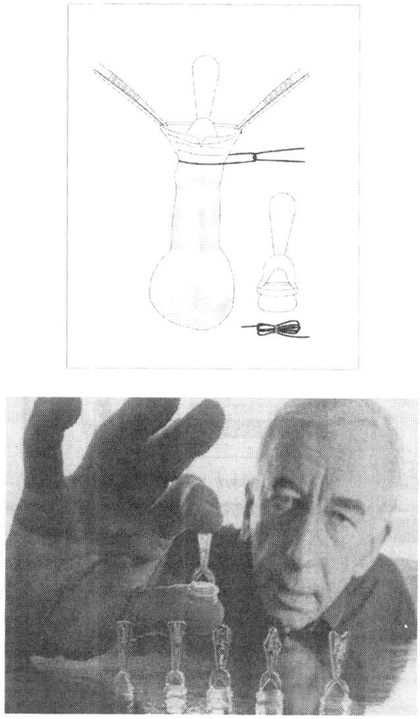

Fig. 7. The Plastibell device is a clear plastic ring with handle and has a deep groove running circumferentially. Upper diagram: How it is used for an infant circumcision (diagram modified from Elder (2007)). Lower image: Dr Terry Russell, Brisbane, Australia, displaying the range of sizes available.

The Plastibell continues to be available in sizes applicable from newborn to early puberty. The metallic precursor, the Ross Ring (Ross, 1939), also came in adult sizes, but adult Plastibell circumcision appears to be unknown. The metallic ring is long discontinued, rendered obsolete by its disposable plastic equivalent. Cosmetic results have met with unanimous parental acceptance (Duncan et al., 2004).

Dr Terry Russell in Brisbane, Australia, developed in 1993 a simple, pain-free method involving 2 hours EMLA cream with the penis wrapped in cling wrap (done by the parents prior to arrival at the clinic), followed by a modified Plastibell circumcision (Russell & Chaseling, 1996). The technique is described in detail on his website (http://www.circumcision.com.au). Dr Russell has used it in 30,000 circumcisions on boys of all ages from neonate to puberty, including 400 older boys every year. More recently he has obtained excellent results with another topically applied anaesthetic cream, LMX4 (4% lidocaine) that is faster acting, more effective and has fewer side effects (C.T. Russell, personal communication). Because complete local anaesthesia is achieved by EMLA or LMX4 cream, Dr Russell reports that no pain is experienced for 5 hours after the Plastibell is applied, so claims the circumcision is completely pain free at all stages. The only major complication in 30,000 circumcisions was one boy who developed mild

methemoglobinaemia (from the EMLA cream) that, after immediate hospital admission, resolved spontaneously overnight, with no medical intervention required.
Prof Roger Short orchestrated the production of a video that teaches the Russell method. Dr Russell featured in this "no scalpel circumcision" video. Also featured was one of Prof Short's students from Botswana, who took it there for teaching purposes. Another, filmed in Vanuatu of a traditional circumcision using a sharpened bamboo, was produced for use in Papua New Guinea (PNG) where, unlike most Pacific Islands, circumcision is uncommon. These were aimed primarily to reduce HIV/AIDS in Botswana and PNG.
Since the simple plastic Plastibell device is now off patent it can be produced at very low cost, but parallel production cannot use the name Plastibell, which remains to this day a Registered Trade Mark. Nevertheless, the device has the potential to help reduce HIV in poor countries (Short, 2004).
Dr. Sam Kunin points out, however, that "the [Plasti]bell techniques leave too much inner skin. Besides the inherent problems of this method with later adhesions and buried penis, allows for possible migration of the bell down the shaft, with ensuing potential damage to the penile skin" (personal communication). A Nigerian study also noted that incorrect technique can lead to proximal migration of the Plastibell in neonatal boys (Bode *et al.*, 2009). Correct training in this method is thus essential. An Iranian study involving 7,510 term neonates found that Plastibell circumcision incorporating thermal cautery of the frenulum reduces bleeding (0.4% versus 0.05%), but led to greater urinary retention (0.03% versus 0.9%) (Kazem *et al.*, 2009). Modifications to the standard procedure by authors in the UK have improved outcomes, particularly the risk of bleeding (Mahomed *et al.*, 2009).
A study in Pakistan found that for babies under 3 months of age, the time taken for the Plastibell to fall off was 8.7 days (Samad *et al.*, 2009). This increased gradually to 16.8 days for children over 5 years.

8.2.5 Mogen Clamp

Inventor:	Bronstein, H.
Primary patent:	US2747576
Patent priority date:	3 Feb 1955
Patient age range:	Full-term neonate to adult
Category:	Tug-&-Chop shield with inbuilt crushing action

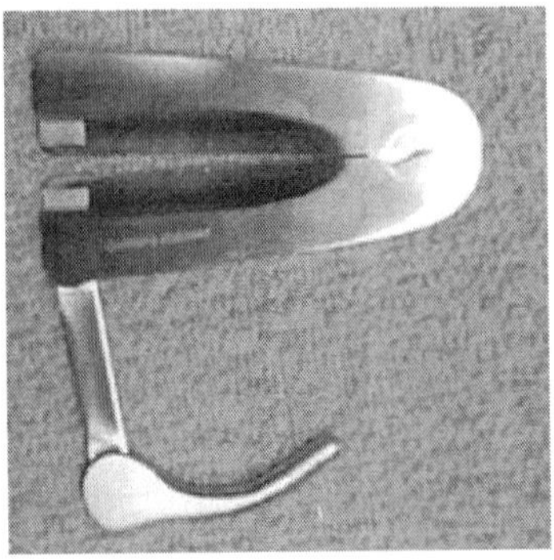

Fig. 8. The Mogen Clamp.

Procedure: Firstly, adhesions between glans and foreskin are divided and a haemostat is placed along the dorsal midline with its tip about 3 mm short of the corona before being locked into place. The Mogen clamp is opened fully. A key step in Mogen circumcision is the safe placement of the clamp. To push the glans out of the way, the surgeon's thumb and index finger pinch the foreskin below the dorsal haemostat. The Mogen clamp is then slid across the foreskin from dorsal to ventral following along the same angle as the corona. The hollow side of the clamp faces the glans. Before locking the clamp shut, the glans is manipulated to be sure it is free of the clamp's jaw. If it is, the clamp is locked. Once locked the foreskin is excised flush with the flat surface of the clamp with a 10 inch blade scalpel. The clamp is left on for a few moments to ensure haemostasis. It is then unlocked and removed. The glans is liberated by thumb-traction at the 3 and 4 o'clock positions that pull the crush line apart.

This device can be and has been used across the whole age range. However, recent safety issues involving the glans being drawn into the clamp are reported to have brought about the bankruptcy of the original manufacturer (Tagami, 2010).

9. Objectives and constraints relating to a campaign of mass circumcision

With the possible exception of the Plastibell, the traditional devices appear not to be well suited to field use by personnel not fully trained as medical professionals. This has led to the development of a number of new designs. Before moving on to consider each in detail, we first address the issue of the design objectives.

Over 30% of the world's male population enters adulthood already circumcised, their foreskins having been removed in infancy, childhood or around puberty, either as a prophylactic measure for prevention of disease, for hygiene reasons, family tradition, cultural reasons, religious requirements, or treatment of foreskin-related medical conditions (World Health Organisation, 2007b). That still leaves hundreds of millions of uncircumcised males who are (or later in life will become) sexually active, but lack the baseline protection provided by MC against a wide range of STIs and other adverse medical conditions.

Valiant MC scale-up efforts are in progress in sub-Saharan Africa. It is, however, unrealistic to expect existing surgical resources to be diverted to the task of circumcising these millions of men worldwide. Such expertise is already fully committed elsewhere. What is required is an *ad hoc* contingent of circumcisers, a cohort of people with sufficient training to carry out circumcisions safely, effectively, with a good cosmetic outcome and minimum disturbance to lifestyle. Given the vast numbers involved, recruitment from outside the pre-existing medical profession is inevitable. Such a need has, moreover, been recognized by those "on the ground" in sub-Saharan Africa (Sahasrabuddhe & Vermund, 2007; Sharlip, 2008; Wamai *et al.*, 2008; World Health Organization, 2008b).

Herein lies the justification for introducing newer methods of circumcision reliant on advances in biomedical engineering. What is needed is a device and method that de-skills the surgical process to the point where it can be safely and effectively undertaken by people whose prior educational achievement would not otherwise have admitted them to the medical profession. Then, and only then, can a campaign of mass circumcision take place without major poaching of skilled personnel from other healthcare programmes.

Prudent planning nevertheless envisages a fully qualified person to be nearby, acting as supervisor and capable of completing by conventional surgery any circumcision that goes wrong when attempted by ordinary members of the task force using de-skilled methodology. Dispensing totally with such supervision and backup would, in the authors' opinions, be too risky.

No matter what method is used, adequate training in technique is crucial. To this end a low-cost penile model has been developed as a teaching aid for use in low-resource settings (Kigozi *et al.*, 2011).

As with previous global public health campaigns such as the one that successfully achieved the eradication of smallpox, it is imperative to bring MC services to the people rather than expect the people to visit distant facilities. Take the example of the peasant farmer. He cannot leave his livestock and his family unattended for days on end whilst he travels, probably on foot, to a clinic many miles away. Hence our second requirement for the ideal new MC device: It must be suitable for use in conditions of limited asepsis. A clean consulting room in a village health clinic would be a luxury, as would a mobile facility built into a shipping container and driven around by truck. Think more in terms of a clean cloth draped over a table in a bamboo or mud hut, with village elders in attendance waving their ceremonial fly whisks and the circumciser arriving on foot with all necessary equipment in a small rucksack. No roads, no electricity, no running water. The 2nd author, Chris Eley, saw exactly this at a religiously-motivated circumcision in Seram, Indonesia, in 1987 (Operation Raleigh expedition 11E, led by the late Major Wandy Swales TD). On that occasion the surgery was done freehand by a well-qualified and highly proficient Egyptian doctor, using injected local anaesthesia, forceps, surgical scissors and sutures.

One obvious consequence of such remoteness is that facilities for re-sterilizing equipment are non-existent. Therefore the ideal device should be single-use. That applies not only to the clamp itself, but also to all ancillary equipment such as any tool needed to close it, plus syringes, forceps and so on. Think here of a whole single-use kit packaged as one, not just a clamping device on its own.

Against this outline of medical objectives, social and logistical background, we can begin to construct a checklist of the design parameters to be met by candidate devices.

Already mentioned:

- Suitable for use by persons without recognised medical qualifications, with limited supervision.
- Suitable for field use; no requirement for an aseptic environment.
- Single use / disposable.

To this list must be added:

- *Cost:* Rather obviously this needs to be minimized, but the raw cost of the device is only a small part of the total financial commitment. Staffing, provisioning and transport in remote areas can dwarf the cost of the circumcision device that the team intends to fit. The design of the device nevertheless remains crucial. For example, does it need a trained attendant to remove it? If so, staffing costs may straight away have escalated in comparison with a rival device not routinely requiring such follow-up.
- *Simplicity:* The ideal device should be easy to comprehend. Not only does that simplify training, it also simplifies the obtaining of each prospective patient's informed consent. Simplicity also reduces the possibility of user error. This implies minimizing the number of components, avoiding all possibility of mis-assembly (such as getting something the wrong way round) and misuse (such as making a scalpel cut on the wrong side of a clamping ring). Enter what we politely refer to here as "The Law of the Inevitable Cussidness of Inanimate Objects", better known as Sod's (or Murphy's) Law

(http://en.wikipedia.org/wiki/Murphy's_law). If something possibly can go wrong, it will. Botched circumcisions cause immense psychological distress. The duty of care owed is of the highest order. One good measure of simplicity is the number of components in a device, the lower that number the better.

- *Size range:* Where the intent is to produce a single design for the whole male population, the smallest device should fit a full-term neonate and the largest should fit the most well-endowed male. But what about those in-between? There is a balance to be struck here between, on the one hand, having a device that is precisely sized so that it is correct for each patient and, on the other hand, needing to carry a vast stock of different sizes. A certain latitude in sizing is needed, such that an acceptable circumcision results even if the device is a few millimetres off the ideal. This is not merely a matter of stockholding; critical sizing invites increased error due to the use of mis-selected devices and it also increases waste arising when an incorrect size is selected and removed from its sterile packaging but discarded before use.
- *Sterility:* Delivery to remote locations requires robust packaging, but that is only half the story. Not all sterilization processes can be applied to all materials. There are known pitfalls with many plastics. Cobalt-60 exposure (gamma irradiation) is a very effective way of sterilizing, but is totally unsuited to a number of plastics; many discolour and become brittle when irradiated. Full consideration of this materials science issue is beyond the scope of the present chapter; just note and beware! The present alternative is the environmentally questionable Ethylene Oxide method. In time, it may become possible to use ultra-high voltage electrostatic fields on an industrial scale, but that is still in the future (Wang *et al.*, 1992; Meijer, 2008).
- *Suitable materials:* Devices that are intended to remain in contact with body tissue for an extended period must be hypoallergenic. Factors such as contact time and plasticizer residues must be scrutinized. The device supply chain should be secure against pirate copies and adulteration of the original specification.
- *Disposability:* Waste disposal must be managed, not just in respect of the usual medical sharps, but also in respect of sloughed-off clamps and associated necrotic tissue. In some societies the payment of a bounty for the return of the spent device might be appropriate as a way of bringing about proper disposal.
- *No fraudulent re-use:* Single-use devices should be exactly that. A key question might be "Does the device self-destruct at the end of the procedure?".
- *Avoidance of wound dehiscence:* "Clip-&-Wear" clamps with an exceptionally narrow clamping ring can bring about wound dehiscence, especially when the circumcision style is tight such that the shaft skin is significantly stretched. What was intended merely to grip takes on the potential to cut, doing so proximally to the intended scar line and thus forcing remedial action that results in a tighter circumcision than originally envisaged. This problem appears to be age-related and gives rise to some criticism of the widespread use of ischaemic necrosis techniques in adults (Vernon Quaintance, The Gilgal Society, personal communication). There may be good cause for separating out older sexually-active adults and providing them with conventional surgery. Local factors appear to intrude here, especially nutritional status, a well-known determinant of wound healing capacity.
- *Even and adequate clamping pressure:* Devices using the process of ischaemic necrosis need to apply their strangulation pressure evenly right around the intended scar line.

Unless effective counter-measures are taken, pressure discontinuities can arise, especially at hinge positions and/or latch positions. This gives rise to the possibility of continued marginal blood flow at these points. In terms of infection, such marginal leaking is exceptionally dangerous. A good design for an ischaemic necrosis clamp is one that has no discontinuity in the clamping ring and which, throughout the wear period, maintains an absolutely even pressure sufficient to bring about total cessation of blood flow across the whole of the intended scar line.

- *Resistance to premature removal by a meddlesome patient:* Premature removal of an ischaemic necrosis clamp can precipitate a clinical emergency. Therefore it is vital that the latching mechanism of the clamp should be secure against tampering. The risk of such tampering is greatest when dealing with post-infancy paediatric patients.
- *Minimum requirement for pre-treatment:* In the world of veterinary medicine, immunization against tetanus is recommended when ischaemic necrosis is used for procedures such as tail docking of lambs by means of the Elastrator device (Thedford, 1983). We commend the idea of similar pre-treatment before any ischaemic necrosis procedure is used for MC.
- *Cultural acceptability:* A whole raft of issues can arise here, any one of which might scupper a proposal to use a particular design of clamp in a particular area. For example, is a device invented in Israel assured of acceptance in Islamic Republics that do not even acknowledge the existence of the Jewish state? Will circumcision ever be accepted by Hindus, many of whom value their foreskins as evidence of not being Muslim? During the partition of India in 1947, strangers suspected of being of the opposite faith were disrobed and put to death on no more evidence than their circumcision status (Kamra, 2002). Rather less dramatically, there is the question of whether a clip-&-wear clamp protrudes beyond the end of the penis during the wear period. Not a problem in societies where loose, flowing robes are normal attire, but an entirely different matter when the male is habitually dressed in tight jeans.

10. Resulting new designs for circumcision devices

The authors are aware of eight products designed to fulfil the demand for a field-use device, all being either in full production or in the final stages of development and testing. These are now considered individually, in alphabetical order of trade name. Only the original patents or patent applications *in the inventor's country of residence* are listed; increments may exist in the same country as well as there being patents elsewhere.

It should be noted that some clamps have been the subject of ongoing development after their initial market launch. Care is needed when reading reports of field trial results. Early criticisms may have been rendered obsolete by subsequent design changes.

10.1 AccuCirc

Inventor:	Tomlinson, D.R.
Primary patent:	US2005/022404
Patent priority date:	25 Jun 2004
Patient age range:	Full-term neonate only
Website:	http://www.accucirc.com
Category:	Automated cutter

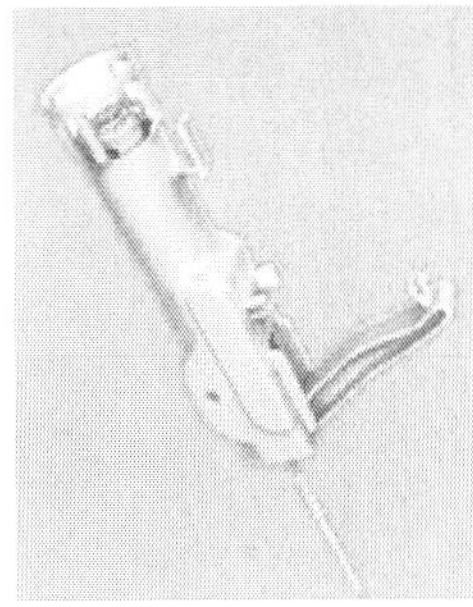

Fig. 9. The AccuCirc device.

Procedure: The AccuCirc uses two innovative components, a Foreskin Probe/Shielding Ring that ensures the glans is protected with the foreskin properly aligned and a Single-Action Clamp that ensures adequate haemostasis and the precise delivery of the protected, circular blade. These work together to protect the infant from injury. This device simplifies the circumcision procedure and eliminates the need for a dorsal slit, as well as removing potential for mismatching of parts. It comes in a self-contained kit. This is completely disposable and no part is retained on the infant.

10.2 Ali's Klamp

Inventor:	Canoğlu, V.A.
Primary patent:	TR2003/00403
Patent priority date:	28 Mar 2003
Patient age range:	Full-term neonate to adult (experimental in adult sizes)
Website:	http://www.alisklamp.com
Category:	Ischaemic necrosis device

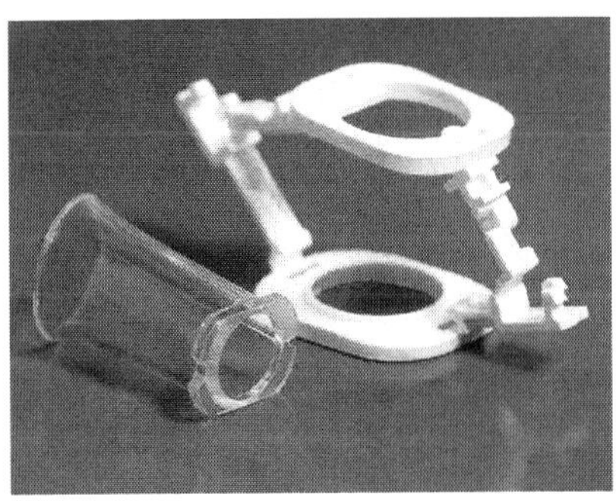

Fig. 10. Ali's clamp.

Procedure: The Ali's Klamp (a.k.a. "Alisklamp" and "Ali's clamp"; Telif Haklari ABAGROUP Ltd) is a single-use ischaemic necrosis device; the foreskin is crushed between two plastic surfaces. The recommended procedure includes severing of the excess tissue. During that process, the tube protects the glans from accidental injury. Note that the final scar line forms at the position of the clamping ring, not at the position of the scalpel cut. In theory the user could dispense with the scalpel cut, leaving the whole foreskin to necrotise. The procedure is illustrated in a two-part video available on the manufacturer's website.

The Ali's Klamp differs from the SmartKlamp (below) only in one significant respect: The clamping ring is angled to match the typical slant of the coronal rim of the glans. In theory this achieves better capture of inner foreskin ventrally. The Ali's clamp apparently shares with the SmartKlamp one notable design weakness. An unwilling or meddlesome patient could, in theory, open the clamp by placing a flat object such as a table knife between the tube and the locking arms and then twisting. Additionally, such action would render the device liable to unscrupulous re-use several times over, until such time as the nominally single-use latching mechanism wore out.

A review of 7,500 boys who underwent circumcision with this device under local anaesthesia concluded that cosmetic appearance was better than conventional circumcision of 5,700 boys (Senel *et al.*, 2010). Duration was 4.5 ± 1.5 minutes versus 23 ± 4 minutes, respectively. Complications were seen in 2% of Ali's clamp versus 10.4% for conventional circumcision, the most common for the Ali's clamp being buried penis (1.04%), followed by infection (0.6%), bleeding (0.4%). A mass circumcision of 2,013 male infants, children, adolescents and adults (mean age 7.8 ± 2.5 years) over a 7-day period, noted a duration of 3.6 ± 1.2 minutes and complication rate of 2.93% in those < 2 years of age, mostly from buried penis (0.98%) and excessive foreskin (0.98%) (Senel *et al.*, 2011). In older children, adolescents and adults complication rate was 2.39%, 2.51% and 2.40%, respectively. Overall, excessive foreskin (0.7%) was ther most common complication, followed by bleeding (0.60%), infection (0.55%), wound dehiscence (0.25%), buried penis (0.25%), and urine retention (0.10%). There was no effect on erectile function and libido, and a 96% satisfaction rate was recorded.

Originally available only for children, adult sizes reportedly now exist for use on a trial basis. Correspondence received mid-February 2011 from Dr. Ali Canoğlu claims a successful field trial in Africa. At the time of writing official independent reports have not yet been published.

10.3 Ismail Klamp

Inventor:	Salleh, I.
Primary patent:	MY2008/000195
Patent priority date:	16 Jan 2008
Patient age range:	Full-term neonate to puberty
Website:	http://www.ismailclamp.com/
Category:	Ischaemic necrosis device

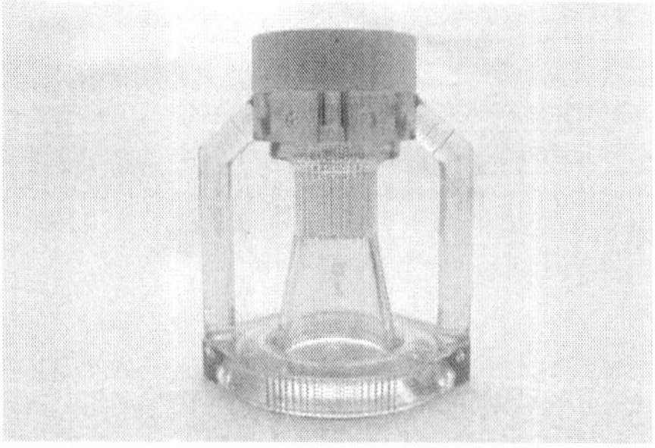

Fig. 11. The Ismail Klamp.

Procedure: The Ismail Klamp is another single-use ischaemic necrosis device, functioning in the same way as the Ali's Klamp, SmartKlamp and Tara KLamp. The distinguishing feature of Dr. Ismail Salleh's device is that the clamping ring can be loosened as well as tightened during the process of application. This the manufacturer describes as "Reversible Clamping". Such a feature is undoubtedly an advantage if a tight style of circumcision is required; it gives greater scope for clamp adjustment. Against that advantage must be offset two risks: A meddlesome patient might loosen the clamp during the healing period and the clamp might be re-used unscrupulously.

10.4 PrePex

Inventors:	Fuerst, O., Kilemnick, I. and Shohat, S.
Primary patent:	(Application:) IL2010/000568
Patent priority date:	16 Jul 2009
Patient age range:	Adult only at present
Website:	http://www.prepex.com/
Category:	Ischaemic necrosis device

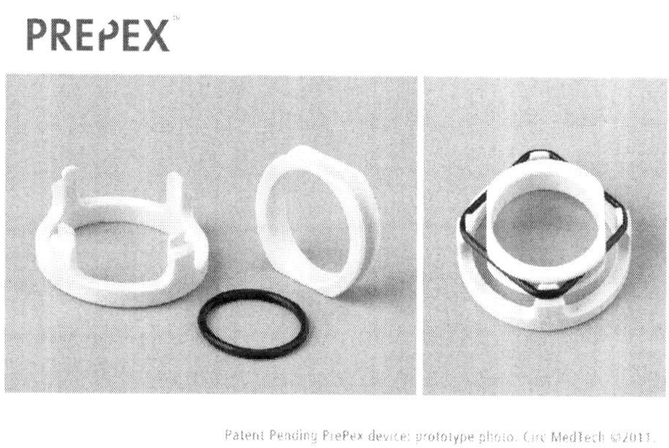
PREPEX
Patent Pending PrePex device: prototype photo. Circ MedTech ©2011.

Fig. 12. The PrePex device. (Photo supplied by Circ MedTech ©2011)

Developed in 2009/10 by Dr. Oren and Tzameret Fuerst, Ido Kilemnick & Shaul Shohat (Fuerst *et al.*, 2009) and marketed by a company called Circ MedTech Limited (incorporated in the British Virgin Islands), this device is designed for use in non-sterile environments by minimally trained healthcare professionals.

Possibly unique for modern clamps, publicized abstracts of safety and efficacy trials held in Rwanda found it to be suitable for use without anaesthesia. Four hundred milligrams of oral Brufen is routinely offered 30 minutes after placement of the clamp, but no other drug use is involved. Whilst the surplus foreskin can be severed, in these trials the foreskin was left to necrotize intact thus facilitating a quick and bloodless procedure that can be handled by minimally trained healthcare professionals in non-sterile settings. The company affirms that there have been no complications to the urine stream as a result of the necrotized foreskin being left *in situ*.

In common with other ischaemic necrosis clamps, the PrePex device requires no sutures.

Procedure: After sizing and marking of the circumcision line based on the circumcision style desired (high/low), the Elastic Ring, loaded on to the Delivery Ring, is placed at "deploy-ready" position on the penis base (proximal). The foreskin tip is stretched open to allow insertion of the Inner Ring, directly under the coronal sulcus. The Elastic Ring is then deployed within the Inner Ring groove, initiating the ischaemic process and the Delivery Ring is removed. The patient resumes his activities with only the Elastic Ring visible. After 7 days, the device is removed by flicking the Elastic Ring out of the groove and extracting the inner ring with fingers or a standard medical spatula.
Regulatory issues (as declared by the manufacturer): "The device has a CE mark and is manufactured using USP Class VI biocompatible elastomeric materials compliant to ISO_13485 Medical Devices (Quality Management systems) and FDA, 21_CFR177.2600."
Declared contra-indication: The device is contraindicated for patients with phimosis if the chosen procedure leaves the foreskin intact.
Once evidence of the style of circumcision achieved by this device is made public, this latecomer to the design contest is expected to show significant advantages over its competitors - especially if the claim of suitability for routine use without anaesthesia is validated in more extensive trials.

10.5 Shang Ring

Inventor:	Shang, J.
Primary patent:	CN2003/000903
Patent priority date:	20 Oct 2003
Patient age range:	Full-term neonate to adult
Website:	http://www.snnda.com/enindex.asp
Category:	Ischaemic necrosis device

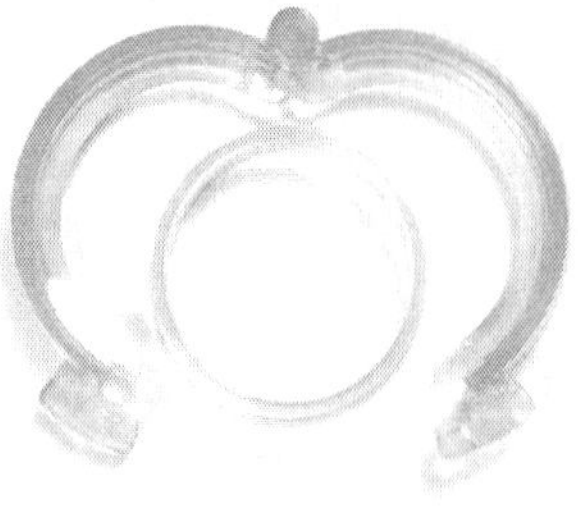

Fig. 13. The Shang Ring device.

Procedure: The "Shenghuan Disposable Minimally Invasive Circumcision Anastomosis Device", developed in China by Jianzhong Shang, involves minimal tissue manipulation and is said to give a simpler, quicker and safer circumcision than conventional techniques (Masson *et al.*, 2010). It consists of two concentric plastic rings that sandwich the foreskin of the penis, allowing circumcision without stitches or notable bleeding. As well as substantially reduced operating times, MC using this device is associated with a low complication rate, and the technique can easily be taught to both physicians and non-physicians. The Shang Ring is produced by Wuhu Snnda Medical Treatment Appliance Technology Co. Ltd, Wuhu City, China.

When tested on 1,200 patients aged 5 to 95 years operating time was 2.5 minutes for patients with excessive foreskin and 3.5 minutes for those with phimosis (Peng *et al.*, 2008). After application it is worn for a week, with no incidents of device dislocation or damage to the frenulum. Peng *et al.* describe the use of oral diethylstilbestrol (at a dosage of 2 mg/night) as a way to prevent nocturnal erections during the wear period. We do not find favour with this, due to the known environmental persistence of DES and the long-term effects of this synthetic oestrogen (Newbold *et al.*, 2006). In this study by Peng *et al.* the incision healed in 96.3%, leaving minimal inner foreskin, with no scarring and good cosmetic results. Antibiotics were not used, and only 0.67% got an infection. After removal, of the device 0.58% had some minimal bleeding around the incision and 2.4% had wound dehiscence of the incision caused by nocturnal erection, but this could be prevented by continuation of diethylstilbestrol for 3 days. It was treated by simply closing the incised rim with a butterfly adhesive plaster, followed by topical disinfectant; no stitches were required. Patients reported less pain than occurs for conventional methods.

Use of the Shang Ring has become a method of choice in the People's Republic of China. Evaluation of a standardized surgical protocol for its use, involving 328 men, showed an operating time of 4.7 ± 1.3 minutes, pain scores of 0.2 ± 0.6 during the surgery, 1.6 ± 1.0 24 hours postoperatively, 1.7 ± 1.1 twenty four hours prior to ring removal, and 2.7 ± 1.4 during ring removal (Cheng *et al.*, 2009). In this study, complications included infection in 0.6%, bleeding in 0.6% and wound dehiscence in 0.6%; none of the latter required suturing. Penile oedema occurred in 4.9%. The time for complete wound healing was 20.3 ± 6.7 days. Satisfaction was 99.7%.

A study in 824 boys with phimosis or redundant foreskin found duration was 2.6 ± 1.2 minutes (Yan *et al.*, 2010). Wounds healed and rings were removed at 13.4 ± 5.8 days revealing a well-smoothed incision and good cosmetic results. Complications were low and included infection in 0.6%, oedema in 3.2%, delayed removal of the ring in 1.5%, and redundant and asymmetric mucosa attributable to performance in 0.9%.

Another study in China, of 402 patients, found duration (4.7 ± 1.3) minutes, blood loss (2.6 ± 1.8 ml), and postoperative satisfaction (99.5%) for Shang Ring circumcision were significantly better than conventional circumcision, and International Index of Erectile Dysfunction (IIEF-5; not "IIRF-5" as stated in the paper) was no different (Li *et al.*, 2010). In 351 males aged 4 to 58 (mean 31) circumcised for phimosis or redundant foreskin using the Shang Ring, infection was seen in 1.4%, mild oedema in 2.6%, moderate oedema in 1.4%, and wound dishescence in 1.7%, with no postoperative bleeding being observed (Peng *et al.*, 2010b).

A proof of concept study in Kenya for the roll-out of MC for HIV prevention found a time of 4.8 ± 2.0 minutes for the procedure and 3.9 ± 2.6 minutes for device removal, with 6 mild adverse events in the 40 men who underwent Shang Ring circumcision (Barone *et al.*, 2011). These included 3 penile skin injuries, 2 cases of oedema and one infection, all of which resolved with conservative management. Partial ring detachment occurred in 3 between days 2 to 7, none of which required treatment or ring removal. Erections with the ring were well tolerated. By day 2, eighty percent of the men had returned to work, and at 42 days all said they were very satisfied with their circumcision and would recommend it to others.

Aside from the matter of diethylstilbestrol use, without which there appears to be a danger of an erection displacing the device, possible further criticisms relate to the discontinuity of the clamping ring at both the hinge and clasp. It should also be noted that it gives no protection whatsoever to the glans during the severing of the prepuce.

The same inventor has also obtained a patent in respect of another, more recent but very different design. The relevant patent is CN2009/000406. It is unclear whether the later design is intended to supersede the original, or compete with it.

10.6 SmartKlamp

Inventor:	Ten Have, H.F.
Primary patent:	MY0100375
Patent priority date:	30 Jan 2001
Patient age range:	Full-term neonate to mid-puberty
Website:	http://smartcircumcision.com/index.html
Category:	Ischaemic necrosis device

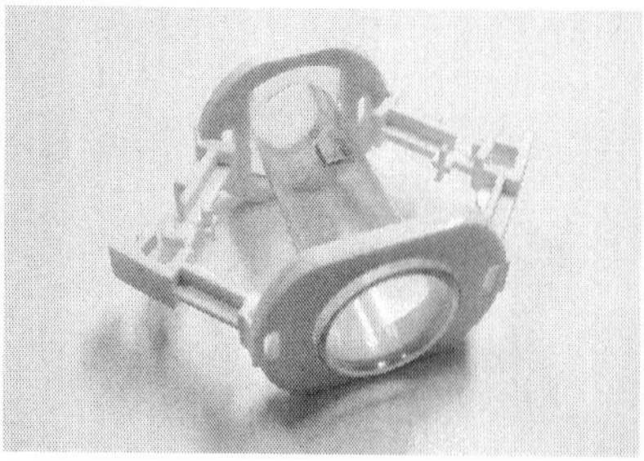

Fig. 14. The SmartKlamp.

Procedure: The SmartKlamp is an ischaemic necrosis device functioning in broadly the same way as the Ali's Klamp, Ismail Klamp and Tara KLamp.

Since its invention by Henri Ferdinand Ten Have, the commercial history of the SmartKlamp has to some extent interfered with its development and availability. Originally produced only in child sizes by the Dutch company Circumvent BV (Hengelo, The Netherlands), supply ceased when Circumvent BV went into liquidation, having apparently over-spent on research and development of the adult model. It should perhaps be noted that Circumvent's experimental adult device had an angled clamping ring similar in principle to that now found in the Ali's Klamp.

The apparently identical product in child sizes has now appeared in Malaysia, marketed by a supplier called Smartcircumcision. Aldemir and co-workers described the device thus: "This fits on the penis much as the others do. After 4 days the connection between its inner tube and casing is cut and removed. The inner tube is then left to fall off spontaneously in time. Median operative time is 8 minutes, compared with 18 minutes for conventional dissection, and cosmetic result, judged blinded by a urologist, was better. Parents' satisfaction scores were the same" (Aldemir *et al.*, 2008).

The SmartKlamp differs from the Ali's Klamp only in one significant respect: The clamping ring is not angled to match the typical slant of the coronal rim of the glans. In theory this achieves less satisfactory capture of inner foreskin ventrally, but the original manufacturer claimed it is possible to adjust the foreskin to compensate. The SmartKlamp apparently shares with the Ali's Klamp one notable design weakness. An unwilling or meddlesome patient could, in theory, open the clamp by placing a flat object such as a table knife between the tube and the locking arms and then twisting. Additionally, such action would render the

device liable to unscrupulous reuse several times over, until such time as the nominally single-use latching mechanism wore out.
A training video is available for purchase from the current supplier's website.

10.7 Sunathrone

Inventor:	Surat, T.b.
Primary patent:	(Application:) MY2006/000281
Patent priority date:	23 Jan 2006
Patient age range:	Full-term neonate to adult
Website:	http://www.sunathrone.com/
Category:	Ischaemic necrosis device

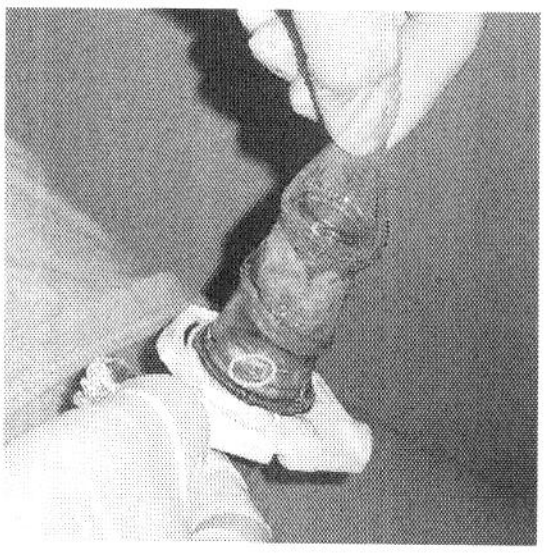

Fig. 15. The Sunathrone device.

Procedure: The Sunathrone clamp differs markedly from the other ischaemic necrosis devices considered here, in that the crushing action is achieved by means of a wrap-around "cuff" rather than concentric rings. Nominally this introduces a problem of pressure discontinuity at the hinge and latch, but Dr. Tasron bin Surat's design overcomes that by means of springy cuff extensions that bridge these gaps.
In order to achieve sufficient pressure between the cuff and the tube, a special tool called a "Sunalever" is required to close the Sunathrone clamp. This is a large item, sized according to the device being applied to the patient. It can be seen in use on the web page http://www.circlist.com/instrstechs/sunathrone.html. In the absence of on-site sterilization facilities, one Sunalever would have to be packaged with each clamp. This has implications in terms of cost, package size and waste disposal.
Two points in favour of this design are that the latching mechanism is highly tamper-resistant and, once the bayonet joint of the tube (ringed in yellow in the image above) is unplugged, nothing protrudes beyond the tip of the glans. The manufacturers claim suitability for use in cases of buried penis, the relatively large diameter of the cuff preventing the glans from withdrawing into the abdomen and forming adhesions during the healing period.

10.8 Tara KLamp

Inventor:	Singh, G.S.T.
Primary patent:	US5649933
Patent priority date:	20 Apr 1992
Patient age range:	Full-term neonate to adult

Website: Tara Medic does not have its own website. See instead: http://www.circlist.com/instrstechs/taraklamp.html

Category: Ischaemic necrosis device

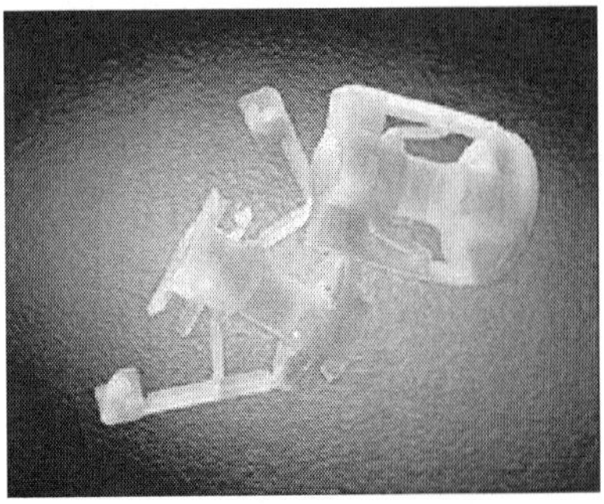

Fig. 16. The Tara KLamp.

Procedure: The Tara KLamp is the original single-use "clip-&-wear" ischaemic necrosis device to have gone into commercial production. Procedure for use is substantially the same as for the Ali's Klamp, Ismail Klamp and SmartKlamp. Since its invention nearly 20 years ago by Gurchran Singh Tara Singh, the Tara KLamp has undergone a number of design changes the most notable of which relates to its size, which has reduced considerably, thus making the current version more convenient to wear than the original.

The latching mechanism of the Tara KLamp is especially secure, making this design suitable for use on unwilling, meddlesome or autistic boys.

Considerable criticism of the Tara KLamp has arisen in consequence of a paper published by Lagarde and associates (Lagarde *et al.*, 2009). The authors of the present chapter are in possession of documentary evidence apparently proving that Lagarde's team did not attend Tara Medic's training course relating to use of the Tara KLamp. Furthermore, these documents also appear to show that Lagarde's team departed from the procedure set down in the package insert. If true, we suggest the resulting criticism of the Tara KLamp to be unfair and possibly unwarranted. Unpublished studies by the Health Department of KwaZulu-Natal apparently failed to replicate the problems and the Tara KLamp has now been accepted as the "preferred device" for use in Kwa-Zulu Natal.

We suggest that, at the very least, Lagarde's findings should be set aside pending further investigation. Safety and efficacy trials of the Tara KLamp should be repeated by a different team. Such a trial might usefully address one further issue: Whether or not the Tara KLamp can be successfully used without the foreskin being severed, instead leaving it to necrotise *in situ* as is done with the PrePex device.

11. World Health Organisation's preference?

Early in 2011 the World Health Organisation formed a Technical Advisory Group (TAG) with a remit to look at evidence and make recommendations to WHO regarding choice of circumcision clamp, but to date the TAG has not published any recommendations (Personal correspondence between co-author C. Eley and the co-Chairman on 21 Feb 2011). It is to be hoped that, when they do, it will be a shortlist for local consideration rather than a recommendation favouring one particular device globally. It is the considered opinion of the present authors that it would be inappropriate for there to be a single winner in this contest. The best clamp in any given situation is likely to be a function of local factors.

12. Conclusions

MC can be performed at any age, but infancy is the ideal time for reasons of safety, procedural simplicity, convenience, minimal risk and cost (Wiswell & Geschke, 1989; Wiswell & Hachey, 1993; Wiswell, 1995; Wiswell, 1997; Wiswell, 2000). The benefits in respect of UTIs and penile cancer are, moreover, maximized if circumcision takes place in infancy. Circumcising prior to onset of sexual activity rather than later also means a completely healed penis, so that risk of infection, such as by HIV, during the healing period is reduced.

Thus the present campaigns to circumcise adults should be seen as a mere catching-up exercise, making good past omissions to circumcise pre-puberty. The ultimate aim should be to make infant MC a global norm, the health rewards being too great to overlook (Morris, 2007; World Health Organisation, 2007a,b; Tobian *et al.*, 2009; Cooper et al., 2010).

MC has no long-term adverse consequences (Morris, 2007; Smith et al., 2010; Tobian et al., 2010). Good quality research studies that include thermal imaging show similar sensation during arousal for the circumcised and uncircumcised penis (Payne *et al.*, 2007). The lack of any diminution in sexual function, satisfaction or sensation is now backed up by evidence from large RCTs (Bailey et al., 2007; Krieger et al., 2008). In fact 64% of the men in one of the trials reported an increase in their penile sensitivity and 54% reported greater ease in reaching orgasm (Krieger et al., 2008). This did not mean an increase in premature ejaculation. The fact that circumcision does not impair, and for many may enhance, a man's sensation and sexual pleasure, should reassure men considering whether to get circumcised (Sharlip, 2008). MC is preferred by most women for reasons of hygiene, sexual activity, reduced STI risk, and greater enjoyment of intercourse (Williamson & Williamson, 1988; Badger, 1989a,b; Moses *et al.*, 1998; Nnko *et al.*, 2001; Kigozi *et al.*, 2009a).

Biomedical engineering clearly has its place in delivering MC, despite the existence of methods and traditions that are many thousands of years old. Recent progress in instrumentation design has resulted in devices that have begun to address the need for circumcisions that are quick, safe and convenient, and that can be used in "field" settings. Such advances in biomedical engineering are essential in ensuring a safe and practical way of dealing with the numbers of males of all ages in the modern world who need to be circumcised.

13. References

Alanis, M.C. & Lucidi, R.S. (2004). Neonatal circumcision: A review of the world's oldest and most controversial operation. *Obstet Gynecol Surv* 59, 379-395.

Aldemir, M., Cakan, M. & Burgu, B. (2008). Circumcision with a new disposable clamp: Is it really easier and more reliable? *Int Urol Nephrol* 40, 377-381.

Auvert, B., Taljaard, D., Lagarde, E., Sobngwi-Tambekou, J., Sitta, R. & Puren, A. (2005). Randomized, controlled intervention trial of male Circumcision for reduction of HIV infection risk: The ANRS 1265 Trial. *PLoS Med* 2 (e298), 1112-1122.

Badger, J. (1989a). The great circumcision report part 2. *Australian Forum* 2 (12), 4-13.

Badger, J. (1989b). Circumcision. What you think. *Australian Forum* 2 (11), 10-29.

Baeten, J.M., Donnell, D., Inambo, M., John-Stewart, G., Kapiga, S., Manongi, R., Ronald, A., Vwakila, B. & Celum, C. (2009). Male circumcision and risk of male-to-female HIV-1 transmission: A multinational prospective study. *5th International AIDS Society Conference, Cape Town, South Africa*, LBPEC06.

Baeten, J.M., Donnell, D., Kapiga, S.H., Ronald, A., John-Stewart, G., Inambao, M., Manongi, R., Vwalika, B. & Celum, C. (2010). Male circumcision and risk of male-to-female HIV-1 transmission: a multinational prospective study in African HIV-1-serodiscordant couples. *AIDS* 24, 737-744.

Bailey, R.C., Moses, S., Parker, C.B., Agot, K., Maclean, I., Krieger, J.N., Williams, C.F., Campbell, R.T. & Ndinya-Achola, J.O. (2007). Male circumcision for HIV prevention in young men in Kisumu, Kenya: a randomised controlled trial. *Lancet* 369, 643-656.

Bailey, R.C., Moses, S., Parker, C.B., Agot, K., Maclean, I., Krieger, J.N., Williams, C.F. & Ndinya-Achola, J.O. (2008). The protective effect of male circumcision is sustained for at least 42 months: results from the Kisumu, Kenya Trial. *XVII International AIDS Conference, 2008*, THAC05.

Bailey, R.C. & Mehta, S.D. (2009). Circumcision's place in the vicious cycle involving herpes simplex virus type 2 and HIV. *J Infect Dis* 199, 923-925.

Bailey, R.C., S. Moses, S., C.B. Parker, C.B., Agot, K., MacLean, I., Krieger, J.N., Williams, C.F.M. & Ndinya-Achola, J.O. (2010). The protective effect of adult male circumcision against HIV acquisition is sustained for at least 54 months: results from the Kisumu, Kenya trial. *XVIII International AIDS Confernece, Jul 18-23, 2010, Vienna*, Abstract#FRLBC1.

Balkan, C., Karapinar, D., Aydogdu, S., Ozcan, C., Ay, Y., Akin, M. & Kavakli, K. (2010). Surgery in patients with haemophilia and high responding inhibitors: Izmir experience. *Haemophilia* 16, 902-909.

Barone, M.A., Ndede, F., Li, P.S., Masson, P., Awori, Q., Okech, J., Cherutich, P., Muraguri, N., Perchal, P., Lee, R., Kim, H.H. & Goldstein, M. (2011). The Shang Ring device for adult male circumcision: A proof of concept study in Kenya. *J Acquir Immune Defic Syndr.*, Feb 21 [Epub ahead of print].

Ben Chaim, J., Livne, P.M., Binyamini, J., Hardak, B., Ben-Meir, D. & Mor, Y. (2005). Complications of circumcision in Israel: a one year multicenter survey. *Isr Med Assoc J* 7, 368-370.

Ben, K.L., Xu, J.C., Lu, L., Lü, N.Q., Cheng, Y., Tao, J., Liu, D.K., Min, X.D., Cao, X.M. & Li, P.S. (2009). [Male circumcision is an effective "surgical vaccine" for HIV prevention and reproductive health](in Chinese). *Zhonghua Nan Ke Xue* 15, 395-402.

Bode, C.O., Ikhisemojie, S. & Ademuyiwa, A.O. (2010). Penile injuries from proximal migration of the plastibell circumcision ring. *J Pediatr Urol* 6, 23-27

Boggiano, C. & Littman, D.R. (2007). HIV's vagina travelogue. *Immunity* 26, 145-147.

Bronstein, H. (1955). United States Patent US2747576 (Mogen clamp). (Priority date Feb 3,1955).

Caballero-Hoyos, R. & Villasenor-Sierra, A. (2001). [Socioeconomic strata as a predictor factor for constant condom use among adolescents] (Spanish). *Rev Saude Publica* 35, 531-538.

Cameron, B.E., Simonsen, J.N., D'Costa, L.J., Ronald, A.R., Maitha, G.M., Gakinya, M.N., Cheang, M., Dinya-Achola, J.O., Piot, P., Brunham, R.C. & Plummer, F.A. (1989). Female to male transmission of human immunodeficiency virus type 1: risk factors for seroconversion in men. *Lancet* ii, 403-407.

Cathcart, P., Nuttall, M., van der Meulen, J., Emberton, M. & Kenny, S.E. (2006). Trends in paediatric circumcision and its complications in England between 1997 and 2003. *Br J Surg* 93, 885-890.

Chekmarev, V.M. (1989). Union of Soviet Socialist Republics Patent SU1683702 (Laser Shield; Uzbek). (Priority date Jul 19,1989).

Cheng, D., Hurt, L. & Horon, I.L. (2008). Neonatal circumcision in Maryland: a comparison of hospital discharge and maternal postpartum survey data. *J Pediatr Urol* 4, 448-451.

Cheng, W. & Saing, H. (1997). A prospective randomized study of wound approximation with tissue glue in circumcision in children. *J Paediatr Child Health* 33, 515-516.

Cheng, Y., Peng, Y.F., Liu, Y.D., Tian, L., Lü, N.Q., Su, X.J., Yan, Z.J., Hu, J.S., Lee, R., Kim, H.H., Sokal, D.C. & Li, P.S. (2009). [A recommendable standard protocol of adult male circumcision with the Chinese Shang Ring: outcomes of 328 cases in China] [Article in Chinese]. *Zhonghua Nan Ke Xue* 15, 584-592.

Christakis, D.A., Harvey, E., Zerr, D.M., Feudtner, C., Wright, J.A. & Connell, F.A. (2000). A trade-off analysis of routine newborn circumcision. *Pediatrics* 105, 246-249.

Cilento, B.G.J., Holmes, N.M. & Canning, D.A. (1999). Plastibell complications revisited. *Clin Pediatr* 38, 239-242.

Coates, T.J., Richter, L. & Caceres, C. (2008). Behavioural strategies to reduce HIV transmission: how to make them work better. *Lancet* 372, 669-684.

Cohen, B. (2002). United States Patent US7080984 (Circumcision training aid). (Priority date Apr 29, 2002).

Cooper, D.A., Wodak, A.D. & Morris, B.J. (2010). The case for boosting infant male circumcision in the face of rising heterosexual transmission of HIV. *Med J Aust* 193, 318-319.

D'Arcy, F.T. & Jaffry, S.Q. (2011). A review of 100 consecutive sutureless child and adult circumcisions. *Ir J Med Sci* 180, 51-53.

de Witte, L., Nabatov, A., Pion, M., Fluitsma, D., de Jong, M.A., de Gruijl, T., Piguet, V., van Kooyk, Y. & Geijtenbeek, T.B. (2007). Langerin is a natural barrier to HIV-1 transmission by Langerhans cells. *Nat Med* 13, 367-371.

Decastro, B., Gurski, J. & Peterson, A. (2010). Adult template circumcision: a prospective, randomized, patient-blinded, comparative study evaluating the safety and efficacy of a novel circumcision device. *Urology* 76, 810-814.

Donovan, B. & Ross, M.W. (2000). Preventing HIV: determinants of sexual behaviour (review). *Lancet* 355, 1897-1901.

Duncan, N.D., Dundas, S.E., Brown, B., Pinnock-Ramsaran, C. & Badal, G. (2004). Newborn circumcision using the Plastibell device: an audit of practice. *West Indian Med J* 53, 23-26.

Elder, J.S. (2007). Surgery illustrated: circumcision. *BJU Int* 99, 1553-1564.

Elemen, L., Seyidov, T.H. & Tugay, M. (2010). The advantages of cyanoacrylate wound closure in circumcision. *Pediatr Surg Int*, Oct 13 [Epub ahead of print].

Elmore, J.M., Smith, E.A. & Kirsch, A.J. (2007). Sutureless circumcision using 2-octyl cyanoacrylate (Dermabond): appraisal after 18-month experience. *Urology* 70, 803-806.

Erikson, S.S. (1999). A model for teaching newborn circumcision. *Obstet Gynecol* 93, 783-784.

Fahrbach, K.M., Barry, S.M., Anderson, M.R. & Hope, T.J. (2010). Enhanced cellular responses and environmental sampling within inner foreskin explants: implications for the foreskin's role in HIV transmission. *Mucosal Immunol* 3, 410-418.

Fergusson, D.M., Boden, J.M. & Horwood, L.J. (2008). Neonatal circumcision: Effects on breastfeeding and outcomes associated with breastfeeding. *J Paediatr Child Health* 44, 44-49.

Ferrante, P., Delbue, S. & Mancuso, R. (2005). The manifestation of AIDS in Africa: an epidemiological overview. *J Neurovirol* 11 (suppl 1), 50-57.

Fette, A., Schleaf, J., Haberlik, A. & Seebacher, U. (2000). Circumcision in paediatric surgery using an ultasound dissection scalpel. *Technol Hlth Care* 8, 75-79.

Fiore, A.E., David K. Shay, D.K., Penina Haber, P., Iskander, J.K., Uyeki, T.M., Mootrey, G., Bresee, J.S. & Cox, N.J. (2007). Prevention and Control of Influenza. Recommendations of the Advisory Committee on Immunization Practices (ACIP), 2007. *Centers for Disease Control and Prevention - Mortality and Morbidity Weekly Report* 56, 1-54.

Freeman, E.E., Weiss, H.A., Glynn, J.R., Cross, P.L., Whitworth, J.A. & Hayes, R.J. (2006). Herpes simplex virus 2 infection increases HIV acquisition in men and women: systematic review and meta-analysis of longitudinal studies. *AIDS* 20, 73-83.

Fuerst, O., Kilemnick & Shohat, S. (2010). Israel Patent Application IL2010/000568 (PrePex). (Priority date Jul 16, 2009).

Ganor, Y., Zhou, Z., Tudor, D., Schmitt, A., Vacher-Lavenu, M.C., Gibault, L., Thiounn, N., Tomasini, J., Wolf, J.P. & Bomsel, M. (2010). Within 1 h, HIV-1 uses viral synapses to enter efficiently the inner, but not outer, foreskin mucosa and engages Langerhans-T cell conjugates. *Mucosal Immunol* 3, 506-522.

Ganor, Y. & Bomsel, M. (2011). HIV-1 transmission in the male genital tract. *Am J Reprod Immunol*, 65, 284-291.

Gao, X. & Ni, J. (1999). People's Republic of China Patent CN2351094 (Gao's Laser Shield). (Priority date Jan 16, 1999).

Gebremedhin, S. (2010). Assessment of the protective effect of male circumcision from HIV infection and sexually transmitted diseases: evidence from 18 demographic and health surveys in sub-Saharan Africa. *Afr J Reprod Health* 14, 105-113.

Gee, W.F. & Ansell, J.S. (1976). Neonatal circumcision: A ten-year overview, with comparison of the Gomco clamp and the Plastibell device. *Pediatrics* 58, 824-827.

Gnassingbé, K., Akakpo-Numado, K.G., Anoukoum, T., Songne, B., Lamboni, D., Kokoroko, E.K. & Tékou, H.A. (2010). [The circumcision in newborn and infant in the operating room of the Lomé Teaching Hospital: technique using Gomco clamp versus technique using only the grips]. (Article in French). *Prog Urol* 20, 532-537.

Goldstein, A.A. (1939). United States Design Patent USD119180 (Gomco Clamp). (Priority date Mar 16,1939).

Goubet, N., Rattaz, C., Pierrat, V., Bullinger, A. & Lequien, P. (2003). Olfactory experience mediates response to pain in preterm newborns. *Dev Psychobiol* 42, 171-180.

Goubet, N., Strasbaugh, K. & Chesney, J. (2007). Familiarity breeds content? Soothing effect of a familiar odor on full-term newborns. *J Dev Behav Pediatr* 28, 189-194.

Gray, R.H., Kigozi, G., Serwadda, D., Makumbi, F., Watya, S., Nalugoda, F., Kiwanuka, N., Moulton, L.H., Chaudhary, M.A., Chen, M.Z., Sewankambo, N.K., Wabwire-Mangen, F., Bacon, M.C., Williams, C.F., Opendi, P., Reynolds, S.J., Laeyendecker, O., Quinn, T.C. & Wawer, M.J. (2007). Male circumcision for HIV prevention in men in Rakai, Uganda: a randomised trial. *Lancet* 369, 657-666.

Gray, R.H., Wawer, M.J., Kigozi, G. & Serwadda, D. (2008). Commentary: Disease modelling to inform policy on male circumcision for HIV prevention. *Int J Epidemiol* 37, 1253-1254.

Haghpanah, S., Vafafar, A., Golzadeh, M.H., Ardeshiri, R. & Karimi, M. (2011). Use of Glubran 2 and Glubran tissue skin adhesive in patients with hereditary bleeding disorders undergoing circumcision and dental extraction. *Ann Hematol* 90, 463-468.

Hallett, T.B., Alsallaq, R.A., Baeten, J.M., Weiss, H., Celum, C., Gray, R. & Abu-Raddad, L. (2011). Will circumcision provide even more protection from HIV to women and men? New estimates of the population impact of circumcision interventions. *Sex Transm Infect*, 2010 87, 88-93

Halperin, D.T., Steiner, M.J., Cassell, M.M., Green, E.C., Hearst, N., Kirby, D., Gayle, H.D. & Cates, W. (2004). The time has come for common ground on preventing sexual transmission of HIV. *Lancet* 364, 1913-1915.

Herschel, M., Khoshnood, B., Ellman, C., Maydew, N. & Mittendorf, R. (1998). Neonatal circumcision. Randomized trial of a sucrose pacifier for pain control. *Arch Pediatr Adolesc Med* 152, 279-284.

Hirbod, T., Bailey, R.C., Agot, K., Moses, S., Ndinya-Achola, J., Murugu, R., Andersson, J., Nilsson, J. & Broliden, K. (2010). Abundant expression of HIV target cells and C-type lectin receptors in the foreskin tissue of young Kenyan men. *Am J Pathol* 176, 2798-2805.

Hladik, F., Sakchalathorn, P., Ballweber, L., Lentz, G., Fialkow, M., Eschenbach, D. & McElrath, M.J. (2007). Initial events in establishing vaginal entry and infection by human immunodeficiency virus type-1. *Immunity* 26, 257-270.

Holman, J.R., Lewis, E.L. & Ringler, R.L. (1995). Neonatal circumcision techniques. *Am Fam Physician* 52, 511-520.

Howard, C., Howard, F., Garfunkel, L., de, B. & Weitzman, M. (1998). Neonatal circumcision and pain relief: Current training practices. *Pediatrics* 101, 423-8.

Howard, C.R., Howard, F.M., Fortune, K., Generalli, P., Zolnoun, D., ten Hoopen, C. & de Blieck, E. (1999). A randomized, controlled trial of a eutectic mixture of local anesthetic cream (lidocaine and prilocaine) versus penile nerve block for pain relief during circircumcision. *Am J Obstet Gynecol* 181, 1506-1511.

Jadack, R.A., Yuenger, J., Ghanem, K.G. & Zenilman, J. (2006). Polymerase chain reaction detection of Y-chromosome sequences in vaginal fluid of women accessing a sexually transmitted disease clinic. *Sex Transm Dis* 33, 22-25.

Johnson, K.E., Sherman, M.E., Ssempiija, V., Tobian, A.A., Zenilman, J.M., Duggan, M.A., Kigozi, G., Serwadda, D., Wawer, M.J., Quinn, T.C., Rabkin, C.S. & Gray, R.H. (2009). Foreskin inflammation is associated with HIV and herpes simplex virus type-2 infections in Rakai, Uganda. *AIDS* 23, 1807-1815.

Kamra, S. (2002). *Bearing Witness.* Calgary, University of Calgary Press.

Kang, M., Rochford, A., Johnston, V., Jackson, J., Freedman, E., Brown, K. & Mindel, A. (2006). Prevalence of Chlamydia trachomatis infection among 'high risk' young people in New South Wales. *Sex Health* 3, 253-254.

Karaman, M.I., Zulfikar, B., Caskurlu, T. & Ergenekon, E. (2004). Circumcision in hemophilia: a cost-effective method using a novel device. *J Pediatr Surg* 39, 1562-1564.

Kariher, D.H. & Smith, T.W. (1955). United States Patent US3056407 (Plastibell). (Priority date May 18, 1955).

Kaufman, G.E., Cimo, S., Miller, L.W. & Blass, E.M. (2002). An evaluation of the effects of sucrose on neonatal pain with 2 commonly used circumcision methods. *Am J Obstet Gynecol* 186, 564-568.

Kazem, M.M., Mehdi, A.Z., Golrasteh, K.Z. & Behzad, F.Z. (2010). Comparative evaluation of two techniques of hemostasis in neonatal circumcision using plastibell device. *J Pediatr Urol*, 6, 258-260

Kelly, H., Carville, K., Grant, K., Jacoby, P., Tran, T. & Barr, I. (2009). Estimation of influenza vaccine effectiveness from routine surveillance data. *PLoS One* 4 (7 pages), e5079.

Kigozi, G., Lukabwe, I., Kagaayi, J., Wawer, M.J., Nantume, B., Kigozi, G., Nalugoda, F., Kiwanuka, N., Wabwire-Mangen, F., Serwadda, D., Ridzon, R., Buwembo, D., Nabukenya, D., Watya, S., Lutalo, T., Nkale, J. & Gray, R.H. (2009a). Sexual satisfaction of women partners of circumcised men in a randomized trial of male circumcision in Rakai, Uganda. *BJU Int* 104, 1698-1701.

Kigozi, G., Wawer, M., Ssettuba, A., Kagaayi, J., Nalugoda, F., Watya, S., Mangen, F.W., Kiwanuka, N., Bacon, M.C., Lutalo, T., Serwadda, D. & Gray, R.H. (2009b). Foreskin surface area and HIV acquisition in Rakai, Uganda (size matters). *AIDS* 23, 2209-2213.

Kigozi, G., Nkale, J., Wawer, M., Anyokorit, M., Watya, S., Nalugoda, F., Kagaayi, J., Kiwanuka, N., Mwinike, J., Kighoma, N., Nalwoga, G.K., Nakigozi, G.F., Katwalo, H., Serwadda, D. & Gray, R.H. (2011). Designing and usage of a low-cost penile model for male medical circumcision skills training in Rakai, Uganda. *Urology*, Feb 4 [Epub ahead of print].

Kong, X., Kigozi, G., Ssempija, V., Serwadda, D., Nalugoda, F., Makumbi, F., 2, T Lutalo, T, , Watya, S., Wawer, M. & R Gray, R. (2011). Longer-term effects of male circumcision on HIV incidence and risk behaviors during post-trial surveillance in Rakai, Uganda. *18th Conference on Retroviruses and Opportunistic Infections, Boston, Feb 27-Mar 2, 2011*, Abstract#36.

Krieger, J.N., Bailey, R.C., Opeya, J.C., Ayieko, B.O., Opiyo, F.A., Omondi, D., Agot, K., Parker, C., Ndinya-Achola, J.O. & Moses, S. (2007). Adult male circumcision outcomes: experience in a developing country setting. *Urol Int* 78, 235-240.

Krieger, J.N., Mehta, S.D., Bailey, R.C., Agot, K., Ndinya-Achola, J.O., Parker, C. & Moses, S. (2008). Adult male circumcision: Effects on sexual function and sexual satisfaction in Kisumu, Kenya. *J Sex Med* 5, 2610-2622.

Kunin, S.A. (2007a). Improved newborn circumcision utilizing dorsal foreskin local anesthesia (DFLA) with Gomco clamp. *Western Section Urological meeting Oct 28-Nov 1, Scottsdale, Arizona*, http://www.samkuninmd.com/docinfo/Improved_GOMCO_Circumcision_abstract.pdf.

Kunin, S.A. (2007b). Dorsal foreskin local anesthesia (DFLA), a new rapid and safe method for infant circumcision anesthesia. *Western Section Urological meeting Oct 28-Nov 1, Scottsdale, Arizona,* http://www.samkuninmd.com/docinfo/Dorsal_Foreskin_Local_Anesthesia.pdf.

Kurtis, P.S., DeSilva, H.N., Bernstein, B.A., Malakh, L. & Schrechter, N.L. (1999). A comparison of the Mogen and Gomco clamps in combination with dorsal penile nerve block in minimizing the pain of neonatal circumcision. *Pediatrics* 103, E23.

Lagarde, E., Taljaard, D., Puren, A. & Auvert, B. (2009). High rate of adverse events following circumcision of young male adults with the Tara KLamp technique: a randomised trial in South Africa. *S Afr Med J* 99, 163-169.

Lane, V., Vajda, P. & Subramaniam, R. (2010). Paediatric sutureless circumcision: a systematic literature review. *Pediatr Surg Int* 26, 141-144.

Langer, J.C. & Coplen, D.E. (1998). Circumcision and pediatric disorders of the penis. *Pediatr Clin N Am* 45, 801-812.

Leibowitz, A.A., Desmond, K. & Belin, T. (2009). Determinants and policy implications of male circumcision in the United States. *Am J Public Health* 99, 138-145.

Li, H.N., Xu, J. & Qu, L.M. (2010). [Shang Ring circumcision versus conventional surgical procedures: comparison of clinical effectiveness]. (Article in Chinese). *Zhonghua Nan Ke Xue* 16, 325-327.

Lopman, B., Nyamukapa, C., Mushati, P., Mupambireyi, Z., Mason, P., Garnett, G.P. & Gregson, S. (2008). HIV incidence in 3 years of follow-up of a Zimbabwe cohort--1998-2000 to 2001-03: contributions of proximate and underlying determinants to transmission. *Int J Epidemiol* 37, 88-105.

Mahomed, A., Zaparackaite, I. & Adam, S. (2009). Improving outcome from Plastibell circumcisions in infants. *Int Braz J Urol* 35, 310-313.

Masson, P., Li, P.S., Barone, M.A. & Goldstein, M. (2010). The ShangRing device for simplified adult circumcision. *Nat Rev Urol* 7, 638-642.

McCoombe, S.G. & Short, R.V. (2006). Potential HIV-1 target cells in the human penis. *AIDS* 20, 1491-1495.

Mehta, S.D., Krieger, J.N., Agot, K., Moses, S., Ndinya-Achola, J.O., Parker, C. & Bailey, R.C. (2010). Circumcision and reduced risk of self-reported penile coital injuries: Results from a randomized controlled trial in Kisumu, Kenya. *J Urol* 184, 203-209.

Meijer, J.M. (2008). New electrostatic sanitation method could have medical device sterilization uses, from http://jmmeijer.wordpress.com/2008/12/17/electrostatic-sterilization-method/.

Méndez-Gallart, R., Estévez, E., Bautista, A., Rodríguez, P., Taboada, P., Armas, A.L., Pradillos, J.M. & Varela, R. (2009). Bipolar scissors circumcision is a safe, fast, and bloodless procedure in children. *J Pediatr Surg* 44, 2048-2053.

Morris, B.J., Castellsague, X. & Bailis, S.A. (2006). Re: Cost analysis of neonatal circumcision in a large health maintenance organization. E. J. Schoen, C. J. Colby and T. T. To. J Urol, 175: 1111-1115, 2006. *J Urol* 176, 2315-2316.

Morris, B.J. (2007). Why circumcision is a biomedical imperative for the 21st century. *BioEssays* 29, 1147-1158.

Morris, B.J., Bailis, S.A., Waskett, J.H., Wiswell, T.E. & Halperin, D.T. (2009). Medicaid coverage of newborn circumcision: a health parity right of the poor. *Am J Public Health* 99, 969-971.

Morris, B.J. (2010). Circumcision: an evidence-based appraisal - medical, health and sexual. [Review]. http://www.circinfo.net (over 1,000 references).

Morris, B.J. & Castellsague, X. (2011). The role of circumcision in the prevention of sexually transmitted infections. *Sexually Transmitted Diseases*. Gross, G.E. & Tyring, S. Heidelberg, Springer: 715-739

Morris, B.J., Gray, R.H., Castellsague, X., Bosch, F.X., Halperin, D.T., Waskett, J.H. & Hankins, C.A. (2011). The strong protection afforded by circumcision against cancer of the penis. (Invited Review). *Adv Urol*, (21 pages): in press.

Moses, S., Bailey, R.C. & Ronald, A.R. (1998). Male circumcision: assessment of health benefits and risks. *Sex Transm Inf* 74, 368-373.

Mousa, G.S. (2007). *Surgery training video "Circumcision: Dissection Method" made for the Faculty of Medicine, Tanta University, Egypt, Jan 16, 2007.*

Munro, H.L., Pradeep, B.S., Jayachandran, A.A., Lowndes, C.M., Mahapatra, B., Ramesh, B.M., Washington, R., Jagannathan, L., Mendonca, K., Moses, S., Blanchard, J.F. & Alary, M. (2008). Prevalence and determinants of HIV and sexually transmitted infections in a general population-based sample in Mysore district, Karnataka state, southern India. *AIDS* 22 (suppl 5), S117-S125.

Naimer, S.A. & Trattner, A. (2000). Are sterile conditions essential for all forms of cutaneous surgery? The case of ritual neonatal circumcision. *J Cutan Med Surg* 4, 177-180.

Newbold, R.R., Padilla-Banks, E. & Jefferson, W.N. (2006). Adverse effects of the model environmental estrogen diethylstilbestrol are transmitted to subsequent generations. *Endocrinology* 147 (Suppl), S11-S17.

Nnko, S., Washija, R., Urassa, M. & Boerma, J.T. (2001). Dynamics of male circumcision practices in Northwest Tanzania. *Sex Transm Dis* 28, 214-218.

O'Farrell, N., Quigley, M. & Fox, P. (2005). Association between the intact foreskin and inferior standards of male genital hygiene behaviour: a cross-sectional study. *Int J STD AIDS* 16, 556-559.

O'Farrell, N., Morison, L., Moodley, P., Pillay, K., Vanmali, T., Quigley, M., Hayes, R. & Sturm, A.W. (2006). Association between HIV and subpreputial penile wetness in uncircumcised men in South Africa. *J Acquir Immune Defic Syndr* 43, 69-77.

Ozkan, K.U., Gonen, M., Sahinkanat, T., Resim, S. & Celik, M. (2005). Wound approximation with tissue glue in circumcision. *Int J Urol* 12, 374-377.

Patterson, B.K., Landy, A., Siegel, J.N., Flener, Z., Pessis, D., Chaviano, A. & Bailey, R.C. (2002). Susceptibility to human immunodeficiency virus-1 infection of human foreskin and cervical tissue grown in explant culture. *Am J Pathol* 161, 867-873.

Payne, K., Thaler, L., Kukkonen, T., Carrier, S. & Binik, Y. (2007). Sensation and sexual arousal in circumcised and uncircumcised men. *J Sex Med* 4, 667-674.

Peng, Y., Masson, P., Li, P.S., Chang, Y., Tian, L., Lee, R., Kim, H., Sokal, D.C. & Goldstein, M. (2010a). No-needle local anesthesia for adult male circumcision. *J Urol* 184, 978-983.

Peng, Y.F., Cheng, Y., Wang, G.Y., Wang, S.Q., Jia, C., Yang, B.H., Zhu, R., Jian, S.C., Li, Q.W. & Geng, D.W. (2008). Clinical application of a new device for minimally invasive circumcision. *Asian J Androl* 10, 447-454.

Peng, Y.F., Yang, B.H., Jia, C. & Jiang, J. (2010b). [Standardized male circumcision with Shang Ring reduces postoperative complications: a report of 351 cases]. (Article in Chinese). *Zhonghua Nan Ke Xue* 16, 963-966.

Peters, K.M. & Kass, E.J. (1997). Electrosurgery for routine pediatric penile procedures. *J Urol* 157, 1453-1455.

Peterson, A.C., Joyner, B.D. & Allen, R.C., Jr. (2001). Plastibell template circumcision: a new technique. *Urology* 58, 603-604.

Ponsky, L.E., Ross, J.H., Knipper, N. & Kay, R. (2000). Penile adhesions after neonatal circumcision. *J Urol* 164, 495-496.

Rattaz, C., Goubet, N. & Bullinger, A. (2005). The calming effect of a familiar odor on full-term newborns. *J Dev Behav Pediatr* 26, 86-92.

Richters, J., Smith, A.M., de Visser, R.O., Grulich, A.E. & Rissel, C.E. (2006). Circumcision in Australia: prevalence and effects on sexual health. *Int J STD AIDS* 17, 547-554.

Ross, C.J. (1939). United States Patent US2272072 (Ross Ring). (Priority date May 22, 1939).

Russell, C.T. & Chaseling, J. (1996). Topical anaesthesia in neonatal circumcision: a study of 208 consecutive cases. *Aust Fam Physician* 25 (suppl 1), 30-34.

Sahasrabuddhe, V.V. & Vermund, S.H. (2007). The future of HIV prevention: control of sexually transmitted infections and circumcision interventions. *Infect Dis Clin North Am* 21, 241-257.

Samad, A., Khanzada, T.W. & Kumar, B. (2010). Plastibell circumcision: A minor surgical procedure of major importance. *J Pediatr Urol* 6, 28-31

Sanchez, T., Finlayson, T., Drake, A., Behel, S., Cribbin, M., Dinenno, E., Hall, T., Kramer, S. & Lansky, A. (2006). Human immunodeficiency virus (HIV) risk, prevention, and testing behaviors--United States, National HIV Behavioral Surveillance System: men who have sex with men, November 2003-April 2005. *MMWR Surveill Summ* 55, 1-16.

Sansom, S.L., Prabhu, V.S., Hutchinson, A.B., An, Q., Hall, H.I., Shrestha, R.K., Lasry, A. & Taylor, A.W. (2010). Cost-effectiveness of newborn circumcision in reducing lifetime HIV risk among U.S. males. *PLoS One* 5, e8723.

Schoen, E.J. (2005). Circumcision for preventing urinary tract infections in boys: North American view. *Arch Dis Child* 90, 772-773.

Schoen, E.J., Colby, C.J. & To, T.T. (2006). Cost analysis of neonatal circumcision in a large health maintenance organization. *J Urol* 175, 1111-1115.

Schoen, E.J. (2007a). Male circumcision. *Male Sexual Dysfunction. Pathophysiology and Treatment.* Kandeel, F.R.Lue, T.F.Pryor, J.L. & Swerdloff, R.S. New York, Informa: 95-107.

Schoen, E.J. (2007b). Circumcision as a lifetime vaccination with many benefits. *J Men's Hlth Gender* 382, 306-311.

Schwartz, O. (2007). Langerhans cells lap up HIV-1. *Nat Med* 13, 245-246.

Senel, F.M., Demirelli, M. & Oztek, S. (2010). Minimally invasive circumcision with a novel plastic clamp technique: a review of 7,500 cases. *Pediatr Surg Int*, 739-745.

Senel, F.M., Demirelli, M. & Pekcan, H. (2011). Mass circumcision with a novel plastic clamp technique. *Urology*, Feb 8 [Epub ahead of print].

Sewefy, A.M.H. (2004). Egyptian Patent EG2004/000050 (Haemophilic Circumcisor). (Priority date Apr 18, 2004).

Sharlip, I. (2008). Circumcision and the risk of HIV transmission in Africa. *J Sex Med* 5, 2481-2484.

Short, R.V. (2004). Male circumcision: a scientific perspective. *J Med Ethics* 30, 241.

Short, R.V. (2006). New ways of preventing HIV infection: thinking simply, simply thinking. (Review). *Philos Trans R Soc Lond B Biol Sci* 361, 811-820.

Siegfried, N., Muller, M., Deeks, J.J. & Volmink, J. (2009). Male circumcision for prevention of heterosexual acquisition of HIV in men. *Cochrane Database Syst Rev* CD003362 (38 pp).

Siegfried, N., Muller, M., Deeks, J.J. & Volmink, J. (2010). Male circumcision for preventing heterosexual acquisition of HIV in men. *Int J Epidemiol* 39, 968-972.

Slaymaker, E. (2004). A critique of international indicators of sexual risk behaviour. *Sex Transm Infect* 80 (Suppl 2), ii13-ii21.

Smith, D.K., Taylor, A., Kilmarx, P.H., Sullivan, P., Warner, L., Kamb, M., Bock, N., Kohmescher, B. & Mastro, T.D. (2010). Male circumcision in the United States for the prevention of HIV infection and other adverse health outcomes: Report from a CDC consultation. *Public Health Reports* 125 (Suppl 1), 72-82.

Stang, H., Snellman, L., Condon, L., Conroy, M., Liebo, R., Brodersen, L. & Gunnar, M. (1997). Beyond dorsal penile nerve block: A more humane circumcision. *Pediatrics* 100, http://www.pediatrics.org/cgi/content/full/100/2/e3.

Stang, H.J. & Snellman, L.W. (1998). Circumcision practice patterns in the United States. *Pediatrics* 101, E51-E56.

Subramaniam, R. & Jacobsen, A.S. (2004). Sutureless circumcision: a prospective randomised controlled study. *Pediatr Surg Int* 20, 783-785.

Szabo, R. & Short, R.V. (2000). How does male circumcision protect against HIV infection? *Brit Med J* 320, 1592-1594.

Taddio, A., Stevens, B., Craig, K., Rastogi, P., Bendavid, S., Shennan, A., Mulligan, P. & Koren, G. (1997). Efficacy and safety of lidocaine-prilocaine cream for pain during circumcision. *N Engl J Med* 336, 1197-1201.

Taeusch, H.W., Martinez, A.M., Partridge, J.C., Sniderman, S., Armstrong-Wells, J. & Fuentes-Afflick, E. (2002). Pain during Mogen or PlastiBell circumcision. *J Perinatol* 22, 214-218.

Tagami, T. (2010). Atlanta lawyer wins $11 million lawsuit for family in botched circumcision. *The Atlanta Journal-Constitution* (http://www.ajc.com/news/nation-world/atlanta-lawyer-wins-11-573890.html).

Thedford, T.R. (1983). *Sheep Health Handbook. A Field Guide for Producers with Limited Veterinary Services.* Little Rock Arkansas, Winrock International.

Tobian, A.A., Gray, R.H. & Quinn, T.C. (2010). Male circumcision for the prevention of acquisition and transmission of sexually transmitted infections: the case for neonatal circumcision. *Arch Pediatr Adolesc Med* 164, 78-84.

Tobian, A.A.R., Serwadda, D., Quinn, T.C., Kigozi, G., Gravitt, P.E., Laeyendecker, O., Charvat, B., Ssempijja, V., Riedesel, M., Oliver, A.E., Nowak, R.G., Moulton, L.H., Chen, M.Z., Reynolds, S.J., Wawer, M.J. & Gray, R.H. (2009). Male circumcision for the prevention of HSV-2 and HPV infections and syphilis. *N Engl J Med* 360, 1298-1309.

Turville, S.G., Cameron, P.U., Handley, A., Lin, G., Pohlmann, S., Doms, R.W. & Cunningham, A.L. (2002). Diversity of receptors binding HIV on dendritic cell subsets. *Nat Immunol* 3, 975-983.

USPTO. United States Patent and Trademark Office database category 606/118. From http://www.uspto.gov.

Uthman, O.A., Popoola, T.A., Yahaya, I., Uthman, M.M. & Aremu, O. (2011). The cost-utility analysis of adult male circumcision for prevention of heterosexual acquisition of HIV in men in sub-Saharan Africa: a probabilistic decision model. *Value Health* 14, 70-79.

Wamai, R.G., Weiss, H.A., Hankins, C., Agot, K., Karim, Q.A., Shisana, O., Bailey, R.C., Betukumesu, B., Bongaarts, J., Bowa, K., Cash, R., Cates, W., Diallo, M.O., Dludlu, S., Geffen, N., Heywood, M., Jackson, H., Kayembe, P.K., Kapiga, S., Kebaabetswe, P., Kintaudi, L., Klausner, J.D., Leclerc-Madlala, S., Mabuza, K., Makhubele, M.B., Miceni, K., Morris, B.J., de Moya, A., Ncala, J., Ntaganira, I., Nyamucherera, O.F., Otolorin, E.O., Pape, J.W., Phiri, M., Rees, H., Ruiz, M., Sanchez, J., Sawires, S., Seloilwe, E.S., Serwadda, D.M., Setswe, G., Sewankambo, N., Simelane, D., Venter, F., Wilson, D., Woelk, G., Zungu, N. & Halperin, D.T. (2008). Male circumcision is an efficacious, lasting and cost-effective strategy for combating HIV in high-prevalence AIDS epidemics: Time to move beyond debating the science. *Future HIV Ther* 2, 399-405.

Wan, J. (2002). GOMCO circumcision clamp; an enduring and unexpected success. *Urology* 59, 790-794.

Wang, X., Wu, Y., Ni, X., Xia, B., Xu, J. & Du, Q. (1992). [Research on sterilization of pathogens by high electrostatic voltage method]. (Article in Chinese). *Zhongguo Zhong Yao Za Zhi (China J Chinese Materia Medica)* 17, 604-606.

Wawer, M.J., Makumbi, F., Kigozi, G., Serwadda, D., Watya, S., Nalugoda, F., Buwembo, D., Ssempijja, V., Kiwanuka, N., Moulton, L.H., Sewankambo, N.K., Reynolds, S.J., Quinn, T.C., Opendi, P., Iga, B., Ridzon, R., Laeyendecker, O. & Gray, R.H. (2009). Circumcision in HIV-infected men and its effect on HIV transmission to female partners in Rakai, Uganda: a randomised controlled trial. *Lancet* 374, 229-237.

Wawer, M.J., Tobian, A.A.R., Kigozi, G., Kong, X., Gravitt, P.E., Serwadda, D., Nalugoda, F., Makumbi, F., Ssempiija, V., Sewankambo, N., Watya, S., Eaton, K.P., Oliver, A.E., Chen, M.Z., Reynonds, S.J., Quinn, T.C. & Gray, R.H. (2011). Effect of circumcision of HIV-negative men on transmission of human papillomavirus to HIV-negative women: a randomised trial in Rakai, Uganda. *Lancet* 377, 209-218.

Weiss, H.A., Thomas, S.L., Munabi, S.K. & Hayes, R.J. (2006). Male circumcision and risk of syphilis, chancroid, and genital herpes: a systematic review and meta-analysis. *Sex Transm Infect* 82, 101-109.

Weiss, H.A., Halperin, D., Bailey, R.C., Hayes, R.J., Schmid, G. & Hankins, C.A. (2008). Male circumcision for HIV prevention: from evidence to action? (Review). *AIDS* 22, 567-574.

Weiss, H.A., Hankins, C.A. & Dickson, K. (2009). Male circumcision and risk of HIV infection in women: a systematic review and meta-analysis. *Lancet Infect Dis* 9, 669-677.

Williams, B.G., Lloyd-Smith, J.O., Gouws, E., Hankins, C., Getz, W.M., Hargrove, J., de Zoysa, I. & Dye, C. (2006). The potential impact of male circumcision on HIV in Sub-Saharan Africa. *PLoS Med* 3, e262: 1032-1040.

Williamson, M.L. & Williamson, P.S. (1988). Women's preferences for penile circumcision in sexual partners. *J Sex Educ Ther* 14, 8-12.

Wiswell, T.E. & Geschke, D.W. (1989). Risks from circumcision during the first month of life compared with those for uncircumcised boys. *Pediatrics* 83, 1011-1015.

Wiswell, T.E. & Hachey, W.E. (1993). Urinary tract infections and the circumcision state: An update. *Clin Pediat* 32, 130-134.

Wiswell, T.E. (1995). Neonatal circumcision: a current appraisal. *Focus Opin Pediat* 1, 93-99.

Wiswell, T.E. (1997). Circumcision circumspection. *N Engl J Med* 36, 1244-1245.

Wiswell, T.E. (2000). The prepuce, urinary tract infections, and the consequences. *Pediatrics* 105, 8602.

World Health Organisation and UNAIDS. (2007a). New data on male circumcision and HIV prevention: policy and programme implications., http://who.int/hiv/mediacentre/MCrecommendations_en.pdf.

World Health Organisation and UNAIDS. (2007b). Male circumcision: Global trends and determinants of prevalance, safety and acceptability. http://whqlibdoc.who.int/publications/2007/9789241596169_eng.pdf. Geneva, World Health Organization.

WHO/UNAIDS/JHPIEGO. (2008). Manual for male circumcision under local anaesthesia. http://www.malecircumcision.org/programs/documents/WHO_MC_Manual_Local_Anaesthesia_v2-5C_Jan08.pdf

Xu, F., Markowitz, L.E., Sternberg, M.R. & Aral, S.O. (2007). Prevalence of circumcision and herpes simplex virus type 2 infection in men in the United States: the National Health and Nutrition Examination Survey (NHANES), 1999-2004. *Sex Transm Dis* 34, 479-484.

Yahya-Malima, K.I., Matee, M.I., Evjen-Olsen, B. & Fylkesnes, K. (2007). High potential of escalating HIV transmission in a low prevalence setting in rural Tanzania. *BMC Public Health* 7, 103 (10 pages).

Yan, B., You, H., Zhang, K., Tang, H.Y., Mao, W., He, G.H. & Yin, Z.G. (2010). [Circumcision with the Chinese Shang Ring in children: outcomes of 824 cases]. (in Chinese). *Zhonghua Nan Ke Xue* 16, 250-253.

Yellen, H.S. (1935). Bloodless circumcision of the newborn. *Am J Obstet Gynecol* 30, 1.

Yilmaz, D., Akin, M., Ay, Y., Balkan, C., Celik, A., Ergün, O. & Kavakli, K. (2010). A single centre experience in circumcision of haemophilia patients: Izmir protocol. *Haemophilia* 16, 888-889.

Zhenyuan, L. (1989). People's Republic of China Patent CN2045993 (Laser Shield (Chinese)). (Priority date Mar 21, 1989).

15

Trends in Interdisciplinary Studies Revealing Porphyrinic Compounds Multivalency Towards Biomedical Application

Radu Socoteanu[1] et al.*
[1]*Ilie Murgulescu Institute of Physical Chemistry, Romanian Academy, Romania*

1. Introduction

Porphyrins are a unique class of compounds widely present in nature. Due to their distinct chemical and photophysical properties they have a variety of applications, the most important being presented in Fig. 1.

Porphyrin chemistry and their applications have undergone a renaissance in the last years reflected in the 20 volumes of the recent comprehensive work giving an overview of the field (Kadish K.M et al., 2002). Despite the impressive volume of data, the question about the actual trends and future involvement of porphyrins in biomedical applications is still a hot topic as reflected by the number of publications on photodynamic therapy (Fig.2).

In the last decades a great deal of efforts from the scientific community focused on developing new therapeutic and diagnosis approaches in major diseases, like cancer and infection. One of the most dynamic fields of investigation is photodynamic therapy (PDT), which takes advantage of controlled oxidative stress for destroying pathogens.

This article aims at reviewing major topics related to biomedical engineering, porphyrins for PDT and photodiagnosis (PDD). We do not intend to provide an exhaustive display and comment of the porphyrinoid structures, as a huge number on papers and reviews dealing with the subject have already been published. We emphasize herein that porphyrins are also among the most promising candidates to be used as fluorescent near infrared (NIR) probes for non-invasive diagnosis and this opens the possibility to perform simultaneously tumor imaging and treatment in the same approach. It is worth mentioning that, besides their medical applications, porphyrins are used in industrial and analytical applications as

* Rica Boscencu[2], Anca Hirtopeanu[3], Gina Manda[4], Anabela Sousa Oliveira[5,6], Mihaela Ilie[2] and Luis Filipe Vieira Ferreira[6].
1 *Ilie Murgulescu Institute of Physical Chemistry, Romanian Academy, Romania,*
2 *Carol Davila University of Medicine and Pharmacy, Faculty of Pharmacy, Romania,*
3 *Costin Nenitescu Institute of Organic Chemistry, Romanian Academy, Romania,*
4 *Victor Babes National Institute, Romania,*
5 *Centro Interdisciplinar de Investigação e Inovação, Escola Superior de Tecnologia e Gestão, Instituto Politécnico de Portalegre, Portugal,*
6 *Centro de Química-Física Molecular, Institute of Nanosciences and Nanotechnology, Instituto Superior Técnico, Portugal.*

sensitized solar cells, pigments, in electrocatalysis, as electrodes in fuel cells, and as chemical sensors, but these issues are not the subject of this paper. Therefore the present chapter will only address the medical applications of porphyrins and metalloporphyrins with a special emphasis on photodynamic therapy.

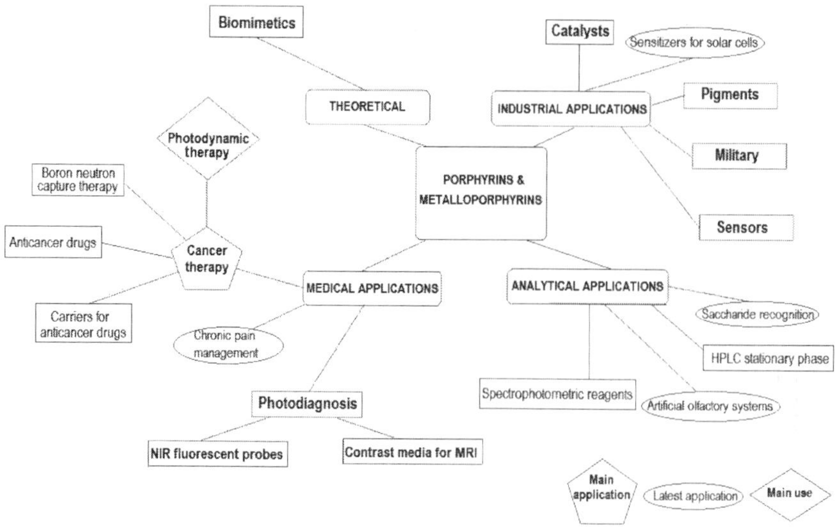

Fig. 1. Applications of porphyrins and metalloporphyrins

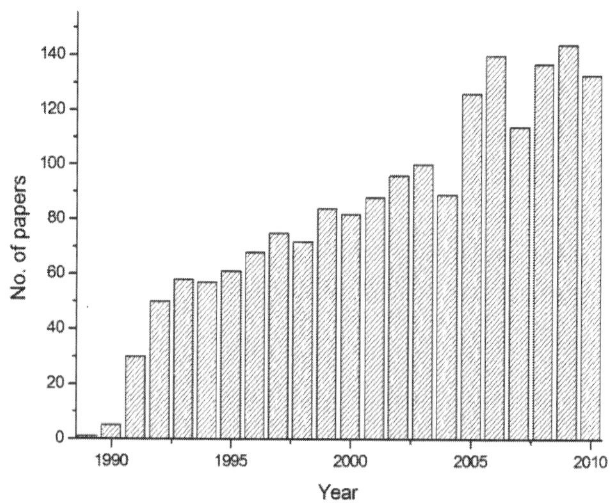

Fig. 2. Ascendant trend of publications on the topic of porphyrins involved in photodynamic therapy, as indexed by ISI Web of Knowledge

We summarize herein basic concepts in the field, stressing out theoretical and technological limitations that currently restrict multidisciplinary research for improving /enlarging theoretical and technological approaches in PDT and PDD using porphyrins. Special emphasis will be given to the development of novel porphyrinic structures related or derived from already confirmed structures and to put them in connection with PDT and PDD applications, focusing on symmetrical vs. asymmetrical molecular structures and on classical vs. more recent synthetic methods. Dosimetry issues for controlling and characterizing related processes, interdisciplinary approaches (chemistry, physics, biochemistry and biomedicine) will be also highlighted.

The major role played by porphyrinoid systems in biomedical applications is due to their photochemical (energy and exciton transfer), redox (electron transfer, catalysis) and coordination properties (metal and axial ligand binding) and their conformational flexibility (functional control) (Senge et al., 2010). The issue of PDT will be extensively adressed in the next section, while other medical applications, some of them very recent, will be described in section 4.

2. Photodynamic therapy - main medical application of porphyrins

PDT typically combines a photosensitizer, molecular oxygen and light to destroy cancer cells and microorganisms by oxidative stress (Bonnett R., 2000). Briefly, PDT is based on the ability of photosensitisers, including porphyrins, to selectively accumulate and kill tumour cells (Dougherty, 1987) by singlet oxygen ($^1O_2$) (Berenbaum & Bonnett, 1990), upon guided light activation with a particular wavelength (usually via laser endoscopy). Reactive oxygen species (ROS) produced by phagocytes underly physiological defense mechanisms against microorganisms, which are highly controlled to destroy pathogens, whilst minimally affecting the surrounding healthy tissues (Witko-Sarsat et al., 2000). As reviewed by Manda et al. (2009) cancer cells show an intrinsic oxidative phenotype, which makes them more sensitive to the deleterious action of additional oxidative stress generated for therapeutical purposes either by radiotherapy, PDT or even chemotherapy.

PDT has gained increasing attention in the past decade as a targeted and less invasive treatment regimen for a number of medical conditions, spanning from various types of cancers and dysplasias to neoangiogenesis, macular degeneration, as well as bacterial infections. The advantage is that PDT provides a localized action rather than a systemic one, when compared to other cancer therapies which are more harmful to the patient. PDT for cancer treatment has been extensively reviewed (Allison & Sibata, 2010; Capella M.A.M. & Capella L.S., 2003; Dickson, 2003; Dolmans, 2003; Dougherty, 1998; O'Connor et al., 2009; Vrouenraets, 2003; Wilson B.C., 2002). The huge effort in PDT development is highlighted by 1074 papers in the field reviewed in PubMed in the last 2 years, while 72 clinical trials in PDT were ongoing in March 2011 (http://clinicaltrials.gov).

2.1 Mechanism of action

As summarized in Fig. 3, there are two recognized mechanisms of action for PDT. The first mechanism (***type I***) involves light induced excitation of the photosensitizer, promoting an electron to a higher energy state. At this point a variety of reactions can take place. For example, the photosensitizer in the excited state can act as a reducing agent in the reaction to create ROS. Conversely, the excited photosensitizer may act as an oxidizing agent by filling the hole vacated by the excited electron. The second mechanism (***type II***) also involves excitation of the photosensitizer with light, but energy is transferred in this case to the triplet ground state of molecular oxygen, resulting in excited singlet state oxygen which is highly cytotoxic (Otsu K et al., 2005). In ***type I*** mechanism, oxygen is not always necessary for the photodynamic action to take place; however, in ***type II*** mechanism, oxygen is essential. Differences in the triplet and singlet states reflect ways in which two eectrons can be placed in degenerate orbitals and, as such, provide an ideal system to examine processes that give rise to Hund's rules for orbital occupancy. Also, the near IR transition between the 8 triplet and singlet states, at 1270 nm, is not very probable and provides an excellent example of selection rules based on changes in spin and orbital angular momentum, symmetry, and parity.

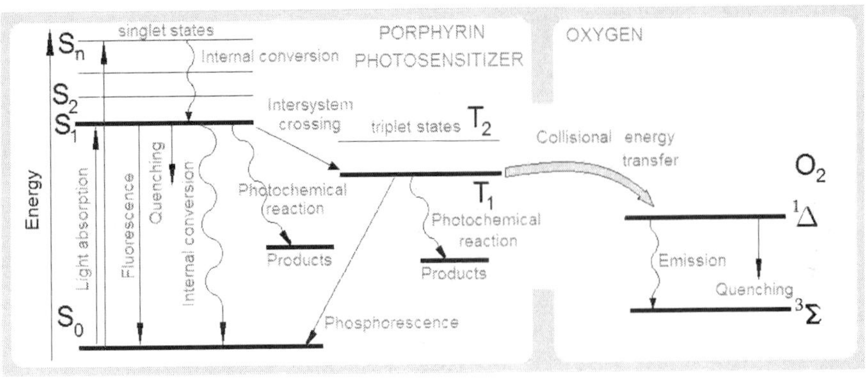

Fig. 3. Photophysical processes involving porphyrinic sensitizer in the presence of oxygen in a modified Jablonski diagram

The photophysical processes required for photodynamic therapy evidentiate the relevant properties for the photosensitizer: wavelength of absorbed light, molar absorbance, fluorescent quantum yield, intersystem crossing quantum yield, singlet oxygen quantum yield and photobleaching quantum yield. These properties depend on the chemical structure of the photosensitizer and will be discussed in paragraph 3.1.

2.2 PDT, ROS and targeted cell death

A prominent feature of PDT relies in focusing light and consequent localized photoactivation of the sensitizer. This spares normal tissue from the deleterious action of ROS generated during PDT reactions. Moreover, selective accumulation of sensitizer in tumors was demonstrated, which relies in physiological differences between tumors and normal tissues; among them can be cited: tumors have a larger interstitial volume than normal tissues, often contain a larger fraction of phagocytes, contain a large amount of newly synthesized collagen, have a leaky microvasculature and poor lymphatic drainage. Additionally, the extracellular pH is low in tumors. Generally cationic sensitizers localize in both the nucleus and mitochondria, lipophilic ones tend to stick to membrane structures, and water-soluble drugs are often found in lysosomes. Not only the lipid/water partition coefficient is important but also other factors such as molecular weight and charge distribution (linked to symmetry/asymmetry of the photosensitizer structure). In some cases, light exposure leads to a relocalization of the sensitizers (Moan & Berg, 1992; Moan & Peng, 2003; Spikes, 1989).

Singlet oxygen is a highly reactive ROS that interacts with proteins, nucleic acids and lipids. Singlet oxygen has a short lifetime within the cell and can migrate in tissues less than 20 nm after its formation. Therefore, the induced injury by singlet oxygen action is highly localized. Nevertheless, generation of about 9×10^8 molecules of singlet oxygen per tumor cell significantly reduces the cell surviving fraction (Dysart et al., 2005).

PDT leads to a molecular interplay between cell death pathways, balancing between apoptosis, necrosis and autophagy (Dewaele et al., 2010). Generally, photosensitizers which specifically target mitochondria induce ROS-mediated cell death by apoptosis (Oleinick et al., 2002), while autophagy occurs during PDT protocols involving sensitizers that localize to the endoplasmic reticulum (ER) (Buytaert, 2006; Kessel, 2006). Nonetheless, Pavani et al. (2009) demonstrated that photodynamic efficiency is directly proportional to membrane binding and is not totally related to mitochondrial accumulation. The presence of zinc in the photosensitizer decreases mitochondrial binding and increases membrane interactions, leading to improved PDT efficiency.

Recent evidence points out that mitochondria and ER associated with B-cell lymphoma 2 are among the cellular targets damaged in PDT protocols, impacting both apoptosis and autophagy. Autophagy may function as a prosurvival or a death pathway in PDT. The former function is obvious at low-dose PDT conditions, whereas the latter one contributes to the killing of cells exhibiting a phenotype that precludes the development of an apoptotic response, or of those cells that surviving to the initial wave of apoptosis after high-dose PDT (Kessel 2007; Pattingree, 2005). Apoptosis dominates as a mechanism of cell death in those cells having a fully competent apoptotic machinery, whereas autophagy seems to be responsible for cell death when apoptosis is compromised (Xue et al., 2007).

ROS are biologically multifaceted molecules, despite their simple chemical structure. Depending on the magnitude and profile of ROS generation in biological systems, on cellular location and on the redox balance, ROS can elicit cell death or cell proliferation. On one hand, aerobic organisms adapted themselves to the injurious oxidative attack and even learned how to use ROS in their own favor, as signaling molecules. On the other hand, ROS proved to be powerful weapons in fighting against infection or as therapeutic armentarium exploiting oxidative stress. Radiotherapy is one of the clearest examples of anti-cancer treatment, whose mechanism relies primarily on ROS, combining the properties of an extremely efficient DNA-damaging agent with high spatial focusing on tumor. Radiotherapy limitation derives mainly from the carcinogenic potential of the ionizing radiation and from the deleterious side-effect associated with the inflammatory response triggered by necrosis. Radiation memory underlies long-lasting effects of radiotherapy in tumors, but also contributes to persistent damage and dysfunctions of bystander normal cells. Taking also advantage of ROS cytotoxic potential, but with significantly less side-effects than radiotherapy, PDT is a fascinating example of biomedical engineering, combining and targeting towards diseased tisssues a photosensitizer, light and oxygen. It is an interdisciplinary approach involving chemistry, physics, biology and medicine for synergizing and fine-tuning all the three above mentioned components towards an efficient and highly targeted treatment regimen.

Although other classes of molecules have been tested and used as photosensitizers, porphyrins and porphyrin-like structures are undoubtly the most relevant for biomedical applications. Porphyrins and porphyrin-like structures have long been of interest for PDT due to their low intrinsic toxicity, the ability to accumulate into tumors and to generate highly ROS only when photoactivated at convenient wavelengths, adequate for deep tissue penetration.

2.3 PDT in oncology

It is now obvious that PDT can work as well as surgery or radiation therapy in treating certain kinds of cancers and dysplasias, having clear advantages over these treatment approaches: no long-term side effects when properly used, less invasive than surgery, can be targeted more precisely, can be repeated many times at the same site, if needed, and finally it is often less expensive than other cancer treatments.

The evidence in the published peer-reviewed scientific literature (Awan, 2006; Fayter, 2010; Rees, 2010) supports PDT as a safe and effective treatment option for selected patients with Barrett's esophagus, esophageal cancer, and non-small cell lung cancer. Although PDT has been proposed for the treatment of various other types of cancers (e.g., head and neck, cholangiocarcinoma, prostate), there is still insufficient evidence in the form of well-designed large, randomized controlled trials. PDT is also successful in the treatment of actinic keratoses, Bowen's disease and basal cell carcinoma.

PDT limitations are mainly related to drug and light accessibility. Although the photosensitizer travels throughout the body, PDT only works at the area exposed to light. This is why PDT cannot be used to treat leukemias and metastasis. Also, PDT leaves patients very sensitive to light, therefore special precautions must be taken after photosensitizers are used. PDT cannot be used in people who have *acute intermittent porphyria* or people who are allergic to porphyrins.

More aggressive local therapies are often necessary to eradicate unresectable tumor cells that invade adjacent normal tissue (i.e., malignant glioma), and this might be achieved by combining PDT and boron neutron capture therapy (BNCT) (Barth et al., 2005). Both are bimodal therapies, the individual components being non-toxic, but tumoricidal in combination. Boronated porphyrins are promising dual sensitizers for both PDT and BNCT, showing tumor affinity by the porphyrin ring, ease of synthesis with a high boron content, low cytotoxicity in dark conditions, strong light absorption in the visible and NIR regions, ability to generate singlet oxygen upon light activation and also ability to display fluorescence (Vicente et al., 2010). Several boronated porphyrins have been synthesized and evaluated in cellular and animal studies (Renner, 2006; Vicente, 2010).

Besides more precise photosensitizer targeting, either by specific cellular function-sensitive linkages or via conjugation to macromolecules (Verma S. et al., 2007), recent approaches aim to combine PDT and a second treatment regimen to either increase the susceptibility of tumor cells to PDT or to mitigate molecular responses triggered by PDT. As an example, Anand et al. (2009) demonstrated both *in vitro* and *in vivo* that low, non-toxic doses of methotrexate can significantly and selectively enhance PDT with aminolevulinic acid in skin cancers. Banerjee et al (2001) showed that meso-substituted porphyrins could impact directly in the radiotherapy outcome, when labeled with beta(-) emitters like 186/188Re.

2.4 PDT and immunomodulation

In contrast with systemic chemo- or radiotherapy, PDT is a local treatment in which the treated tumor remains *in situ*, while the immune response is only locally affected and has the capability to recover by recruitment of circulating immune cells.

Generally, immune cells are found in the tumor stroma, separated from tumor cells by extracellular matrix and basal membrane-like structures which hinder the development of an efficient anti-tumor immune response. By destroying the structure of the tumor, PDT facilitates direct interaction between immune and tumor cells, resulting in a local or systemic immune response, as shown in both preclinical as well as clinical settings (Gollnick, 2002). Nonetheless, the efficiency of the *in situ* vaccination triggered by PDT is still debatable (van Duijnhoven et al., 2003).
As reviewed by Garg et al (2010), PDT is capable of eliciting various effects in the tumor microenvironment thereby affecting tumor-associated immune cells and the activation of different immune reactions e.g. acute-phase response, complement cascade and production of cytokines/chemokines (Garg et al., 2010). The ability of PDT to induce exposure/release of certain damage-associated molecular patterns (DAMPs) like HSP70, opens new perspectives in PDT and PDT-like photoimmunotherapy (Garg et al., 2010).
PDT, by evoking oxidative stress at specific subcellular sites through light-activation of organelle-associated photosensitizers, may be unique in combining tumor cells destruction and antitumor immune response in one therapeutic paradigm (Garg et al., 2011).

2.5 Antimicrobial PDT

The very success of antibiotics limited their efficiency by rendering microorganisms resistant (Hancock R.E.W., 2007). PDT seems to be a viable alternative, proving to be efficient against bacteria (including drug-resistant strains), yeasts, viruses and protozoa. In addition to destroying microorganisms, PDT can induce immune stimulatory reactions (Castano et al., 2006; Hryhorenko et al., 1998), and consequently has the potential to improve the overall host response to infections.
The positive charge of photosensitizers appears to promote a tight electrostatic interaction with negatively charged sites at the outer surface of any species of bacterial cells (Maisch et al., 2004). Moreover, drug-resistant microorganisms are as susceptible to PDT as their native counterparts (Maisch, 2009), or even more susceptible (Tang et al., 2009). It is considered less likely that the bacteria will develop resistance towards PDT (Jori & Coppellotti, 2007; Konopka & Goslinski, 2008), presumably because of the short-lived ROS produced by the photodynamic effect and the non-specific nature of the photooxidative damage that leads to cell death.
It is known that gram-positive bacteria species are much more sensitive to photodynamic inactivation than gram-negative species (Merchat et al., 1996). Efforts have therefore been made to design photosensitizers capable of attacking gram-negative strains. This can be achieved if photosensitizers are coadministrated with outer membrane disrupting agents such as calcium chloride, EDTA or polymixin B nonapeptide, that are able to promote electrostatic repulsion and consequent alteration of the cell wall structure.
As reviewed by Alves et al. (2009), porphyrins can be transformed into cationic entities through the insertion of positively charged substituents in the peripheral positions of the tetrapyrrole macrocycle, which affect the kinetics and extent of binding to microorganisms. The hydrophobicity of porphyrins can be modulated by the number of cationic moieties (up to four in *meso*-substituted porphyrins) or by the introduction of hydrocarbon chains of different length on the amino nitrogens.
Antimicrobial PDT is making rapid advances towards clinical applications in oral infections, periodontal diseases, healing of infected wounds and treatment of *Acne vulgaris*. The first product to be applied in the oral cavity came on the market in Canada in 2005 (Periowave™,

Ondine) and several products for the treatment of infected wounds are under clinical trial. Antimicrobial PDT requires topical applications of the photosensitizers, selective for the microorganism, without causing significant damage to the host tissue. The possibility of adverse effects on host tissues has often been raised as a limitation of antimicrobial PDT. However, studies have shown that the photosensitizers are more toxic against microbial species than against mammalian cells, and that the concentration of photosensitizer and light energy dose necessary to kill the infecting organism has little effect on adjacent host tissues.

Photoactivated disinfection of blood samples and surfaces like benches and floors is also introduced as a promising application of antimicrobial PDT. The group of Parsons (2009) developed a method for concentrating PDT effect at a material surface to prevent bacterial colonization by attaching a porphyrin photosensitizer at, or near to that surface. Anionic hydrogel copolymers were shown to permanently bind a cationic porphyrin through electrostatic interactions as a thin surface layer. The mechanical and thermal properties of the materials showed that the porphyrin acts as a surface cross-linking agent, and renders surfaces more hydrophilic. Importantly, *Staphylococcus epidermidis* adherence was reduced by up to 99% relative to the control in intense light conditions and 92% in the dark. As such, candidate anti-infective hydrogel-based intraocular lens materials were developed for improving patient outcomes in cataract surgery.

3. Porphyrins as PDT photosensitizers

Porphyrins are involved as sensitizers in PDT because of their ability to localize in tumors and of their capacity to be activated by irradiation (see Fig 3).

The main basic architectures of the porphyrinoid compounds used as photosensitizers are presented in Fig. 4 highlighting the minor differences between them. Porphyrins and porphyrin-related dyes used in PDT may have substituents in the peripheral positions of the pyrrole rings or on the four methine carbons (*meso*-positions).

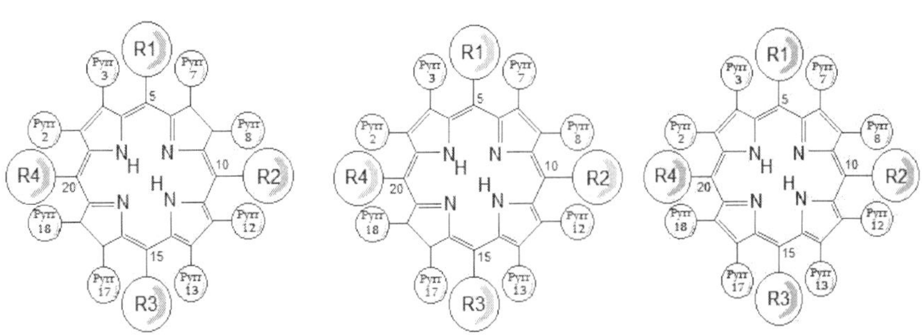

Dihydroporphyrin (Bacteriochlorin) Tetrahydroporphyrin (Chlorin) Porphyrin

Fig. 4. Basic architectures of porphyrinoid photosensitizers

These derivatives are synthesized to influence the water/lipid solubility, amphiphilicity, pKa and stability of the compounds since these parameters determine their pharmacokinetics.

Porphyrins can also coordinate metal ions by replacing the hydrogen atoms on nitrogen; the metal ion and its electronic properties are of importance for their photocytotoxic potential as photosensitisers. Several metallophotosensitizers have been developed for clinical purposes. Although in most cases, they have lower quantum yields for cell inactivation than they would have in the absence of metal ions, they have other properties like improved solubility and stability, which makes them interesting as therapeutic substances. The metals used include Zn, Pd, Sn, Ru, Pt and Al.

3.1 Properties of porphyrins relevant for their biomedical applications

The use of porphyrins in biomedical applications including PDT is tightly connected to their physical - chemical characteristics. Among these, most important are their electronic molecular absorption and emission properties, but solubility and stability must also be taken into account.

3.1.1 Absorption properties

Porphyrinoids have a large range of absorption wavelengths together with a large range of molar absorbtion coefficients as shown in Fig. 5. Although the absorption of porphyrins does not cover the entire PDT window, they compensate that with their ability to localize in tumors and their chemical versatility.

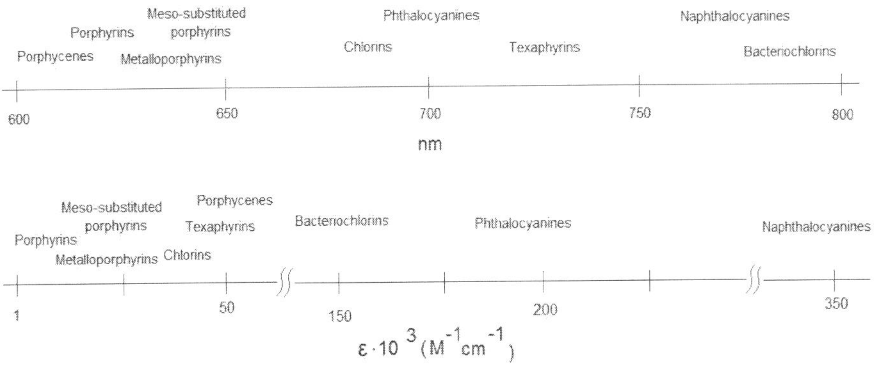

Fig. 5. Chart of one exclusive pair criteria for photosensitizers suitable for PDT: absorption maxima vs. intensity (ε)

The electronic absorption spectrum of the free-base porphyrins is dominated by a typical intense Soret band and four weaker Q bands, located in the spectral range 415-650 nm, which are monotonously decreasing in intensity (Kadish et al., 2002). The Q bands of the free base porphyrins consist of four absorption peaks which are typical to the Qx(0,0), Qx(0,1), Qy(0,0), Qy(0,1) transitions in the free base porphyrin (D_{2h} symmetry). Upon complexation with a metal ion, the number of Q bands decreases due to the enhancement of the molecular symmetry from D_{2h} to D_{4h} (Boscencu et al., 2008; Boscencu et al., 2010). The molecular electronic absorption spectra are usually used for the quantitative determination of compounds, but in the case of porphyrinic compounds they give real "fingerprints" that can be used to predict the usefulness of a certain compound as photosensitizer. This is explained by the fact that the peripheral substitution does not significantly disturb the inner π electron ring of the porphyrinic macrocycle, which is responsible for the active electronic transitions in the above mentioned spectral range.

3.1.2 Emission properties

Photodetection for tissue characterization in cancer is not new, the first study being reported by Policard in 1924, who noticed the fluorescence of a tumor under illumination with UV light. This fluorescence was considered to originates from tumor's endogenous porphyrins (Masilamani et al., 2004). Some of the most important aspects of metaloporphyrins are connected to the photophysical characteristics of porphyrins in different media: fluorescence quantum yields (Φ_f) and fluorescence lifetimes (τ_f).

Fluorescence emission characteristics of porphyrinic compounds are also important features for the biomedical use of porphyrins. In case of their use in photodiagnosis, emission characteristics as fluorescence quantum yields and/or fluorescence lifetimes are of importance to differentiate the signal of the fluorescent marker from the fluorescence of the environmental matter. In case of PDT, all deactivation processes (fluorescence, phosphorescence, internal conversion, collisional quenching) play an important role in the very process of ROS generation (Fig. 3).

Despite significant advantages, the porphyrinic compounds as photosensitizers have limitations. Due to the large π conjugate systems, they easily form aggregates, which have a significantly lower ability to form reactive oxygen species and consequently decrease the photodynamic activity. In recent years, nanostructured materials such as liposomes, nanoparticles and micelles have been considered as potential carriers for porphyrinic compounds that may resolve the aforementioned problems. The presence of polar headgroups and hydrophobic chains in micellar structures allows the study of the potential affinity of a porphyrinic structure to cell-membrane type structures.

3.2 Main features for an efficient photosensitizer

There is a great deal of interest in design and synthesis of new photosenzitizers with porphyrinoid structures, with improved characteristics that make worth their investigation as possible new PDT drugs. The general characteristics of a good sensitizer, displayed as basic requirements, are presented in Table 1. For photosensitizers designed to kill cancer or other mammalian cells, it has been found that their intracellular localization is another important parameter. For example, the photosensitizers which localize in mitochondria seem to be more powerful in killing cells than those locating in lysosomes (Mroz et al., 2009).

Porphyrins are essential constituents of important biological systems. The porphyrin-type nucleus, along with metal ions, is found in cytochromes, peroxidases and catalases. Other biologically important porphyrins that occur in nature and in the human body are hemin (an iron porphyrin - the prosthetic group of hemoglobin and myoglobin), chlorophyll (magnesium porphyrin-like compound involved in plant photosynthesis), and vitamin B12 (cobalt porphyrin-like compound, commonly known as cobalamine). As a result of their vital role in biologic processes, metallo-porphyrins have always attracted chemist's attention. Porphyrins proved to be valuable photosensitizers since they are non-toxic, are selectively retained in tumors, are cleared in a reasonable time from the body and skin, and thus photosensitive reactions are minimized. Moreover, porphyrins have got convenient amphiphilicity which renders them more photodynamically active than symmetrically hydrophobic or hydrophilic molecules.

Required features	Details
Purity	Substance of known composition, stable at room temperature
Toxicity, overdosage, and side effects	- Minimal toxicity in the absence of light - Cytotoxic in the presence of light of defined wavelength - Non- toxic metabolites; - Minimal side effects
Absorption, distribution, metabolism and excretion (ADME)	Optimum ADME properties
Activation and wavelength	Activation in the phototherapeutical window (600 to 850 nm)
Singlet oxygen quantum yield	High singlet oxygen generation quantum yield ($\Phi\Delta$)
Cost and availability	Inexpensive Commercially available to allow extensive utilization
Selectivity	- Good tumour/healthy tissue localization ratio - Favourable subcellular localization to induce an apoptotic rather than a necrotic mode of cell death
Mutagenicity/ Carcinogenicity	Non-mutagenic Non-carcinogenic
Painless	No pain during the procedure or in the following treatment stages
Combined treatment	No adverse interactions with other drugs or medical procedures
Multisession	Possibility for application in repeated sessions, without immunosuppressive effects
Carriers	Possibile formulation with different carriers
Multivalency Marker and molecular beacon	Multiple effects desired (antitumoral and antimicrobial, antitumor and diagnosis) Marker or beacon
Upgradable chemical structures	The structure can be easily improved by simple chemical reactions

Table 1. Required features for an efficient photosensitizer

3.3 Timeline in the development of porphyrinoid photosensitizers

Porphyrins were identified in the mid-nineteenth century, but it was not until the early twentieth century that they were used in medicine.

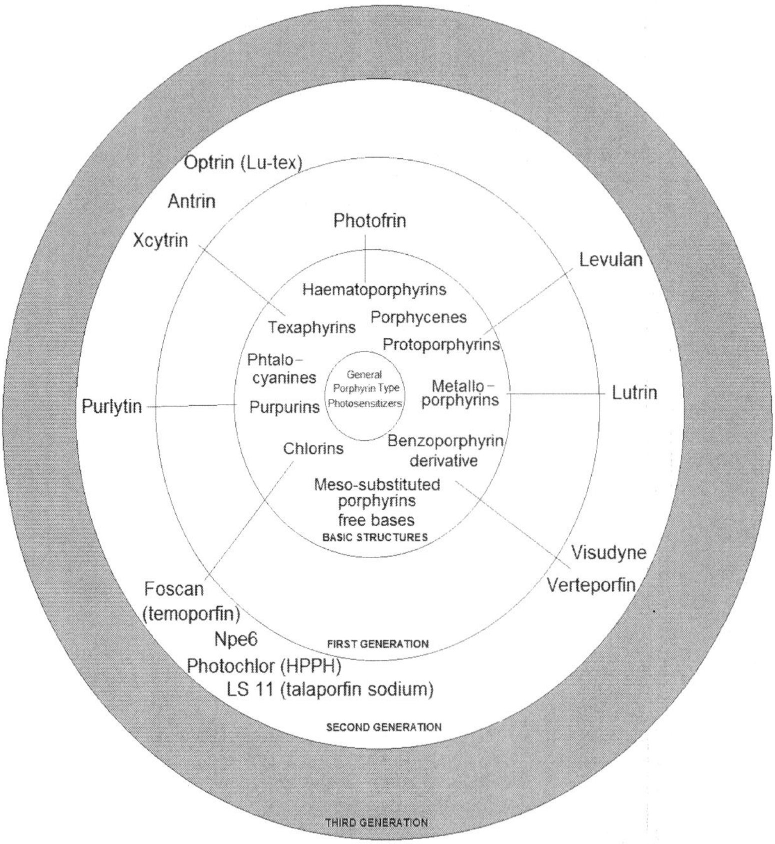

Fig. 6. General frame of the porphyrin type structures involved in biomedical studies

Porphyrinoid photosensitizers are classified as belonging to the first, second or third generation of photosensitizers as shown in Figure 6, or depending on the platform to which they belong (porphyrin, chlorophyll, dyes) (Allison R.R. et al., 2004). They could also be classified according to their primary mechanism of action and/or according to their use (type of cancer, photodiagnosis or therapy).

The first generation of photosensitizers consists only of hematoporphyrin derivatives and was developed during the 70's. Photosensitizers belonging to the second generation are porphyrin derivatives or synthetics made from the late '80s on. Second generation 10 photosensitizers are improved compared to the first generation: they have a definite structure (which means they are no more a combination of monomers, dimers and oligomers), absorb light at longer wavelengths and cause less skin photosensitization.

Third generation photosensitizers use available drugs and then modify them with different carriers in order to obtain tailored characteristics.

Examples of clinically available porphyrin sensitizers are presented in Table 2.

Brand names	**Substance (structure)**	**Substance Name (abbreviation)**	**Substance chemical name**	**Activation wavelength (nm)**	**Manufacturer**
Photofrin	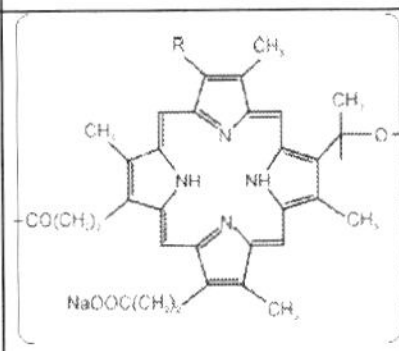	HpD	Hematoporphyrin	630	Axcan Pharma, Inc.
Levulan	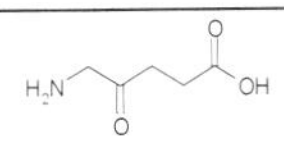	ALA	5-Aminolevulinic acid	630	DUSA Pharmaceuticals, Inc.
Metvix Metvixia	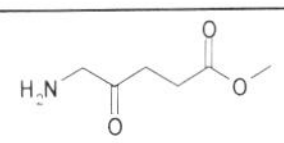	M-ALA	Methyl-5-Aminolevulinic acid	634	PhotoCure ASA Galderma, Dallas, TX
Visudyne	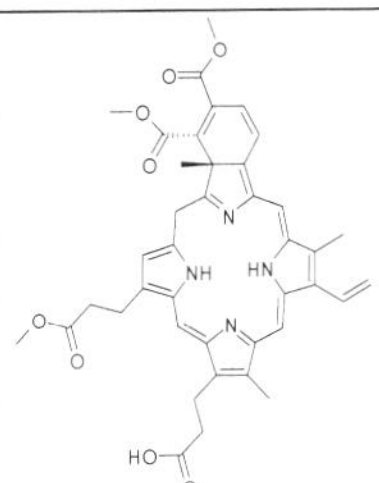	Verteporfin		690	Novartis Pharmaceuticals
Foscan	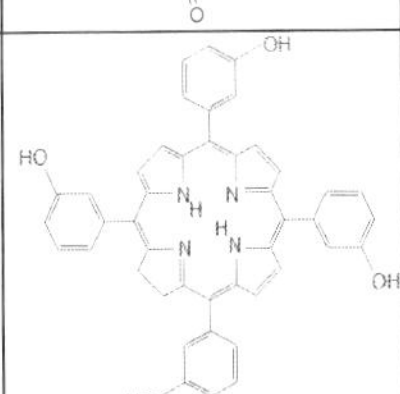	Temoporfin	5,10,15,20-tetrakis (3-hydroxyphenyl)-chlorin	652	Biolitec Pharma Ltd.
LS11 NPe6 Laserphyrin	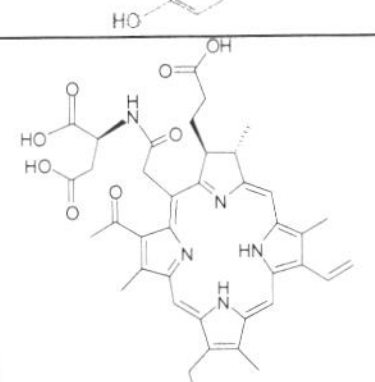	Talaporfin	mono-L-aspartyl chlorine e6	664	Light Science
Photochlor	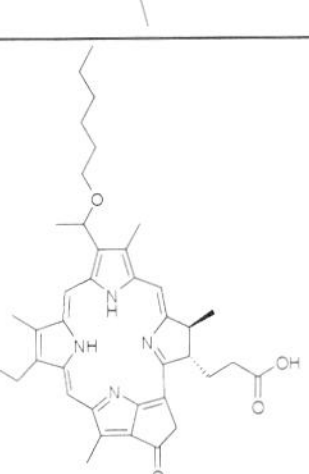	HPPH	2-(1-Hexyloxyethyl) -2-devinyl pyropheophorbide-a	665	RPCI

Table 2. Clinically available porphyrin sensitizers (adapted from Allison et al., 2004)

Photofrin® (HpD) has the longest clinical history and patient track record being the first commercial photosensitiser. It is actually a combination of monomers, dimers, and oligomers derived from chemical manipulation of hematoporphyrin (HpD). The complex mixture is required for clinical activity. In the US, Photofrin® is FDA approved for early and late endobronchial lesions as well as Barrett's esophagus and esophageal obstructing lesions. The drug is approved worldwide for a number of additional uses, such as for treatment of bladder cancer.

5-Aminolevulinic acid (ALA) is a prodrug, a naturally occurring amino acid which is converted enzymatically to protoporphyrin. By topical administration the treatment can be selectively performed without associated light sensitization of the untreated regions. Systemic administration does not have this built in selectivity. The drug is active at 630 nm, which should give adequate depth penetration; however, when topically administered, the drug has a limited penetration capacity and therefore is less efficient for treating deep

	First generation photosensitizers	**Second generation photosensitizers**	
Porphyrin sensitizer molecular structure	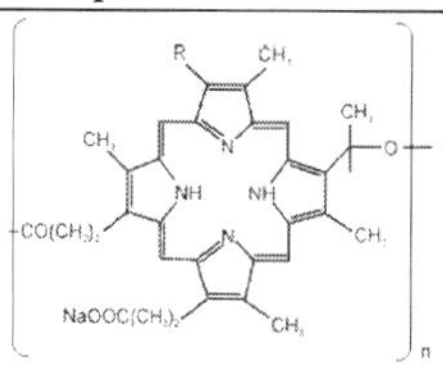	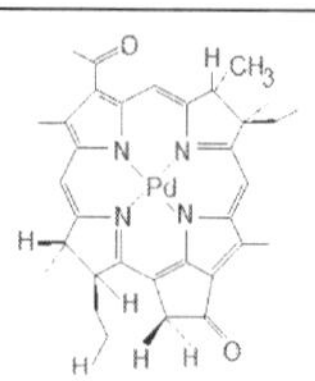	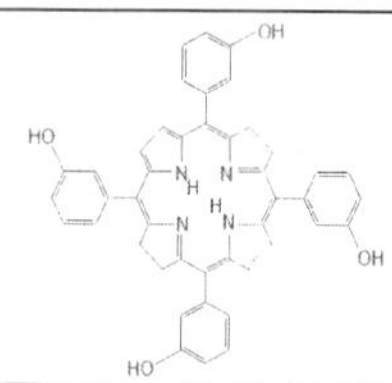
Porphyrin sensitizer name	Photofrin	Tookad	Foscan
Absorption (nm)	630	763	652
Localization	Golgi apparatus plasma membrane	Vasculature	Endoplasmic reticulum (ER) Mitochondria
Primary mechanism of action	Vascular damage ischemic tumor cell necrosis	Vascular damage Direct tumor cytotoxicity	Vascular damage
Most commonly light time irradiation interval	24-48 h	15 min	96 h
Status:	Approved	Clinical trials	Approved
Applications	Esophageal cancer, lung cancer, gastric cancer, cervical dysplasia and cancer	Prostate cancer	Head and Neck cancer
Local side effects	Mild to moderate erythema	-	Swelling, bleeding, ulceration scarring
Systemic side effects	Photosensitivity, mild constipation	-	-

Table 3. Examples of porphyrin sensitizers and their characteristics (adapted from O'Connor et al., 2009)

lesions. ALA is not highly active, so relatively high light doses or long time treatments are needed. Despite using topical anesthetics, ALA PDT can be painful. ALA has been successful for esophageal treatment and with the oral form of drug this is convenient. Dysplastic epithelium can be reliably destroyed by ALA PDT.

The methylated form of ALA (M-ALA), known commercially as Metvix® in Europe and Metvixia® in the US, has FDA approval for the treatment of non-hyperkeratotic actinic keratoses of the face and scalp, using a red-light source. Metvix also has EU approval for the treatment of superficial basal cell carcinomas. Both ALA and its methylated form proved clinical efficacy in the treatment of actinic keratoses and have also been used for photorejuvenation and inflammatory *acne vulgaris*.

Verteporfin, known commercially as Visudyne, is a benzoporphyrin derivative, which is clinically active when formulated with liposomes. The photosensitizer is active at 690 nm, allowing deep tissue penetration and light activation. The drug is rapidly accumulated and cleared, so that skin photosensitization is minimal. Most of the clinical response induced by Verteporfin is based on vascular disruption and therefore, this drug seems ideal for lesions depending on neovasculature.Verteporfin has been successful as treatment for choroidal neovascularization due to serous chorioretinopathy.

Table 3 presents some of the clinically available sensitizers together with their most relevant features in order to emphasize the influence of the chemical changes (among others, free base versus metallated form) on the characteristics and applications.

3.4 Selected aspects of the synthesis

Synthesis of porphyrins has been extensively reviewed in literature (Kadish K., 2002).

The hematoporphyrin derivatives (HpD) were the start line for the porphyrinic photosensitizers, the result consisting in several commercial products, as Photofrin®, which is a mixture of oligomers formed by ether and ester linkages of several porphyrin units, delivered as sodium porphimer. Their efficacy is linked also to the different proportions of monomers, dimers and oligomers (Mironov et al., 1990). The porphyrinic ring is β-pyrrolic substituted in this case. By changing the substitution on the *meso* positions, new photosensitizers can be generated, such as the tetraphenylsulphonated structures (TSPP or TSPP4-meso-tetrakis(4-sulfonatophenyl)porphyrin). Despite a few advantages, as solubility and low cost, the neurotoxicity, cytoskeletal abnormalities and nerve fiber degeneration in systemic administration, has oriented the compound only to topical use (Lapes M. et al., 1996; Winkelman J.W. et al., 1987).

Meso-substituted porphyrins (Fig. 7) are more attractive compared to the naturally occurring beta substituted porphyrins for different applications including the biomedical field. Their synthesis is an ongoing subject of research (Halime Z. et al., 2006; Senge M.O., 2010, 2005; Lindsey J.S. 2010) being directed toward increasing efficacy in obtaining unsymmetric ABCD substituted structures, in larger quantities. One approach is the use of microwave (MW) irradiation which offers excellent yields within minutes.

As shown in figure 7, the porphyrin ring can be substituted in its 5, 10, 15 and 20 positions respectively with R_1, R_2, R_3 and R_4. If the substituents are all hydrogen atoms, the structure is a symmetrical porphin; if the substituents are not hydrogens, but are identical to each other, the structure is a symmetrical *meso* porphyrin. Whenever one or more of R_1 to R_4 is not hydrogen, the structure is an unsymmetrical porphyrin. Porphyrins are said to have type A unsymmetrical structure when only R_1 is not hydrogen; type A,B - 5, 10 or type A,B - 5, 15 when either R_1 and R_2 or R_1 and R_3 are not hydrogens; type ABC if only R_4 is hydrogen and type ABDC when none of the substituents is hydrogen. Whenever unsymmetrical, porphyrins posses an amphiphilic character.

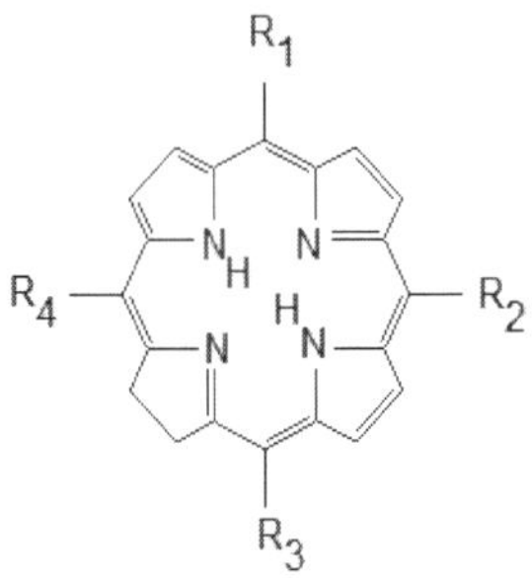

Symmetrical	
$R_1 = R_2 = R_3 = R_4 = H$	Porphin
$R_1 = R_2 = R_3 = R_4$	*meso-*
Unsymmetrical	
$R_1;\ R_2 = R_3 = R_4 = H$	type A
$R_1; R_2;\ R_3 = R_4 = H$	type AB - 5,10
$R_1; R_3;\ R_2 = R_4 = H$	type AB - 5,15
$R_1; R_2; R_3;\ R_4 = H$	type ABC
$R_1; R_2; R_3; R_4$	type ABCD

Fig. 7. Substitution patterns for porphyrins

The quest for viable structures, able to compete with Foscan (also known as Temoporfin, see Table 2), has included as spearhead the *meso-* substituted amphiphilic porphyrins. The desirable hydrophilic configurations give short singlet oxygen lifetime, unsuitable to PDT (Bonnett R., 2000). Controlled equilibrium in terms of hydrophilic-hydrophobic character was obtained in structures where porphyrinic periphery was mainly achieved by synthesizing a large number of asymmetrical structures, with all R_x (1 to 4) different (i.e., an ABCD unsymmetrical structure) (Rao et al., 2000; Wiehe et al., 2005). For increased targeted delivery and enhancement of phototoxicity by raising the level of the accumulation in pathologic cells, several carboplatin-containing porphyrins were synthesized (Brunner et al., 2004).
New structures were synthesized by several methods. The conjugation approach, coupled with photophysical studies and biological evaluation was reported for several compounds, from folic acid (Schneider et al., 2005) to Pt(II)-containing structures (Song et al., 2002).
The posibility to add functional groups to the substituted porphyrin recommends this type of compounds for multiple biomedical purposes.

3.4.1 Classical synthesis

Since the 20's, with the work of Nobel laureates H.Fischer and R. Willstätter on porphyrins as haemoglobin, chlorophyll and other pigments, followed later by R.B Woodward and A. Eschenmoser with the synthesis of vitamin B12, considered at the time as impossible, porphyrin synthesis has been continuously leading to complex structures. The Rothemund process is considered as classical (Rothemund, 1936, 1939) with the contributions of Adler - Longo (Longo, 1969; Adler, 1976) and those of Lindsey (Lindsey, 1986, 1987).
Some of the complex porphyrinic structures were obtained by adding various substituents in all peripheral positions (Fig. 4), others by expanding the core- beginning with five pyrrole units: sapphyrin (Chmielewski et al., 1995) and smaragdyirin (Sessler et al., 1998) to the turcasarin (Sessler et al., 1994) as relevant extreme examples.

The general synthetic methods for meso-porphyrins are presented in Figure 8.

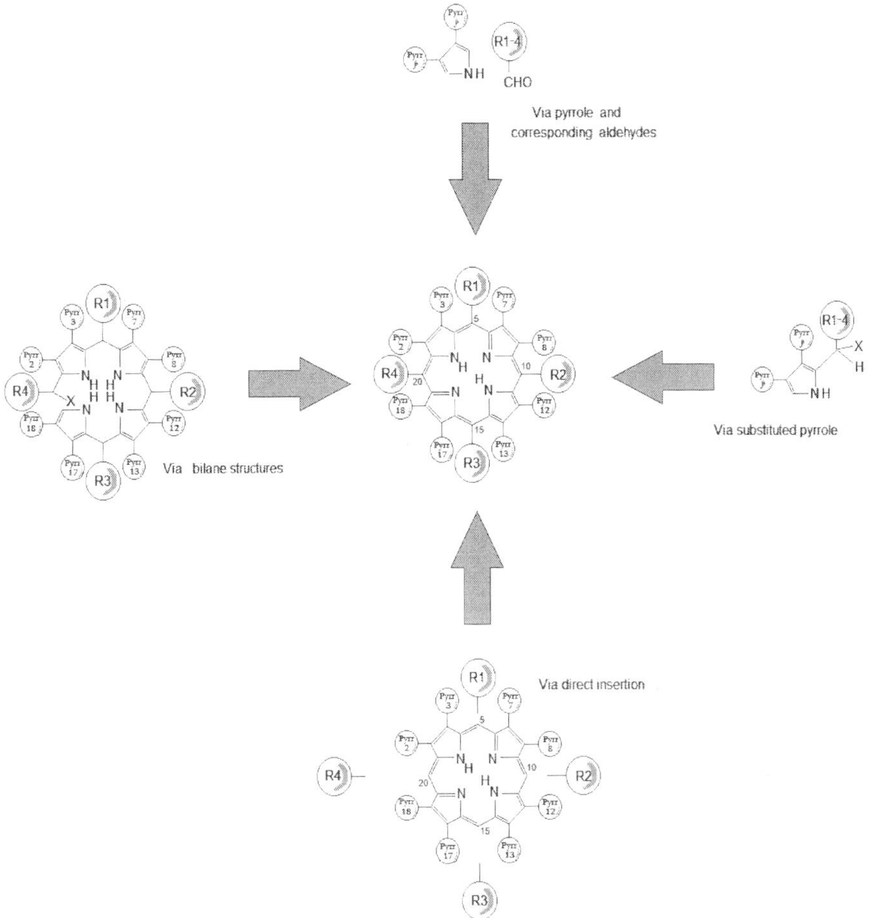

Fig. 8. Theoretical synthetic approach for the peripheral substitution on meso- porphyrins

Four pathways are generally available (according to Fig. 8): the condensation process involving pyrrole and various aldehydes, reaction mixture involved also in MW assisted procedures, the combination of substituted pyrroles carrying the desired future porphyrin substituents or via bilane structure; this last option was successfully applied on ABCD substituted porphyrins via synthesis of a protected acylbilane (by acid-catalyzed condensation of a acyldipyrromethane and protected dipyrromethane-n-carbinol) (Dogutan et al., 2007) and insertion of the substituents in meso positions in the already formed porphyrin core.
The unsymmetrical porphyrins were chosen as our main synthetic target (Boscencu, 2008, 2009, 2010; Oliveira, 2009) because

a. they are easy to prepare either via the Adler route (Adler et al., 1976) or by microvawe (MW) irradiation
b. the phenolic hydroxy group is a suitable site on which to build a different substituent (Milgrom LR, 1983)
c. the 4-methoxycarbonyl side-chains of the other meso-substituents may be de-esterified to convert a hydrophobic porphyrin into a hydrophilic one.

3.4.2 Synthesis by microwave irradiation

Microwave-assisted procedure is now a valid method to synthesize various type of compounds, including porphyrins and related structures, with significant advantages, from eco-friendliness to fastness and selectivity (Loupi et al., 2001). Since the first successful attempt for the *meso*-5,10,15,20 tetraphenylporphyrin (Petit et al., 1992), a wide range of compounds were obtained using either professional or domestic microwave ovens. The metalloporphyrins can also be obtained via MW methods (Mark et al., 2005).
Microwave-assisted procedures have become increasingly important in chemical synthesis in the last two decades due to several already proved important advantages over conventional heating pathways (table 4).
The position of the microwave irradiation stage in preliminary *evaluation- synthetic process- purification- analysis* chain is just by replacing classical Rothemund method with no additional operations (Fig. 9.)

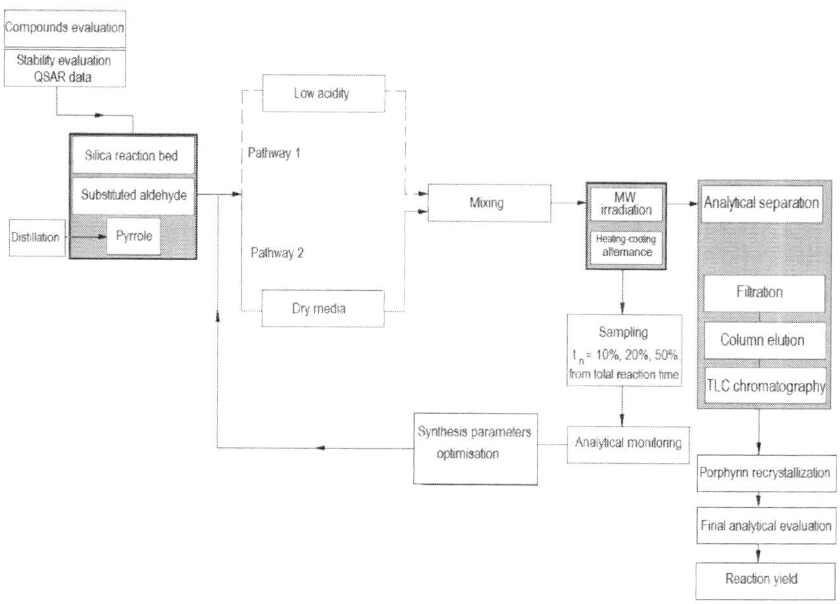

Fig. 9. Synthesis strategy for obtaining porphyrinic compounds including both classical and MW irradiation methods

The microwave-assisted cyclocondensation of benzaldehyde and pyrrole in dry media or in propionic acid (Chauhan et al., 2001) produces 5,10,15,20-tetraaryl porphyrins type with excellent yields.

Characteristics	Classical Method	MW Method
Reaction environment (starting materials)	Complex (reactants in greater number)	Simple
Conditions	Difficult (pressure, temperature, Nitrogen atmosphere)	Easy
Experimental	Precautions (adding reagents under special conditions)	No restrictions
Reaction yield	Small-Average	Average-High
Time	Hours-Days	Minutes
Toxicity	Average	Average-Low
Secondary reaction products	High (separation in several steps)	Few (easier separation)
Chlorine (related structure)	Present	Absent

Table 4. Characteristics of the MW vs. classical synthetic method

The pathway towards improved photosensitizers imposed extended interdisciplinary studies. The second generation of photosensitizers will provide a large volume of "starting material" for future clinical tests, considering that the present synthetic methods can provide almost all types of substituted porphyrinoid systems.

4. Other medical applications of porphyrins

Porphyrins and metalloporphyrins have applications in cancer therapy, in photodiagnosis and more recently in chronic pain management and in the emerging field called theranostics which is actually a combination between therapy and diagnosis (Ray et al., 2010).

4.1 Cancer therapy

4.1.1 Boron neutron capture therapy

Boron neutron capture therapy (BNCT) is a binary radiation therapy approach, bringing together two components which, when kept separate, have only minor effects on cells. The first component is a stable isotope of boron (boron-10) that can be concentrated in tumor cells by attaching it to tumor-seeking compounds. The second is a beam of low-energy neutrons. Boron-10 into or adjacent to the tumor cells disintegrates after capturing a neutron producing high energy heavy charged particles which destroy only the cells in close proximity, primarily cancer cells, leaving adjacent normal cells largely unaffected. Clinical interest in BNCT has focused primarily on the treatment of high-grade gliomas and either cutaneous primaries or cerebral metastases of melanoma, most recently, head, neck and liver cancer. Neutron sources for BNCT are limited to nuclear reactors and these are available in the US, Japan, several European countries, and Argentina (Bregadze et al., 2001; Evstigneeva et al., 2003; Fronczek et al., 2005; Ol'shevskaya et al., 2006; Vicente et al., 2003). Boron-containing porphyrins have excellent tumor-localizing properties (Vicente, 2001) and have been proposed for dual application as boron delivery agents and photosensitizers for PDT in brain tumors (Rosenthal, 2003).

4.1.2 Anticancer drugs

A series of interesting gold(III) meso-tetraarylporphyrin complexes with relevant antiproliferative effects on CNE1 human cancer cell lines were described by Che et al. (2003). Among them, the complex Au(III)(*p*-H-TPP)]Cl was found to be more cytotoxic for CNE1 than cisplatin. The lack of cross-resistance suggested that gold(III) porphyrins and cisplatin induced cytotoxicity through different mechanisms. Replacement of Au(III) with Zn(II) drastically reduced the drug potency.

Cationic Mn porphyrins may be advantageous compared to other anti-cancer drugs, owing to their ability to afford pain management in cancer patients (Rabbani et al., 2009).

4.1.3 Carriers for anti-cancer drugs

The tumor-affinity of porphyrins has been exploited for designing porphyrin–anticancer drug conjugates. Brunner et al. created a series of porphyrin–platinum conjugates by combining porphyrin with cytotoxic platinum complexes (Brunner, 2004; Lottner, 2002). Zhou reported some porphyrin - DNA-alkylation-agent conjugates (Zhou, 2006) and Guo et al. (2003, 2004) prepared conjugates by linking porphyrin with other nitrogen heterocyclic species. However none of the conjugates mentioned above may be considered as a prodrug, since they do not release the actual drug. The first example of a porphyrin anticancer prodrug was reported in 2008 and consists of three parts: a porphyrin, a photocleavable *o*-nitrobenzyl moiety as a light-triggered group, and a parent anticancer drug Tegafur (Lin et al., 2008). The prodrug is significantly less toxic than its parent anticancer drug Tegafur, which is released upon photoactivation.

Combined with the up-to-date medical fiber optic technique, the light-triggered porphyrin anticancer prodrugs may find useful applications in chemotherapy to minimize side effects of anticancer drugs and in the light-controllable anticancer drug dosing (McCoy et al., 2007).

4.2 Chronic pain management

Severe pain syndromes reduce the quality of life of patients with inflammatory and neoplastic diseases, partly because reduced analgesic effectiveness of chronic opiate therapy leads to escalating doses and distressing side effects. Peroxynitrite ($ONOO^-$) and its reactive oxygen precursor superoxide ($O_2^{\bullet -}$), are critically important in the development of pain.

Metalloporphyrins have the highest rate constants for scavenging $O_2^{\cdot}-$ and ONOO− and were shown to alleviate conditions originating from oxidative stress, such as diabetes, cancer, radiation injury, and central nervous system injuries, including morphine antinociceptive tolerance (Salvemini & Neuman, 2010, Salvemini et al., 2011). The most potent ONOO− scavengers and superoxide dismutase mimics reported so far are cationic Mn(III) N-alkylpyridylporphyrins (Fig. 10) (Batinić-Haberle et al, 1999; Rebouças et al., 2008a; Rebouças et al., 2008b).

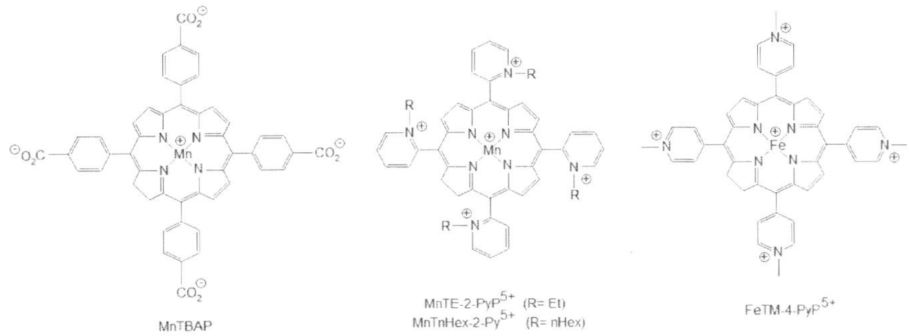

Fig. 10. Metalloporphyrins reported as radical scavengers

4.3 Photodiagnosis

The intriguing "tumor-localization" nature of porphyrins prompted the development of porphyrin-based diagnostic pharmaceuticals for different imaging modalities (Lipson, 1961; Nelson, 1991) or radioactive tracers (Nakajima et al., 1993) for tumor detection with encouraging results (Lee et al., 2010).

4.3.1 Contrast media for MRI

Magnetic resonance imaging (MRI) with molecular probes offers the potential to monitor physiological parameters with high spatial and temporal resolution, but the construction of cell-permeable imaging agents remains a challenge. Membrane permeability, optical activity, and high relaxivity of porphyrin-based contrast agents offer exceptional functionality for *in-vivo* imaging. It was recently shown that a porphyrin-based MRI molecular imaging agent, Mn-(DPA-C_2)$_2$-$TPPS_3$, effectively penetrates cells and persistently stains living brain tissue in intracranially injected rats. Due to cromogenicity, its distribution can also be observed by histology (Chen, 1984; Lee, 2010; Shahbazi-Gahrouei, 2001).

Porphyrin-based complexes were also identified as necrosis-avid contrast agents (NACAs) for noninvasive MRI identification of acute myocardial infarction, assessment of tissue or organ viability, and therapeutic evaluation after interventional therapies (Ni, 2008).

4.3.2 NIR fluorescent probes

The NIR region of the spectrum offers considerable opportunities for diagnosis because of the lack of interference with endogenous absorbers such as haeme pigments and melanin. In this region, light is able to penetrate deeper into tissue, thus offering routes to the therapy of blood vessel disorders and larger or deeper seated malignancies.

Although the greatest activity in the synthesis of NIR-absorbing compounds for therapeutic intent has come from the porphyrin area, with bacteriochlorins and texaphyrins being promising derivatives, none of them is yet in everyday use (Wainwright M., 2010).

5. Current limitations and future trends

Only a small part of the impressive number of synthesized porphyrinic compounds is highly efficient in PDT, so the quest for the ideal photosensitizer still continues.

5.1 Coupling with light sources

Several porphyrin related photosensitizers are currently on the market. Unfortunately, they have several limitations. The perfect balance and fulfilment of the criteria displayed in Table 1, is not reached at this stage of development. The light sources, especially lasers, are increasingly acquiring improved characteristics, so more and more photosynthetizers can be used in biomedical applications and consequently an increased number of tumors are targeted. Future developments in porphyrinic-type photosensitizers will be oriented toward interdisciplinary applications. The improvement of lasers, mainly with increased tissue penetrability, will be associated with the significant development of new photosensitizers, not necessarily related to porphyrins.

5.2 Dosimetry of PDT

Despite promising in vitro studies, many attempts to use PDT in the clinic have led to inadequate tumor response or unacceptable side-effects, and this is partially due to the complexity of PDT mechanisms and the associated dosimetry problems. We must take into account that the local concentration of photosensitizer varies within the body and inter-individual variability is registered. The penetration of light into the target depends on the specific optical properties of particular tissues. If the tissue is hypoxic, or becomes hypoxic due to PDT, the yield of singlet oxygen will be lower than expected. Therefore, development of accurate modeling tools, definition of PDT "dose" and *in vivo* measurements are nowadays major challenges in PDT.

5.3 Oxygen and singlet oxygen

Target tissue oxygenation is one of the essential factors coupled with the photosensitizers behavior (Patterson M.S. & Mazurek E., 2010; Ogilby P.R., 2010; Wilson et al., 2007). Oxygen can be measured invasively using implanted oxygen electrodes. But, as demonstrated in radiotherapy studies, the spatial distribution can be highly non-uniform. Non-invasive methods based on magnetic resonance or optical absorption spectroscopy can provide indirect measures of oxygen concentration, and were associated with porphyrins and related structures (Yu et al., 2005).

Singlet oxygen remains at the cutting-edge of modern science, particularly in photosensitised systems. Singlet oxygen brings together seemingly disparate issues such as nanoparticle-dependent surface plasmon resonances and genetically engineered protein tagging experiments.

The conventional method used for direct singlet oxygen measurement is the detection of the weak phosphorescence emitted at 1270 nm when singlet oxygen returns to the ground state. Upon laser excitation the singlet oxygen emission decay is detected at a 90° geometry with a germanium photodiode working at room temperature. Luminescence intensity at a time, t, after laser pulse is measured for the compound under study and for a reference compound with known singlet oxygen quantum yield on the desired solvent and matched optical density. Accurate calibration curves, with linear dependence of singlet oxygen emission intensity versus laser energy are obtained and a comparison of the slopes for the sample and those of the reference yields the singlet oxygen quantum yield. (Oliveira A.S. et al. 2009 and Santos P.F. et al. 2003, 2004, 2005). Nowadays it is already possible to "see" the spectra of singlet oxygen emission in the NIR region using a cooled IndiumGaliumArseniate (InGaAs) Carged Coupled Device (CCD) detector in the arrangement above described (Oliveira A.S. et al. 2011).

The cumulative singlet oxygen signal measured during PDT of cell suspensions correlated well with cell survival over a range of treatment conditions. Unfortunately, local concentration of singlet oxygen is in the picomolar range due to its rapid reaction with biomolecules (emission of only about 10^8 photons cm^{-3} s^{-1}) and the biological microenvironment might influence the real 1270 nm emission. Accordingly, the instrumentation for detecting such weak luminescence is relatively complex and expensive. Lately, an effective method, Singlet Oxygen Luminescence Dosimetry (SOLD) for quantitative PDT related photobiological studies was evaluated and considered as optimal tool to evaluate photosensitizers in correlation with delivery methods (Jarvi et al., 2006).

The group of Zhang (2008) increased the generation of singlet oxygen via electric-field metal-photosensitizer interactions, taking advantage of near-field interactions of fluorophores with metallic nanoparticles, a phenomenon called metal-enhanced fluorescence (MEF). Nonradiative energy transfer occurs from excited distal fluorophores to the surface plasmon electrons on noncontinuous films. The surface plasmons in turn radiate the photophysical characteristics of the coupling fluorophores. However, additional work is required to optimize or control the amount of singlet oxygen generation from photosensitizers in proximity to metal nanoparticles.

Molecular Probes (Invitrogen Inc.) developed the Singlet Oxygen Sensor Green reagent, which is highly selective for singlet oxygen. It exhibits initially weak blue fluorescence, with excitation peaks at 372 and 393 nm and emission peaks at 395 and 416 nm. In the presence of singlet oxygen, it emits a green fluorescence similar to that of fluorescein (excitation/ emission maxima ~504/525 nm). Unfortunately, the reagent has only in vitro applications and is used only for cumulative measurements.

Price et al (2009) showed that 3'-*p*- (aminophenyl) fluorescein (APF) is adequate for the detection of singlet oxygen and hydroxyl radical under conditions relevant to PDT, in cell-free studies and in cultured L1210 cells photosensitized with benzoporphyhrin. Studies have to be performed in the presence and absence of DMSO to eliminate hydroxyl radical contribution.

The group of Lee S (2010) developed two instruments, an ultra-sensitive singlet oxygen point sensor and a 2D imager, as real-time dosimeters for PDT researchers. The 2D imaging system can visualize in vitro and in vivo spatial maps of both the singlet oxygen production and the localization of the photosensitizer in a tumor during PDT.

5.4 Photosensitizer delivery

Penetration of the photosensitizer into tissues is the major limiting factor in PDT. Porphyrin-like molecules are polycyclic, often heavily charged and in many cases insoluble in both hydrophilic and lipophilic media. In addition, porphyrins and their analogues are known to self-aggregate, which is facilitated by a flat, wide, and electron-rich surface, creating van der Waals, π–π stacking, charge-transfer interactions (Andrade et al., 2008). Therefore, finding adequate drug delivery systems is crucial in improving bioavailability, target specificity and cellular localization of photosensitizers in PDT. Drug targeting from parenteral administration of photosensitizers has been achieved by using liposomes, oil emulsions, microspheres, micellar nanoparticles, proteins and monoclonal antibodies, but the ideal formulation has not yet been developed.

Polymeric nanoparticles offer numerous advantages over the conventional drug delivery systems including high drug loading, controlled release, and a large variety of carrier materials and pharmaceutical formulations (Konan, 2002).

In the development of new drug delivery principles and devices, one may take advantage of the very basics of PDT, namely photoactivation. The method provides a broad range of adjustable parameters (e.g., wavelength, intensity, duration, spatial and temporal control) that can be optimized to suit a given application. Photoactivated drug delivery can be used to control the release rate of the active principle from a dosage form (i.e., a carrier system), to activate a drug molecule that is already present at the site of action in an inactive form (e.g., a photosensitizer or a prodrug), or it can combine the two (i.e., photocontrolled drug release and drug activation). While photoactivation of sensitizers is well established, the application of photoactivated carrier systems offers new opportunities, including photoresponsive hydrogels, microcapsules, liposomes, nanoparticles and oligonucleotides (Sortino, 2008).

As shown recently by Kishwar et al. (2010), ZnO nanorods proved to be an efficient light system attached to a photosensitizer for intracellular necrosis. Zinc oxide (ZnO) has many advantageous properties like direct band gap of 3.37 eV, large exciton binding energy of 60 eV at room temperature and deep level defects emissions that cover the whole visible range. The UV and green emission part of the white light of ZnO can be used for the activation of photosensitizers in PDT. The family of ZnO nanostructures is the richest known so far and the growth of these nanostructures is facilitated by the self organized growth property of this material. Being a bio-safe and bio-compatible material, ZnO is an attractive candidate for biomedical applications. ZnO nanorods grown on the femto tip were shown to deliver the photosensitizer to breast cancerous cells and cause necrosis within few minutes. Topical pain caused by the conventional PDT method can be reduced by this technique.

5.5 Increased fluorescence for photodiagnosis

There is a tremendous need for developing novel non-invasive or minimally invasive diagnostic tools for assessing cell/tissue metabolism and functions, in order to discriminate pathological disturbances in early disease stages. The capability to visualize pathologic tissues as first step before surgical procedure or therapy, may clearly increase treatment efficacy.

Intensive research is done to get probes with appropriate fluorescence characteristics (high quantum yield, large Stokes shifts, reduced photolability and great suitability for cells and tissues, i.e., well-balanced amphiphyllic character, low or no intrinsic toxicity, higher excitation wavelengths to prevent spectral interferences due to the auto fluorescence of the biological samples). Due to the adequacy of their properties, the use of porphyrins and metalloporphyrins as near infrared probes (NIR probes) in biomedical applications increased exponentially. Porphyrinic structures, either in solution or in restricted nanometric geometries, typically display long decay times, and this can be used as an extra discrimination advantage for fluorescence imaging (long lifetime probes for lifetime based sensing). We believe that nowadays the analysis of porphyrins and porphyrin-like structures from the point of view of their fluorescence properties is crucial for developing minimally invasive fluorescent tools for diagnosis.

Several studies on fluorescent photosensitizers show them as markers and beacons and point toward their dual utility for "*seeing and treating*" (Chen et al., 2005; Cló et al., 2007). Theranostic nanomedicine, integrating nano-platforms which can diagnose, deliver targeted therapy and monitor response to therapy, is best illustrated in PDT. Photosensitizers will not only kill pathologic cells when light-activated, but being inherently fluorescent they can be used for imaging and locating disease as photosensitizers selectively accumulate within diseased tissue. The use of lasers and minimally invasive fiber optic tools, along with the development of new agents that respond to NIR wavelengths for better tissue penetration, makes direct targeting of deep tissues possible, enabling imaging and treatment of several pathologies. Alongside, nanoprobes have been developed for in vivo optical imaging, which include quantum dots, up-converting nanophosphors, gold and silica nanoparticles, and photosensitizers containing nanoparticulate carriers. This approach is becoming of increasing interest for oncological applications, addressing the challenges of cancer heterogeneity and adaptability.

5.6 Nano PDT

The general advances in medicine and the progress in the use of photosensitizers for PDT directed the research towards the development of photoactive nanoparticles which can be used for cancer therapy, as sensors for tumor indication and imaging and for other applications of PDT such as vascular disorders (Paszko et al., 2011). The effectiveness of PDT could be maximised by using nanoparticles which can improve the photosensitizer solubility in aqueous media, its formulation properties and selectivity to the target tissue. Selectivity improvement can be achieved by nano-formulating the photosensitizers with liposomes or by modifying them using dendrimers, nanotubes (Zhu, 2008) or fullerenes; such liposomal formulation of Foscan (Foslip®) is currently under investigation (Buchholz, cited by Lassale et al., 2008).

6. Conclusions

Porphyrins have a well-defined place among the substances used in biomedical engineering as medical devices (as defined by the European Council directives No. 93/42/EEC and 98/79/EC, completed by the associated MEDDEV guidance documents) as they can be used effectively as both diagnosis and treatment tools.

<table>
<tr><th>No</th><th>Target</th><th>Drug/Procedure/ Device</th><th>Theme</th><th>Status</th></tr>
<tr><td>1.</td><td>Colorectal Cancer</td><td>Optical Fluoroscopy</td><td>Colorectal Cancer Detection by Means of Optical Fluoroscopy</td><td rowspan="3">Recruiting</td></tr>
<tr><td>2.</td><td>Porphyria Cutanea Tarda</td><td>Exjade</td><td>Safety and Efficacy of Oral Deferasirox in Patients With Porphyria Cutanea Tarda</td></tr>
<tr><td>3.</td><td>Glioma</td><td>5-Aminolevuline Acid</td><td>Safety Study of Aminolevulinic Acid (ALA) to Enhance Visualization and Resection of Malignant Tumors of the Brain</td></tr>
<tr><td>4</td><td>Lung Cancer</td><td>CyPath</td><td>Sputum Labeling Utilizing Synthetic Meso Tetra (4-Carboxyphenyl) Porphine (TCPP) for Detection of Lung Cancer</td><td>Active</td></tr>
<tr><td>5.</td><td>Acne Vulgaris</td><td>Visonac</td><td>Photoactive Porphyrins (PAP) Levels After Topical Visonac Application in Acne Patients</td><td rowspan="7">Completed</td></tr>
<tr><td>6.</td><td>Basal Cell Carcinoma</td><td>PDT with Metvix 160 mg/g cream
PDT with placebo cream</td><td>Photodynamic Therapy (PDT) With Metvix Cream 160 mg/g Versus PDT With Placebo Cream in Patients With Primary Nodular Basal Cell Carcinoma</td></tr>
<tr><td>7.</td><td>Basal Cell Carcinoma</td><td>PDT with Metvix 160 mg/g cream and Placebo cream</td><td>PDT With Metvix 160 mg/g Cream Versus PDT With Placebo Cream in Patients With Primary Nodular Basal Call Carcinoma</td></tr>
<tr><td>8.</td><td>Porphyria</td><td>Heme arginate;
Tin mesoporphyrin</td><td>Phase I/II Study of Heme Arginate and Tin Mesoporphyrin for Acute Porphyria</td></tr>
<tr><td>9.</td><td>Healthy Subjects</td><td>Eltrombopag;
Ciprofloxacin; Placebo</td><td>Study In Healthy Subjects To Evaluate The Photo-Irritant Potential Of Eltrombopag</td></tr>
<tr><td>10.</td><td>Basal Cell Carcinoma</td><td>Procedure: PDT with Metvix 160 mg/g cream</td><td>Metvix PDT in Patients With "High Risk" Basal Cell Carcinoma</td></tr>
<tr><td>11.</td><td>Porphyria</td><td>Heme arginate;
Tin mesoporphyrin</td><td>Studies in Porphyria III: Heme and Tin Mesoporphyrin in Acute Porphyrias</td></tr>
</table>

Table 5. Current status of medical trials involving porphyrins (source: *ClinicalTrials.gov*)

To underline the importance of porphyrinic compounds and to reveal again their multivalency toward biomedical applications we present the current status (2011, April) of their involvement in a wide range of medical trials of the U.S. National Institutes of Health (see Table 5).

7. Acknowledgements

The work was performed within the frame of MNT-Era-Net projects No. 7-030/ 2010 (CNMP), 0003/2009 and 0004/2009 (FCT).

8. References

*** ClinicalTrials, available on http://clinicaltrials.gov/

*** Directive 98/79/EC of the European Parliament and of the Council of 27 October 1998 on *in vitro* diagnostic medical devices

*** European Council directive 93/42/EEC of 14 June 1993 concerning medical devices

*** Molecular Probes Handbook, available on http://www.invitrogen.com/site/us/en/home/brands/Molecular-Probes.html

Adler A.D, Longo F.R, Finarelli J.D, Goldmacher J, Assour J, Korsakoff L (1976). *Journal of Organic Chemistry* Vol. 32 No.2 (February), pp. 476-476, ISSN 1434-193X, doi: 10.1021/jo01288a053

Allison R.R., Downie G.H., Cuenca R., Hu X.H., Childs C.J.H., Sibata C.H. (2004). Photosensitizers in clinical PDT. *Photodiagnosis and Photodynamic Therapy* Vol. 1, pp. 27 – 42, ISSN 0031-8655, doi: 10.1016/S1572-1000(04)00039-0.

Allison R., Sibata C. (2010). Oncologic photodynamic therapy photosensitizers: A clinical review. *Photodiagnosis and Photodynamic Therapy*, Vol. 7 No.2 (June), pp. 61-75, ISSN 0031-8655 doi: 10.1016/j.pdpdt.2010.02.001

Alves E., Costa L., Carvalh C.M.B., Tomé J.P.C., Faustino M.A., Neves M.G.P.M.S., Tomé A.C., Cavaleiro J.A.S., Cunh Â., Almeida A. (2009). Charge effect on the photoinactivation of Gram-negative and Gram-positive bacteria by cationic meso-substituted porphyrins. *BMC Microbiology* Vol. 9:70, ISSN 1471-2180, doi:10.1186/1471-2180-9-70

Anand S., Honari G., Hasan T., Elson P., Maytin E.V. (2009). Low-dose Methotrexate Enhances Aminolevulinate-based Photodynamic Therapy in Skin Carcinoma Cells In vitro and In vivo. *Clinical Cancer Research* Vol. 15 No. 10 (May 15), pp. 3333–3343, ISSN: 1078-0432, doi: 10.1158/1078-0432.CCR-08-3054

Andrade S.M., Teixeira R., Costa S.M.B., Sobral A.J.F.N. (2008). Self-aggregation of free base porphyrins in aqueous solution and in DMPC vesicles. *Biophysical Chemistry* Vol. 133 No 1-3 (March), pp 1–10, ISSN 0301-4622, doi: 10.1016/j.bpc.2007.11.007

Awan M.A., Tarin S.A.(2006). Review of photodynamic therapy. *The Surgeon*. Vol.4 No.4 (August) pp. 231-236, ISSN 1479-666X, doi: 10.1016/S1479-666X(06)80065-X.

Banerjee S., Das T., Samuel G., Sarma H.D., Venkatesh M., Pillai M.R. (2001). A novel [186/188Re]-labelled porphyrin for targeted radiotherapy. *Nuclear Medicine Communication* Vol. 22 No. 10 (October), pp. 1101-1107, ISSN 0143-3636.

Barth R.F., Coderre J.A., Vicente M.G., Blue T.E. (2005). Boron neutron capture therapy of cancer: Current status and future prospects. *Clinical Cancer Research* Vol. 11 No. 11, pp. 3987–4002, ISSN: 1078-0432.

Batinić-Haberle, I.; Benov, L.; Spasojević, I.; Hambright, P.; Crumbliss, A. L., Fridovich I. (1999). The relationship between redox potentials, proton dissociation constants of pyrrolic nitrogens, and in vitro and in vivo superoxide dismutase activities of manganese(III) and iron(III) cationic and anionic porphyrins. *Inorganic Chemistry* Vol. 38 No. 18 (August 17), pp 4011–4022, ISSN 0020-1669, doi: 10.1021/ic990118k

Berenbaum M.C. & Bonnett, R. (1990). in *Photodynamic Therapy of Neoplastic Disease*, Kessel, D. (Ed.), Vol. 2, pp. 169, CRC Press, ISBN 978-0849358166, Boca Raton, Boston.

Bonnett, R. (2000). *Chemical aspects of Photodynamic Therapy*, Gordon & Breach Publishers, ISBN 9056992481 Amsterdam

Boscencu R., Socoteanu R, Oliveira A.S., Vieira Ferreira L.F., Nacea V., Patrinoiu G. (2008). Synthesis and Characterization of Some Unsymmetrically-substituted Mesoporphyrinic Mono-Hydroxyphenyl Complexes of Copper(II). *Polish Journal of Chemistry* Vol 82, No. 3, pp. 509–521, ISSN 0137-5083

Boscencu R., Socoteanu R., Ilie M., Oliveira A. S., Constantin C., Vieira Ferreira L. F. (2009). Synthesis, spectral and biological evaluation of some mesoporphyrinic Zn(II) complexes, *Revista de Chimie* Vol. 60 No. 10, pp 1006-1011, ISSN 0034-7752

Boscencu R., Ilie M., Socoteanu R., Oliveira A. S., Constantin C., Neagu M., Manda G., Vieira Ferreira L. F. (2010). Microwave Synthesis, Basic Spectral and Biological Evaluation of Some Copper (II) Mesoporphyrinic Complexes, *Molecules* Vol. 15 No.5, pp. 3731-3743, ISSN 1420-3049, doi:10.3390/molecules15053731

Bregadze V.I., Sivaev I.B., Gabel D., Wohrle D. (2001). Polyhedral boron derivatives of porphyrins and phthalocyanines. *Journal of Porphyrins & Phthalocyanines* Vol. 5 No. 11 (November), pp. 767-781, ISSN 1088-4246, doi: 10.1002/jpp.544.

Brunner H., Gruber N. (2004). Carboplatin-containing porphyrin–platinum complexes as cytotoxic and phototoxic antitumor agents, *Inorganica Chimica Acta* Vol. 357, No. 15 (December 1), pp. 4423-4451, ISSN 0020-1693, doi: 10.1016/j.ica.2004.03.061

Buytaert E., Callewaert G., Hendrickx N., Scorrano L., Hartmann D., Missiaen L., Vandenheede J.R., Heirman I., Grooten J., Agostinis P. (2006). Role of endoplasmic reticulum depletion and multidomain proapoptotic BAX and BAK proteins in shaping cell death after hypericin-mediated photodynamic therapy. *FASEB J* Vol. 20 No.6 (April), pp.756–758, ISSN 0892-6638, doi: 10.1096/fj.05-4305fje

Capella M.A.M., Capella L.S. (2003). A light in multidrug resistance: Photodynamic treatment of multidrug-resistant tumors. *Journal of Biomedical Science* Vol. 10 No.4, pp 361–366, ISSN 1021- 7770, doi: 10.1007/BF02256427

Castano A.P., Mroz P., Hamblin M.R. (2006). Photodynamic therapy and anti-tumour immunity. *Nature Reviews. Cancer* 2006; Vol 6 (July), pp 535-545, ISSN 1474-175X, doi: 10.1038/nrc1894.

Chauhan S.M. S., Sahoo B.B., Srinivas K.A. (2001). Microwave-Assisted Synthesis of 5,10,15,20-Tetraaryl Porphyrins. *Synthetic Communications: An International Journal for Rapid Communication of Synthetic Organic Chemistry*, Vol. 31, No. 1 pp. 33 - 37, ISSN 0039-7911, doi: 10.1081/SCC-100000176

Che C.M., Sun R.W., Yu W.Y., Ko C.B., Zhu N., Sun H. (2003). Gold(III) porphyrins as a new class of anticancer drugs: cytotoxicity, DNA binding and induction of apoptosis in human cervix epitheloid cancer cells. *Chemical Communications* Vol. 21, No.14 pp. 1718 – 1719 ISSN 1359-7345, doi: 10.1039/B303294A.

Chen C., Cohen J.S., Myers C.E., Sohn M. (1984). Paramagnetic metalloporphyrins as potential contrast agents in NMR imaging. *FEBS Letters* Vol. 168 No.1 (March12), pp. 70-74, ISSN 0014-5793 , doi: 10.1016/0014-5793(84)80208-2.

Chen Y., Gryshuk A., Achilefu S., Ohulchansky T., Potter W., Zhong T., Morgan J., Chance B., Prasad P.N., Henderson B.W., Oseroff A., Pandey R.K. (2005). A novel approach to a bifunctional photosensitizer for tumor imaging and phototherapy. *Bioconjugate Chemistry* Vol. 16 No. 5, pp. 1264-1274, ISSN 1043-1802, doi: 10.1021/bc050177o

Chmielewski P.J.; Latos-Grażyński L., Rachlewicz K. (1995). 5,10,15,20-Tetraphenylsapphyrin - Identification of a Pentapyrrolic Expanded Porphyrin in the Rothemund Synthesis. *Chemistry. A European Journal* Vol. 1 No.1 (April), pp. 68-73, ISSN 0947-6539, doi: 10.1002/chem.19950010111

Cló E., Snyder J.W., Ogilby P.R., Gothelf K.V. (2007). Control and selectivity of photosensitized singlet oxygen production: challenges in complex biological systems. *Chembiochem* Vol. 8 No. 5, pp 475-81, ISSN 1439-7633, doi: 10.1002/cbic.200600454.

Dewaele M., Verfaillie T., Martinet W., Agostinis P. (2010). Death and survival signals in photodynamic therapy. *Methods in Molecular Biology* Vol. 635 pp. 7-33, ISSN 1064-3745, doi: 10.1007/978-1-60761-697-9_2

Dickson E.F.G., Goyan R.L., Pottier R.H. (2002) New directions in photodynamic therapy. *Cellular and Molecular Biology* Vol. 48 No.8, pp. 939–954, ISSN 0145-5680.

Dogutan D.K., Zaidi S.H.H., Thamyongkit P., Lindsey J. S. (2007). New Route to ABCD-Porphyrins via Bilanes. *Journal of Organic Chemistry* Vol. 72 No. 20 (September), ISSN 1434-193X, doi: 10.1021/jo701294d

Dolmans D., Fukumura D., Jain R.K. (2003). Photodynamic therapy for cancer. *Nature Reviews. Cancer* Vol. 3 No.5, pp. 380–387, ISSN 1474-175X, doi: 10.1038/nrc1071

Dougherty T.J. (1987). Photosensitizers: therapy and detection of malignant tumors *Photochemistry and Photobiology,* Vol. 45, Supplement 1 (May) pp. 879–889, ISSN 0031-8655, doi: 10.1111/j.1751-1097.1987.tb07898.x

Dougherty T.J., Gomer C.J., Henderson B.W., Jori G., Kessel D., Korbelik M., Moan J., Peng Q. (1998). Photodynamic therapy. *Journal of the National Cancer Institute* Vol. 90, No. 12, pp 889–905, ISSN 0027-8874.

Dysart J.S., Singh G., Patterson M.S. (2005). Calculation of singlet oxygen dose from photosensitizer fluorescence and photobleaching during mTHPC photodynamic therapy of MLL cells. *Photochemistry and Photobiology* Vol. 81, No 1 (January), pp 196-205, ISSN 0031-8655, doi: 10.1111/j.1751-1097.2005.tb01542.x

Evstigneeva R.P., Zaitsev A.V., Luzgina V.N., Ol'shevskaya V.A., Shtil A.A. (2003). Carboranylporphyrins for boron neutron capture therapy of cancer. *Current Medicinal Chemistry - Anti-Cancer Agents* Vol. 3 No. 6 (November), pp. 383-392, ISSN 1568-0118.

Fayter D., Corbett M., Heirs M., Fox D., Eastwood A. (2010). A systematic review of photodynamic therapy in the treatment of pre-cancerous skin conditions, Barrett's oesophagus and cancers of the biliary tract, brain, head and neck, lung, oesophagus and skin. *Health Technology Assessment* Vol. 14 No. 37 (July), pp. 1-288, ISSN 1366-5278, doi: 10.3310/hta14370

Garg A.D., Nowis D., Golab J., Agostinis P. (2010). Photodynamic therapy: illuminating the road from cell death towards anti-tumour immunity. *Apoptosis*. Vol. 15 No. 9 (September), pp 1050-71, DOI: 10.1007/s10495-010-0479-7

Garg A.D., Krysko D.V., Vandenabeele P., Agostinis P. (2011). DAMPs and PDT-mediated photo-oxidative stress: exploring the unknown. *Photochemical & Photobiological Sciences* ISSN 1474-905X, doi: 10.1039/C0PP00294A (Epub ahead of print)

Gollnick S.O., Vaughan L., Henderson B.W. (2002). Generation of effective antitumor vaccines using photodynamic therapy, *Cancer Research Vol.* 62 No.6 (March 15), pp. 1604-8, ISSN 0008-5472.

Gottumukkala V., Luguya R., Fronczek F.R., Vicente M.G.H. (2005). Synthesis and cellular studies of an octa-anionic 5,10,15,20-tetra[3,5(nidocarboranylmethyl)phenyl]porphyrin (H2OCP) for application in BNCT. *Bioorganic & Medicinal Chemistry* Vol. 13 No. 5 (March 1), pp. 1633-1640, ISSN 09680896, doi: 10.1016/j.bmc.2004.12.016.

Guo C.C., Li H. P., Zhang X. B. (2003). Study on synthesis, characterization and biological activity of some new nitrogen heterocycle porphyrins. *Bioorganic & Medicinal Chemistry*, Vol. 11 No. 8 (April), pp. 1745–1751, ISSN 09680896, doi: 10.1016/S0968-0896(03)00027-0.

Guo C.C., R. B. Tong, K. L. Li (2004). Chloroalkyl piperazine and nitrogen mustard porphyrins: synthesis and anticancer activity. *Bioorganic & Medicinal Chemistry*, Vol. 12 No. 9 (April), pp. 2469–2475, ISSN 09680896, doi: 10.1016/j.bmc.2004.01.045.

Halime Z., Belieu S, Lachkar M., Roisnel T., Richard P., Boitrel B. (2006). Functionalization of Porphyrins: Mechanistic Insights, Conformational Studies, and Structural Characterizations, *Eur. J. Org. Chem.* 2006, Nr. 5, 1207–1215, ISSN 1099-0690; DOI: 10.1002/ejoc.200500685

Hancock R.E.W. (2007). The end of an era? *Nature Reviews Drug Discovery*, Vol. 6 No. 28 (January), ISSN 1474-1776, doi: 10.1038/nrd2223.

He H., Zhou Y., Liang F., Li D., Wu J., Yang L., Zhou X., Zhang X., Cao X. (2006). Combination of porphyrins and DNA-alkylation agents: Synthesis and tumor cell apoptosis induction *Bioorganic & Medicinal Chemistry*. Vol. 14 No.4 (February), pp. 1068–1077, ISSN 09680896, doi: 10.1016/j.bmc.2005.09.041.

Hryhorenko E.A., Oseroff A.R., Morgan J., Rittenhouse-Diakun K. (1998). Antigen specific and nonspecific modulation of the immune response by aminolevulinic acid based photodynamic therapy. *Immunopharmacology* Vol. 40 No. 3 (November), pp. 231-240, ISSN 0892-3973, doi: 10.1016/S0162-3109(98)00047-2.

Jarvi M. T., Niedre M.J., Patterson M.S., Wilson B.C. (2006). Singlet Oxygen Luminescence Dosimetry (SOLD) for Photodynamic Therapy: Current Status, Challenges and Future Prospects. *Photochemistry and Photobiology* Vol. 82 No. 5 (September), pp. 1198–1210, ISSN 0031-8655, doi: 10.1562/2006-05-03-IR-891.

Jori G., Coppellotti O. (2007). Inactivation of pathogenic microorganisms by photodynamic techniques: mechanistic aspects and perspective applications. *Anti-infective Agents in Medicinal Chemistry*, Vol. 6 No.2. (April), pp. 119-131, ISSN 1871-5214.

Kadish K., Guilard R., Smith K.M. Eds. 2002 The Porphyrin Handbook Series, Vols. 1-20, Academic Press, available at http://www.icpp.uh.edu/Documents/Porphyrin_Handbook_030305b.pdf

Kessel D., Vicente M.G., Reiners J.J. Jr. (2006). Initiation of apoptosis and autophagy by photodynamic therapy. *Lasers in Surgery & Medicine* Vol.38 No.5 (June), pp. 482–488, ISSN 0196-8092, doi: 10.1002/lsm.20334

Kessel D. & Reiners Jr. J.J. (2007). Apoptosis and Autophagy After Mitochondrial or Endoplasmic Reticulum Photodamage. *Photochemistry & Photobiology* Vol. 83 No.5 (September-October), pp. 1024–1028, ISSN 0031-8655 doi: 10.1111/j.1751-1097.2007.00088.x.

Kishwar S., Asif M.H., Nur O., Willander M., Larsson P.O. (2010). Intracellular ZnO Nanorods Conjugated with Protoporphyrin for Local Mediated Photochemistry and Efficient Treatment of Single Cancer Cell. *Nanoscale Research Letters* Vol. 5 No.10, pp. 1669–1674, ISSN 1556-276X, doi: 10.1007/s11671-010-9693-z.

Konan Y.N., Gurny R., Allemann E. (2002). State of the art in the delivery of photosensitizers for photodynamic therapy. *Journal of Photochemistry and Photobiology B: Biology* Vol. 66 No. 2 (March), pp. 89–106, ISSN 1011-1344, doi: 10.1016/S1011-1344(01)00267-6

Konopka K., Goslinski T. (2007). Photodynamic therapy in dentistry. *Journal of Dental Research.* Vol. 86 no. 8 (August), pp. 694-707, ISSN 0022-0345, doi: 10.1177/154405910708600803.

Konopka K., Goslinski T. (2008). Prospects for photodynamic therapy in dentistry. *Biophotonics International,* Vol 15 No. 7 (July), pp. 32-35, ISSN 1081-8693.

Lapes M., Petera J., Jirsa M. (1996). Photodynamic therapy of cutaneous metastases of breast cancer after local application of meso-tetra-(para-sulphophenyl)-porphyrin (TPPS4) *Journal of Photochemistry & Photobiology B: Biology* Vol. 36 No. 2 (November), pp. 205-207, ISSN 1011-1344, doi: 10.1016/S1011-1344(96)07373-3

Lassalle H.P., Wagner M., Bezdetnaya L., Guillemin F., Schneckenburger H. (2008). Fluorescence imaging of Foscan® and Foslip in the plasma membrane and in whole cells. *Journal of Photochemistry and Photobiology B: Biology* Vol. 92 No.1 (July 24), pp 45-73, ISSN 1011-1344, doi:10.1016/j.jphotobiol.2008.04.007

Lee S., Galbally-Kinney K.L., Murphy B.A., Davis S.J., Hasan T., Spring B., Yupeng T., Pogue B.W., Isabelle M.E., O'Hara J.A. (2010). In vivo PDT dosimetry: singlet oxygen emission and photosensitizer fluorescence. *Progress in biomedical optics and imaging* Vol. 11 No.4, ISSN 1605-7422

Lee T., Zhang X., Dhar S., Faas H., Lippard S.J., Jasanoff A. (2010). In Vivo Imaging with a Cell-Permeable Porphyrin-Based MRI Contrast Agent. *Chemistry & Biology,* Vol. 17 No 6 (June 25), pp. 665-673, ISSN 1074-5521, doi: 10.1016/j.chembiol.2010.05.009.

Lin W., Peng D., Wang B., Long L., Guo C., Yuan J. (2008). A Model for Light-Triggered Porphyrin Anticancer Prodrugs Based on an o-Nitrobenzyl Photolabile Group. *European Journal of Organic Chemistry* No. 5 (February), pp 793–796, ISSN 1434-193X, doi: 10.1002/ejoc.200700972.

Lindsey J.S. (2010). Synthetic Routes to meso-Patterned Porphyrins, *Accounts of Chemical Research,* Vol. 43, No. 2 (October), pp. 300-311, doi 10.1021/ar900212t

Hsu H.C., Schreiman I.C. (1986). Synthesis of Tetraphenylporphyrins Under Very Mild Conditions, *Tetrahedron Letters* Vol. 27, No. 41, pp. 4969–4970, ISSN 0040-4039, doi: 10.1016/S0040-4039(00)85109-6.

Lindsey J.S., Schreiman I.C., Hsu H.C., Kearney P.C., Marguerettaz A.M. (1987). Rothemund and Adler-Longo Reactions Revisited: Synthesis of Tetraphenylporphyrins Under

Equilibrium Conditions, *Journal of Organic Chemistry*, Vol. 52 No.5, 827-836 , ISSN 1434-193X, doi: 10.1021/jo00381a022.

Lipson R.L., Baldes E.J., Olsen A.M. (1961). Hematoporphyrin derivative: A new aid for endoscopic detection of malignant disease. *Journal of Thoracic Cardiovascular Surgery*, Vol. 42 (November), pp 623-629, ISSN 0022-5223.

Liu M.O., Tai C.H., Hu A.T. (2005). Synthesis of metalloporphyrins by microwave irradiation and their fluorescent properties. *Materials Chemistry and Physics*, Vol. 92 No. 2-3 (August 15), pp. 322-326, ISSN 0254-0584, doi: 10.1016/j.matchemphys.2004.09.027.

Longo F.R., Finarelli J.D., Kim J. (1969). The synthesis and some physical properties of *ms*-tetra(pentafluorophenyl)-porphin and *ms*-tetra(pentachlorophenyl)porphin. *Journal of Heterocyciclic Chemistry* Vol. 6 No. 6 (December), pp. 927-931, ISSN 0022-152X, doi: 10.1002/jhet.5570060625.

Lottner C., Bart K.C., Bernhardt G., Brunner H. (2002). Hematoporphyrin-Derived Soluble Porphyrin−Platinum Conjugates with Combined Cytotoxic and Phototoxic Antitumor Activity *Journal of Medicinal Chemistry* Vol. 45 No 10 (April 17), pp. 2064–2078, ISSN 0022-2623, doi: 10.1021/jm0110688.

Loupy A., Perreux L., Liagre M., Burle K., Moneuse M. (2001). Reactivity and selectivity under microwaves in organic chemistry. Relation with medium effects and reaction mechanisms. *Pure & Applied Chemistry* Vol. 73 No. 1 pp. 161-166, ISSN: 0033-4545.

Maisch T., Szeimies R.-M., Jori G., Abels C. (2004). *Photochemical & Photobiological Sciences* Vol. 3 No 10 (October), pp. 907-917, ISSN 1474-905X, doi: 10.1039/B407622B

Maisch T. (2009). A new strategy to destroy antibiotic resistant microorganisms: antimicrobial photodynamic treatment. *Mini-Reviews in Medicinal Chemistry* Vol. 9 No.8, pp 974-983, ISSN 1389-5575.

Manda G., Nechifor M.T., Neagu T.M. (2009). Reactive Oxygen Species, Cancer and Anti-Cancer Therapies. *Current Chemical Biology*, Vol 3 No.1 (January 1), pp. 342-366, ISSN 1872-3136.

Masilamani V., Al-Zhrani K., Al-Salhi M., Al-Diab A., Al-Ageily M. (2004). Cancer diagnosis by autofluorescence of blood components. *Journal of Luminescence* Vol. 109 No. 3-4 (September), pp.143–154, ISSN 0022-2313, doi: 10.1016/j.jlumin.2004.02.001.

McCoy C.P., Rooney C., Edwards C.R., Jones D.S., Gorman S.P. (2007). Light-Triggered Molecule-Scale Drug Dosing Devices, *Journal of American Chemical Society* Vol 129 No. 31 (July 18), pp. 9572–9573, ISSN 0002-7863, doi: 10.1021/ja073053q.

Merchat M., Bertolini G., Giacomini P., Villaneuva A.· Jori G. (1996). Meso-substituted cationic porphyrins as efficient photosensitizers of gram-positive and gram-negative bacteria, *Journal of Photochemistry & Photobiology B: Biology*, Vol. 32 No 3, pp. 153-157, ISSN 1011-1344, doi: 10.1016/1011-1344(95)07147-4.

Milgrom, L.R. (1983). Synthesis of some new tetra-arylporphyrins for studies in solar energy conversion *Journal of the Chemical Society, Perkin Transactions 1.*, pp. 2535-2539, ISSN 1472-7781, doi: 10.1039/P19830002535.

Mironov A.F., Nizhnik A.N., Nockel A.Y. (1990). Haematoporphyrin derivatives: an oligomeric composition study. *Journal of Photochemistry & Photobiology B: Biology* Vol. 4 No. 3 (January), pp. 297-306, ISSN 1011-1344, doi: 10.1016/1011-1344(90)85035-U

Moan J., Berg K. (1992). Photochemotherapy of cancer: experimental research. *Photochemistry and Photobiology* Vol 55, No.6 (June), pp.145-157, ISSN 0031-8655, doi: 10.1111/j.1751-1097.1992.tb08541.x

Moan J., Peng Q. (2003). An outline of the history of PDT. in *Photodynamic therapy*. Patrice T (Ed.), pp.1-18, The Royal Society of Chemistry, Thomas Graham House, ISBN 978-1-84755-165-8, Science Park, Cambridge, UK.

Mroz P., Bhaumik J., Dogutan D.K., Aly Z., Kamal Z., Khalid L., Kee H.L., Bocian D.F, Holten D., Lindsey J.S., Hamblin M.R. (2009). Imidazole metalloporphyrins as photosensitizers for photodynamic therapy: Role of molecular charge, central metal and hydroxyl radical production. *Cancer Letters*, Vol. 282 No. 1, pp. 63-76, ISSN 0304-3835, doi: 10.1016/j.canlet.2009.02.054.

Nakajima S., Yamauchi H., Sakata I., Hayashi H., Yamazaki K., Maeda T., Kubo Y., Samejima N., Takemura T. (1993). Indium-111-labeled manganese-metalloporphyrin for tumor imaging. *Nuclear Medicine & Biology* Vol. 20 No 2 (February), pp. 231-237, ISSN 0969-8051, doi: 10.1016/0969-8051(93)90120-J

Nelson J.A, Schmiedl U. (1991). Porphyrins as contrast media. *Magnetic Resonance in Medicine*, Vol. 22, No. 2 (December), pp. 366-371, ISSN 0740-3194, doi: 10.1002/mrm.1910220243.

Ni Y. (2008). Metalloporphyrins and Functional Analogues as MRI Contrast Agents *Current Medical Imaging Reviews* Vol. 4 No. 2 (May), pp 96-112, ISSN 1573-4056, doi: 10.2174/157340508784356789.

O'Connor A.E., Gallagher W.M., Byrne A.T. (2009). Porphyrin and Nonporphyrin Photosensitizers in Oncology: Preclinical and Clinical Advances in Photodynamic Therapy. *Photochemistry & Photobiology*, Vol. 85 No. 5 (September/October), pp. 1053-1074, ISSN 0031-8655, doi: 10.1111/j.1751-1097.2009.00585.x.

Ogilby P.R. (2010). Singlet oxygen: there is indeed something new under the sun. *Chemical Society Reviews*, Vol. 39, pp. 3181-3209, ISSN 0306-0012, doi: 10.1039/B926014P

Ol'shevskaya V.A. Zaitsev A.V., Luzgina V.N., Kondratieva T.T., Ivanov O.G., Kononova E.G., Petrovskii P.V., Mironov A.F., Kalinin V.N., Hofmann J., Shtil A.A. (2006). Novel boronated derivatives of 5,10,15,20-tetraphenylporphyrin: Synthesis and toxicity for drug-resistant tumor cells. *Bioorganic & Medicinal Chemistry* Vol.14 No.1(january 1), pp. 109-120, ISSN 09680896, doi: 10.1016/j.bmc.2005.07.067

Oleinick N.L., Morris R.L. & Belichenko I. (2002) The role of apoptosis in response to photodynamic therapy: what, where, why, and how. *Photochemical & Photobiological Sciences*, Vol. 1, pp. 1-21, ISSN 1474-905X, doi: 10.1039/B108586G

Oliveira A.S., Licsandru L., Boscencu R., Socoteanu R., Nacea V., Vieira Ferreira L.V. (2009). A Singlet Oxygen Photogeneration and Luminescence Study of Unsymmetrically Substituted Mesoporphyrinic Compounds. *International Journal of Photoenergy*, Vol. 2009, article ID 413915, DOI: 10.1155/2009/413915

Oliveira A.S, Ferreira D., Boscencu R., Socoteanu R., Ilie M., Constantin C., Manda G., Vieira Ferreira L.F. (2011), Synthesis, Spectral and Cytotoxicity Evaluation of Some Asymmetrical Mesoporphyrinic Compounds with Biomedical Application, in *CIIEM 2011 - International Congress of Energy and Environment Engineering and Management*, pp.144 – 148. ISBN 9052992441

Otsu K., Sato K., Ikeda Y., Imai H., Nakagawa Y., Ohba Y., Fujii J. (2005). An abortive apoptotic pathway induced by singlet oxygen is due to the suppression of caspase activation. *Biochemical Journal*, Vol. 389 Pt 1 (July 1), pp. 197–206, ISSN 0264-6021.

Parsons C., McCoy C.P., Gorman S.P., Jones D.S., Bell S.E.J., Brady C., McGlinchey S.M. (2009). Anti-infective photodynamic biomaterials for the prevention of intraocular lens-associated infectious endophthalmitis. *Biomaterials* Vol.30 No. 4 (February), pp. 597–602, ISSN 0142-9612, doi: 10.1016/j.biomaterials.2008.10.015

Paszko E., Ehrhardt C., Senge M.O., Kelleher D.P, Reynolds J.V. (2011). Nanodrug applications in photodynamic therapy *Photodiagnosis & Photodynamic Therapy*, Vol. 8 No. 1 (March), 14-29, ISSN 1572-1000, doi:10.1016/j.pdpdt.2010.12.001].

Patterson M.S., Mazurek E. (2010). Calculation of Cellular Oxygen Concentration for Photodynamic Therapy In Vitro. In *Photodynamic Therapy. Methods and Protocols* ,Gomer G.J. (ed.), *Methods in Molecular Biology* vol. 635, pp. 195-205, Springer New York Dordrecht Heidelberg London, ISBN 978-1-60761-696-2, doi: 10.1007/978-1-60761-697-9_14.

Pattingre S., Tassa A., Qu X., Garuti R., Liang X.H., Mizushima N., Packer M., Schneider M.D., Levine B. (2005). Bcl-2 Antiapoptotic Proteins Inhibit Beclin 1-dependent Autophagy. *Cell* Vol. 122 No. 6, pp. 927–939, ISSN 0914-7470, doi: 10.1016/j.cell.2005.07.002

Pavani C., Uchoa A.F., Oliveira C.S., Iamamoto Y, Baptista M.S. (2009). Effect of zinc insertion and hydrophobicity on the membrane interactions and PDT activity of porphyrin photosensitizers. *Photochemical & Photobiological Sciences*, Vol. 8 No.2, pp. 233–240, ISSN 1474-905X, doi: 10.1039/B810313E

Petit A., Loupy A., Maillard Ph., Momenteau M. (1992). Microwave Irradiation in Dry Media: A New and Easy Method for Synthesis of Tetrapyrrolic Compounds. *Synthetic Communications: An International Journal for Rapid Communication of Synthetic Organic Chemistry*, Vol. 22 No. 8, pp. 1137-1142, ISSN 0039-7911, doi: 10.1080/00397919208021097.

Price M., Reiners J.J., Santiago A.M., Kessel D. (2009). Monitoring Singlet Oxygen and Hydroxyl Radical Formation with Fluorescent Probes During Photodynamic Therapy. *Photochemistry & Photobiology* Vol. 85 No. 5 (September/October), pp. 1177–1181, ISSN 0031-8655, doi: 10.1111/j.1751-1097.2009.00555.x

Rabbani Z.N., Spasojevic I., Zhang X., Moeller B.J., Haberle S., Vasquez-Vivar J., Dewhirst M.W., Vujaskovic Z., Batinic-Haberle I. (2009). Antiangiogenic action of redox-modulating Mn(III) meso-tetrakis(N-ethylpyridinium-2-yl) porphyrin, MnTE-2-PyP5+, via suppression of oxidative stress in a mouse model of breast tumor. *Free Radical Biology & Medicine* Vol. 47 No.1 (October 1), pp. 992-1004, ISSN 0891-5849, doi: 10.1016/j.freeradbiomed.2009.07.001.

Rai P., Mallidi S., Zheng X., Rahmanzadeh R., Mir Y., Elrington S., Khurshid A., Hasan T. (2010). Development and applications of photo-triggered theranostic agents. *Advanced Drug Delivery Reviews*, Vol. 62 No. 11 (August 30), pp. 1094-1124, ISSN 0169-409X, doi: 10.1016/j.addr.2010.09.002

Rao P.D., Dhanalekshmi S., Littler B. J., Lindsey J. S. (2000). Rational Syntheses of Porphyrins Bearing up to Four Different Meso Substituents, *Journal of Organic Chemistry* Vol. 65 No. 22 (September), pp. 7323–7344, DOI: 10.1021/jo000882k

Rebouças J.S.; DeFreitas-Silva G.; Idemori Y.M., Spasojević I., Benov L., Batinić-Haberle I. (2008a). Impact of electrostatics in redox modulation of oxidative stress by Mn porphyrins: protection of SOD-deficient Escherichia coli via alternative mechanism where Mn porphyrin acts as a Mn carrier. *Free Radical Biology & Medicine* Vol. 45 No 2 (July 15), pp. 201-210, ISSN 0891-5849, doi: 10.1016/j.freeradbiomed.2008.04.009.

Rebouças J.S., Spasojević I., Tjahjono D.H., Richaud A., Mendez F., Benov L., Batinić-Haberle I. (2008b). Redox modulation of oxidative stress by Mn porphyrin-based therapeutics: the effect of charge distribution. *Dalton Transactions*, No.9, pp. 1233-1242, ISSN 1477-9226, doi: 10.1039/B716517J

Rees J.R.E., Lao-Sirieix P., Wong A., Fitzgerald R.C. (2010). Treatment for Barrett's oesophagus. *Cochrane Database of Systematic Reviews* Issue 1. Art. No.: CD004060. doi: 10.1002/14651858.CD004060.pub2

Renner M.W., Miura M., Easson M.W., Vicente M.G.H. (2006). Recent progress in the syntheses and biological evaluation of boronated porphyrins for boron neutron-capture therapy. *Anticancer Agents Medicinal Chemistry* Vol. 6 No.2 (October 31), pp. 145-157, ISSN: 1871-5206, doi: 10.1002/chin.200644231

Rosenthal M.A., Kavar B., Uren S., Kaye A.H. (2003). Promising survival in patients with high-grade gliomas following therapy with a novel boronated porphyrin. *Journal of Clinical Neuroscience* Vol. 10 No. 4 (July), pp. 425-427, ISSN 0967-5868, doi: 10.1016/S0967-5868(03)00062-6.

Rothemund P. (1936). A New Porphyrin Synthesis. The Synthesis of Porphin. *Journal of American Chemists Society*, vol. 58, No. 4 pp. 625-627, ISSN 0002-7863, doi: 10.1021/ja01295a027.

Rothemund, P. (1939). Porphyrin studies. III. The structure of the porphine ring system *Journal of American Chemists Society* Vol. 61 No. 10, pp. 2912-2015, ISSN 0002-7863

Salvemini D., Little J., Doyle T., Neumann W. (2011). Roles of reactive oxygen and nitrogen species in pain. *Free Radical Biology & Medicine*, ISSN 0891-5849, doi:10.1016/j.freeradbiomed.2011.01.026 (Epub ahead of print).

Salvemini D., Neumann W. (2009). Targeting peroxynitrite driven nitroxidative stress with synzymes: A novel therapeutic approach in chronic pain management. *Life Sciences* Vol. 86 No. 15-16 (April 10), pp. 604-614, ISSN 0024-3205, doi: 10.1016/j.lfs.2009.06.011

Santos P.F., Reis L.V., Almeida P., Oliveira A.S., Vieira Ferreira L.F., Singlet oxygen generation ability of squarylium cyanine dyes, *J.Photochem. Photobiol. A: Chem.* 160 (2003) pp. 159-161. ISSN 09380856, doi: 10.1013/j.bmc.2005.03.062

Santos P.F., Reis L.V., Almeida P., Serrano J.P., Oliveira A.S., Vieira Ferreira L.F., Efficiency of singlet oxygen generation of aminosquarylium cyanines, *J.Photochem. Photobiol. A: Chem.* 163 (2004) pp. 267-269. ISSN 0001-4845, 25 doi: 10.1011/ar0300012

Schneider R.; Schmitt F.; Frochot C.; Fort Y.; Lourette N.; Guillemin F.; Müller J.F.; Barberi-Heyob M. (2005). Design, synthesis, and biological evaluation of folic acid targeted tetraphenylporphyrin as novel photosensitizers for selective photodynamic therapy, *Bioorganic & Medicinal Chemistry*, Vol 13 No. 8 (April 15), pp. 2799-808,. ISSN 09680896, doi: 10.1016/j.bmc.2005.02.025

Senge M.O. (2005). Nucleophilic Substitution as a Tool for the Synthesis of Unsymmetrical Porphyrins. *Accounts of Chemical Research* Vol. 38 No. 9, 733-743, ISSN 0001-4842, doi: 10.1021/ar0500012

Senge M.O., Shaker Y.M., Pintea M., Ryppa C., Hatscher S.S., Ryan A., Sergeeva Y., (2010). Synthesis of meso-substituted ABCD-type porphyrins by functionalization reactions. *European Journal of Organic Chemistry* No.2 (January), pp. 237-258, ISSN 1434-193X, doi: 10.1002/ejoc.200901113

Sessler J.L., Weghorn S.J., Lynch V., Johnson M.R. (1994a). Turcasarin, The Largest Expanded Porphyrin Prepared to Date. *Angewandte Chemie International Edition English*, vol. 33, pp. 1509-1512, ISSN. 1433-7851

Sessler J.L.; Brucker E.A.; Weghorn S.J.; Kisters M.; Schäfer M., Lex J., Vogel E. (1994b). Corrphycene: A New Porphyrin Isomer. *Angewandte Chemie International Edition English*, vol. 33, pp. 2308-2312, ISSN. 1433-7851

Sessler J.L., Davis JM, Lynch V. (1998). Synthesis and Characterization of a Stable Smaragdyrin Isomer. *Journal of Organic Chemistry* Vol. 60 No. 23 (September), pp. 7062-7065, ISSN 1434-193X, doi: 10.1021/jo981019b

Shahbazi-Gahrouei D., Williams M., Rizvi S., Allen B.J. (2001). In vivo studies of Gd-DTPA-monoclonal antibody and Gd-porphyrins: potential magnetic resonance imaging contrast agents for melanoma. *Journal of Magnetic Resonance Imaging,* Vol.14 No.2 (August), pp. 169-174, ISSN 1053-1807, doi: 10.1002/jmri.1168.

Song R.; Kim Y.S.; Sohn Y.S. (2002). Synthesis and selective tumor targeting properties of water soluble porphyrin-Pt(II) conjugates, *Journal Inorganic Biochemistry.* Vol. 89 No. 1-2 (April 10) pp.83-88, ISSN 0162- 0134, doi: 10.1016/S0162-0134(01)00413-5.

Sortino S. (2008). Nanostructured molecular films and nanoparticles with photoactivable functionalities. *Photochemical & Photobiological Sciences*, Vol. 7, pp. : 911-924, ISSN 1474-905X, doi: 10.1039/B807353H.

Spikes J.D. (1989). Photosensitization. In *The Science of Photobiology. Photosensitization,* Smith K.S. (Ed.), pp. 79-110. Plenum Press, ISBN 978-0306430596 New York, London.

Tang H.M., Hamblin M.R., Yow C.M. (2007). A comparative *in vitro* photoinactivation study of clinical isolates of multidrug-resistant pathogens. *Journal of Infection and Chemotherapy* Vol 13 No.2 (April), pp. 87-91, ISSN 1341-321X, doi: 10.1007/s10156-006-0501-8.

van Duijnhoven F.H., Aalbers R.I., Rovers J.P., Terpstra O.T., Kuppen P.J. (2003). The immunological consequences of photodynamic treatment of cancer, a literature review. *Immunobiology* Vol. 207 No. 2, pp. 105-113, ISSN 0171-2985, doi: 10.1078/0171-2985-00221.

Verma S., Watt G.M., Mai Z., Hasan T. (2007). Strategies for enhanced photodynamic therapy effects *Photochemistry & Photobiology* Vol 83 No. 5 (September/October) pp. 996-1005, ISSN 0031-8655, doi: 10.1111/j.1751-1097.2007.00166.x

Vicente M.G.H. (2001). Porphyrin-based sensitizers in the detection and treatment of cancer: recent progress. *Current Medicinal Chemistry - Anti-Cancer Agents* Vol. 1, No. 2 (August), pp. 175-194, ISSN 1568-0118.

Vicente M.G.H., Wickramasighe A., Nurco D.J., Wang H.W.H., Nawrocky M.M., Makar M.S., Miura M. (2003). Syntheses, toxicity and biodistribution of two 5,15-di[3,5-(nido-carboranyl-methyl)phenyl]porphyrin in EMT-6 tumor bearing mice.

Bioorganic & Medicinal Chemistry Vol. 11 No. 14 (July 17) pp. 3101-3108, ISSN 09680896, doi: 10.1016/S0968-0896(03)00240-2.

Vicente M.G.H., Sibrian-Vazquez M. (2010). Syntheses of boronated porphyrins and their application in BNCT. In: *The Handbook of Porphyrin Science*. Vol. 4. pp.: 191–248 Kadish K.M., Smith K.M., Guilard R. (Eds.) World Scientific Publishers ISBN 978-981-4280-16-7, Singapore.

Vrouenraets M.B., Visser G.W.M., Snow G.B., van Dongen G.A.M.S. (2003). Basic principles, applications in oncology and improved selectivity of photodynamic therapy *Anticancer Research* Vol. 23 No. 1B, pp. 505–522, ISSN 0250-7005.

Wainwright M. (2010). Therapeutic applications of near-infrared dyes, *Coloration Technology*, Vol. 126, Iss. 3, 115-123, ISSN 1478-4408, doi: 10.1111/j.1478-4408.2010.00244.x

Wiehe A., Shaker Y. M., Brandt J.C., Mebs S., Senge M.O. (2005). Lead structures for applications in photodynamic therapy. Part 1: Synthesis and variation of m-THPC (Temoporfin) related amphiphilic A_2BC-type porphyrins, *Tetrahedron* Vol. 61, No. 23 (June 6), pp. 5535-5564, ISSN 0040-4020, doi: 10.1016/j.tet.2005.03.086

Wilson B.C., Patterson M.S., Lilge L. (1997). Implicit and explicit dosimetry in photodynamic therapy: a New paradigm. *Lasers in Medical Science* Vol. 12, No.3 (October), pp. 182-199, ISSN 0268-8921.

Wilson B.C. (2002). Photodynamic therapy for cancer: Principles. *Canadian Journal of Gastroenterology*, Vol. 16 No.6, pp. 393–396, ISSN 1352-0504.

Winkelman J.W., Collins G.H. (1987). Neurotoxicity of tetraphenylporphinesulfonate TPPS4 and its relation to photodynamic therapy *Photochemistry & Photobiology*, Vol. 46 No. 5 (November), pp. 801-807, ISSN 0031-8655, doi: 10.1111/j.1751-1097.1987.tb04851.x

Witko-Sarsat V., Rieu P., Descamps-Latscha B., Lesavre P., Halbwachs-Mecarelli L. (2000). Neutrophils: molecules, functions and pathophysiological aspects. *Laboratory Investigation* Vol. 80 No.5 (May), pp 617-653, ISSN 0023-6837.

Xue L.Y., Chiu S.M., Azizuddin K., Joseph S., Oleinick N.L. (2007). The death of human cancer cells following photodynamic therapy: Apoptosis competence is necessary for Bcl-2 protection but not for induction of autophagy. *Photochemistry & Photobiology* Vol. 83 No. 5 (Sept-Oct), pp. 1016–1023, ISSN 0031-8655, DOI: 10.1111/j.1751-1097.2007.00159.x

Yu G., Durduran T., Zhou C., Wang H.W., Putt M.E., Saunders H.M., Sehgal C.M., Glatstein E., Yodh A.G., Busch T.M. (2005). Noninvasive monitoring of murine tumor blood flow during and after photodynamic therapy provides early assessment of therapeutic efficacy. *Clinical Cancer Research* Vol 11 No. 9 (May 1), pp. 3543-3552, ISSN 1078-0432, doi: 10.1158/1078-0432.CCR-04-2582.

Zhang Y., Aslan K., Previte M.J.R., Geddes C.D. (2008). Plasmonic engineering of singlet oxygen generation. *Proceedings of the National Academy of Science of the United States of America* vol. 105 no. 6 (February 12), pp. 1798–1802, ISSN 0027-8424, doi: 10.1073/pnas.0709501105

Zhu Z, Tang Z., Phillips J.A., Yang R., Wang H., Tan W. (2008). Regulation of Singlet Oxygen Generation Using Single-Walled Carbon *Journal of American Chemical Society* Vol. 130 No. 33 (August 20), pp. 10856-10857, ISSN 0002-7863, doi: 10.1021/ja802913f

16

The Potential of Genetically Engineered Magnetic Particles in Biomedical Applications

Tomoko Yoshino, Yuka Kanetsuki and Tadashi Matsunaga
Tokyo University of Agriculture and Technology
Japan

1. Introduction

Magnetic particles are currently one of the most important materials in the industrial sector, where they have been widely used for biotechnological and biomedical applications such as carriers for recovery and for detection of DNA, proteins, viruses, and cells (Perez *et al.*, 2002; Kramer *et al.*, 2004; Gonzales and Krishnan, 2005). The major advantage of magnetic particles is that they can be easily manipulated by magnetic force, which enables rapid and easy separation of target molecules bound to the particles from reaction mixtures (Mirzabekov *et al.*, 2000; Gu *et al.*, 2003; Kuhara *et al.*, 2004; Xu *et al.*, 2004). Use of magnetic particles is beneficial for complete automation of steps, resulting in minimal manual labor and providing more precise results (Sawakami-Kobayashi *et al.*, 2003). Biomolecules such as DNA, biotin, and antibodies have been assembled onto magnetic particles and used as recognition materials for target recovery, separation, or detection.

The method chosen for biomolecule assembly is determined by the surface properties of the magnetic particles. Various methods of assembly onto magnetic particles have been reported such as electrostatic assembly (Goldman *et al.*, 2002), covalent cross-linking (Grubisha *et al.*, 2003; Gao *et al.*, 2004) avidin-biotin technology (Gref *et al.*, 2003), membrane integration (Mirzabekov *et al.*, 2000; Tanaka *et al.*, 2004), and gene fusion techniques (Nakamura *et al.*, 1995b; Yoshino *et al.*, 2004; Yoshino and Matsunaga, 2006). The amount and stability of assembled biomolecules and the percentage of active biomolecules among assembled molecules are dependent on the method used for coupling. However, the fabrication techniques have not been standardized. As applications for magnetic particles in the biotechnology field increase, magnetic particles with greater functionality and novel methods for their production are in demand.

Magnetotactic bacteria synthesize uniform, nano-sized magnetite (Fe_3O_4) particles, which are referred to as "bacterial magnetic particles" (BacMPs). A thin lipid bilayer membrane envelops the individual BacMP, which confers high and even dispersion in aqueous solutions as compared to artificial magnetic particles, making them ideal biotechnological materials (Matsunaga *et al.*, 2003). To use these particles for biotechnological applications, it is important to attach functional molecules such as proteins, antibodies, peptides, or DNA. BacMP-specific proteins have been used as anchor proteins, which facilitate efficient localization and appropriate orientation of various functional proteins attached to BacMPs. We have developed several methods for modification and assembly of these functional organic molecules over the surface of BacMPs using chemical and genetic techniques. In this chapter, we describe advanced magnetic particles used in biomedical applications and the methods for bioengineering of these particles. Specific focus is given to the creation of functional BacMPs by magnetotactic bacteria and their applications.

2. Production of functional magnetic particles

Currently, magnetic particles offer vast potential for ushering in new techniques, especially in biomedical applications, as they can be easily manipulated by magnetic force. The important characteristics of these particles include (1) immobilization of higher numbers of probes onto magnetic particles because particle surfaces are wider than those of a flat surface, (2) reduction of reaction times because of good dispersion properties that increase reaction efficiency, (3) facilitation of the bound/free separation step with a magnet, without centrifugation or filtration, and (4) the use of automated robotic systems for all reaction steps. These characteristics offer great benefits for biomedical applications such as rapid and precise measurements or separations of bio-targets. Here, the methods for production of functional magnetic particles are introduced.

2.1 Commercialized magnetic particles

Commercialized magnetic particles are usually composed of superparamagnetic iron oxide nanoparticles (Fe_3O_4 or Fe_2O_3), which exhibit magnetic properties only in the presence of external magnetic fields. These particles are embedded in polymers such as polysaccharides, polystyrene, silica, or agarose. Micro-sized magnetic particles can be easily removed from suspension with magnets and easily suspended into homogeneous mixtures in the absence of an external magnetic field (Ugelstad *et al.*, 1988). Furthermore, functional groups or biomolecules for the recognition of targets are conjugated to the polymer surfaces of magnetic particles (Fig. 1), and targets can be collected, separated, or detected by the magnetic particles.

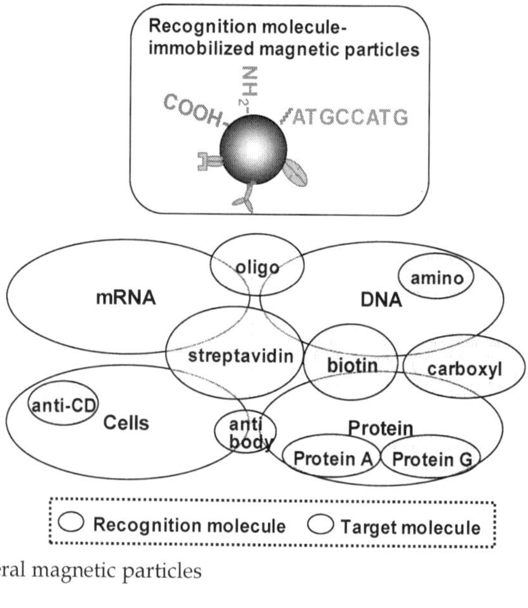

Fig. 1. Use of general magnetic particles

Biotin or streptavidin-assembled magnetic particles, on which complementary nucleic acid strands are immobilized, are widely used for the recovery or extraction of specific nucleic acids and are marketed worldwide. Moreover, magnetic particles can be used as supports for separation or detection of proteins or cells. For example, protein A- or protein G-assembled magnetic particles are suitable for antibody purification and are more efficient than column-purification techniques.

Currently, polymer magnetic particles marketed as Dynabeads® (Invitrogen, co.) are one of the most widely used magnetic particles for biotechnology applications (Sawakami-Kobayashi *et al.*, 2003; Prasad *et al.*, 2003). These particles are prepared from mono-sized macroporous polystyrene particles that are magnetized by an in situ formation of ferromagnetic materials inside the pores. Dynabeads® with diameters of 2.8 μm or 4.5 μm are the most widely used magnetic particles by scientists around the world, particularly in the fields of immunology, cellular biology, molecular biology, HLA diagnostics, and microbiology.

Antibody-immobilized magnetic particles have been used preferentially in target-cell separation of leukocytes (Stampfli *et al.*, 1994; Schratzberger *et al.*, 1997; Schwalbe *et al.*, 2006; Nakamura *et al.*, 2001) for in vitro diagnosis because of the simpler and more rapid methodology as compared to cell sorting using a flow cytometer. These commercially available magnetic particles are chemically synthesized compounds of micrometer and nanometer sizes. Several cell separation systems using nano-sized magnetic particles, such as 50-nm iron oxide particles with polysaccharide- (Miltenyi Biotech, co.) or dextran- (StemCell Technologies Inc.) coated superparamagnetic nanoparticles, are commercially available (Miltenyi, 1995; Wright, 1952). Because these particles are superparamagnetic and are preferred for high-gradient magnetic separation, specially-designed magnetic columns that produce high magnetic field gradients are required for cell separation (Miltenyi, 1995). Nano-sized magnetic particles are advantageous for assay sensitivity, rapidity, and precision. However, it remains difficult to synthesize nano-sized magnetic particles with uniform size and shape that adequately disperse in aqueous solutions. Consequently, advanced techniques and high costs are required for the production of nano-sized magnetic particles.

Magnetic particles are widely used not only as carriers for recovery or detections of bio-molecules, but also used as probes for magnetic detections, or agent for magnetic-field-induced heating. Especially, magnetic particles that have high saturation magnetization are ideal candidates for MRI contrast agents, and various kinds of magnetic particles have been developed and used for diagnoses. Recently, Mulder *et. al.* developed the paramagnetic quantum dots (pQDs) coated with paramagnetic and pegylated lipids which had a high relaxivity. The high relaxivity makes the pQDs contrast agent an attractive candidate for molecular MRI purposes. This nanoparticulate probe makes it detectable by both MRI and fluorescence microscopy (Mulder *et al.*, 2006). It was successful that the synthesis of quantum dots with a water-soluble and paramagnetic micellular coating were used as a molecular imaging probe for both fluorescence microscopy and MRI. The present study uses magnetic nanoparticles as bimodal tools and combines magnetically induced cell labelling and magnetic heating. The particles are used in hyperthermia agents, where the magnetic particles are heated selectively by application of an high frequency magnetic field (Mulder *et al.*, 2006). These magnetic heating treatments using superparamagnetic iron oxide nanoparticles continue to be an active area of cancer research. The research aimed to assess if a selective and higher magnetic nanoparticles accumulation within tumor cells is due to magnetic labeling and consequently a larger heating effect occurs after exposure to an alternating magnetic field in order to eliminate labeled tumor cells effectively (Kettering *et al.*, 2007). Moreover, in recent years magnetic devised like giant magnetoresistive (GMR) sensors have shown a great potential as sensing elements for biomolecule detection (Baselt *et al.*, 1998; Edelstein *et al.*, 2000; Schotter *et al.*, 2004). The GMR biochip based on spin valve sensor array and magnetic nanoparticle probes was developed for inexpensive, sensitive and reliable DNA detection using plasmid-derived samples (Xu *et al.*, 2008). The applications of magnetic particles as probes are increasingly advanced in biomolecule quantitative analysis.

2.2 Magnetic particles produced by magnetotactic bacteria

Magnetotactic bacteria synthesize nano-sized biomagnetites, otherwise known as bacterial magnetic particles (BacMPs), that are enveloped individually by a lipid bilayer membrane (Blakemore, 1983). BacMPs are ultrafine magnetite crystals (50-100 nm in diameter) with uniform morphology produced by *Magnetospirillum magneticum* AMB-1 (Fig. 2).

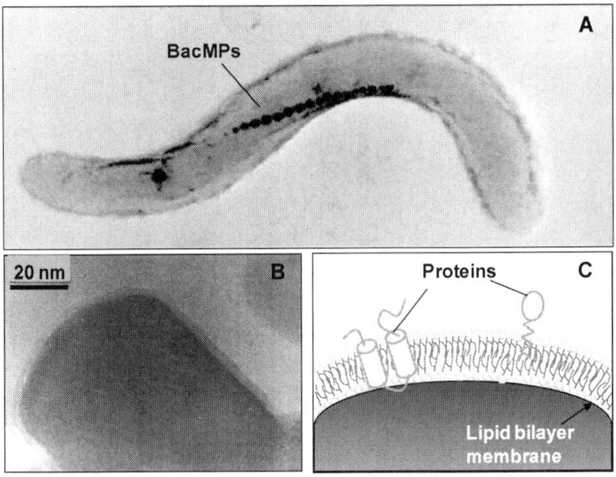

Fig. 2. Transmission electron microscopic (TEM) image and schematic diagram of *Magnetospirillum magneticum* AMB-1 (A), bacterial magnetic particles (BacMPs, B) and schematic diagram of proteins on the BacMPs surface (C).

The molecular mechanism of BacMP synthesis involves a multiple-step process that includes vesicle formation, iron transport, and magnetite crystallization. This mechanism has been studied using genomic, proteomic, and bioinformatic approaches (Matsunaga *et al.*, 2005; Nakamura *et al.*, 1995a; Arakaki *et al.*, 2003; Amemiya *et al.*, 2007) , and a comprehensive analysis provided a clear view of the elaborate regulation of BacMP synthesis.

Techniques for the mass cultivation of magnetotactic bacteria have been developed, allowing for a steady supply of BacMPs for industrial applications. Based on the molecular mechanism of BacMP formation in *M. magneticum* AMB-1, designed functional nanomaterials have also been developed. Through genetic engineering, functional proteins such as enzymes, antibodies, and receptors have been displayed on the surface of BacMPs.

The display of proteins on BacMPs was achieved using a fusion technique involving anchor proteins isolated from magnetotactic bacteria (Nakamura *et al.*, 1995b). Figure 3A shows the procedure for producing functional magnetic particles through genetic engineering of these bacteria. Several proteins involved in the magnetic biosynthetic mechanism are embedded in the BacMP membrane. In *M. magneticum* AMB-1, MagA (46.8 kDa), Mms16 (16 kDa), and Mms13 (13 kDa) proteins have been used as anchor molecules for displaying functional proteins (Nakamura *et al.*, 1995b; Yoshino *et al.*, 2004; Matsunaga *et al.*, 2005; Matsunaga *et al.*, 1999; Matsunaga *et al.*, 2000).

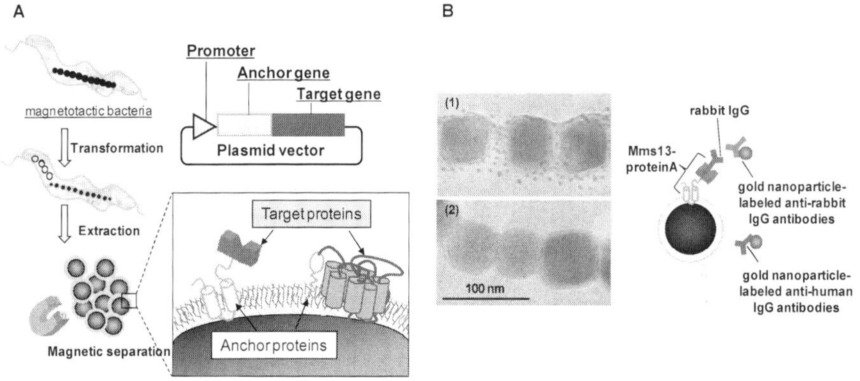

Fig. 3. Preparation of BacMPs displaying functional proteins.
(A) The functional protein gene is fused to an anchor gene for display of a functional protein on BacMPs. A plasmid harboring the fusion gene is introduced into *M. Magneticum* AMB-1.
(B) TEMs of BacMPs displaying protein A which were treated with rabbit IgG after addition of gold nanoparticle (5 nm)-labeled anti-rabbit IgG antibodies (1) or anti-human IgG antibodies (2).

MagA was one of the first proteins experimentally demonstrated to be localized on the surface of BacMPs (Nakamura *et al.*, 1995a; Nakamura *et al.*, 1993). MagA is a transmembrane protein identified from a *M. magneticum* AMB-1 mutant strain generated by transposon mutagenesis (Nakamura *et al.*, 1995a). As proof of localization, luciferase (61 kDa) was fused to the C-terminus of MagA (Nakamura *et al.*, 1995b). This was the first report of protein display on BacMPs using gene fusion techniques. However, the efficiency and stability of proteins displayed on BacMPs were limited, and only a few molecules were displayed on a single BacMP.

As research in this field progressed, a more effective and stable method for protein display was developed. To establish high levels of expressed proteins displayed on BacMPs, strong promoters and stable anchor proteins were identified using *M. magneticum* AMB-1 genome and proteome analysis (Yoshino and Matsunaga, 2005).

An integral BacMP membrane protein, Mms13, was isolated as a stable anchor molecule, and its anchoring properties were confirmed by luciferase fusion studies. The C-terminus of Mms13 was expressed on the surface of BacMPs, and Mms13 was tightly bound to the magnetite directly, permitting stable localization of luciferase on BacMPs. Consequently, the luminescence intensity obtained from BacMPs using Mms13 as an anchor molecule was more than 1,000-times greater than when MagA was used. Furthermore, the IgG-binding domain of protein A was displayed uniformly on BacMPs using Mms13 (Fig. 3B).

Strong promoters and stable anchor proteins allowed efficient display of functional proteins on BacMPs. However, the display of particular proteins remained a technical challenge due to the cytotoxic effects of the proteins when they were overexpressed in bacterial cells. Specifically, transmembrane proteins such as G-protein coupled receptors were still difficult to express in magnetotactic bacteria. An inducible protein expression system is often used to control the expression dose and timing of transmembrane proteins. Recently, we developed a tetracycline-inducible protein expression system in *M. magneticum* AMB-1 to prevent the toxic effects of transmembrane protein expression (Yoshino *et al.*, 2010). This system was implemented to obtain the expression of tetraspanin CD81, where the truncated form of CD81, including the ligand binding site, was successfully expressed on the surface of BacMPs using Mms13 as an anchor protein and the tetracycline-inducible protein expression system. These results suggest that the inducible expression system will be a useful tool for the expression and display of transmembrane and other potentially cytotoxic proteins on the membranes of BacMPs.

Currently, many types of functional proteins can be displayed at high levels on magnetic particles due to the modifications described above. Generally, immobilization of proteins onto magnetic particles is performed by chemical cross-linking; however, this can hinder the activity of some proteins. Because the amine-reactive cross-linker can bind to proteins in a random manner, the target proteins may become inactivated. Furthermore, protein orientation on the solid phase is difficult to control during chemical conjugation. To overcome these difficulties, protein display on magnetic particles produced by magnetotactic bacteria through gene fusion is a promising approach, and the techniques have expanded the number of applications.

3. Applications of magnetic particles

Magnetic iron oxide particles, such as magnetite (Fe_3O_4) and maghemite (γ-Fe_2O_3), are widely used in medical and diagnostic applications such as magnetic resonance imaging (Gleich and Weizenecker, 2005), cell separation (Miltenyi *et al.*, 1990) , drug delivery (Plank *et al.*, 2003), and hyperthermia (Pardoe *et al.*, 2003). To use these particles for biotechnological applications, the surface modification of the magnetic particle with functional molecules such as proteins, peptides, or DNA must be considered. Previously, only DNA- or antibody-immobilized magnetic particles were marketed and used in biotechnology; it was suggested that the techniques for the immobilization of enzymes or receptors were more complicated and time consuming. However, as the methods for assembling functional proteins onto magnetic particles have become simpler and more efficient, the applications of magnetic particles have expanded. Here, the applications of BacMPs displaying functional proteins such as antibody, enzyme, or receptor are described.

3.1 Applications of antibody-magnetic particles

Magnetic particles have been widely used as carriers of antibodies for immunoassay, cell separation, and tissue typing (Herr *et al.*, 2006; Tiwari *et al.*, 2003; Weissleder *et al.*, 2005). The use of magnetic particles is advantageous for full automation, minimizing manual labor and providing more precise results (Sawakami-Kobayashi *et al.*, 2003; Tanaka and Matsunaga, 2000). In particular, immunomagnetic particles have been used preferentially in target cell separation from leukocytes (Stampfli *et al.*, 1994; Schratzberger *et al.*, 1997) for in vitro diagnosis, as this provides a more rapid and simple methodology compared with cell sorting using a flow cytometer.

To immobilize antibody, protein A, which is the antibody-binding protein derived from *Staphylococcus aureus* (Deisenhofer, 1981), has been immobilized on magnetic particles using the sequence of the Z-domain, a synthetic analogue of the IgG-binding B-domain. *Staphylococcus* protein A consists of a cell wall binding region and five domains, termed C, B, A, D, and E, with C next to the cell wall. The molecular interaction of protein A with IgG is well understood, and the binding sites on the Fc domain of IgG1, -2, and -4 have been characterized. X-ray analysis has revealed that the B-domain of protein A has two contact sites that interact with the Fc domain of IgG (Eliasson and Kogelschatz, 1988) . Based on this knowledge, a synthetic Z-domain, which consists of 58 amino acids and is capable of binding the Fc domain, has been constructed (Lowenadler *et al.*, 1987) . IgG can bind the Z-domain on magnetic particles with uniform orientation.

Z-domain was displayed on bacterial magnetic particles using gene fusion techniques and was used to detect human insulin from whole blood by sandwich enzyme immunoassays. The experimental procedure was fully automated using a pipetting robot bearing a magnet (Tanaka and Matsunaga, 2000).

Antibody-conjugated BacMPs also can be utilized for cell separation. In general, nano-sized magnetic particles, rather than micro-sized particles, are preferred for cell separation because separated cells with nano-sized magnetic particles on their surfaces can be used in subsequent flow cytometric analysis (Graepler *et al.*, 1998). Additionally, micro-sized magnetic particles are more likely to have inhibitory effects on cell growth and differentiation after magnetic separation.

Magnetic separation permits target cells to be isolated directly from crude samples such as blood, bone marrow, tissue homogenates, or cultivation media. Compared to other more conventional methods of cell separation, magnetic separation may be considered a sample enrichment step for further chromatographic and electromigratory analysis. To enrich for target cells, cell surface antigens, such as cluster of differentiation (CD) antigens, were used as markers. CD8, CD14, CD19, CD20, and CD34 positive cells were efficiently enriched from peripheral blood (Kuhara *et al.*, 2004; Matsunaga *et al.*, 2006). The separated CD34 positive cells retained the capability of forming colonies as hematopoietic stem cells.

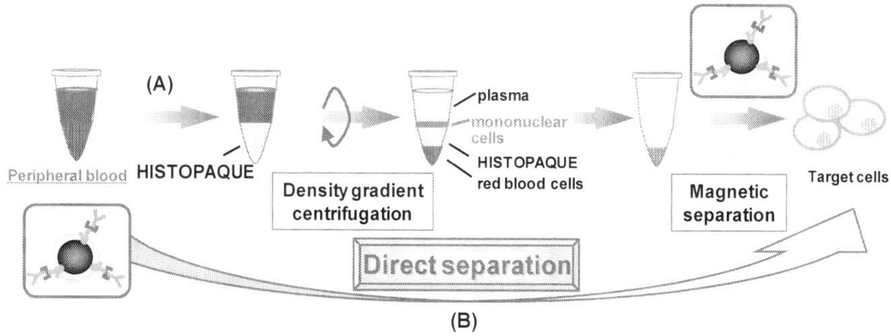

Fig. 4. Schematic illustration of cell separation procedures. (A) The initial separation of peripheral blood mononuclear cells (PBMCs) from whole blood and the subsequent magnetic separation of target cells from PBMCs using magnetic particles followed the common procedure. (B) Target cells were separated directly from whole blood using magnetic particles in the procedure for direct magnetic cell separation.

Protein G from *Streptococcus* sp (Gronenborn *et al.*, 1991) was also displayed on BacMPs, resulting in the expansion of IgG-binding diversity. Direct magnetic separation of immune cells from whole blood using protein G-BacMPs binding anti-CD monoclonal antibodies was demonstrated (Fig. 4). Using this technique, B lymphocytes ($CD19^+$ cells) or T lymphocytes ($CD3^+$ cells) were successfully separated at a high purity.

To increase cell separation efficiency, a novel functional polypeptide, which functions to minimize nonspecific adsorption of magnetic particles to cells, was developed for surface modification of BacMPs (Takahashi *et al.*, 2010). Previous reports had shown that the hydrophilicity or neutral charge of the particle surface was important for the reduction of nonspecific interactions between the nanoparticle and the cell surface (Fang *et al.*, 2009; Patil *et al.*, 2007). The designed polypeptide was composed of multiple units consisting of four asparagines (N) and one serine (S) residue and was referred to as the NS polypeptide. Modification of the surface of a magnetic particle with the NS polypeptide resulted in reduction of non-specific particle-particle and particle-cell interactions. NS polypeptides on magnetic nanoparticle surfaces function as a barrier to block particle aggregation and minimize nonspecific adsorption of cells to the nanoparticles; they also add the ability to recognize and bind to target cells by working as a linker to display protein G on the nanoparticles (Fig. 5). When the NS polypeptide is used in a single fusion protein as a linker to display protein G on magnetic particles, the particle acquires the capacity to specifically bind target cells and to avoid nonspecific adsorption of non-target cells. $CD19^+$ cells represent 4.1% of leukocytes and in peripheral blood were calculated to be less than 0.004% of the total cells. Analysis of magnetically separated cells using flow cytometry revealed that $CD19^+$ cells were separated directly from peripheral blood with greater than 95% purity using protein G-displaying BacMPs bound to anti-CD19 monoclonal antibodies with the NS polypeptide. Purities were approximately 82% when the NS polypeptide was not present.

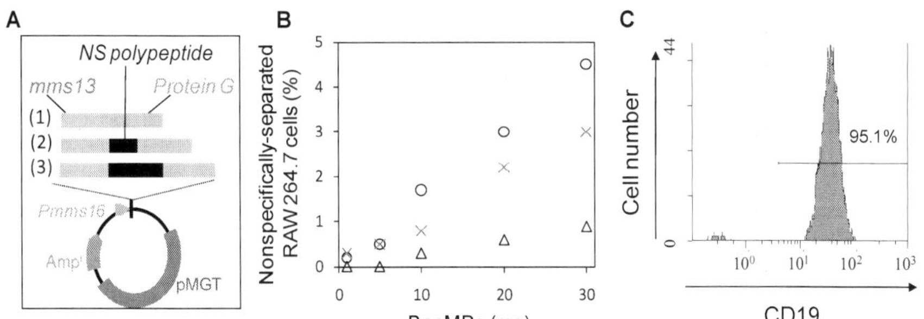

Fig. 5. Effect of NS polypeptide on cell separation.
(A) Schematic diagram of expression vectors for fusion proteins, Mms13-protein G (1), Mms13-$(N_4S)_{10}$-protein G (2), and Mms13-$(N_4S)_{20}$-protein G (3). (B) Correlation between the display of NS polypeptide on BacMPs and nonspecific binding of BacMPs to the cell surface. The number of RAW 264.7 cells separated using BacMPs displaying protein G (○), BacMPs displaying $(N_4S)_{10}$-protein G (×), or BacMPs displaying $(N_4S)_{20}$-protein G (Δ) were counted, and the ratio of nonspecifically separated cells was calculated. (C) Direct magnetic separation of $CD19^+$ cells from whole blood using BacMPs displaying $(N_4S)_{20}$-proteins bound to PE-labeled anti-CD19 mAbs.

Display of fusion proteins (protein G and NS polypeptide) on BacMPs significantly improved recognition of and binding to target cells, and minimized adsorption of non-target cells. These promising results demonstrated that NS polypeptides may be a powerful and valuable tool in various cell associated applications.

3.2 Applications of enzyme-magnetic particles

Enzymes can catalyze various biochemical reactions with high efficiency and specificity and are therefore used in industrial production (Patil *et al.*, 2007). However, the production and purification of recombinant enzymes can be quite time and cost consuming. If enzymes could be immobilized on magnetic particles, they could be reused following magnetic recovery from the reaction mixture. Enzymes and antibodies immobilized on BacMPs using bifunctional reagents and glutaraldehyde have been found to have higher activities than those immobilized on artificial magnetic particles (Matsunaga and Kamiya, 1987). The luciferase gene (luc) was cloned downstream of the MagA promoter and the effect of iron on the regulation of MagA expression was investigated; transcription of MagA was found to be enhanced by low concentrations of iron. As an initial proof-of-concept experiment for the recovery of enzyme-displaying BacMPs, luciferase was assembled onto BacMPs (Nakamura *et al.*, 1995b). The genes for acetate kinase and liciferase were fused to the N- and C-terminus of the MagA anchor protein for simultaneous display of two different enzymes (Matsunaga *et al.*, 2000). Acetate kinase catalyzes the phosphorylation of acetate by ATP. Therefore, this reversible reaction generates ATP in the presence of ADP and acetyl phosphate. The results presented in Fig. 6 are consistent with the hypothesis that ATP is generated in situ by acetate kinase present on BacMPs through phosphorylation of ADP to ATP (Fig. 6). Thus, protein-BacMPs complexes were constructed by joining the luciferase gene to the N- or the C-terminal domains of MagA, and also constructed bifunctional active fusion proteins on BacMPs using MagA as an anchor with acetate kinase and luciferase.

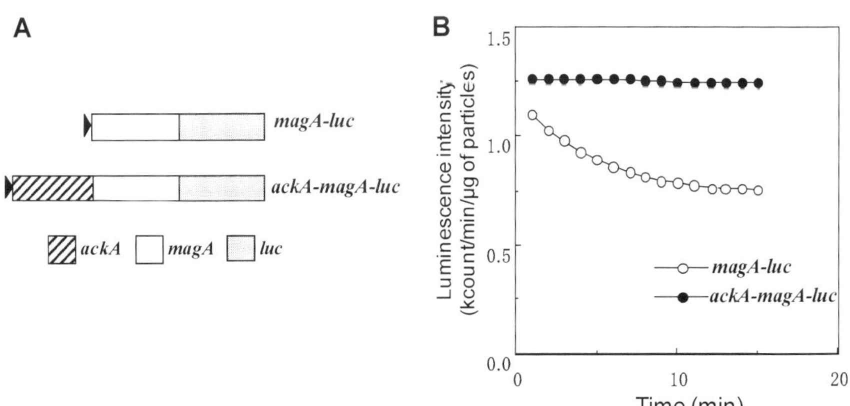

Fig. 6. Simultaneous display of two different enzymes, acetate kinase (ackA) and luciferase (luc), onto BacMPs. (A) Schematic diagram of fusion genes, and (B) luciferase activity on BacMPs

A highly thermostable enzyme, pyruvate phosphate dikinase (PPDK), which converts pyrophosphate PPi to ATP, was also expressed on BacMPs. Pyrosequencing relies on the incorporation of nucleotides by DNA polymerase, which results in the release of PPi. The ATP produced by PPDK-displaying BacMPs can be used by luciferase in a luminescent reaction (Fig. 7). PPDK-displaying BacMPs were employed in a pyrosequencing reaction and a target oligonucleotide was successfully sequenced (Yoshino *et al.*, 2009). The PPDK enzyme was recyclable in each sequence reaction as it was immobilized onto BacMPs which could be manipulated by a magnet. These results illustrate the advantages of using enzyme-displaying BacMPs as biocatalysts for repeat usage. Nano-sized PPDK-displaying BacMPs are useful for the scale-down of pyrosequencing reaction volumes, thus permitting high-throughput data acquisition.

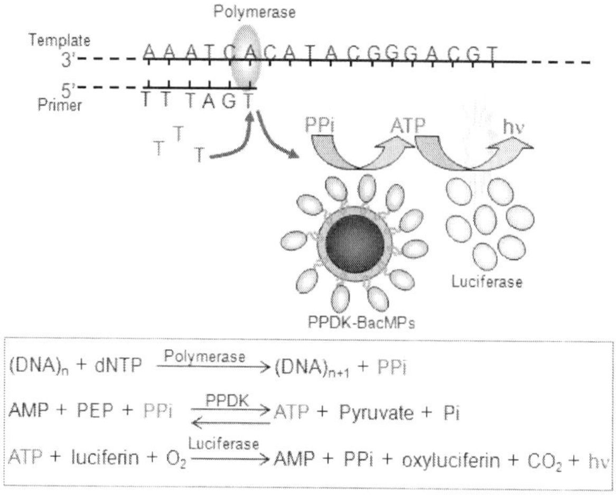

Fig. 7. Schematic diagram of the principle of pyrosequencing using PPDK-BacMPs. PEP: phosphoenolpyruvate, PPi: pyrophosphate, Pi: phosphate, PPDK: Pyruvate phosphate dikinase. PEP : phosphoenolpyruvate, PPi : pyrophosphate, Pi : phosphate, PPDK : Pyruvate phosphate dikinase

3.3 Applications of receptor-magnetic particles

Along with immunoassays and cell separations, ligand-binding assays to study receptor proteins are highly desired applications for magnetic particles. Receptor proteins play critical roles in gene expression, cellular metabolism, signal transduction, and intercellular communication. In particular, nuclear receptors and transmembrane receptors can be major pharmacological targets. These types of receptors have been assembled onto BacMPs.

The estrogen receptor is a nuclear receptor serving as a ligand-inducible transcriptional regulator. In recent decades, it has been suggested that natural and synthetic compounds can act as steroid hormones and adversely affect humans and wildlife through interactions with the endocrine system. These compounds have been broadly referred to as environmental endocrine disrupting chemicals (EDCs). Several chemicals, such as plastic softeners (bisphenol A) or detergents (4-nonylphenol), were originally considered harmless, but now are suspected of having estrogenic effects. It is probable that many unidentified chemical compounds are potential EDCs.

To evaluate and detect these chemical compounds, estrogen receptor ligand-binding domain (ERLBD) was displayed on BacMPs (Yoshino *et al.*, 2005). ERLBD-BacMP complexes can be used for assays based on the competitive binding of alkaline phosphatase conjugated 17β-estradiol (ALP-E2) as a tracer. The dissociation constant of the receptor was 2.3 nM. Inhibition curves were evaluated by the decrease in luminescence intensity resulting from the enzymatic reaction of alkaline phosphatase. The overall simplicity of this receptor binding assay resulted in a method that could be easily adapted to a high-throughput format.

Subsequent-generation evaluation systems for EDCs can distinguish between agonists and antagonists (Yoshino *et al.*, 2008). In one system, ERLBD-displaying BacMPs and green fluorescent protein (GFP)-fused coactivator proteins were used in combination, and ERLBD-displaying BacMPs were incubated with ligands and GFP-coactivators. Binding of the agonist to ERLBD induced a conformational change of ERLBD and promoted binding of the GFP-coactivator to an ERLBD dimer on the BacMP. Binding of the antagonist to ERLBD prevented the GFP-coactivator from binding to the ERLBD-BacMPs. Ligand-dependent recruitment assays of GFP-labeled coactivators to ERLBD-BacMPs were performed by measuring the fluorescence intensity (Fig. 8A). This method was used to evaluate 17β-estradiol (E2) and estriol (E3) as full agonists, octylphenol (OP) as a partial agonist, and ICI 182,780 (ICI) as an antagonist (Fig. 8B). The full agonists showed dose-dependent increases in fluorescence. Octylphenol had lower fluorescence intensity than E2, and ICI 182,780 did not produce fluorescence. The method developed in this study can be used to evaluate the estrogenic potential of chemicals by discriminating whether a chemical is an ER full agonist, a partial agonist, or an antagonist. This novel method has important potential for screening for new EDC candidates and their effects in the environment.

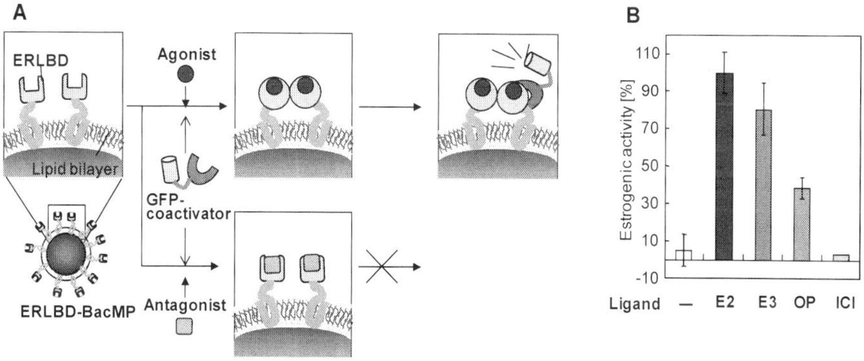

Fig. 8. Schematic diagram of the GFP-coactivator recruitment assay (A) and the assay results (B). Estrogen receptor ligand binding domain (ERLBD)-BacMPs were incubated with ligand and GFP-coactivator. Binding of agonist to ERLBD induced conformation change of ERLBD and promoted binding of GFP-coactivator to ERLBD dimmer on BacMPs. Binding of antagonist to ERLBD prevented GFP-coactivator binding to ERLBD-BacMPs.
E2:17βEstradiol, E3:Estriol, OP:Octylphenol, ICI:ICI 182780

G protein-coupled receptors (GPCRs) play a central role in a wide range of biological processes and are prime targets for drug discovery. GPCRs have large hydrophobic domains, and therefore, purification of GPCRs from cells is frequently time-consuming and typically results in loss of the native conformation. The D1 dopamine receptor, which is a GPCR, was successfully assembled into the lipid membrane of BacMPs (Yoshino *et al.*, 2004). D1 dopamine receptor-displaying BacMPs were simply extracted by magnetic separation from ruptured AMB-1 transformants. This system conveniently retains the native conformation of GPCRs without the need for detergent solubilization, purification, and reconstitution after cell disruption.

Additionally, display of the tetraspanin CD81 was demonstrated using the inducible expression system (Yoshino *et al.*, 2010) described above. CD81 is utilized when hepatitis C virus (HCV) infects hepatocytes and B lymphocytes. Therefore an inhibitor of the human CD81-HCV E2 interaction could possibly prevent HCV infection (Pileri *et al.*, 1998). This interaction was the motivation behind efforts to produce CD81-displaying BacMPs. Consequently, the interaction between BacMPs displaying truncated CD81 and the HCV E2 envelope were detected, suggesting that CD81-displaying BacMPs could be effectively applied to identify inhibitors of the CD81-E2 interaction.

Transmembrane receptors constitute the most prominent family of validated pharmacological targets in biomedicine. Receptor-displaying BacMPs were readily extracted from ruptured AMB-1 transformants by magnetic separation, and after several washings were ready for analysis. Moreover, BacMPs are well-suited for use in a fully automated ligand-screening system that employs magnetic separation. This type of system facilitates rapid buffer exchange and stringent washing, and reduces nonspecific binding.

4. Automated systems

The suitability of magnetic particles for use in fully-automated systems is an important advantage in solid phases of bioassays. Automated robots bearing magnets permit rapid and precise handling of magnetic particles leading to high-throughput analysis. Different types of fully-automated systems have been developed to handle the magnetic particles and to apply them to nucleotide extraction, gene analysis, and immunoassays.

Figures 9-11 show the layout of an automated workstation with which magnetic particles are collected at the bottom of microtiter plates (Maruyama *et al.*, 2004; Tanaka *et al.*, 2003). For fluid handling, the processor is equipped with an automated pipetter (1) that moves in the vertical and horizontal directions. The platform contains a disposable tip rack station (2), a reagent station (3) that serves as reservoirs for wash buffers, and a reaction station (4) for a 96-well microtiter plate, where a magnetic field can be applied using a neodymium iron boron sintered (Nd-Fe-B) magnet on its underside. One pole of the Nd-Fe-B magnet applies a magnetic field to one well (Matsunaga, 2003). Eight poles of the Nd-Fe-B magnet are aligned on iron rods, and 12 rods are set on the back side of the microtiter plate to apply magnetic fields to the 96 wells. The magnetic field can be switched on (magnetic flux density: 318 mT) and off (magnetic flux density: <10 mT) by rotating the rods 180°. The reaction station is combined with a heat block with a range of 4–99°C and is configured to perform the hybridization step. Heating and magnetic separation can be performed simultaneously in one well. This precise thermal control unit is suitable for DNA handling and has been used for DNA extraction, SNP detection in the genes for aldehyde dehydrogenase 2 (ALDH2) (Maruyama *et al.*, 2004) and transforming growth factor (TGF)

(Yoshino *et al.*, 2010), detection of epidermal growth factor receptor (EGFR) mutations in non-small cell lung cancer (NSCLC), and determination of microsatellite repeats in the human thyroid peroxidase (TPOX) gene (Nakagawa *et al.*, 2007).

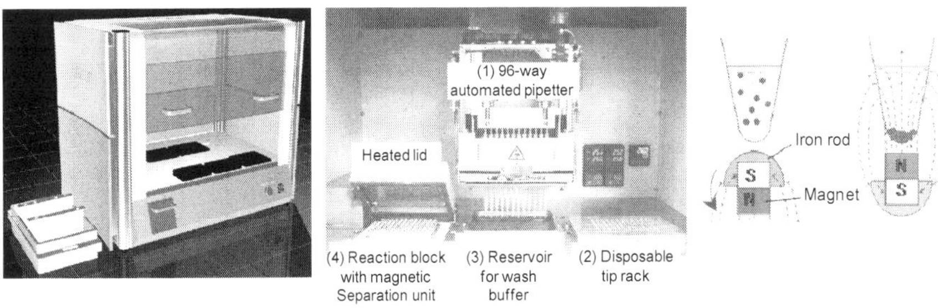

Fig. 9. Automated magnetic separation system, and magnetic separation is achieved in the bottom of microtiter plates.

Figure 10 shows the layout of an automated workstation with which magnetic particles can be separated on the inner surface of pipette tips. The automated system consists of an automated eight-way pipette bearing a retractable magnet mounted close to the pipette tips (1) a tip rack, (2) a reaction station for a 96-well microtiter plate, and (3) a luminescence detection unit. One rack can hold 8 × 3 tips for reactions. For automated magnetic separation, the suspension of magnetic particles is aspirated and dispersed using an automated pipette bearing a magnet. The automated pipette can move horizontally, and magnetic particles collected on the inner surface of pipette tips can be resuspended in the subsequent wells by the pipetting action (Matsunaga *et al.*, 2007). As an advantage, this system can eliminate the carry-over of reaction mixtures to the following reaction steps. Due to precise liquid handling, this workstation is mainly used for highly-sensitive immunoassays, though its throughput capacity is less than the above system. Using this workstation, a fully-automated immunoassay was developed to detect EDCs (Matsunaga *et al.*, 2003; Yoshino *et al.*, 2008), human insulin (Tanaka and Matsunaga, 2000), and a prostate cancer marker (prostate specific antigen).

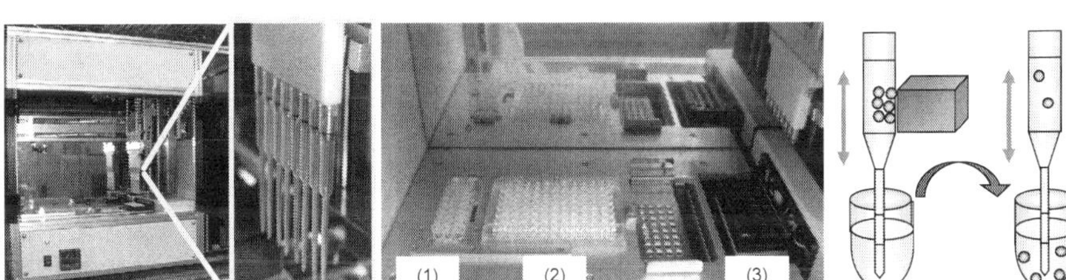

Fig. 10. Automated magnetic separation system, and magnetic separation is achieved on the inner surface of pipette tips.

Figure 11 shows the layout of an automated workstation with which magnetic particles can be collected onto a magnetic rod (Ota *et al.*, 2006). This workstation is equipped with eight automated pestle units and a spectrophotometer that is interfaced with a photosensor amplifier. The magnetic rod that moves in both vertical and horizontal directions is composed of a neodymium-iron-boron (Nd-Fe-B) magnet pole and a covering sheath. DNA concentrations and purities are measured in the cuvette using an absorbance spectrometer that is integrated with the workstation. Light traverses the solution in the cuvette from bottom to top. When magnetic particles are collected from the reaction mixture, the core magnetic pole is sheathed, and then magnetic particles are suspended in the following step by stirring of the sheath without the core rod. The sheath is used as a pestle to gently mix the suspension of magnetic particles and solid samples. Using this system, DNA was directly extracted from dried maize powder using aminosilane-modified BacMPs. Furthermore, the quantitative detection of genetically-modified maize genes was examined by real-time PCR. This system offers rapid assay completion with high DNA yields and qualities comparable to those of conventional detergent-based methods.

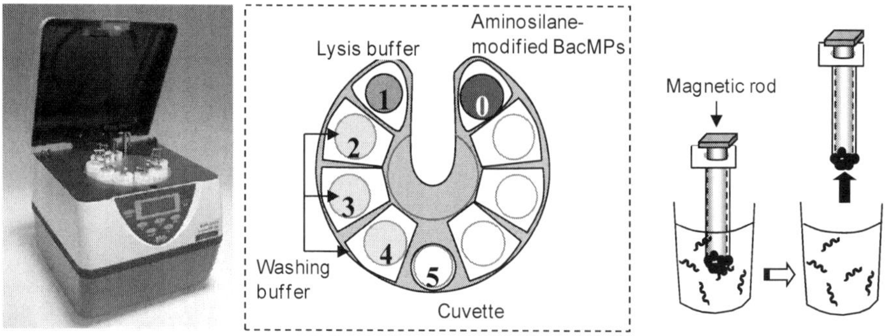

Fig. 11. Automated magnetic separation system, and magnetic separation is achieved onto a magnetic rod.

5. Conclusion

Magnetic particles have been utilized as biomolecule carriers since the 1970s when applied research examined bioreactors using enzyme-immobilized magnetic particles. Since then, various types of synthetic and bioengineered magnetic particles have been produced, modified, and enhanced. These magnetic particles have been widely used in place of centrifugation, filter, and chromatography separations, and applied to purifications of biological matter including target cells, proteins, and nucleic acids. More recent advances in the bioengineering of magnetic particles produced by magnetotactic bacteria have resulted in powerful tools for medical applications as well as basic research. This review focused on the applications of BacMPs for recovery or detections of bio-molecule. BacMPs are also available for other applications such as MRI contrast agents, and carriers for drug delivery systems, and so on. High potential magnetic particles will be developed combining with genetic engineering, and especially it is quite easy to control the kinds and numbers of proteins-displayed on BacMPs. Furthermore, it is possible to display artificially designed proteins or polypeptides onto BacMPs by the same methods. These approaches provide a new innovation in material science. Elucidation of the mechanism of magnetic particle formation in *M. magneticum* AMB-1 has provided a roadmap for designing novel biomaterials useful in multidisciplinary fields.

6. References

Amemiya, Y., Arakaki, A., Staniland, S. S., Tanaka, T. & Matsunaga, T. (2007). Controlled formation of magnetite crystal by partial oxidation of ferrous hydroxide in the presence of recombinant magnetotactic bacterial protein Mms6. *Biomaterials* 28: 5381-5389.

Arakaki, A., Webb, J. & Matsunaga, T. (2003). A novel protein tightly bound to bacterial magnetic particles in Magnetospirillum magneticum strain AMB-1. *Journal of Biological Chemistry* 278(10): 8745-8750.

Baselt, D. R., Lee, G. U., Natesan, M., Metzger, S. W., Sheehan, P. E. & Colton, R. J. (1998). A biosensor based on magnetoresistance technology. *Biosensors & Bioelectronics* 13(7-8): 731-739.

Blakemore, R. (1983). Magnetic bacteria and products derived therefrom. *US4385119*.

Deisenhofer, J. (1981). Crystallographic refinement and atomic models of a human Fc fragment and its complex with fragment B of protein A from Staphylococcus aureus at 2.9- and 2.8-.ANG. resolution. *Biochemistry* 20(9): 2361-2370.

Edelstein, R. L., Tamanaha, C. R., Sheehan, P. E., Miller, M. M., Baselt, D. R., Whitman, L. J. & Colton, R. J. (2000). The BARC biosensor applied to the detection of biological warfare agents. *Biosensors & Bioelectronics* 14(10-11): 805-813.

Eliasson, B. & Kogelschatz, U. (1988). UV excimer radiation from dielectric-barrier discharges. *Applied Physics B-Photophysics and Laser Chemistry* 46(4): 299-303.

Fang, Y. L., Jayaram, H., Shane, T., Kolmakova-Partensky, L., Wu, F., Williams, C., Xiong, Y. & Miller, C. (2009). Structure of a prokaryotic virtual proton pump at 3.2 angstrom resolution. *Nature* 460(7258): 1040-1043.

Gao, X. H., Cui, Y. Y., Levenson, R. M., Chung, L. W. K. & Nie, S. M. (2004). In vivo cancer targeting and imaging with semiconductor quantum dots. *Nature Biotechnology* 22(8): 969-976.

Gleich, B. & Weizenecker, R. (2005). Tomographic imaging using the nonlinear response of magnetic particles. *Nature* 435(7046): 1214-1217.

Goldman, E. R., Anderson, G. P., Tran, P. T., Mattoussi, H., Charles, P. T. & Mauro, J. M. (2002). Conjugation of luminescent quantum dots with antibodies using an engineered adaptor protein to provide new reagents for fluoroimmunoassays. *Analytical Chemistry* 74(4): 841-847.

Gonzales, M. & Krishnan, K. M. (2005). Synthesis of magnetoliposomes with monodisperse iron oxide nanocrystal cores for hyperthermia. *Journal of Magnetism and Magnetic Materials* 293(1): 265-270.

Graepler, F., Lauer, U. & Gregor, M. (1998). Magnetic cell sorting for parietal cell purification using a new monoclonal antibody without influence on cell function. *Journal of Biochemical and Biophysical Methods* 36(2-3): 143-155.

Gref, R., Couvreur, P., Barratt, G. & Mysiakine, E. (2003). Surface-engineered nanoparticles for multiple ligand coupling. *Biomaterials* 24(24): 4529-4537.

Gronenborn, A. M., Filpula, D. R., Essig, N. Z., Achari, A., Whitlow, M., Wingfield, P. T. & Clore, G. M. (1991). A novel, highly stable fold of the immunoglobulin binding domain of streptococcal protein G. *Science* 253(5020): 657-661.

Grubisha, D. S., Lipert, R. J., Park, H. Y., Driskell, J. & Porter, M. D. (2003). Femtomolar detection of prostate-specific antigen: An immunoassay based on surface-enhanced Raman scattering and immunogold labels. *Analytical Chemistry* 75(21): 5936-5943.

Gu, H. W., Ho, P. L., Tsang, K. W. T., Wang, L. & Xu, B. (2003). Using biofunctional magnetic nanoparticles to capture vancomycin-resistant enterococci and other gram-positive bacteria at ultralow concentration. *Journal of the American Chemical Society* 125(51): 15702-15703.

Herr, J. K., Smith, J. E., Medley, C. D., Shangguan, D. & Tan, W. (2006). Aptamer-conjugated nanoparticles for selective collection and detection of cancer cells. *Analytical Chemistry* 78(9): 2918-2924.

Kettering, M., Winter, J., Zeisberger, M., Bremer-Streck, S., Oehring, H., Bergemann, C., Alexiou, C., Hergt, R., Halbhuber, K. J., Kaiser, W. A. & Hilger, I. (2007). Magnetic nanoparticles as bimodal tools in magnetically induced labelling and magnetic heating of tumour cells: an in vitro study. *Nanotechnology* 18(17).

Kramer, R. M., Li, C., Carter, D. C., Stone, M. O. & Naik, R. R. (2004). Engineered protein cages for nanomaterial synthesis. *Journal of the American Chemical Society* 126(41): 13282-13286.

Kuhara, M., Takeyama, H., Tanaka, T. & Matsunaga, T. (2004). Magnetic cell separation using antibody binding with protein a expressed on bacterial magnetic particles. *Analytical Chemistry* 76(21): 6207-6213.

Lowenadler, B., Jansson, B., Paleus, S., Holmgren, E., Nilsson, B., Moks, T., Palm, G., Josephson, S., Philipson, L. & Uhlen, M. (1987). A gene fusion system for generating antibodies against short peptides. *Gene* 58(1): 87-97.

Maruyama, K., Takeyama, H., Nemoto, E., Tanaka, T., Yoda, K. & Matsunaga, T. (2004). Single nucleotide polymorphism detection in aldehyde dehydrogenase 2 (ALDH2) gene using bacterial magnetic particles based on dissociation curve analysis. *Biotechnology and Bioengineering* 87(6): 687-694.

Matsunaga, T. & Kamiya, S. (1987). Use of magnetic particles isolated from magnetotactic bacteria for enzyme immobilization. *Applied Microbiology and Biotechnology* 26(4): 328-332.

Matsunaga, T., Maeda, Y., Yoshino, T., Takeyama, H., Takahashi, M., Ginya, H., Aasahina, J. & Tajima, H. (2007). Fully automated immunoassay for detection of prostate-specific antigen using nano-magnetic beads and micro-poly styrene bead composites, 'Beads on Beads'. *Analytica Chimica Acta* 597(2): 331-339.

Matsunaga, T., Okamura, Y., Fukuda, Y., Wahyudi, A. T., Murase, Y. & Takeyama, H. (2005). Complete genome sequence of the facultative anaerobic magnetotactic bacterium Magnetospirillum sp strain AMB-1. *DNA Research* 12(3): 157-166.

Matsunaga, T., Sato, R., Kamiya, S., Tanaka, T. & Takeyama, H. (1999). Chemiluminescence enzyme immunoassay using ProteinA-bacterial magnetite complex. *Journal of Magnetism and Magnetic Materials* 194(1-3): 126-131.

Matsunaga, T., Takahashi, M., Yoshino, T., Kuhara, M. & Takeyama, H. (2006). Magnetic separation of CD14(+) cells using antibody binding with protein A expressed on bacterial magnetic particles for generating dendritic cells. *Biochemical and Biophysical Research Communications* 350(4): 1019-1025.

Matsunaga, T., Togo, H., Kikuchi, T. & Tanaka, T. (2000). Production of luciferase-magnetic particle complex by recombinant Magnetospirillum sp AMB-1. *Biotechnology and Bioengineering* 70(6): 704-709.

Matsunaga, T., Ueki, F., Obata, K., Tajima, H., Tanaka, T., Takeyama, H., Goda, Y. & Fujimoto, S. (2003). Fully automated immunoassay system of endocrine disrupting chemicals using monoclonal antibodies chemically conjugated to bacterial magnetic particles. *Analytica Chimica Acta* 475(1-2): 75-83.

Matsunaga, T., Yoda, K., Udagawa, Y., Nemoto, E. & Maruyama, K. (2003). Hybridization apparatus and method for detecting nucleic acid in sample using the same. *US20030059823*.

Miltenyi, S. (1995). Methods and materials for improved high gradient magnetic separation of biological materials. *US5411863*.

Miltenyi, S., Muller, W., Weichel, W. & Radbruch, A. (1990). High gradient magnetic cell separation with MACS. *Cytometry* 11(2): 231-238.

Mirzabekov, T., Kontos, H., Farzan, M., Marasco, W. & Sodroski, J. (2000). Paramagnetic proteoliposomes containing a pure, native, and oriented seven-transmembrane segment protein, CCR5. *Nature Biotechnology* 18(6): 649-654.

Mulder, W. J. M., Koole, R., Brandwijk, R. J., Storm, G., Chin, P. T. K., Strijkers, G. J., Donega, C. D., Nicolay, K. & Griffioen, A. W. (2006). Quantum dots with a paramagnetic coating as a bimodal molecular imaging probe. *Nano Letters* 6(1): 1-6.

Nakagawa, T., Maruyama, K., Takeyama, H. & Matsunaga, T. (2007). Determination of microsatellite repeats in the human thyroid peroxidase (TPOX) gene using an automated gene analysis system with nanoscale engineered biomagnetite. *Biosensors & Bioelectronics* 22(9-10): 2276-2281.

Nakamura, C., Burgess, J. G., Sode, K. & Matsunaga, T. (1995a). An iron-regulated gene, magA, encoding an iron transport protein of Magnetospirillum sp. strain AMB-1. *Journal of Biological Chemistry* 270(47): 28392-28396.

Nakamura, C., Kikuchi, T., Burgess, J. G. & Matsunaga, T. (1995b). Iron-regulated expression and membrane localization of the magA protein in Magnetospirillum sp. strain AMB-1. *Journal of Biochemistry* 118(1): 23-27.

Nakamura, C., Sakaguchi, T., Kudo, S., Burgess, J. G., Sode, J. & Matsunaga, T. (1993). Characterization of iron uptake in the magnetic bacterium Aquaspirillum sp. AMB-1. *Applied Biochemistry and Biotechnology* 37(39/40): 169-176.

Nakamura, M., Decker, K., Chosy, J., Comella, K., Melnik, K., Moore, L., Lasky, L. C., Zborowski, M. & Chalmers, J. J. (2001). Separation of a breast cancer cell line from human blood using a quadrupole magnetic flow sorter. *Biotechnology Progress* 17(6): 1145-1155.

Ota, H., Lim, T. K., Tanaka, T., Yoshino, T., Harada, M. & Matsunaga, T. (2006). Automated DNA extraction from genetically modified maize using aminosilane-modified bacterial magnetic particles. *Journal of Biotechnology* 125(3): 361-368.

Pardoe, H., Clark, P. R., St Pierre, T. G., Moroz, P. & Jones, S. K. (2003). A magnetic resonance imaging based method for measurement of tissue iron concentration in liver arterially embolized with ferrimagnetic particles designed for magnetic hyperthermia treatment of tumors. *Magnetic Resonance Imaging* 21(5): 483-488.

Patil, S., Sandberg, A., Heckert, E., Self, W. & Seal, S. (2007). Protein adsorption and cellular uptake of cerium oxide nanoparticles as a function of zeta potential. *Biomaterials* 28: 4600-4607.

Perez, J. M., Josephson, L., O'Loughlin, T., Hogemann, D. & Weissleder, R. (2002). Magnetic relaxation switches capable of sensing molecular interactions. *Nature Biotechnology* 20(8): 816-820.

Pileri, P., Uematsu, Y., Campagnoli, S., Galli, G., Falugi, F., Petracca, R., Weiner, A. J., Houghton, M., Rosa, D., Grandi, G. & Abrignani, S. (1998). Binding of hepatitis C virus to CD81. *Science* 282(5390): 938-941.

Plank, C., Schillinger, U., Scherer, F., Bergemann, C., Remy, J. S., Krotz, F., Anton, M., Lausier, J. & Rosenecker, J. (2003). The magnetofection method: Using magnetic force to enhance gene delivery. *Biological Chemistry* 384(5): 737-747.

Prasad, B. L. V., Stoeva, S. I., Sorensen, C. M., Zaikovski, V. & Klabunde, K. J. (2003). Gold nanoparticles as catalysts for polymerization of alkylsilanes to siloxane nanowires, filaments, and tubes. *Journal of the American Chemical Society* 125(35): 10488-10489.

Sawakami-Kobayashi, K., Segawa, O., Obata, K., Hornes, E., Yohda, M., Tajima, H. & Machida, M. (2003). Multipurpose robot for automated cycle sequencing. *Biotechniques* 34(3): 634-637.

Schotter, J., Kamp, P. B., Becker, A., Puhler, A., Reiss, G. & Bruckl, H. (2004). Comparison of a prototype magnetoresistive biosensor to standard fluorescent DNA detection. *Biosensors & Bioelectronics* 19(10): 1149-1156.

Schratzberger, P., Reinisch, N., Prodinger, W. M., Kahler, C. M., Sitte, B. A., Bellmann, R., FischerColbrie, R., Winkler, H. & Wiedermann, C. J. (1997). Differential chemotactic activities of sensory neuropeptides for human peripheral blood mononuclear cells. *Journal of Immunology* 158(8): 3895-3901.

Schwalbe, M., Pachmann, K., Hoffken, K. & Clement, J. H. (2006). Improvement of the separation of tumour cells from peripheral blood cells using magnetic nanoparticles. *Journal of Physics-Condensed Matter* 18(38): S2865-S2876.

Stampfli, M. R., Miescher, S., Aebischer, I., Zurcher, A. W. & Stadler, B. M. (1994). Inhibition of human IgE synthesis by anti-IgE antibodies requires divalent recognition. *European Journal of Immunology* 24(9): 2161-2167.

Takahashi, M., Yoshino, T. & Matsunaga, T. (2010). Surface modification of magnetic nanoparticles using asparagines-serine polypeptide designed to control interactions with cell surfaces. *Biomaterials* 31(18): 4952-4957.

Tanaka, T., Maruyama, K., Yoda, K., Nemoto, E., Udagawa, Y., Nakayama, H., Takeyama, H. & Matsunaga, T. (2003). Development and evaluation of an automated workstation for single nucleotide polymorphism discrimination using bacterial magnetic particles. *Biosensors & Bioelectronics* 19(4): 325-330.

Tanaka, T. & Matsunaga, T. (2000). Fully automated chemiluminescence immunoassay of insulin using antibody-protein A-bacterial magnetic particle complexes. *Analytical Chemistry* 72(15): 3518-3522.

Tanaka, T., Takeda, H., Kokuryu, Y. & Matsunaga, T. (2004). Spontaneous integration of transmembrane peptides into a bacterial magnetic particle membrane and its application to display of useful proteins. *Analytical Chemistry* 76(13): 3764-3769.

Tiwari, A., Punshon, G., Kidane, A., Hamilton, G. & Seifalian, A. M. (2003). Magnetic beads (Dynabead) toxicity to endothelial cells at high bead concentration: Implication for tissue engineering of vascular prosthesis. *Cell Biology and Toxicology* 19(5): 265-272.

Ugelstad, J., Berge, A., Ellingsen, T., Aune, O., Kilaas, L., Nilsen, T. N., Schmid, R., Stenstad, P., Funderud, S., Kvalheim, G., Nustad, K., Lea, T., Vartdal, F. & Danielsen, H. (1988). Monosized magnetic particles and their use in selective cell separation. *Makromolekulare Chemie-Macromolecular Symposia* 17: 177-211.

Weissleder, R., Kelly, K., Sun, E. Y., Shtatland, T. & Josephson, L. (2005). Cell-specific targeting of nanoparticles by multivalent attachment of small molecules. *Nature Biotechnology* 23: 1418-1423.

Wright, L. D., Cresson, E. L., Skeggs, H. R., Wood, T. R., Peck, R. L., Wolf, D. E. & Folkers, K. (1952). Isolation of crystalline biocytin from yeast extract. *Journal of the American Chemical Society* 74(8): 1996-1999.

Xu, C. J., Xu, K. M., Gu, H. W., Zhong, X. F., Guo, Z. H., Zheng, R. K., Zhang, X. X. & Xu, B. (2004). Nitrilotriacetic acid-modified magnetic nanoparticles as a general agent to bind histidine-tagged proteins. *Journal of the American Chemical Society* 126(11): 3392-3393.

Xu, L., Yu, H., Akhras, M. S., Han, S. J., Osterfeld, S., White, R. L., Pourmand, N. & Wang, S. X. (2008). Giant magnetoresistive biochip for DNA detection and HPV genotyping. *Biosensors & Bioelectronics* 24(1): 99-103.

Yoshino, T., Kaji, C., Nakai, M., Saito, F., Takeyama, H. & Matsunaga, T. (2008). Novel method for evaluation of chemicals based on ligand-dependent recruitment of GFP labeled coactivator to estrogen receptor displayed on bacterial magnetic particles. *Analytica Chimica Acta* 626(1): 71-77.

Yoshino, T., Kato, F., Takeyama, H., Nakai, M., Yakabe, Y. & Matsunaga, T. (2005). Development of a novel method for screening of estrogenic compounds using nano-sized bacterial magnetic particles displaying estrogen receptor. *Analytica Chimica Acta* 532(2): 105-111.

Yoshino, T. & Matsunaga, T. (2005). Development of efficient expression system for protein display on bacterial magnetic particles. *Biochemical and Biophysical Research Communications* 338(4): 1678-1681.

Yoshino, T. &Matsunaga, T. (2006). Efficient and stable display of functional proteins on bacterial magnetic particles using Mms13 as a novel anchor molecule. *Applied and Environmental Microbiology* 72(1): 465-471.

Yoshino, T., Nishimura, T., Mori, T., Suzuki, S., Kambara, H., Takeyama, H. & Matsunaga, T. (2009). Nano-sized bacterial magnetic particles displaying pyruvate phosphate dikinase for pyrosequencing. *Biotechnology and Bioengineering* 103(1): 130-137.

Yoshino, T., Shimojo, A., Maeda, Y. & Matsunaga, T. (2010). Inducible Expression of Transmembrane Proteins on Bacterial Magnetic Particles in Magnetospirillum magneticum AMB-1. *Applied and Environmental Microbiology* 76(4): 1152-1157.

Yoshino, T., Takahashi, M., Takeyama, H., Okamura, Y., Kato, F. & Matsunaga, T. (2004). Assembly of G protein-coupled receptors onto nanosized bacterial magnetic particles using Mms16 as an anchor molecule. *Applied and Environmental Microbiology* 70(5): 2880-2885.

17

Metals for Biomedical Applications

Hendra Hermawan, Dadan Ramdan and Joy R. P. Djuansjah
Faculty of Biomedical Engineering and Health Science, Universiti Teknologi Malaysia
Malaysia

1. Introduction

In modern history, metals have been used as implants since more than 100 years ago when Lane first introduced metal plate for bone fracture fixation in 1895 (Lane, 1895). In the early development, metal implants faced corrosion and insufficient strength problems (Lambotte, 1909, Sherman, 1912). Shortly after the introduction of the 18-8 stainless steel in 1920s, which has had far-superior corrosion resistance to anything in that time, it immediately attracted the interest of the clinicians. Thereafter, metal implants experienced vast development and clinical use.

Type of metal used in biomedical depends on specific implant applications. 316L type stainless steel (316L SS) is still the most used alloy in all implants division ranging from cardiovascular to otorhinology. However, when the implant requires high wear resistance such as artificial joints, CoCrMo alloys is better served. Table 1 summarized the type of metals generally used for different implants division.

Division	Example of implants	Type of metal
Cardiovascular	Stent Artificial valve	316L SS; CoCrMo; Ti Ti6Al4V
Orthopaedic	Bone fixation (plate, screw, pin) Artificial joints	316L SS; Ti; Ti6Al4V CoCrMo; Ti6Al4V; Ti6Al7Nb
Dentistry	Orthodontic wire Filling	316L SS; CoCrMo; TiNi; TiMo AgSn(Cu) amalgam, Au
Craniofacial	Plate and screw	316L SS; CoCrMo; Ti; Ti6Al4V
Otorhinology	Artificial eardrum	316L SS

Table 1. Implants division and type of metals used

Metallic biomaterials are exploited due to their inertness and structural functions; they do not possess biofunctionalities like blood compatibility, bone conductivity and bioactivity. Hence, surface modifications are required. Improving their bone conductivity has been done by coating with bioactive ceramics like hydroxyapatite (Habibovic, 2002), or blood compatibility by coating with biopolymers (Lahann, 1999). Nowadays, large number of metallic biomaterials composed of nontoxic and allergy-free elements are being developed. Even more, a new type of biodegradable metals has been proposed as temporary implants (Hermawan, 2009).

Generally, all metal implants are non-magnetic and high in density. These are important for the implants to be compatible with magnetic resonance imaging (MRI) techniques and to be visible under X-ray imaging. Most of artificial implants are subjected to loads, either static or repetitive, and this condition requires an excellent combination of strength and ductility. This is the superior characteristic of metals over polymers and ceramics. Specific requirements of metals depend on the specific implant applications. Stents and stent grafts are implanted to open stenotic blood vessels; therefore, it requires plasticity for expansion and rigidity to maintain dilatation. For orthopaedic implants, metals are required to have excellent toughness, elasticity, rigidity, strength and resistance to fracture. For total joint replacement, metals are needed to be wear resistance; therefore debris formation from friction can be avoided. Dental restoration requires strong and rigid metals and even the shape memory effect for better results.

In overall, the use of biomaterials in clinical practice should be approved by an authoritative body such as the FDA (United States Food and Drug Administration). The proposed biomaterial will be either granted Premarket Approval (PMA) if substantially equivalent to one used before FDA legislation of 1976, or has to go through a series of guided biocompatibility assessment.

2. Common metals used for biomedical devices

Up to now, the three most used metals for implants are stainless steel, CoCr alloys and Ti alloys. The first stainless steel used for implants contains ~18wt% Cr and ~8wt% Ni makes it stronger than the steel and more resistant to corrosion. Further addition of molybdenum (Mo) has improved its corrosion resistance, known as type 316 stainless steel. Afterwards, the carbon (C) content has been reduced from 0.08 to 0.03 wt% which improved its corrosion resistance to chloride solution, and named as 316L.

Titanium is featured by its light weight. Its density is only 4.5g/cm^3 compared to 7.9g/cm^3 for 316 stainless steel and 8.3g/cm^3 for cast CoCrMo alloys (Brandes and Brook, 1992). Ti and its alloys, i.e. Ti6Al4V are known for their excellent tensile strength and pitting corrosion resistance. Titanium alloyed with Ni, i.e. Nitinol, forms alloys having shape memory effect which makes them suitable in various applications such as dental restoration wiring.

In dentistry, precious metals and alloys often used are Au, Ag, Pt and their alloys. They possess good castability, ductility and resistance to corrosion. Included into dental alloys are AuAgCu system, AuAgCu with the addition of Zn and Sn known as dental solder, and AuPtPd system used for porcelain-fused-to-metal for teeth repairs.

CoCr alloys have been utilised for many decades in making artificial joints. They are generally known for their excellent wear resistance. Especially the wrought CoNiCrMo alloy has been used for making heavily loaded joints such as ankle implants (Figure 1).

Other metals used for implants include tantalum (Ta), amorphous alloys and biodegradable metals. Tantalum which has excellent X-ray visibility and low magnetic susceptibility is often used for X-ray markers for stents. Amorphous alloys featured interesting properties compared to its crystalline counterparts whereas they exhibit higher corrosion resistance, wear resistance, tensile strength and fatigue strength. With low Young's modulus, amorphous alloys like that of Zr-based (Wang, 2011), may miniaturized metal implants. Up to now, metals proposed for biodegradable implants, named as biodegradable metals, are either iron-based or magnesium-based alloys. The Mg-based alloys include MgAl-, MgRE (rare earth)- (Witte, 2005), and MgCa- (Li, 2008) based alloys. Meanwhile, the Fe-based alloys include pure iron (Peuster, 2001) and Fe-Mn alloys (Hermawan, 2008).

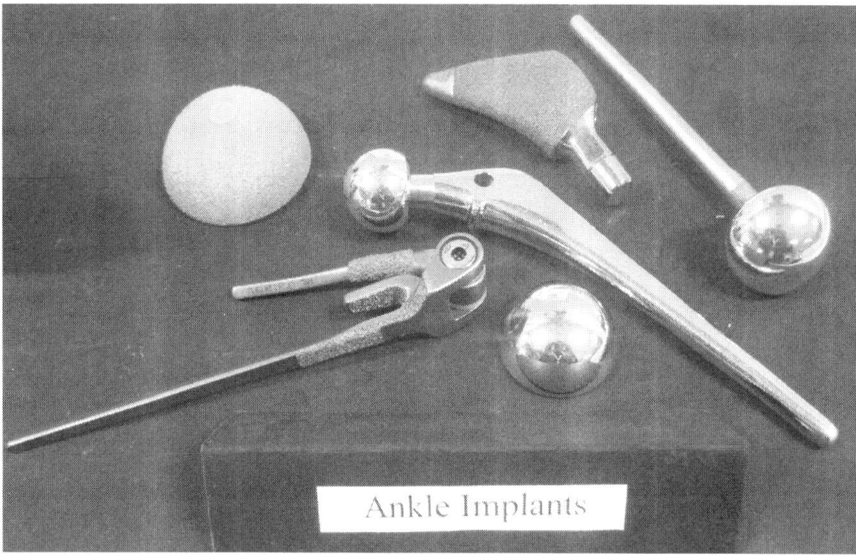

Fig. 1. A set of ankle implants (Courtesy of MediTeg, UTM).

3. Structure and property of metals

3.1 Microstructure of metal and its alloys

When molten metals are cooled into a solid state, the atoms rearrange themselves into a crystal structure. There are three basic crystal structures for most metals: (1) body-centered cubic, (2) face-centered cubic, and (3) hexagonal close-packed. Each structure has different properties and shows distinct behaviour when subjected under loading in the application. Under external force a crystal undergoes elastic deformation. When the force is removed, it returns to its original shape. However, if the force is increased beyond its elastic limit, the crystal undergoes plastic or permanent deformation, and it does not return to its original shape even after the removal of the applied force.

Imperfections usually exist in metals include interstitial atom, impurity, dislocations, grain boundaries, and pores. Dislocation is a defect which could explain the discrepancy between the actual strength of metals and the theoretical calculations based on molecular dynamics. After the invention of electron microscope, many scientists have directly observed the existence of dislocation. Since then, dislocation theory has evolved and explains many of the physical and mechanical phenomena in metals. Another important type of defect is the grain boundary. The mechanical properties of metals are significantly influenced by the size of their grain. At ambient temperature, metals with large grain size generally have a low strength and hardness, and also low in ductility. Since grain boundaries hinder the dislocations movement, they also influence the strain hardening process to increase the strength and ductility of metals.

Pure metals have relatively limited properties; however these properties can be enhanced by alloying the metals. Most of the metals used in engineering applications are in the form of their alloy. Most alloys consist of two or more solid phase in the form of either solid solutions or intermetallic compounds that depend on the alloying composition and temperature. A phase is defined as a homogenous portion in a material that has its own physical and chemical characteristics and properties. Every pure metal is considered as a phase, as also is every solid solution and intermetallic compound. Alloying a metal with finely dispersed particles as a second-phase is one of the important method of strengthening alloys and enhancing their properties. The second-phase particles present as obstacles to the movement of dislocations thus increase the overall strength and hardness of the alloys.

3.2 Physical and mechanical properties of metals

One important criterion in metals selection is the consideration of their physical properties, such as density, melting point, specific heat, thermal conductivity, thermal expansion and corrosion. Density of a metal plays a significant role on the specific strength and specific stiffness, which are the ratio of strength-to-weight and stiffness-to-weight, respectively.

For many applications, one of the most important considerations is their deterioration by corrosion. Corrosion of metal depends on the metals composition and the corrosive media in the surrounding environment. The most common and easiest way of preventing corrosion is the careful selection of metals once the corrosion environment has been characterized. Nonferrous metals, stainless steel, and non-metallic materials generally have high corrosion resistance due to the presence of protective passive layer. Titanium develops a film of titanium oxide, TiO_2. A similar phenomenon also occurs in stainless steels due to the presence of chromium in the alloy that develops chromium oxide layer on the surfaces. If the protective film is broken and exposes the metal underneath, a new oxide film begins to form for further protection.

Unlike the physical properties, mechanical properties of metal are the behaviour of metals that measured under the effect of external forces. Tension test is the most common method to determine the mechanical properties of materials, such as strength, ductility, toughness, elastic modulus, and strain hardening capability. The specimen used in this test usually is prepared according to ASTM specifications. Another important mechanical property of metal is the hardness which gives a general indication of its resistance to localize plastic deformation. Several test methods which use different indenter materials and shapes have been developed to measure the hardness of metals.

Table 2 shows mechanical properties of some alloys used for implant. It also shows chemical composition of the alloy which is a determined factor for the formation of microstructure and phases, thus their properties, i.e. mechanical properties. For example, the addition of Al and V into pure Ti greatly increase its tensile strength. Beside composition, metallurgical state and synthesis process of the metals change their mechanical properties, i.e. annealed condition has better ductility than that of cold worked and cast metal implants usually possess lower strength than those made by forging.

Different from the breakdown in the tension test where the specimen is subjected under gradual increase of loading until fractures, failure of a component practically occurs after a lengthy period of repeated stress or strain cycling. This phenomenon is called fatigue failure and responsible for the majority of failures in many mechanical components. To avoid this kind of failure, the stress level should be reduced to a level which the material can be subjected without fatigue failure, regardless of the number of cycle. The maximum level of loading stress is known as the endurance limit or fatigue limit.

Metals	Main alloying composition (wt%)	Mechanical properties*			
		YS (MPa)	UTS (MPa)	YM (GPa)	Max elongation (%)
Stainless steel: 316L type (ASTM, 2003)	Fe; 16-18.5Cr; 10-14Ni; 2-3Mo; <2Mn; <1Si; <0.003C	190	490	193	40
CoCr alloys:					
CoCrWNi (F90) (ASTM, 2007a)	Co; 19-21Cr; 14-16W; 9-11Ni	310	860	210	20
CoNiCrMo (F562) (ASTM, 2007b)	Co; 33-37Ni; 19-21Cr; 9-10.5Mo	241	793	232	50
Ti and its alloys:					
Pure Ti grade 4 (F67) (ASTM, 2006)	Ti; 0.05N; 0.1C; 0.5Fe; 0.015H; 0.4O	485	550	110	15
Ti6Al4V (F136) (ASTM, 2008)	Ti; 5.5-6.75Al; 3.5-4.5V; 0.08C; 0.2O	795	860	116	10
Degradable metals:					
Pure iron (Goodfellow, 2007)	99.8Fe	150	210	200	40
WE43 magnesium alloy (ASTM, 2001)	Mg; 3.7-4.3Y; 2.4-4.4Nd; 0.4-1Zr	150	250	44	4

*under annealed condition except for WE43 which was solution heat-treated and artificially aged (T6). YS = yield strength, UTS = ultimate tensile strength, YM = Young's modulus.

Table 2. Example of metals used for implants and their mechanical properties

3.3 Biocompatibility of metals

The understanding of biocompatibility has been focused for long-term implantable devices, which biologically inactive and chemically inert so that they give no harmful effect to the human tissues. However, with recent development in biotechnology, some level of biological activity is needed in particular research area, such as tissue engineering, drug and gene delivery systems, where direct interactions between biomaterials and tissue components are very essential.

One of the recent definition of biocompatibility is "the ability of a biomaterial to perform its desired function with respect to a medical therapy, without eliciting any undesirable local or systemic effects in the recipient or beneficiary of that therapy, but generating the most appropriate beneficial cellular or tissue response in that specific situation, and optimising the clinically relevant performance of that therapy" (Williams, 2008). In metals, biocompatibility involves the acceptance of an artificial implant by the surrounding tissues and by the body as a whole. The metallic implants do not irritate the surrounding structures, do not incite an excessive inflammatory response, do not stimulate allergic and immunologic reactions, and do not cause cancer. Other functional characteristics that are important for metallic device include adequate mechanical properties such as strength, stiffness, and fatigue properties; and also appropriate density.

Since many applications of metallic devices are for the structural implant, metal biocompatibility is of considerable concern since metals can corrode in an *in vivo* environment. The corrosion of metallic implant gives adverse effects to the surrounding tissues and to the implant itself. It produces chemical substances that harmful for human organs and deteriorates the mechanical properties of the implant. Therefore, corrosion resistance of a metallic implant is an important aspect of its biocompatibility. Even though, in special cases, metals which can degrade are proposed for temporary implants but certainly without ignoring the biocompatibility requirement (Hermawan, 2010, Witte, 2009).

4. Processing of metals

4.1 Primary processes

In general, primary process of metals include the processing ingot to mill products in the case of wrought alloys, and casting process in the case of cast alloy. In addition, the primary products of metals can also be produced by powder metallurgy. Processing of implant alloys is thought to be a very expensive process, which involves complex process of production, especially for the case of Ti alloy. The main reason for this condition is due to the high reactivity of the alloys, therefore special handlings are required to perform their process of production. These conditions also induce the necessity in developing new material which is easier to be processed (Zhuka, 2007).

Thermo-mechanical process (TMP) is the most implemented primary fabrication process to convert ingot into mill products. It serves two functions; to produce certain shape of product such as slab, bloom and billet, and to improve the mechanical properties of the initial ingot materials by grain size refinement and the production of more uniform microstructure (Weiss, 1999). TMP of Ti alloys and similarly with other alloys involves several stages of processes. Forging is typically become the first process prior to other TMP. The selection of the type of TMP after forging depends on the mill product which is going to be produced, whether it is a billet, bar, plate or sheet (Campbel, 2006).

Determination of temperature is a crucial step for TMP (Liu, 1995, Germain, 2008, Ming-Wei, 2007), which determine the properties of the alloys and therefore different alloy will be treated at different temperature. As example, during 304 stainless steels's TMP, instability bands were found when the process temperature are below 1100°C, 1000°C, 800°C after hammer forging, rolling and press forging, respectively. It was suggested that the ideal process can be performed at 1200°C to obtain a defect-free microstructure (Venugopal, 1995). Other important parameters are degree of deformation and phase composition. It was reported that increase in degree of plastic deformation during forging of dual phase Ti alloys results in lower fatigue strength (Kubiak, 1998). However the decrease in the fatigue strength is smaller for the case of forging process in the beta range as compared to (α+β) range. In the case of phase composition, it has long been recognized that different phase has different ability to be deformed, therefore different phase composition will have different performance during and after TMP. As an example, it was reported that the flow-ability of dual phase Ti alloys depends on the beta phase grain size and volume fraction (Hu, 1999).

As mentioned earlier, casting process of implant alloy is relatively more difficult than TMP of wrought alloys. The reason is due to the high reactivity of the alloys, especially for the case of Ti alloys, which easily reacts with both the atmosphere and the cast mold (Campbel, 2006). However recent progress shows the used of investment casting has increased which is followed with hot iso-static pressing (HIP) process as the primary process for the production of implant alloys. In addition, different with other alloys, cast products of Ti alloys are generally comparable with the wrought products and in certain case can be superior (ASM, 1998a). On the other hand, Co base alloys are considered to have a better cast-ability than both Ti and stainless steel alloys. These alloys shows several important characteristics for casting process such as good fluidity, low melting points, freedom from dissolved-gas defects and low alloy losses due to oxidation (ASM, 1998c). Improvement of cast-ability and cast product of this alloy can be achieved by additional alloying element such as carbon and vacuum melting process. It was reported that additional carbon content up to 0.5wt% lower the melting temperature (increase cast-ability) and in turn produce finer grain size as compared to binary CoCr alloys (Black, 1998).

Another primary fabrication process of metal implant is powder metallurgy. The process includes blending and mixing of ingredient materials, compaction, sintering and in most cases followed with HIP process. This process is relatively expensive; therefore it is suitable for the production of highly loaded implants like femoral stems of total hip prostheses (Black, 1998). One of the important requirements for implant materials is porosity which is expected in the range between 20-50% volume fractions (Dewidar, 2007). This condition can be achieved by controlling the sintering process parameters. In addition, improvement in the mechanical properties of implant by this method can be achieved by conducting HIP process after sintering by decreasing defects like gas or shrinkage pores.

4.2 Advanced processes

There are several processes which can be considered as advanced processes in the manufacturing of implant materials, such as superplastic deformation, isothermal forging and directed metal deposition. They offer an improvement in the process of production as well as achieveing a better quality of product. Superplastic deformation (SPD) is an advanced forming process where higher degree of deformation applied to form complex shape of product whereas low rate forming process is required (Krishna, 1997). Dual phase materials have potential to be treated by SPD process with the additional requirement that the materials have ultra-fine grain structure. This superplasticity, i.e. in duplex stainless steel, is due to dynamic recrystallization assisted grain boundary sliding (Han, 1999) where different rate of sliding for the different type of grain boundary is required in order to achieve an optimum superplasticity (Miyamoto, 2001). Ultra-fine grain structure can be produced by several methods of severe plastic deformation processes, such as equal channel angular pressing (ECAP), accumulative roll-bonding (ARB), high pressure torsion (HPT) and others similar processes (Azushima, 2008). At the present time superplasticity is used for superplastic deformation and diffusion bonding processes (Huang, 1999).

Another advanced process is isothermal forging where the dies is maintained at higher temperature and therefore reduces die chill and increases metal flow (Campbel, 2006). Relatively low strain rate condition is preferable in order to provide superplasticity condition and therefore high degree uniform deformation can be achieved after the process. This process offers a more uniform microstructure, longer lifetime of dies, and reduces the step of process to obtain near net shape of product. However initial cost of the process is high due to the usage of high temperature dies materials which is more expensive than dies for conventional forging process.

Another near net shape process is directed metal deposition which use focus laser beam that melt metal powder on metal substrate plate. This process reduces the cost of production of

Ti parts especially by the saving in the material utilized through the process. The material saving is higher in the case of production complex shape of product.

4.3 Surface treatment

Surface treatment or surface modification is considered as one major concern on recent developments in metallic biomaterials (Kohn, 1998). The treatment includes surface morphological modification and chemical modification. Surface morphology such as roughness, texture and porosity are important characteristics of implant since it influences the ability of cells to adhere to solid substrate (Peckner, 1977). For the case of chemical modification, the objective of the modification is to provide specific biological response on the metallic surface and increase the stability of bio-molecules.

An appropriate surface roughness can be achieved by applying electro-polishing where an improvement in the corrosion resistance of stainless steels can be achieved. Surface grain refinement, by a process similar to SPD but only employed on the surface, improves fatigue life of stainless steel alloys since ultra fine grain boundary of surface can impede the dislocation movement, whereas the compressive residual stress on the surface can delay the crack initiation (Roland, 2006). In addition, improvement on the corrosion resistance is also observed since more grain boundaries results in the more active site for diffusion of chromium (Mordyuk, 2007). The surface of material can also be modified by using laser where an improvement in the corrosion resistance of stainless steel was reported (Kwok, 2003). This improvement is believed due to the dissolution or refinement of carbide particles and the presence of retained austenite after the process.

Chemical modification on the stainless steel alloys by hybrid plasma surface alloying process using nitrogen and methane gas mixtures below 450°C was reported (Sun, 2008). The formed dual layer of hard nitrogen-enriched on the hard carbon enrich-layer improves the corrosion resistance of the alloy. Another chemical modification was also reported by nitrogen ion beam processing on stainless steel alloy (Williamson, 1998). A relatively low-energy beam of nitrogen ions was used with the substrate temperature was held at 400°C during a 15 minutes treatment to introduce nitrogen onto the surface of the alloy and form N-rich layer that improve the surface hardness of the alloy.

By applying cyclic potentiodynamic polarisation to a 316LVM stainless steel between the potential of hydrogen and oxygen evolution, it was found that the passive surface film formed will possess very good resistance to general corrosion and pitting (Bou-Saleh, 2007). Cyclic potentiodynamic polarisation in sodium nitrate or phosphate also significantly beefs up the pitting corrosion resistance of the same steel, because the density of oxygen vacancies, which may act as initiation sites for pits, in the passive film formed in this way is lowered (Shahryari, 2008).

4.4 Coating

Ti6Al4V offers excellent corrosion resistance and ability to be deformed superplastically that make it preferable to substitute complex shape hard tissue. However, Ti6Al4V alone does not fully satisfy biocompatibility requirements as implant product. Therefore ceramic bio-apatite such as hydroxyapatite (HAP) or carbonated apatite (CAP), normally are coated on this alloy. Bio-apatite deposited on Ti implants shows good fixation to the host bone and increases bone ingrowth to the implant (Adell, 1981). This improved biocompatibility is due to the chemical and biological similarity of bio-apatite to hard tissues (Ratner, 1993). Beside biocompatibility, coated implant also shows improvement on the mechanical properties due to the combination of hard surface and ductile substrate.

Numerous coating methods have been employed to improve bio-compatibility of metal implant including plasma spray (Schrooten, 2000) and sol-gel (Nguyen, 2004). Among the processes, plasma spray has been the most popular method for the coating process of bio-apatite on Ti substrate. Process parameters such as temperature and pressure play important role on the bonding strength of the coating. Composition of the alloy was also reported to play important role on the bonding strength of ceramic dental on CoCr alloys (Chan, 2010). Pre-treatment such as sand blasting process on the alloy substrate is also required to enhance the bonding strength (Kern, 1993).

A combination of deformation in superplastic condition and coating process was reported in (Ramdan, 2008). Here, carbonated apatite was deposited using continuous pressing at elevated temperature, which can be considered as superplastic deformation-like method. Beside diffusion process from thermal energy at elevated temperature, continuous pressing is expected to give additional energy that forces the bio-apatite to move inside the substrate and in turn enhance good bonding properties of bioapatite on the substrate.

4.5 Sterilization and cleaning

In order to avoid bacteria contamination which could be transferred to patients, sterilization and cleaning are important requirements on metal implant. Descaling is a method to clean metal implant surface which can be done mechanically, chemically or by combination of both of the methods. Mechanically it can be done with sand blasting process and chemical cleaning can be done by pickling using strong acid such as NaOH and H_2SO_4.

On the other hand sterilization can be done by several processes such as autoclaving, glow discharge Ar plasma treatment and γ-irradiation (Serro, 2003). Beside serves as a method to clean any contaminant from the surface, sterilization methods are also considered to play an important role in the bio-mineralization of Ti alloys.

5. Failure of metals for biomedical devices

5.1 Corrosion

Metal implant is prone to corrosion during its services due to corrosive medium of implantation site and in most cases subjected to cyclic loading. Types of corrosion that frequently found in implant applications are fretting, pitting and fatigue. Fretting corrosion most frequently happens in hip joint prostheses due to small movement in corrosive aqueous medium (Geringera, 2005).

Fretting corrosion refers to corrosion damage at the small area of contact surface due to repeated load, the mechanism of which frequently refers to corrosion which is activated by friction (Tritschler, 1999). Corrosive medium, chemical composition of alloy and level of stress at the contact surfaces are among important parameters that determine fretting corrosion behavior of metallic implant (Aparicioa, 2003). It was reported that the presence of chlorides influences the degradation acceleration of the stainless steel surface (Tritschler, 1999). On the other hand it was observed that corrosion resistance of Ti15Mo alloy is strongly depend on the concentration of fluoride ions for dental application (Kumar, 2008).

Prevention of corrosion will be greatly assisted by evaluation of corrosion behavior using methods which resemble the services condition of the metal implants. Since stress and corrosive medium play an important role, special devices that combine these two factors should be developed. Ultrasonic frequency was used in corrosive medium in order to evaluate the fatigue corrosion of metallic implant which enables the application of very-high stress cycle within reasonable testing period (Papakyriacou, 2000). On the other hand the fretting corrosion behavior of metallic implant can be evaluated by a typical pin-on disc method in an artificial physiological medium (Tritschler, 1999, Kumar, 2010). Parameters that are needed to be set include concentration of corrosive medium, load or friction forces, frequency and number of fretting cycles. In the case of pitting corrosion, it can be evaluated with the absences of applied forces. It was reported that a good example of pitting corrosion evaluation was obtained in a buffered saline solution using anodic polarisation and electrochemical impedance measurements (Aziz-Kerrzo, 2001).

Titanium nitride coating on the metallic implant has been a popular method to improve corrosion resistance of metallic implant such as Ti alloy and Co based alloy by physical vapor deposition, plasma spray process, etc. Modification of metallic implant surface by electropolishing, sand blasting or shot peening method were also reported to improve the corrosion resistance of the implant (Aparicioa, 2003). It is known that a significant improvement of corrosion resistance can be achieved for the electropolished surfaces and sand blasted surfaces, where the former surfaces are corroded most slowly. The modification of corrosion resistance properties by the two methods are considered due to the increasing surface area and the introduction of compressive stress on the surface. In addition, chemical composition modification is also possible by sand blasting process with the introduction of sand particle that form certain layer on the surface being blasted.

5.2 Fatigue and fracture

During its service most of metallic implants are subjected to cyclic loading inside the human body which leads to the possibility for fatigue fracture. Factors determine the fatigue behavior of implant materials include microstructure of the implant materials. It was reported that Ti6Al4V with equiaxed structure has a better fatigue strength properties than the elongated structure (Akahori, 1998). Another important parameter is the frequency of the cyclic loading or the cycling rate (Karla, 2009, Lee, 2009) whereas a different fatigue behavior was found for the sample subjected to cyclic loading at 2 Hz than 38 Hz.

Design of the implants also plays an important role on the fatigue failure characteristics. It was reported that fatigue failure of femoral screw had initiated near a keyway, and suggestion on design improvement has been proposed by the lengthening the barrel around the lag screw (Amis, 1987). In addition, beside the type of fluid medium of the implant, the existence of other substances such as protein was also reported to have significant influence on the surface reaction and fatigue resistance of Ti implant (Fleck, 2010).

Since fatigue failure is generally accompanied with corrosion process, thus in addition to cyclic loading, corrosive medium is needed to be introduced in order to evaluate the fatigue properties of implant materials. One of the methods to conduct implant fatigue test was reported by (Leinenbach, 2004) which used rotating bending in physiological media. This method gives a reliable detection on the initial crack growth for the fatigue failure. In most cases, fatigue failure is indicated by the appearance of beach marks and fatigue striation on the failed surfaces as observed by scanning electron microscope (Triantafylldis, 2007). Depend on the stress concentration factor, in certain case such as in the cast of CoCrMo alloys, fracture was observed locally at the (111) faceted fractures (Zhuang, 1988).

Similar with the corrosion failure, various surface modification methods give beneficial influences in improving the fatigue resistance of implant materials. These surface modifications include shot blasting and shot peening (Papakyriacou, 2000) that were observed to work well in any medium or environment. Beside improvement in the fatigue resistance, this method was also observed to improve the osseointegration on the implant materials.

5.3 Wear

Together with corrosion process, wear is among the surface degradation that limits the use of metallic implant such as Ti alloy (Dearnley, 2004). Removal of dense oxide film which naturally formed on the surface of this metallic implant in turn caused wear process (Komotori, 2007). In fact, the major factor that causing premature failure of hip prostheses is due to the wear process with multiple variables interact and thus increase the resultant wear rates (Buford, 2004).

A common method to measure the wear behavior of metallic implant is by pin on disc method which enables lubrication with artificial human body fluid. There are several variables which determine the performance of wear test such as contact stresses, lubricants and clearance, surface hardness and roughness, type of articulation due to motion, number of cycles, oxidation of materials, and surface abrasions (Buford, 2004). Volume of material removed was measured to characterize the wear rate as a function of the contact loads and surface stress state (Mitchell, 2007). It was reported that a critical level of contact stresses is required to initiate wear of the CoCr surface and increase this parameter value will increase the wear rate process. On the other hand the formation of thick oxide layer on Ti alloy after thermal-treatment for 36 h at 625°C was reported to significantly reduce the corrosion and wear of Ti alloy due to the significant increasing of hardness over 1000 HV (Dearnley, 2004). Since wear is type of failure due to surface contact, thus surface modification is an appropriate method to improve wear resistance. An improvement on the wear properties of Ti alloy was reported due to titanium nitride coating on hip implant (Harman, 1997). Another way to avoid the catastrophic wear failure can be done by proper material selection. For the case of joint materials in knee replacement, it was reported that changing implant material from UHMWPE (ultra-high molecular weight polyethylene) to CoCrMo implant alloys significantly reduces the wear debris process (Harman, 1997). Similar condition was also reported that metal-on-metal arthroprostheses show better wear performance than metal-on-UHMPWE (Spriano, 2005).

5.4 Metal ions release

It is realized that high strength alloys possess good mechanical strength but has relatively poor corrosion resistance properties. In most situations it is worst if metal ion release follow corrosion process which can be a toxic contaminant inside human body. As an example, the vanadium ions release on Ti alloys that is preceded with corrosion process (Morais, 2007, Ferrari, 1993). Similar condition was found on CoCrMo alloys which are used as orthopedic implant materials, that these alloys release Co, Cr, Mo ions to host tissues (Öztürk, 2006). There are several factors which play important role on the metal ion release. First, the existence of passive oxide films where once it is broken, metal ions release will be easier to occur (Hanawa, 2004). Second, pH factor where ion release in both stainless steel and Co are affected by pH of the body fluid at a degree that higher for stainless steel (Okazaki, 2008). Similar situation was reported in (Brune, 1986) that Co based alloys show less ion released during the test using natural and synthetic saliva for dental alloys.

In order to reduce the metal ion release from metallic implant, coating is the appropriate method to reduce this process. Nitrogen ion implantation on the CoCrMo alloys enables modification of near surface region of this alloy by forming protective layer on the surface (Öztürk, 2006). Titanium nitride layer was found to have an excellent biocompatibility and the formation of hard nitride layer showed a lower ion release on the metallic implant (Ferrari, 1993). Therefore coating of titanium nitride has been implemented on the Ti alloy and Co based alloy (Ferrari, 1993). Hydroxyapatite coating was also reported to decrease the metal ion release (Browne, 2000). On the other hand significant improvement was also reported by Ti coating on Co base alloy using plasma spraying method (Reclarua, 2005). One point to be noted here is the morphology and surface roughness of the coating layer also determine the corrosion resistance and in turn the metal ion release behavior. Therefore proper coating process as well as substrate preparation is required to obtain optimum results.

6. Recent developments in metals for biomedical devices

Along with the advances in biomedical technology and tissue engineering, biomaterials are desired to exhibit low elastic modulus, shape memory effect or superelasticity, wear resistance, superplasticity and workability. In addition, they are required to eliminate all possibility of toxic effects from leaching, wear and corrosion. One of the concerns is avoiding the use of Ni in fabricating metal alloys. This demand leads to the development of new generation of metallic biomaterials and their novel processing

6.1 New generation of metallic biomaterials

Stainless steels for metal implants have been further developed to be Ni-free. Replacing Ni with other alloying elements while maintaining the stability of austenitic phase, corrosion resistance, magnetism and workability, has lead to the use of nitrogen creating FeCrN, FeCrMoN and FeCrMnMoN systems. The high strength which has been achieved opens the possibility for reduction of implant sizes where limited anatomical space is often an issue, for example, coronary stents with finer meshes (Yang, 2010).

In CoCr alloys system, maximizing C content to its upper limit and addition of Zr and N with optimal precipitation hardening permit the formation of fine and distributed carbides and the suppression of σ-phase which in turn improves the wear resistance of cast CoCr alloy (Lee, 2008). Contrary, for wrought CoCr alloys, addition of N and suppression of carbides and intermetallics results into the desired better workability (Chiba, 2009).

β-type Ti alloy exhibits a lower elastic modulus than α type and α+β type which makes it considered to be the first candidate for low elastic modulus metallic biomaterials (Narushima, 2010). In Ti-Nb systems such as Ti29Nb13Ta4.6Zr (Kuroda, 1998) and Ti35Nb4Sn (Matsumoto, 2005), the elastic moduli can be reduced to 50-60 GPa which are closer to that of cortical bone (10-30 GPa).

Metallic glasses are novel class of metals which currently gets attention from biomaterialist (Schroers, 2009). As represented by some Ni-free Zr based bulk metallic glasses, they show interesting properties in term of higher tensile strength, lower elastic modulus and higher corrosion resistant compared to those of crystalline alloys (Chen, 2010).

Besides, the development in alloy's composition and microstructure, the processing technology for metallic biomaterials is also progressed. Porous structure further reduces elastic modulus to get closer to that of cortical bone. This structure can be obtained through powder sintering, space holder methods, decomposition of foaming agents and rapid prototyping (Ryan, 2006). A combination of rapid prototyping with investment casting (Lopez-Heredia, 2008), with powder sintering (Ryan, 2008), with 3D fibre deposition (Li,

2007) and with selective laser melting (Hollander, 2006) are some of promising process for the development of porous metal structure for biomedical implants.

6.2 Biodegradable metals

Degradable biomaterials can be defined as materials used for medical implants which allow the implants to degrade in biological (human body) environments (Hermawan, 2009). They are expected to provide a temporary healing support for specific clinical problems (disease/trauma) and progressively degrade thereafter. Degradable implants made of metal can be considered as a novel concept which actually opposes the established paradigm of "metallic biomaterials must be corrosion resistant". In term of mechanical property, biodegradable metals are more suitable compared to biodegradable polymers when a high strength to bulk ratio is required such as for internal bone fixation screws/pins and coronary stents.

Metal, metallurgical condition and its composition (wt%)	Density (g/cm^3)	YS (MPa)	UTS (MPa)	YM (GPa)	Max elongation (%)
316L SS, annealed plate (ASTM, 2003)* Fe, 16-18.5 Cr, 10-14 Ni, 2-3 Mo, <2 Mn, <1 Si, <0.03 C	8.00	190	490	193	40
Iron, annealed plate (Goodfellow, 2007) 99.8 Fe	7.87	150	210	200	40
Fe35Mn alloy, powder sintering+thermomechanical treatment (Hermawan, 2008) Fe, 35.5 Mn, 0.04 C	N/A	235	550	N/A	32
FeMnPd alloy, cast+heat treatment (Schinhammer, 2009) Fe, 10.2 Mn, 0.92 Pd, 0.12 C	N/A	850	1450	N/A	11
Magnesium, annealed sheet (ASM, 1998b) 99.98 Mg	1.74	90	160	45	3
WE43 magnesium alloy, temper T6 (ASTM, 2001) Mg, 3.7-4.3 Y, 2.4-4.4 Nd, 0.4-1 Zr	1.84	170	220	44	2
MgZnMnCa alloy, cast (Zhang, 2008) Mg, 0.5 Ca, 2.0 Zn, 1.2 Mn	N/A	70	190	N/A	9
MgCa alloy, extruded (Li, 2008) Mg, 1 Ca	N/A	140	240	N/A	11

* Non-degradable, taken for comparison purpose. The values shown here are the minimum requirements by ASTM. YS = yield strength, UTS = ultimate tensile strength, YM = Young's modulus.

Table 3. Comparative mechanical properties of proposed degradable metallic biomaterials compared to 316L SS

Table 3 shows a comparison on mechanical properties of proposed biodegradable metals versus SS316L. Basically, magnesium- and iron-based alloys are two classes of metals which have been proposed. Among Mg-based alloys have been studied, include MgAl- (Heublein, 2003, Witte, 2005, Xin, 2007), MgRE- (Di Mario, 2004, Peeters, 2005, Witte, 2005, Waksman, 2006, Hänzi, 2009) and MgCa- (Zhang, 2008, Li, 2008) based alloys. Meanwhile, for Fe-based alloys, pure iron (Peuster, 2001, Peuster, 2006) and FeMn alloys (Hermawan, 2008, Schinhammer, 2009) have been investigated mainly for cardiovascular applications.
Among the most advanced studies on biodegradable metals is the development of stents. Figure 2 shows a prototype of biodegradable stent made of iron. The potentiality of biodegradable metal stents for use in treating cardiovascular problem has been assessed by the three level of biological assessment from *in vitro, in vivo* and clinical trials. However, more explorations to understand some fundamental aspects involving the interaction between cells (tissue) - material (degradation product), which was never considered for inert materials, are strongly necessary.

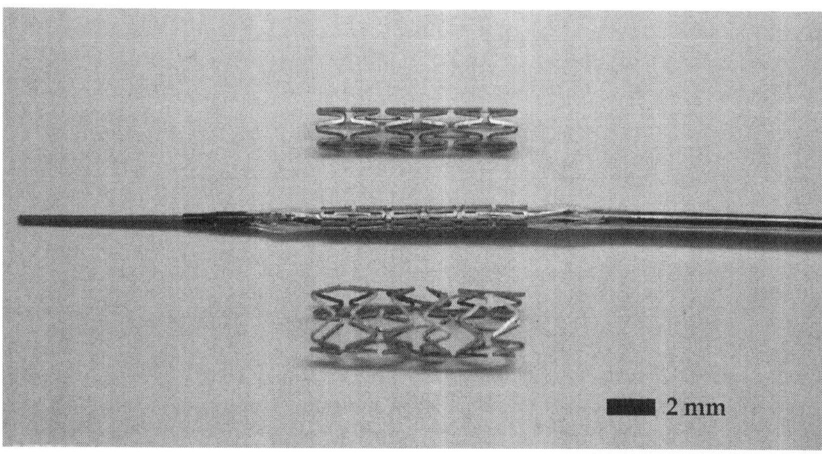

Fig. 2. Prototype of biodegradable stent; (up) as fabricated, (middle) crimped onto a balloon catheter, and (bellow) expanded to 3mm by 6 atm pressure.
(Courtesy of Cordynamics, SA)

7. Conclusion

Nowadays, some metal implants have been replaced by ceramics and polymers due to their excellent biocompatibility and biofunctionality. However, for implants which require high strength, toughness and durability, they are still made of metals. On the other side, clinical use of the promising research in using bioactive polymers and ceramics in regenerative medicine is still far away from practice. With further improvement on novel biofunctionalities and revolutionary use of metal such as for biodegradable implants, it is with a confidence to say that metals will continue to be used as biomaterials in the future.
The future trend seems to combine the mechanically superior metals and the excellent biocompatibility and biofunctionality of ceramics and polymers to obtain the most desirable clinical performance of the implants.

8. Acknowledgment

Authors would like to acknowledge the kind assistantship from Medical Implant Technology Research Group (MediTeg), Universiti Teknologi Malaysia (UTM). This work was supported by the UTM's Research Grant Schemes.

9. References

Adell, R., Lekholm, U., Rockler, B., & Branemark, P.I. (1981). A 15-year study of osseointegrated implants in the treatment of the edentulous jaw. *Intl J Oral Surg*, 10, 387.

Akahori, T., & Niinomi, M. (1998). Fracture characteristics of fatigued Ti6Al4V ELI as an implant material. *Mater Sci Eng A*, 243, 237.

Amis, A.A., Bromagen, J.D., & Lazvin, M. (1987). Fatigue fracture of a femoral sliding compression screw-plate device bone union. *Biomaterials*, 8, 153.

Aparicioa, C., Gil, F.J., Fonseca, C., Barbosa, M., & Planell, J.A. (2003). Corrosion behaviour of commercially pure Ti shot blasted with different materials and sizes of shot particles for dental implant applications. *Biomaterials*, 24, 263.

ASM (1998a). *ASM Handbook Vol. 2, Properties and Selection Nonferrous Alloys and Special-Purpose Materials*, Materials Park, ASM Internaional.

ASM (1998b), *ASM Handbook Vol. 7, Powder Metals Technologies and Applications*, Materials Park, ASM International.

ASM (1998c), *ASM Handbook Vol. 15, Casting*, Materials Park, ASM International.

ASTM (2001). *ASTM B 80: Standard Specification for Magnesium-Alloy Sand Castings*, West Conshohocken, ASTM International.

ASTM (2003). *ASTM F 138: Standard Specification for Wrought 18chromium-14nickel-2.5molybdenum Stainless Steel Bar and Wire for Surgical Implants (UNS S31673)*, West Conshohocken, ASTM International.

ASTM (2006). *ASTM F 67: Standard Specification for Unalloyed Titanium, for Surgical Implant Applications (UNS R50250, UNS R50400, UNS R50550, UNS R50700)*, West Conshohocken, ASTM International.

ASTM (2007a). *ASTM F 90: Standard Specification for Wrought Cobalt-20Chromium-15Tungsten-10Nickel Alloy for Surgical Implant Applications (UNS R30605)*, West Conshohocken, ASTM International.

ASTM (2007b). *ASTM F 562: Standard Specification for Wrought 35Cobalt-35Nickel-20Chromium-10Molybdenum Alloy for Surgical Implant Applications (UNS R30035)*, West Conshohocken, ASTM International.

ASTM (2008). *ASTM F 136: Standard Specification for Wrought Titanium-6 Aluminum-4 Vanadium ELI (Extra Low Interstitial) Alloy for Surgical Implant Applications (UNS R56401)*, West Conshohocken, ASTM International.

Aziz-Kerrzo, M., Conroy, K.G., Fenelon, A.M., Farrell, S.T., & Breslin, C.B. (2001). Electrochemical studies on the stability and corrosion resistance of Ti-based implant materials, *Biomaterials*, 22, 1531-1539.

Azushima, A., Kopp, R., Korhonen, A., Yang, D.Y., Micari, F., Lahoti, G.D., Groche, P., Yanagimoto, J., Tsuji, N., Rosochowski, A., & Yanagida, A. (2008). Severe plastic deformation (SPD) processes for metals, *CIRP Annal Manuf Technol*, 57, 716.

Black, J., & Hastings, G. (1998). *Handbook of Biomaterial Properties*, Chapman Hall.

Bou-Saleh, Z., Shahryari, A., & Omanovic, S. (2007). *Thin Sol Film*, 515, 4727.

Brandes, E.A. & Brook, G.B. (1992). Smithells Metals Reference Book. 7th ed. Oxford, Butterworth-Heinemann.

Browne, M., & Gregson, P.J. (2000). Effect of mechanical surface pretreatment on metal ion release. *Biomaterials*, 21, 385.

Brune, D. (1986). Metal release from dental biomaterialsm, *Biomaterials*, 7, 163.

Buford, A., & Goswami, T. (2004). Review of wear mechanisms in hip implants: Paper I - General. *Mater Des*, 25, 385.

Campbel, F.C. (2006). *Manufacturing Technology for Aerospace Structural*, Elsevier.

Chan S.Y., Park, C.H., & Moriwaki. T. (2010). Mirror finishing of CoCrMo alloy using elliptical vibration cutting. *Prec Eng*, 34, 784.

Chen, Q., Liu, L. & Zhang, S.-M. (2010). The potential of Zr-based bulk metallic glasses as biomaterials. *Front Mater Sci China*, 4, 34.

Chiba, A., Lee, S.-H., Matsumoto, H. & Nakamura, M. (2009). Construction of processing map for biomedical Co28Cr6Mo0.16N alloy by studying its hot deformation behavior using compression tests. *Mater Sci Eng A*, 513-514, 286.

Dearnley, P.A., Dahma, K.L., & Çimenoglu, H. (2004). The corrosion-wear behaviour of thermally oxidised CP-Ti and Ti6Al4V. *Wear*, 256, 469.

Dewidar, M.M., Khalil, K.A, & Lim J.K. (2007). Processing and mechanical properties of porous 316L stainless steel for biomedical applications, *Trans Nonferrous Met Soc China*, 17, 468.

Di Mario, C., Griffiths, H., Goktekin, O., Peeters, N., Verbist, J., Bosiers, M., Deloose, K., Heublein, B., Rohde, R., Kasese, V., Ilsley, C. & Erbel, R. (2004). Drug-eluting bioabsorbable magnesium stent. *J Interv Cardiol*, 17, 391.

Ferrari, F., Miotello, A., Pavloski, L., Galvanetto, E., Moschini, G., Galassini, S., Passi, P., Bogdanovie, S., Fazini, S., Jaksi, M., & Valkovi, V. (1993). Metal-ion release. from Ti and TiN coated implants in rat bone. *Nuclear Instr Meth Phys Res B*, 79, 421.

Fleck, C., & Eifler, D. (2010). Corrosion, fatigue and corrosion fatigue behaviour of metal implant materials, especially Ti alloys. *Intl J Fatigue*, 32, 929.

Geringera, J., Foresta, B., & Combrade, P. (2005). Fretting-corrosion of materials used as orthopaedic implants, *Wear*, 259, 943.

Germain, L., Gey, N., Humbert, M., Vob, P., Jahazi, M., & Bocher, P. (2008). Texture heterogeneities induced by subtransus processing of near a Ti alloys. *Acta Mater*, 56, 4298.

Goodfellow (2007). Iron (Fe) - Material information. Goodfellow Corporation.

Habibovic, P., Barrère, F., Blitterswijk, C.A.V., Groot, K.D. & Layrolle, P. (2002). Biomimetic hydroxyapatite coating on metal implants. *J Am Ceram Soc*, 83, 517.

Han, Y.S., & Hong, S.H. (1999). Microstructural changes during superplastic deformation of Fe24Cr7Ni3Mo0.14N duplex stainless steel. *Mater Sci Eng A*, 266, 276.

Hanawa, T. (2004). Metal ion release from metal implants, *Mater Sci Eng C*, 24, 745.

Hänzi, A.C., Sologubenko, A.S. & Uggowitzer, P.J. (2009). Design strategy for microalloyed ultra-ductile magnesium alloys for medical applications. *Mater Sci Forum*, 618-619, 75.

Harman, M.K., Banks, S.A., & Hodge, W.A. (1997). Wear analysis of a retrieved hip implant with titanium nitride coating. *J Arthroplast*, 12, 938.

Hermawan, H. & Mantovani, D. (2009). Degradable metallic biomaterials: The concept, current developments and future directions. *Minerv Biotecnol*, 21, 207.

Hermawan, H., Alamdari, H., Mantovani, D. & Dubé, D. (2008). Iron-manganese: New class of degradable metallic biomaterials prepared by powder metallurgy. *Powder Metall*, 51, 38.

Hermawan, H., Dubé, D. & Mantovani, D. (2010). Developments in metallic biodegradable stents. *Acta Biomater*, 6, 1693.

Heublein, B., Rohde, R., Kaese, V., Niemeyer, M., Hartung, W. & Haverich, A. (2003). Biocorrosion of magnesium alloys: A new principle in cardiovascular implant technology? *Heart*, 89, 651.

Hollander, D.A., Von Walter, M., Wirtz, T., Sellei, R., Schmidt-Rohlfing, B., Paar, O. & Erli, H.-J. (2006). Structural, mechanical and in vitro characterization of individually structured Ti6Al4V produced by direct laser forming. *Biomaterials*, 27, 955.

Hu, Z.M., Brooks, J.W., & Dean, T.A. (1999). Experimental and theoretical analysis of deformation and microstructural evolution in the hot-die forging of Ti alloy aerofoil sections. *J Mater Proc Technol*, 88, 251.

Huang, J.C., & Chuang, T.H. (1999). Progress on superplasticity and superplastic forming in Taiwan during 1987-1997. *Mater Chem Phys*, 57, 195.

Karla, M., & Kelly, J.R. (2009). Influence of loading frequency on implant failure under cyclic fatigue conditions. *Dent Mater*, 25, 1426.

Kern, M., & Thompson, V.P. (1993). Sandblasting and silica-coating of dental alloys: volume loss, morphology and changes in the surface composition. *Dent Mater*, 9, 155.

Kohn, D.H. (1998). Metals in medical applications, *Curr Op Solid State Mater Sci*, 3, 309.

Komotori, L.J., Hisamori, N., & Ohmoric, Y. (2007). The corrosion/wear mechanisms of Ti6Al4V alloy for different scratching rates. *Wear*, 263, 412.

Krishna, V.G., Prasad, Y.V.R.K., Birla, N.C., & Rao, G.S. (1997). Processing map for the hot working near-alpha Ti alloy 685. *J Mater Proc Technol*, 71, 377.

Kubiak, K., & Sieniaski, J. (1998). Development of the microstructure and fatigue strength of two phase Ti alloys in the processes of forging and heat treatment. *J Mater Proc Technol*, 78, 117.

Kumar, S., & Narayanan, T.S.N.S. (2008). Corrosion behaviour of Ti15Mo alloy for dental implant applications. *J Dentist*, 36, 500.

Kumar, S., Narayanan, T.S.N.S., Raman, S.G.S., & Seshadri, S.K. (2010). Evaluation of fretting corrosion behaviour of CP-Ti for orthopaedic implant applications, *Tribol Intl*, 43, 1245.

Kuroda, D., Niinomi, M., Morinaga, M., Kato, Y. & Yashiro, T. (1998). Design and mechanical properties of new [beta] type Ti alloys for implant materials. *Mater Sci Eng A*, 243, 244.

Kwok, C.T., Cheng, F.T., & Man, H.C. (2003). Effect of processing conditions on the corrosion performance of laser surface-melted AISI 440C martensitic stainless steel. *Surf Coat Technol*, 166, 221.

Lahann, J., Klee, D., Thelen, H., Bienert, H., Vorwerk, D. & Hocker, H. (1999). Improvement of haemocompatibility of metallic stents by polymer coating. *J Mater Sci Mater Med*, 10, 443.

Lambotte, A. (1909). Technique et indication des prothèses dans le traitement des fractures. *Presse Med*, 17, 321.

Lane, W.A. (1895). Some remarks on the treatment of fractures. *Brith Med J*, 1, 861.

Lee, C.K., Karl, M., & Kelly, J.R. (2009). Evaluation of test protocol variables for dental implant fatigue research. *Dent Mater*, 25, 1419.

Lee, S.H., Nomura, N. & Chiba, A. (2008). Significant improvement in mechanical properties of biomedical CoCrMo alloys with combination of N addition and Cr-enrichment. *Mater Trans*, 49, 260.

Leinenbach, C., Fleck, C., & Eifler, D. (2004). The cyclic deformation behaviour and fatigue induced damage of the implant alloy TiAl6Nb7 in simulated physiological media. *Intl J Fatigue*, 26, 857.

Li, J.P., Habibovic, P., Van Den Doel, M., Wilson, C.E., De Wijn, J.R., Van Blitterswijk, C.A. & De Groot, K. (2007). Bone ingrowth in porous Ti implants produced by 3D fiber deposition. *Biomaterials*, 28, 2810.

Li, Z., Gu, X., Lou, S. & Zheng, Y. (2008). The development of binary Mg-Ca alloys for use as biodegradable materials within bones. *Biomaterials*, 29, 1329.

Liu, Y., & Baker, T.N. (1995). Deformation characteristics of IMI685 Ti alloy under β isothermal forging conditions. *Mater Sci Eng A*, 197, 125.

Lopez-Heredia, M.A., Sohier, J., Gaillard, C., Quillard, S., Dorget, M. & Layrolle, P. (2008). Rapid prototyped porous Ti coated with calcium phosphate as a scaffold for bone tissue engineering. *Biomaterials*, 29, 2608.

Matsumoto, H., Watanabe, S. & Hanada, S. (2005). Beta TiNbSn alloys with low Young's modulus and high strength. *Mater Trans*, 46, 1070.

Ming-Wei, W., Li-Wen, Z., Ji-Bin, P., Li Chen, P., & Fan, H. (2007). Effect of temperature on vacuum hot bulge forming of BT20 Ti alloy cylindrical work piece. *Trans Nonferrous Met Soc China*, 17, 957.

Mitchell, A., & Shrotriya, P. (2007). Onset of nanoscale wear of metallic implant materials:Influence of surface residual stresses and contact loads. *Wear*, 263, 1117.

Miyamoto, H., Mimaki, T., & Hashimoto, S. (2001). *Mater Sci Eng A*, 319-321, 779.

Morais, L.S., Serra, G.G., Muller, C.A., Andrade, L.R., Palermo, E.F.A., Elias, C.N., & Meyers, M. (2007). Titanium alloy mini-implants for orthodontic anchorage: Immediate loading and metal ion release. *Acta Biomater*, 3, 331.

Mordyuk, B.N., Prokopenko, G.I. Vasylyev, M.A., & Iefimov, M.O. (2007). Effect of structure evolution induced by ultrasonic peening on the corrosion behavior of AISI-321 stainless steel. *Mater Sci Eng A*, 458, 253.

Narushima, T. (2010). New-generation metallic biomaterials. IN NIINOMI, M. (Ed.) *Metals for Biomedical Devices*. Cambrigde, Woodhead Publishing.

Nguyen, H.Q., Deportera, D.A., Pilliara, R.M., Valiquettea, N., & Yakubovich, R. (2004). The effect of sol-gel-formed calcium phosphate coatings on bone ingrowth and osteoconductivity of porous-surfaced Ti alloy implants. *Biomaterials*, 25, 865.

Okazaki, Y., & Gotoh, E. (2008). Metal release from stainless steel, CoCrMoNiFe and NiTi alloys in vascular implants. *Corr Sci*, 50, 3429.

Öztürk, O., Türkan, U., & Ahmet, E.E. (2006). Metal ion release from nitrogen ion implanted CoCrMo orthopedic implant material. *Surf Coat Technol*, 200, 5687.

Papakyriacou, M., Mayer, H. Pypen, C., Plenk Jr, H., & Stanzl-Tschegg, S. (2000). Effects of surface treatments on high cycle corrosion fatigue of metallic implant materials. *Intl J Fatigue*, 22, 873.

Peckner, D., & Bernstein, I.M. (1977). *Handbook of Stainless Steels*, McGraw-Hill Inc.

Peeters, P., Bosiers, M., Verbist, J., Deloose, K. & Heublein, B. (2005). Preliminary results after application of absorbable metal stents in patients with critical limb ischemia. *J Endovasc Ther*, 12, 1.

Peuster, M., Hesse, C., Schloo, T., Fink, C., Beerbaum, P. & Von Schnakenburg, C. (2006). Long-term biocompatibility of a corrodible peripheral iron stent in the porcine descending aorta. *Biomaterials*, 27, 4955.

Peuster, M., Wohlsein, P., Brugmann, M., Ehlerding, M., Seidler, K., Fink, C., Brauer, H., Fischer, A. & Hausdorf, G. (2001). A novel approach to temporary stenting: Degradable cardiovascular stents produced from corrodible metal-results 6-18 months after implantation into New Zealand white rabbits. *Heart*, 86, 563.

Ramdan, R.D., Jauhari, I., Hasan, R., & Nik Masdek, N.R. (2008). The role of strain rate during deposition of CAP on Ti6Al4V by superplastic deformation-like method using high-temperature compression test machine. *Mater Sci Eng A*, 477, 300.

Ratner, B.D. (1993). New ideas in biomaterials science-A path to engineered biomaterials. *J Biomed Mater Res*, 27, 837.

Reclarua, L., Eschlera, P., Lerf, R., & Blatter, A. (2005) Electrochemical corrosion and metal ion release from CoCrMo prosthesis with Ti plasma spraycoating, *Biomaterials*, 26, 4747.

Roland, T., Retraint, D., Lu, K., & Liu, J. (2006) Fatigue life improvement through surface nanostructuring of stainless steel by means of surface mechanical attrition treatment. *Script Mater*, 54, 1949.

Ryan, G.E., Pandit, A.S. & Apatsidis, D.P. (2008). Porous Ti scaffolds fabricated using a rapid prototyping and powder metallurgy technique. *Biomaterials*, 29, 3625.

Ryan, G., Pandit, A. & Apatsidis, D.P. (2006). Fabrication methods of porous metals for use in orthopaedic applications. *Biomaterials*, 27, 2651.

Schinhammer, M., Hänzi, A.C., Löffler, J.F. & Uggowitzer, P.J. (2010). Design strategy for biodegradable Fe-based alloys for medical applications. *Acta Biomater*, 6, 1705.

Schroers, J., Kumar, G., Hodges, T., Chan, S. & Kyriakides, T. (2009). Bulk metallic glasses for biomedical applications. *J Mater*, 61, 21.

Schrooten, J., & Helsen, J.A. (2000). Adhesion of bioactive glass coating to Ti6Al4V oral implant. *Biomaterials*, 21, 1461.

Serro, A.P., & Saramago, B. (2003). Influence of sterilization on the mineralization of Ti implants induced by incubation in various biological model fluids. *Biomaterials*, 24, 4749.

Shahryari, A., Omanovic, S., & Szpunar, J.A. (2008). Electrochemical formation of highly pitting-resistant passive films on biomedical grade 316LVM stainless steel surface. *Mater Sci Eng C*, 28, 94.

Sherman, W.O. (1912). Vanadium steel bone plates and screws. *Surg Gynecol Obstet*, 14, 629.

Spriano, S., Vernè, E., Faga, M.G., Bugliosi, S., & Maina, G., Surface treatment on an implant cobalt alloy for high biocompatibility and wear resistance. *Wear*, 259, 919.

Sun, Y., & Haruman, E. (2008) Influence of processing conditions on structural characteristics of hybrid plasma surface alloyed austenitic stainless steel. *Surf Coat Technol*, 202, 4069.

Triantafylldis, G.K., Kazantzis, A.V., & Karageorgiou, K.T. (2007). Premature fracture of a stainless steel 316L orthopaedic plate implant by alternative episodes of fatigue and cleavage decoherence. *Eng Failure Anal*, 14, 1346.

Tritschler, B., Forest, B., & Rieu, J. (1999). Fretting corrosion of materials for orthopaedic implants: a study of a metal/polymer contact in an artificial physiological medium. *Tribol Intl*, 32, 587.

Venugopal, S., Sivaprasad, P.V., Vasudevan, M., Mannan, S.L., Jha, S.K., Pandey, P., & Prasad, Y.V.R.K. (1995). Validation of processing maps for 304L stainless steel using hot forging, rolling and extrusion. *J Mater Proc Technol*, 59, 343.

Waksman, R., Pakala, R., Kuchulakanti, P.K., Baffour, R., Hellinga, D., Seabron, R., Tio, F.O., Wittchow, E., Hartwig, S., Harder, C., Rohde, R., Heublein, B., Andreae, A., Waldmann, K.-H. & Haverich, A. (2006). Safety and efficacy of bioabsorbable Mg alloy stents in porcine coronary arteries. *Catheter Cardiovasc Interv*, 68, 606.

Wang, Y.B., Zheng, Y.F., Wei, S.C. & Li, M. (2011). In vitro study on Zr-based bulk metallic glasses as potential biomaterials. *J Biomed Mater Res*, 96B, 34.

Weiss, I., & Semiatin, S.L. (1999). Thermomechanical processing of alpha Ti alloys—An overview. *Mater Sci Eng A*, 263, 243.

Williams, D.F. (2008). On the mechanisms of biocompatibility. *Biomaterials*, 29, 2941.

Williamson, D.L., Davis, J.A., & Wilbur, P.J. (1998). Effect of austenitic stainless steel composition on low-energy, high-flux, nitrogen ion beam processing. *Surf Coat Technol*, 103-104, 178.

Witte, F., Hort, N., Vogt, C., Cohen, S., Kainer, K.U., Willumeit, R. & Feyerabend, F. (2009). Degradable biomaterials based on magnesium corrosion. *Curr Op Solid State Mater Sci*, 12, 63.

Witte, F., Kaese, V., Haferkamp, H., Switzer, E., Linderberg, A.M., Wirth, C.J. & Windhagen, H. (2005). In vivo corrosion of four magnesium alloys and the associated bone response. *Biomaterials*, 26, 3557.

Xin, Y., Liu, C., Zhang, X., Tang, G., Tian, X. & Chu, P.K. (2007). Corrosion behavior of biomedical AZ91 magnesium alloy in simulated body fluids. *J Mater Res*, 22, 2004.

Yang, K. & Ren, Y. (2010). Nickel-free austenitic stainless steels for medical applications. *Sci Technol Adv Mater*, 11, 1.

Zhang, E. & Yang, L. (2008). Microstructure, mechanical properties and biocorrosion properties of MgZnMnCa alloy for biomedical application. *Mater Sci Eng A*, 497, 111.

Zhuang, L.Z., & Langer, E.W. (1988). Effects of the range of the stress intensity factor on the appearance of localized fatigue fracture in cast CoCrMo alloy used for surgical implants. *Mater Sci Eng A*, 102, L9.

Zhuka, H.V., Kobryn, P.A., & Semiatin, S.L. (2007). Influence of heating and solidification conditions on the structure and surface quality of electron-beam melted Ti6Al4V ingots. *J Mater Proc Technol*, 190, 387.

18

Orthopaedic Modular Implants Based on Shape Memory Alloys

Daniela Tarnita[1], Danut Tarnita[2] and Dumitru Bolcu[1]
[1]*University of Craiova,*
[2]*University of Medicine and Pharmacy, Craiova,*
Romania

1. Introduction

Intelligent materials are those materials whose physical characteristics can be modified not only through the charging factors of a certain test, but also through diverse mechanisms involving a series of additional parameters like luminous radiation, temperature, magnetic or electric fields etc. The use of intelligent materials in medical sciences offers to the economic medium the safest way to launch effective, highly-feasible and especially biocompatible products on the internal and international markets. The most important alloy used in biomedical applications is Ni-Ti, Nitinol (Nickel Titanium Naval Ordinance Laboratory), an alloy of an almost equal mixture of nickel and titanium, which is able to fulfil functional requirements related not only to their mechanical reliability but also to its chemical reliability and its biological reliability. Superelastic Nitinol alloys are becoming integral to the design of a variety of new medical products. The very big elasticity of these alloys is the most important advantage afforded by this material, but by no means the only or most important one. To highlight the value of superelastic Nitinol to the medical industry, we can present other properties: biocompatibility, kink resistance, constancy of stress, physiological compatibility, shape-memory deployment, dynamic interference, fatigue resistance hysteresis, and MRI compatibility (Duerig et al., 1999; Friend & Morgan, 1999; Mantovani, 2000; Pelton et al., 2000; Ryhanen et al., 1999). These properties were used for manufacturing medical products including stents, filters, retrieval baskets, and surgical tools.
There are many metals exhibit superelastic effects, but only Nitinol based alloys is biologically and chemically compatible with the human body (Kapanen et al., 2002; Raghubir et al., 2007; Shabalovskaya, 1995; Yeung et al., 2007). In vivo testing and experience indicates that Nitinol is highly biocompatible, more so than stainless steel. The extraordinary compliance of Nitinol clearly makes it the metal that is most similar mechanically to biological materials. This improved physiological similarity promotes bony ingrowths and proper healing by sharing loads with the surrounding tissue, and has led to applications such as hip implants, bone spacers, bone staples, and skull plates. NiTi applications in orthopaedics currently include internal fixation by the use of fixatives, compression bone stables used in osteotomy and fracture fixation, rods for the correction of scoliosis (Yang et al., 1987), shape memory expansion staples used in cervical surgery (Sanders et al., 1993), staples in small bone surgery (Mei et al., 1997), and fixation systems for suturing tissue in minimal invasive surgery (Musialek et al., 1998). Several types of

shape memory orthopaedic staples and plates for recovery of bones are used to accelerate the healing process of bone fractures, exploiting the shape memory effect.

2. AO classification of human bones fractures

In the AO classification system (Muller et al., 2006), for each long bone or bone group a number from 1 to 9 is assigned (Fig.1). The human long bones are: humerus-1; radius/ulna-2; femur-3 and they are divided in three segments, designated by a number 1, 2 or 3; tibia/fibula-4 are divided in four segments, designated by 1, 2, 3, 4. A fracture is classified morphologically into three types in accordance with all the segments of the bone. The type of fracture is indicated by one of the following letters: A, B, C. Each type is divided into three groups: 1, 2 or 3 and each group is also divided into three subgroups, designated by: .1, .2, and .3. There are nine groups (Al, A2, A3 - B1, B2, B3 - C1, C2, C3) for each segment of the bone. The nine groups are organized according to severity criteria, as a function of the morphological complexity, the difficulty of the treatment and the prognosis, the gravity increasing from A1 (the most simple fracture) to C3 (the most complex and grave fracture). For exemple, the groups and the subgroups of tibial diaphyseal fractures are (Figure 3):
42. A1. Simple spiroid fracture; 42. A2. Simple oblique fracture (>30°); 42. A3. Simple transversal fracture (<30°)

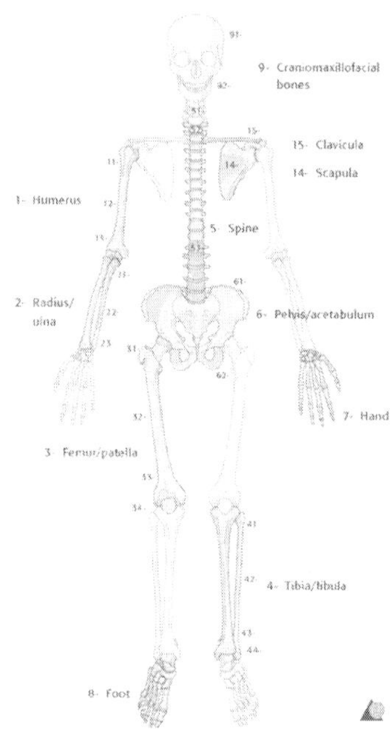

Fig. 1. AO system for numbering the anatomical location of a fracture in three bone segments (proximal=1, diaphyseal=2, distal=3); where the assigned numbers for human bones are: humerus-1; radius/ulna-2; femur-3; tibia/fibula-4; spine-5, pelvis-6, fand-7, foot-8, craniomaxillofacial-9 [Muller et al., 2006]

The anatomical location of the fractures for long bones is presented in Fig.2 and the AO classification of the type A tibial diaphyseal fractures is presented in Fig.3 (www.aofoundation.org).

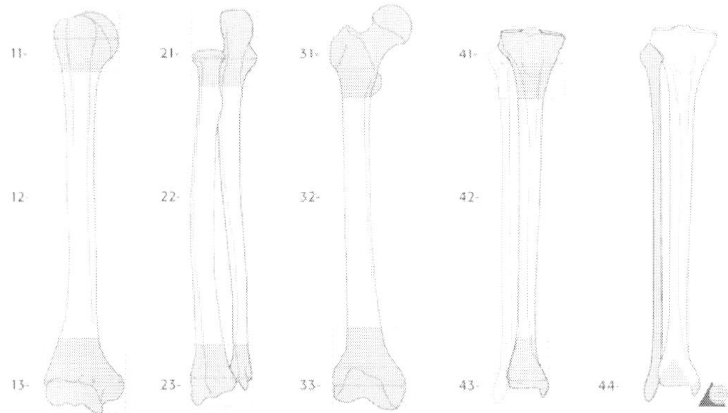

Fig. 2. Anatomical location of a fracture is designated by two numbers: one for the bone and one for its segment: 1.1. proximal humerus; 1.2. diaphyseal humeru; 1.3. distal humerus; ulna and radius are regarded as one bone: 2.1. proximal radius+ulna; 2.2. diaphyseal radius +ulna, 2.3. distal radius +ulna); 1.1. proximal femur; 1.2. diaphyseal femur; 1.3. distal femur; 4.1. proximal tibia+fibula; 4.2. diaphyseal tibia+fibula, 4.3. distal tibia+fibula;

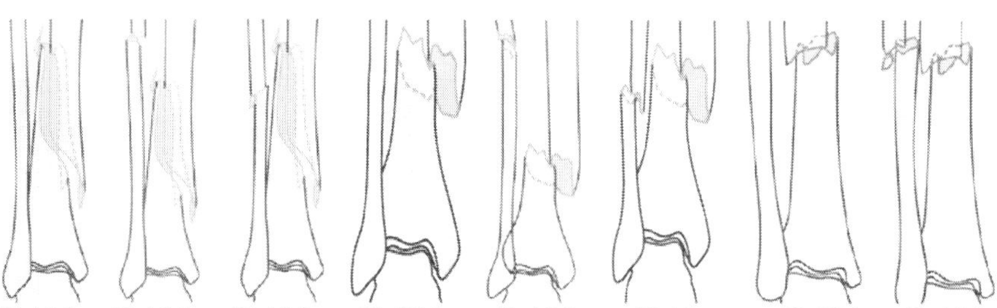

42-A1.1; 42-A1.2; 42-A1.3; 42-A2.1; 42-A2.2; 42-A2.; 42-A3.1; 42-A3.3

Fig.3. AO classification of the type A tibial diaphyseal fractures: A1- Simple spiroid fracture; A2-Simple oblique fracture; A3-Simple transversal fracture; 42-A1.1 Fibula intact; 42-A1.2; Fibula fractured at other level; 42-A1.3 Fibula fractured at the same level; 42-A2.1 Fibula intact; 42-A2.2 Fibula fractured at other level; 42-A2.3 Fibula fractured at the same level; 42-A3.1 Fibula intact; 42-A3.3 Fibula fractured at the same level

A comparative analysis of 2700 diaphyseal bone fractures shows that each type of fracture occurs with similar incidence in the case of the four bones: A type: 61% for humerus, 65% for radius/ulna, 53% for femur and 45% for tibia/fibula; B type: 32% for humerus, 29 for radius/ulna, 34% for femur and 46% for tibia/fibula; C type: 7% humerus, 6% radius/ulna, 13% femur and 9% tibia/fibula. The fracture groups have a similar distribution for humerus, femur and tibia/fibula. For example, the spiroid fractures take 27% from the humeral fractures, 23% from the femoral fractures and 25% from tibial fractures (Muller et al., 2006).

3. Three dimensional virtual models for human bones

The geometry and mechanical properties of the bone system vary naturally by individual which can create great difficulties in biomechanical research. The dimensions, form, mechanical properties, elastic constants, physical constants of the bone are different for different individuals. They depend on: age, sex, height, profession etc. The geometrical aspects of the bone systems modelling are dominated by the necessity of using some spatial models because most of the bone elements have complicated geometrical forms in space. The creation of the virtual 3D model of the human bones and the numerical simulations require:

a. Three-dimensional modelling of the bones -using parametrical CAD software, SolidWorks or Catia.
b. Mesh generation of each virtual model of human bones in finite elements (using tetrahedral 3D elements).
c. Establishment of the contour conditions
d. Introduction of the mechanical parameters for each material (cortical and spongy) of the bones
e. Finite element method analysis and simulation with dedicated software (ANSYS, VisualNastran)

To obtain the three-dimensional virtual models, bones from dead persons, kept in the Laboratory of Anatomy from the University of Medicine and Pharmacy, Craiova were used. To obtain the bone cross sections a PHILIPS AURA CT tomograph installed in the Emergency Hospital from Craiova was used. The obtained images were re-drawn in AutoCad over the real tomographies and the drawings were imported in SolidWorks (a parametrical CAD software), section by section, in parallel planes. Solidworks allows the creation of a solid by "unifying" the sections drawn in parallel planes (www.solidworks.com). The feature we used the Loft Shape and it defines the solid starting with the sections and using a Guide Curve defined automatically by the software. Finally, we obtained the spatial virtual models of the studied bones. The bones have been modelled, mainly, through a cylinder of compact bone tissue having a central canal called medullar cavity which penetrates the extremities where the model narrows due to some lamellar systems. The extremities of the bone are made from a thin layer of compact bone substance (cortical) at the exterior and a spongy material at the interior.

For the next step we used the ANSYS program to obtain the mesh structure with finite elements method of the spatial structure of bones (Tarnita et al., 2009). The three-dimensional modelling of the bone structures has been succeeded by the introduction of a series of physiological and morphological parameters in order to allow a corresponding study of the bones at different stresses and deformations that characterise both normal situations and accidents.

The next step was to apply the material properties to the virtual models by introducing the elastic constants (elasticity modules and Poisson coefficient) by considering the nature of the bone material: a composite material made from cortical and spongy. The values for the longitudinal elasticity modules and Poisson coefficient have been chosen from the literature.The work hypotheses are:

a. Even though the material of the bone is an-isotropic and not homogeneous, in the modelling, the bone was considered homogeneous and isotropic, for a zone of solicitation that does not exceed certain limits.
b. The bone is made by two kinds of materials, compact and spongy, like a composite material.

c. The average values considered for the longitudinal modulus of elasticity, E, are: 18.500 N/mm^2 for the compact bone, situated in the exterior zone of the bone and 2 N/mm^2 for the spongy bone, situated in the interior zone. The value of the Poisson coefficient was 0.3.

d. The virtual central canal is realized in accordance with the obtained tomographies, so the complex spatial structure is ensured.

Ulna: The ulna is a long bone of the forearm, broader proximally, and narrower distally. Proximally, the ulna has a bony process, the olecranon process, a hook-like structure that fits into the olecranon fossa of the humerus. This prevents hyperextension and forms a hinge joint with the trochlea of the humerus (Gray, 2000). There is also a radial notch for the head of the radius, and the ulnar tuberosity to which muscles can attach. Distally (near the hand), there is a styloid process. The long, narrow medullary cavity is enclosed in a strong wall of compact tissue which is thickest along the interosseous border and dorsal surface. At the extremities the compact layer thins. The compact layer is continued onto the back of the olecranon as a plate of close spongy bone with lamellae parallel. The sections of ulna bone realized in SolidWorks are presented in Figure 4b. Finally, it is obtained the virtual model of the ulna bone (Figure 4c).

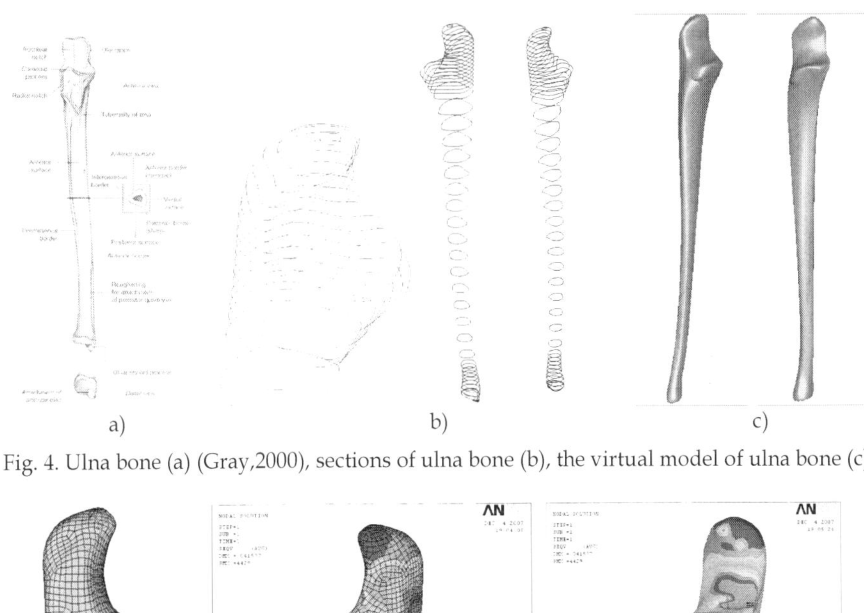

a) b) c)

Fig. 4. Ulna bone (a) (Gray,2000), sections of ulna bone (b), the virtual model of ulna bone (c)

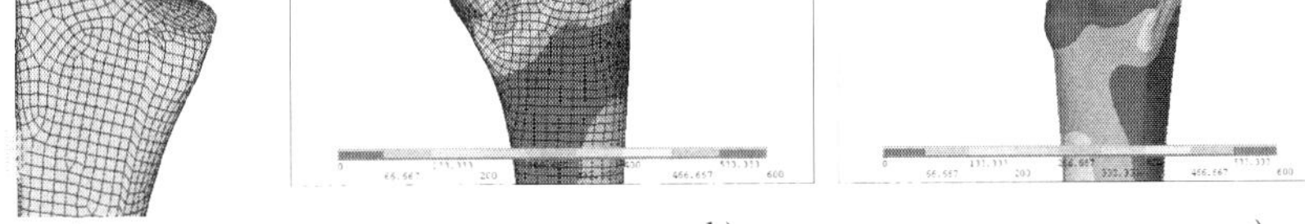

a) b) c)

Fig. 5. The loading forces (a) and the resulted stress maps (b and c) for the first case

The mesh structure is presented in Fig. 5a. The bone is considered leaned on its metaphyseal area. The geometrical model was subjected to a solicitation equal to a force of 1000N, in two cases, like in Fig. 5a, and Fig.6a.
In Fig.5b and Fig.5c the stresses diagram for first loading case were obtained. In Fig.6 are presented the stress diagrams for the second loading case. We can see that the maximum values of stresses appear in the articular portion of the proximal ulna. They may involve the olecranon process or the coronoid process. This area is the most solicited part of the bone which is more likely to be involved in fractures.

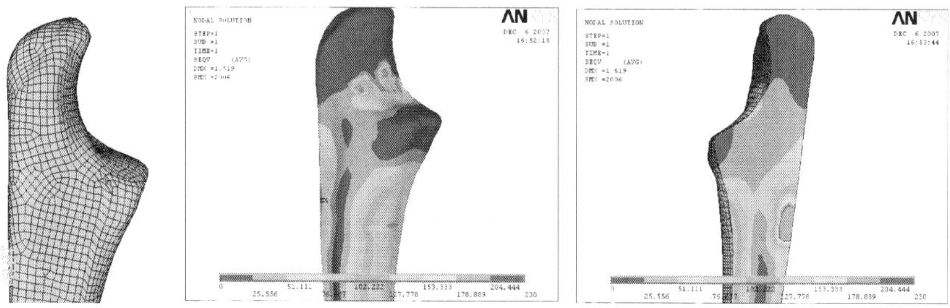

a) b) c)

Fig. 6. The loading forces (a) and the obtained stress maps (b and c) for the second loading case

Tibia. In the first case the tibia bone was subjected to a torsion couple on the top surface (Fig.7a.). The bone is supported on its inferior base. We obtained the resultant stress distribution for the torsion solicitation for the entire bone (Fig.7b). and for a section made in this bone (Fig.7c). In the second case the bone was supposed to the bending by a normal force equal with 180N distributed on the middle of tibia bone. The bone is leaned in his both heads. We obtained the resultant stress distribution for the bending solicitation (Fig.8a.). In third case the bone was supposed to a compression force distributed on the both superiors condils (Fig.8b.). Finally, we obtained the resultant stress distribution for the compression solicitation (Fig.8c.).

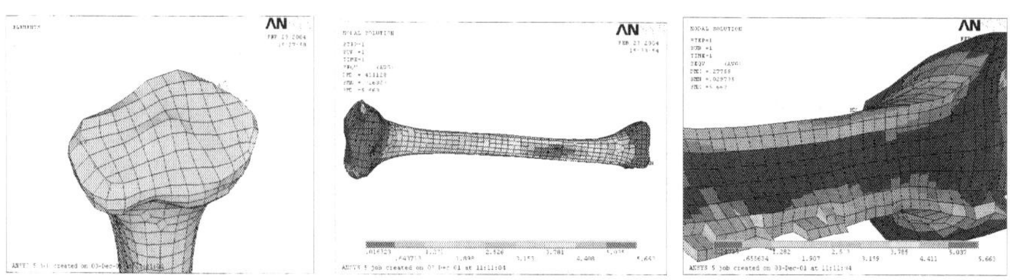

Fig. 7. The torsion solicitation (a) and the stress diagram obtained for the entire bone (b) and for a section of the bone (c)

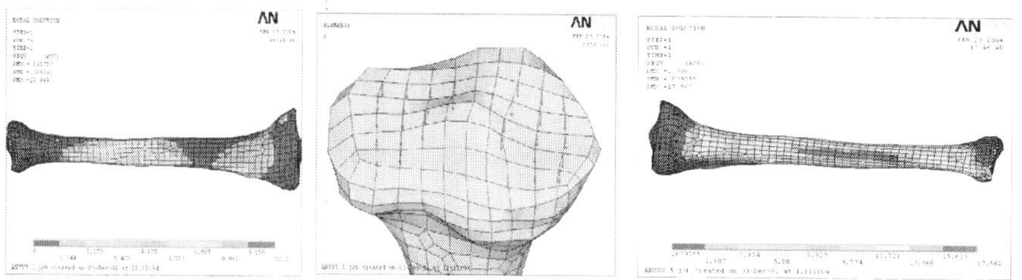

(a) b) c)

Fig. 8. The stress map for the second case(a), the loading force in the third case (b) and the stress map obtained for the third case (c)

Metacarpi: The virtual model of the bone was subjected to:

- traction with a force evenly distributed on the head of the metacarpal bone surface, while the basis is the fixation surface. The stresses diagram can be observed in Figure 9a and the displacements diagram in Figure 9b.
- torsion with a moment applied at the metacarpal head, the basis of the bone being fixed. The tension diagram is given in Figure 9c and Figure 9d.

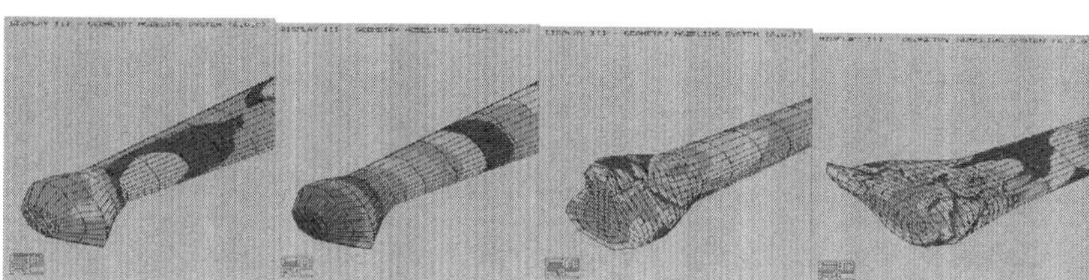

a) b) c) d)

Fig. 9. The stresses diagram (a), the displacements diagram (b) for traction and stresses diagram for torsion solicitation of the metacarpi bone (c and d)

Clavicle: Two loading cases have been taken into consideration:

1. compression with an evenly distributed force equal with 4 N/mm^2 applied on the extreme surface of the clavicle while the basis is the fixation surface (results in Figure 10a and Figure 10b).
2. flexion given by 400 N of force distributed on the lateral surface of the clavicle (results in Fig.10c and Fig.10d)

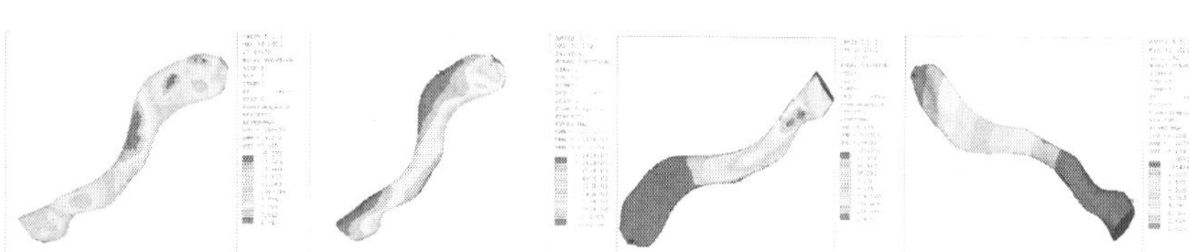

a) b) c) d)

Fig. 10. The normal tension map for clavicle (a), the linear deformations for the clavicle bone in the first case (b), and tension map (c) and deformation map (d) in the second case

Phalanx: The virtual model of the phalanx has been tested to:

1. compression with a force evenly distributed on the superior surface of the phalanx head, while the bone is fixed at the basis (Fig 11 a- The stress diagram; Fig 11 b- The displacements diagram);
2. bending given by a force which acts at the middle of the bone, both extremities (proximal and distal) being fixed (Fig 11 c- The stress diagram; Fig 11 d- The displacements diagram);

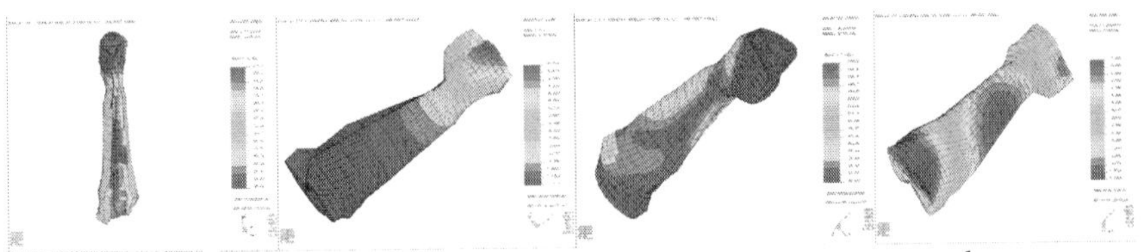

a. b. c. d.

Fig. 11. The results obtained by numerical simulations for the above considered loading cases for the phalanx bone

Radius: In Fig. 12.a. we present the mesh structure of the virtual model of the radius bone. In Fig.12.b, a longitudinal section through radius is presented. The virtual model was tested with a moment of 4.8 Nm (torsion) applied on the surface of the radius head. The bone is fixed at the inferior side. The virtual stress is given by a set of forces placed at the extremities of the radius head in a plane normal to the longitudinal axis of the bone. The stress diagrams are shown in Fig.12.c, while the deformations diagrams in Fig.12.d.

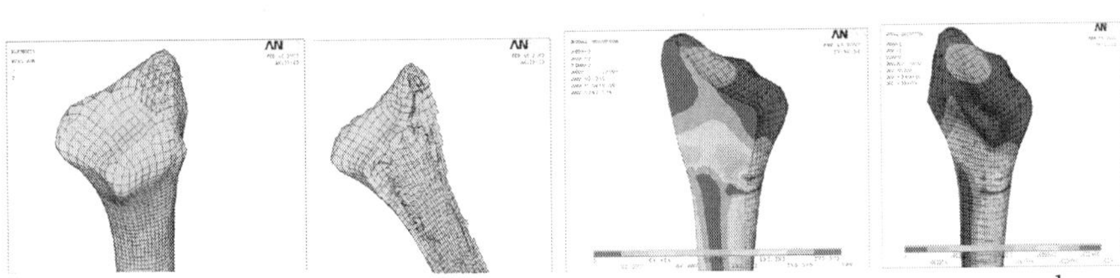

a. b. c. d.

Fig. 12. The virtual model of the radius (a), longitudinal section through radius (b) the stress map (c) and deformation map (d)

Analysis of stresses and deformations of the fracture areas is carried out with the Finite Element Method which allows: accuracy of the complex bony structure geometry, variation of designing parameters, and combination with other bone modelling algorithms leading to various types of analyses. The software allows the determination of the stress and displacements distribution in some particular cases which determine the breaking of the ulna. The correspondence between the clinical observations, virtual simulations and the results obtained from the experimental tests using the universal testing machine EDZ20 certify the accuracy and the fidelity of the spatial geometry, but also of the bone structure, of the mechanical properties of the bone.

4. Orthopaedic modular implants based on shape memory alloys

Treatment of bone fractures depends on the stability of the fracture configuration. The fixation of the fracture must sometimes accomplish a reduction of the fragments and to spare the vasculature of these fragments as much as possible. It is well known that stable fixation and compression are the two main factors in obtaining union between two bony fragments. The choice of fracture treatment, orthopaedic or surgical and also the type of surgical treatment must take into account the type of fracture, the importance of displacements, the skin condition, patient age and also the patient's possibilities and his willingness to cooperate. A stable fracture can be adequately managed with cast immobilization. An unstable fracture may require surgical fixation. In many cases, the treatment of fractures involves surgical intervention to stabilize the fracture. The traditional method of open reduction and plate fixation requires wide exposure of the fracture site with stripping of the soft tissues which may devascularize the fracture fragments (Heim & Pfeiffer, 1988). This may contribute to the necrosis caused by trauma and increase the risks of delayed healing and infection.
In selecting the optimum technique, the surgical complexity, mechanical performance, and biological response should be considered. Typically, a fractured or cut bone is treated using a fixation device, which strengthens the bone and keeps it aligned during the healing process. Mechanically, the fixation should provide sufficient stability. Biologically, the treatment should be minimally invasive, the implants well tolerated, and the resulting bone stresses optimal for fracture healing. Even if it's well known how important the integrity of soft tissues is during surgical fracture treatment, by plate-screw fixation, trauma surgeons have always had a tendency to reach maximum biomechanical stability, regardless of the impact on bone vasculature. The conflict between the anatomical needs to reduce the distance of the fracture and the desire to keep the vascularisation of all bone fragments is the reason for the appearance of minimal invasive surgical techniques. Techniques of minimally invasive surgery were developed to avoid wide exposures of the fracture site and minimize soft tissue damage (Farouk et al., 1999). They are described for some fractures in the lower extremity (Kregor at al., 2001). The implants of classical materials have the following disadvantages, clinically observed, in time, by the orthopaedic specialists:

1. Relatively large dimensions of implants due to respecting resistance conditions to materials' breaking norms, classical materials have break-resistance values much more inferior to alloys' values with shape memory;
2. The augmentation of the implants dimensions determines large incisions with large blood and soft tissues losses, and aggravating conditions of the bone, which lead to consolidation delays but also to increased infection risk;
3. The healing process becomes complicated due to lack of fracture components' compaction, fact which often leads to consolidation delays and even pseudo-arthrosis;
4. Multiple holes where implant-fixing screws are introduced represent tension concentration which leads to bones' fragility and appearance of new fracture focuses;
5. They are supplied with differently typo-sizes, separately for each type of bone, for each bone area for each fracture type and size separately
6. Using compaction devices designed to improve the rate of healing percentage when plate screwed fixation is used, cause scarring even longer and destruction of soft tissues greater than plate screwed fixation without compaction.

7. Because of cortex sponging the boards need to be extracted (which means a second surgery). By extracting, there is a fracture risk of one of the holes for screws, causing peri-fracture tissue damage and peri-implant as big as or bigger than the implant operation. In order to eliminate or at least reduce inconveniences caused by the lack of compaction, plates with screws with compacting or self compacting have been created. These plates, however, fail to achieve a satisfactory compaction and, in addition, require larger incisions and with greater tissue damage, higher blood loss and increased exposure to infections and scarring are larger and more unsightly and compaction in this case is achieved with the bone fixation and not continuously, as with the model proposed by us.
8. All inconveniences, besides prolonging patient's suffering, increase the number of hospital days as well as the number of disability days at work, leading to high social costs.

4.1 Orthopaedic modular plates based on shape memory alloys

The classical bone plates with screws prevent bone compaction and do not allow application of axial forces caused by muscle tension in normal bones which leads to the delay of fracture focus consolidation or leads to a non-union (pathological neo-articulation). The classical metal plate used as an implant must be sufficiently large to achieve solid fixation of the fracture fragments. Current orthopaedic plates use titanium or special steel, materials which are subject to electrolytic action of the biological environment, without allowing a pseudo- elastic behaviour similar to bone structure. Because the lengths of the classical plates are big, the surgery for metallic implant mounting needs large incisions with great tissue damage, with great loss of blood, tissues with high exposure to the environment, which increases the risk of infections, with big risks in their propagation to the bone (bone infections are incurable) and obtain scarring. Internal tissues are exposed to foreign microbial increasing the danger of infecting the wound. The implant has a large contact surface with the biological environment which increases the risk of rejection by the body or occurrence of inflammatory phenomena. These requests affect the process of bone recovery leading to the appearance of a bony callus formed incorrectly, to structural goals or to geometrical deformations of fractured bone. Another disadvantage is related to plates' reduced adaptability to the specific particularities of each fracture case occurred in practice. The only degree of adaptability allowed to the current plate-type implants is provided by using additional holes which allow fixing screws depending on the size of fracture/fractures.

For modelling the optimum implant shape according to the type of fracture, it is taken into consideration the simulation with Finite Element Method of the various areas where the implants are to be placed. Studies continue with modelling various implant shapes and their experimentation in virtual environment in order to determine optimum shapes to provide perfect interweaving of fractured bony structures. The optimum shape has to take into consideration the implant insertion technique as well. The proposed implants have a modular design, with memory shape as elements of module coupling. The design of proposed modular implant involves a minimal invasive implantation, small dimensions, which can be coupled intra-operatory, in order to obtain modular plates of various lengths and configurations appropriate to the fracture.

The modular structures for implants are used for the osteosynthesis of diaphyseal and metaphyseal fractures of long bones. These are based on the making of identical modules-completely interchangeable, made of titanium or biocompatible stainless steel 316L, after which Nitinol elements are interconnected. The shape memory effect in the case of a staple is connected with a contraction of the fixative, enabling not only reduction or elimination of a gap between the bone fragments to be joined, but also appropriate compression. This system includes a multitude of identical linear modules which correspond to the diaphyseal area of the bone, as well as a multitude of nonlinear modules with different dimensions corresponding to the epiphyseal areas of the bone. These modules can be manufactured in shapes and dimensions compatible with the area of the bone undergoing surgical intervention. They have a particular type of shape which allows for an initial coupling by translation, the final coupling and fracture compacting being aided by memory shape staples. The shape and the dimension of the plates can be adjusted to fit any bone type and fracture location, allowing the surgeon to improve the alignment of the fractured bones and the distance between them.
Modular plates have the task of fixing and stabilizing the fracture centre and can be mounted on the bones via a well established procedure. The surgeon must: 1) select the appropriate module, 2) reduce the fracture fragments; 3) secure the plate modules onto the two fragments on either side of the fracture with screws and 4) compact the fracture by coupling the modules using memory shape elements. The modules are made from biocompatible materials with adequate mechanical properties (titanium and titanium alloys, cobalt, stainless steel, ceramic materials). The plate axis coincides with the bone axis. The length and/or width of the modules can be different from one application to another. Generally, the modules are linear, for using on the diaphyseal portion of long bones, but they can also be nonlinear for the bone heads, being configured and dimensioned in a nonlinear shape which best suites the epiphyseal bone areas. These nonlinear modules have a transversal portion of corresponding shape and dimensions and an axial portion to ensure the attachment with a linear module to the diaphyseal portion of the bone.

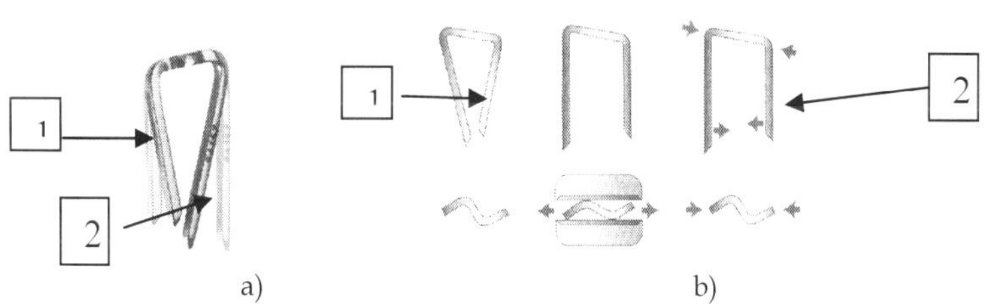

Fig. 13. The schema process of staple shape transformation: a) the two positions of the staple: 1)-initial and 2)-final; b) the transition process from the austenitic stage 1) (high temperature) to the martensitic stage 2) (low temperature)

The U-shaped staple has two straight sides and a middle "active" section pre-deformed by tensile stress. The connection of the modules is made by inserting the staple pins in their open form (at low temperature, in the martensitic state) in the channels of the modules. After implantation, the staples return to their initial form under the influence of body heat, thus closing the space between bone fragments. The open structure is designed to stabilize and stiffen the montage and allows for a sliding motion along the longitudinal axis of the bone which coincides with the plate axis and allows for the compacting process for the two bone fragments. The schema process of staple shape memory transformation is presented in Figure 13 (www.groupe-lepine.com) Due to its pseudo-elastic property, a memory-alloy staple maintains a compressive effect ensuring a constant compressive force between the two modules and, thus, between the two bone fragments. This way, the staple forces a bone alignment very close to the normal anatomical alignment of the bone, which is highly conducive to cellular regeneration and healing. After the fracture is healed, the staple can be cooled, thus returning to its open form, allowing for an easy extraction. The modules may also be extracted easily by the surgeon.

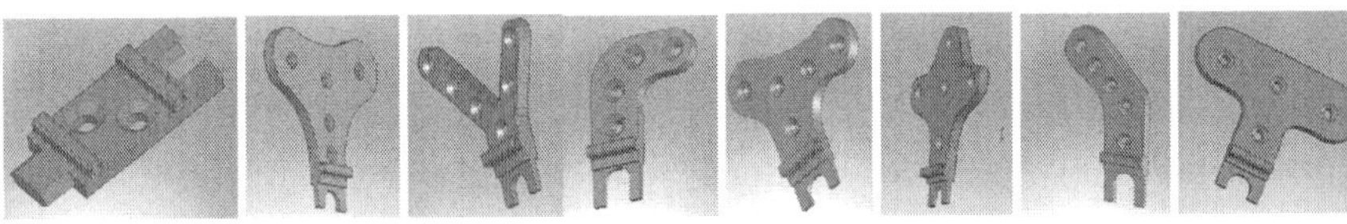

Fig. 14.Various diaphyseal and epiphyseal modules

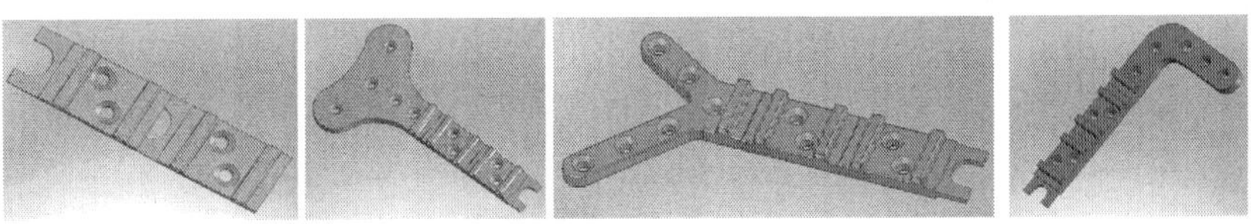

Fig. 15. Various types of modular plates for diaphyseal fractures (a) and for metaphyseal and epiphyseal fracturesa (b,c, d)

Using specialized software as VisualNastran [18-19], and the principle of the von Mises stress, the numerical simulations movies of the assembly fractured tibia-modular plate are obtained. In materials science and engineering the von Misses yield criterion (von Mises, 1913) can be formulated in the following way: a material is said to start yielding when its von Misses stress reaches a critical value known as the yield strength. The von Misses stress is used to predict yielding of materials under any loading condition from results of simple uniaxial tensile tests.

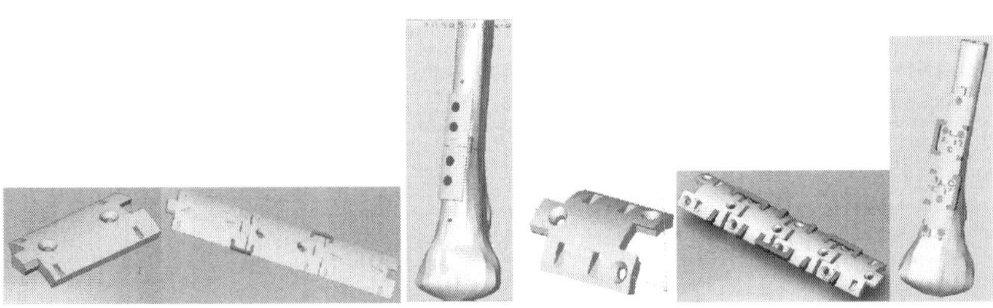

Fig. 16. Modules, plates and tibia-modular plate assembly for diaphyseal fractures

A compression force of 54 N was applied on the extremities of the staples which connects the modules. In Fig. 17 the stress maps and the displacements maps for two succesives moments of the implant assembly are presented

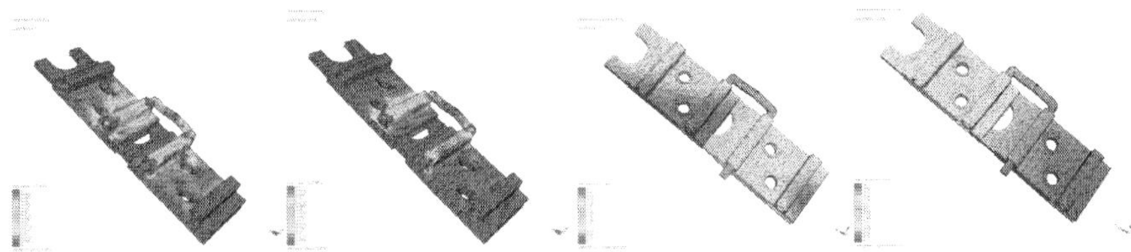

a) b)

Fig. 17. The stress (a) and displacements (b) maps for the implant assembly

In Figure 18 a)-c) are presented three different stages of the numerical simulation movie of the assembly tibia bone-virtual modular plate for each kind of diagram: von Mises stress diagram [Pa], displacements diagram [mm] and von Mises strain diagram [mm/mm]. In Fig.18 d) two stages of the von Mises stress diagram for the staple are presented. These diagrams show the variation of the values during the simulation of the staple shape transformation from the martensitic stage to the austenitic stage.

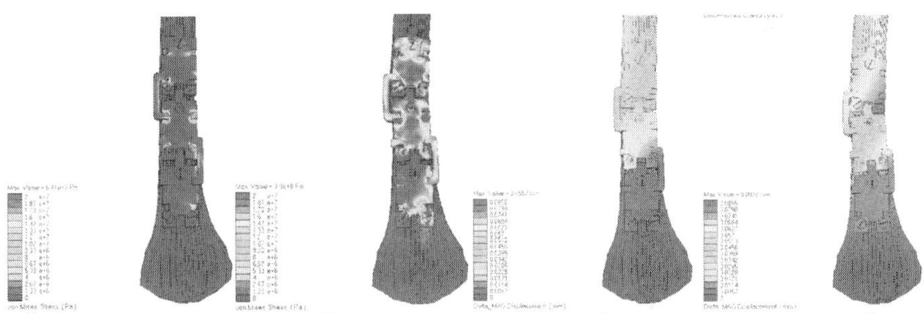

a) b) c) d)

Fig. 18. Two stages of the simulation movie: for the virtual assembly (fractured tibia and modular plate): a) the von Mises stress diagrams [Pa]; b) the displacement diagrams [mm];

The human femur osteosynthesis process using modular adaptive plates based on shape memory alloys can be numericaly simulated with the help of ANSYS software packages, following 3 steps. Used materials: Cortical bone: E=18000 MPa, Poisson's Coefficient=0,3; Spongious bone: E=50 MPa, Poisson's Coefficient=0,25; Plates: (Titanium); Fixing screws - (Titanium). The holding elements: Nitinol - simulated material in ANSYS using the material model "shape memory alloy".To highlight the use of nitinol for the holding elements it is necessary to follow three steps.

For the simulation of the nitinol elements behavior and for the study of their effects, we have considered only the surface placed in the proximity of the humeral head. The small plates were placed both ways of the longitudinal axis of the bone, proximate under its head, following the curve and dip of the bone surface geometry. There were simulated the screws for fixing the small plates and the bone. On a bone area situated on the region of the intermediate plates the bone was interrupted (on a distance of 1-2 mm), obtaining two bone segments that are about to be joined using the small plates and the nitinol holding elements. The plates are not fixed in an initial position, they can move 2 mm. The stress and displacements diagrams for bone, for plate modules and for staples, for each of the three process steps are obtained.

Step 1. The upper and lower plates are fixed with screws on the bone. It simulates the mounting of head off for holding elements on the fixed plates on the bone, the holding elements having the other head already mounted in the middle plates (common nodes). The temperature of all the elements and of the holding elements is 23^0 C. Resultant displacements in plate modules and resultant displacements in femur bone are presented.

Step 2. The ends of the nitinol elements are considered mounted in plates, considering the pretension of step 1, eliminating imposed movements, and realizing the state of tension for mounting the implant.

Step 3. Starting from the final state of tension obtained in step 2 we are simulating the increase of temperature for holding elements from room temperature to body temperature 36.5^0 C. Resultant displacements in plate modules, Von Mises stress in Nitinol staples and resultant displacements in femur bone are presented.

The use of nitinol elements makes contact pressure between the two bone segments to grow by 58%. The values of maximum tensions on the plates and on the fixing screws are placed below the limit of proportionality.

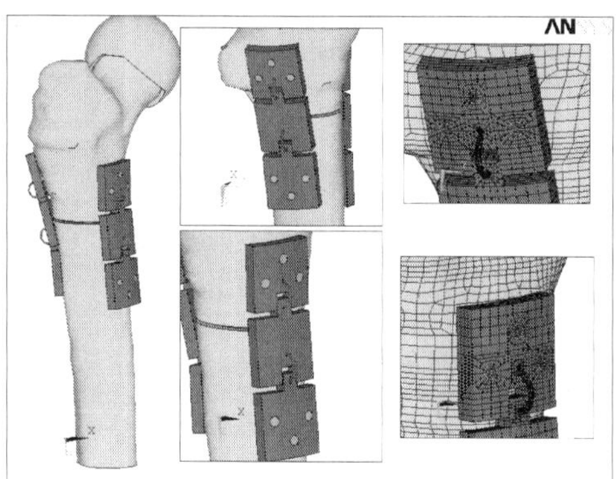

Fig. 19. The finite element model of the femur-implant assembly

Step 1

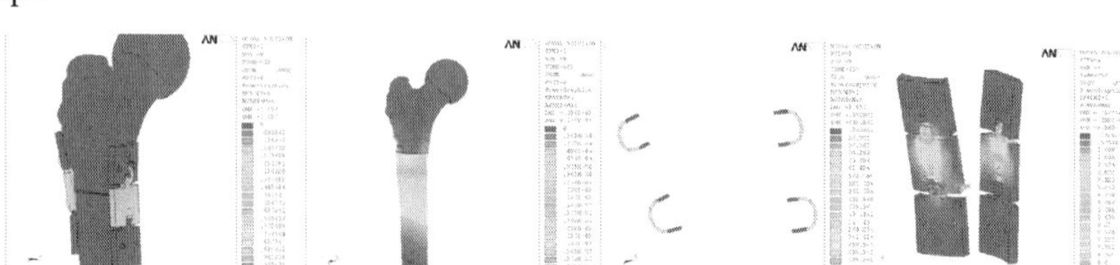

Fig. 20. Total displacements of the second module (a), total displacements for the femur (b), von Mises stress in the element (c), von Mises stress in the plates (d)

Step 2

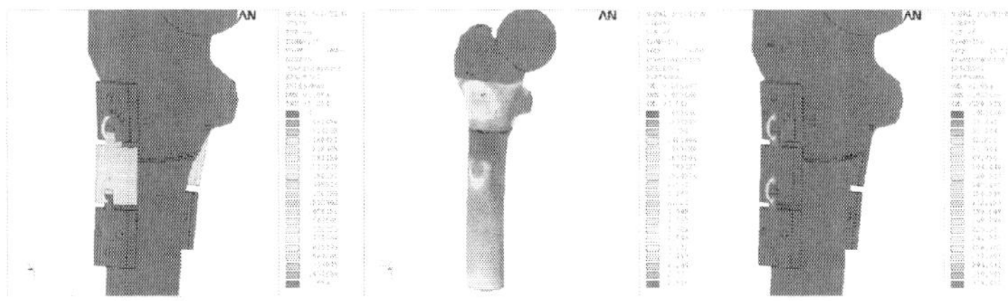

Fig. 21. Total displacements in the bone-implant assembly (a), von Mises stress in femur (b), von Mises in the element (c)

Step 3

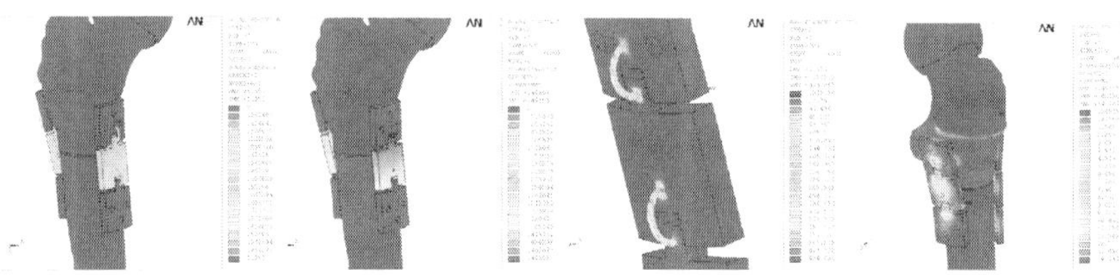

Fig. 22. Total displacements in the bone-implant assembly (a), total displacements in the plates (b), von Mises stress in the element (c) and von Mises stress in the plates (d)

4.2 Orthopaedic modular centro-medullar rods based on shape memory alloys

Centro-medullar rods can be used only for diaphyseal fracture fixation of long bones (femur, tibia, and humerus) which limit their use. They make a good centring but compaction is quite poor. When these rods are blocked by passing a proximal screw and a distal one, transversely, trough the bone and rod, it results in the cancellation of compaction forces and implicitly the delay of consolidation, with the development of pseudarthrosis.

Disadvantages of classical centro-medullar rods are that their shape and length do not adapt to the bone channel and that they allow rotation of bone fragments from fractures (the main cause of pseudarthrosis). The rods also get stuck in the medullar canal of the bone and they are difficult to extract after the reduction of the fracture centre and bone healing. If the centro-medullar rod is not well calibrated, it does not prevent rotation of bone fragments and, therefore, does not always permit a good compaction of the fragments, causing pseudoarthrosis. Also in the fracture centre, micro-movements can occur leading to fatigue of the rod's material and, implicitly, to breaking. Centro-medullar rods that have mobility can cause important degenerative-dystrophic injuries at the interface with the fracture centre.

The technical solution consists in designing and execution of a centro-medullar rod whose dimensional characteristics (length and diameter) can be adapted to the medullar canal of the bone.

The total length of the centro-medullar rod can be adjusted by simply substituting the two modules which can be adapted for different bone lengths. Also, two modules may slide partially or wholly on the part of the extreme deformation module through the grooves made on these surfaces. The central module is made of a shape memory material which, under the influence of temperature, will deform, allowing the surface of the rod to mold to the medullar canal of the bone.

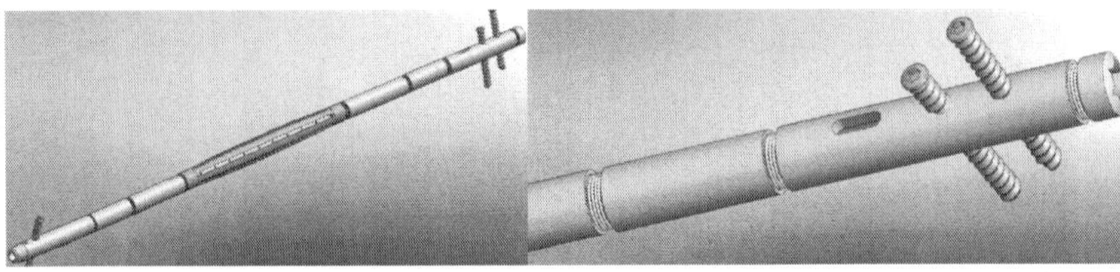

Fig. 23. The first variant of the intramedullary rod system

The second variant: the device is composed of an actuation rod 1 which inserts the steel clips 4 into the bone through the holes made in the modules 2, thus fixing the device into the medullar canal of the bone (in total, the intramedullar rod system has four steel clips). The device is based on the Nitinol module 3 which expands when the intramedullary nail is inserted into the bone (by increasing the temperature to the level of the body temperature). In addition, to better link the device to the medullar canal we use the Nitinol wires 5 which are placed on the distal segment of the device. The modules 2 can slide over the two extreme surfaces of the Nitinol module 3, thus enhancing the versatility of the device (i.e. ensuring various types and dimensions of the bone from one individual to another).

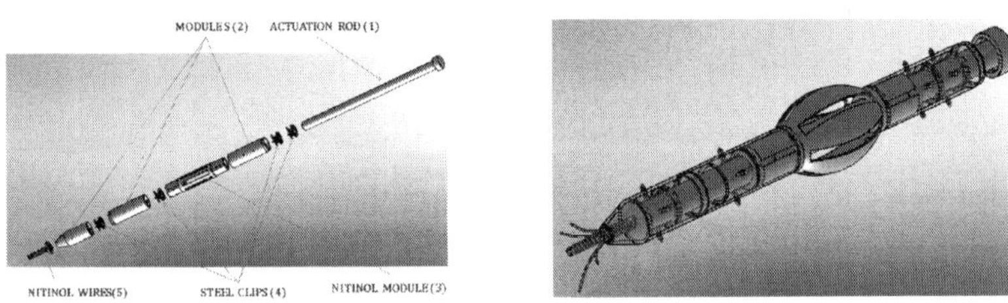

Fig. 24. An exploded view of the intramedullary rod system and the intramedullary nail system in the active state

In the passive state, the Nitinol module and wires are not activated by the rise of the temperature in the human body, the biocompatible steel clips having the legs close together. By contrast, in the active state, the Nitinol module and wires expands and the actuation rod forces the steel clips to penetrate the bone and firmly lock the intramedullary nail to the medullar channel (Fig. 24). The centro-medullar rod based on intelligent materials avoids the disadvantages of conventional centro-medullar rods aforesaid and solves their problems, in that:

- The rod is modular (composed of several components with suitable lengths and diameters which are assembled together) and adaptable to any type of shaft of long bone fracture (shape memory elements are used for a good cohesion between the centro-medullar channel and the centro-medullar rod),

- Easy to manufacture thanks to components with simple shapes, most components having two threaded surfaces which are used to assemble the next components.
- Easy to extract by cooling the shape memory material
- Provide good compaction of the bone fragments, lowering or eliminating the risk of non-union (pseudo-arthrosys);
- does not allow micro-movements between bone fragments found in fracture centre
- Motion stability is ensured by continuous inter-fragmentary compression
- Avoid the appearance of important degenerative-dystrophic lesions on the contact surface of the fracture centre.

4.3 External fixator actuated by shape memory alloys elements

In the open fractures with important coetaneous lesions (type III) using the osteosynthesis materials (plates, centro-medullar rods) is a real danger for infection. In these cases one can use the external fixator which comprises threaded rods or Kirschner brooch which are fixated in the bone fragments at a certain distance above and below the fracture centre, passing through the healthy tissue. These structures are linked externally with rods or circles. In the case of an external fixator, the resistance required to stabilize and consolidate the fracture changes in time, the initial fixation must be rigid enough in order to withstand the mechanical stress that appear once the patient can walk, without fracture disequilibrium. In the same time, the fixator rigidity has to be under certain limits in order to allow the development of pressures at the fracture centre which stimulate the callus formation. In order to obtain the highest resistance for the fixator, several requests must be fulfilled: the distance between the rod and bone to be reduced, the pins diameter to be augmented, the pins located near fracture to be close one to other, the pins thread to be totally inserted in the bone.

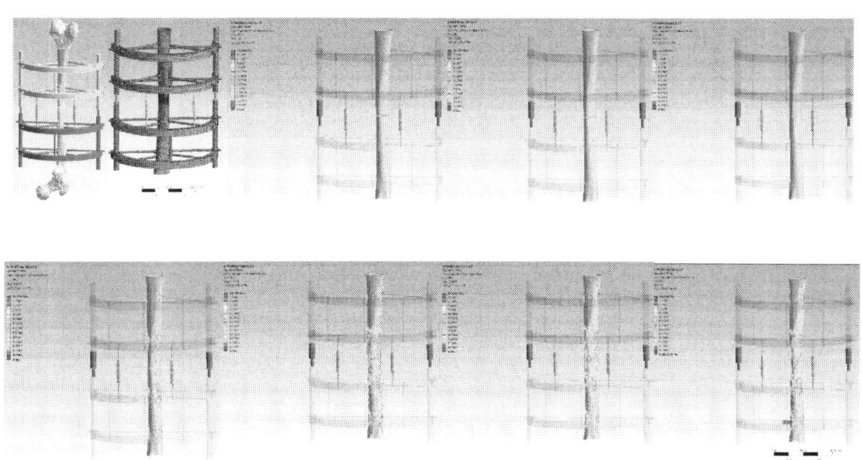

Fig. 25. Sequential frames of the femur external fixator - showing the osteosynthesis process

The management of bone fractures using an external fixator, adjustment of the bone segment is often necessary to reduce residual deformities. Proposed unilateral external retainer is composed of bone pins inserted into the proximal and distal segment, four semi-circular frames, two telescopic side rods, and two of Nitinol compression springs that are designed to compact fracture, the effect of compression on bone fragments interested. It was also simulated femoral shaft osteotomy. In addition to studies of adjustability of the retainer, this model is used to investigate the rigidity of the retainer for evaluating device performance. Transverse fracture was simulated on the axis of the femur and bone segments were modelled as rigid. Were analyzed several cases of bone fragment alignment study using ANSYS software, based on finite Elements Method. Different sequences are generated.This is an example of the need for practical study and application of clinically relevant biomechanical analysis of the results.

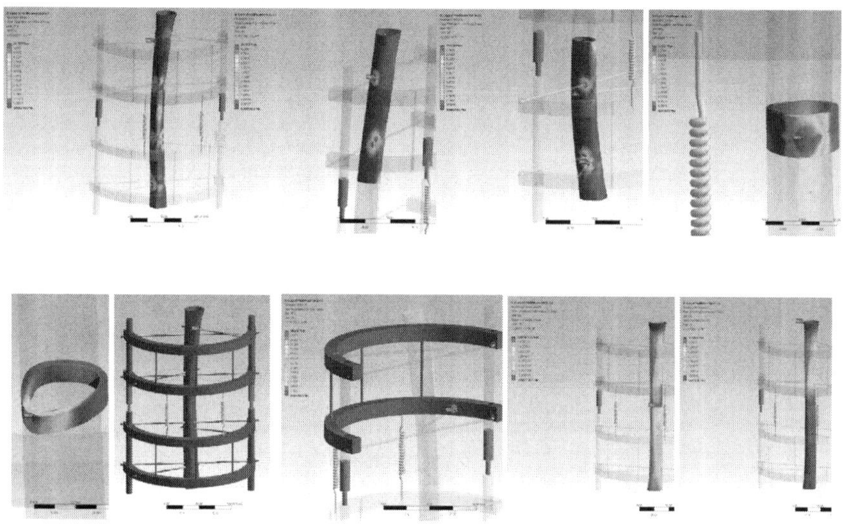

Fig. 26. Stress and deformation maps recorded in the femur-external fixator assembly, when the NiTi springs are placed towards the symmetry axis of the assembly

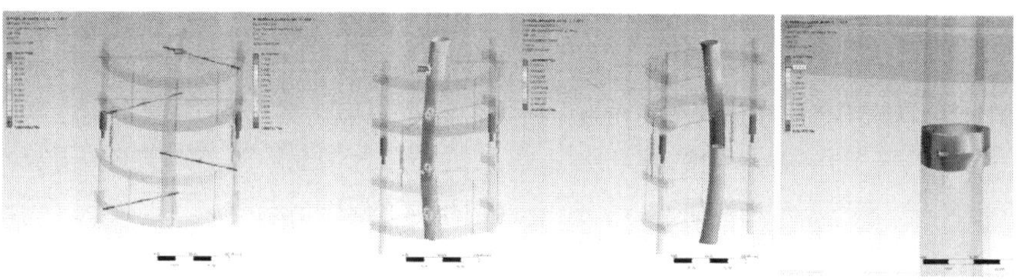

Fig. 27. Stress and deformation maps in the femur-external fixator assembly, the case when NiTi springs are placed towards the lateral rods of the fixator

4.4 Orthopaedic implants used for osteoporotic bones fractures

Osteoporosis is a disease which leads to the reduction of the bone minerals and is directly related to the age of the patient. Therefore, osteoporosis can cause fractures to the spine and to the femur extremities and, especially, to the humeral head. In comparison to the patients who have normal bone density, patients with osteoporosis can suffer fractures of the spine or long bones from low magnitude forces or minor trauma. The most frequent compression fractures of the osteoporotic spine are located at the thorax and lumbar vertebrae level. These fractures can cause acute pain of the back at the level of the fractured vertebra. Once a spinal fracture caused by osteoporosis has occurred the risk of another is increased fourfold compared to the case of non-osteoporotic patients.

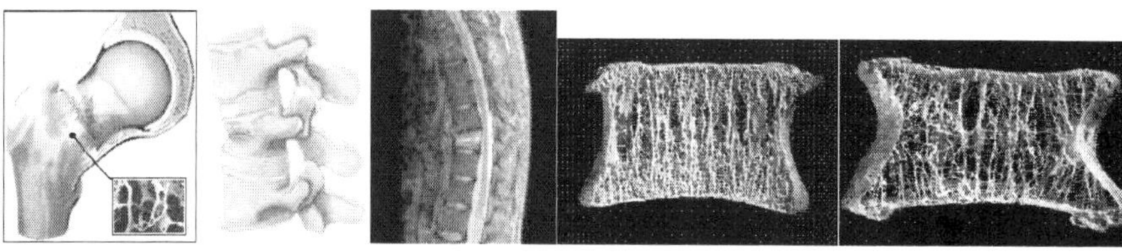

Fig. 28. The humeral head and vertebra fracture and the structure of the normal bone and osteoporotic spongy bone

The numerical simulation of osteoporosis in the case of the femoral head is based on the hypothesis according to which the effect of the osteoporosis is equivalent to the change in the mechanical characteristics of the bone, more exactly, of the osteoporotic spongy tissue. These mechanical characteristics are the longitudinal elasticity module (E) and the Poisson coefficient. In the case of the bone structure we have considered the material as orthotropic, having different values of the mechanical characteristics on the Ox, Oy and Oz axis. The purpose of this simulation is to visualize the influence of osteoporosis in the whole mass of the bone and spongy tissue in order to draw some conclusions regarding:

- the most dangerous zones in which the mechanical properties are diminished;
- the degree of osteoporosis at which the bone cannot support the loads;
- the influence of osteoporosis on the mechanical resistance of the bone.

From the presented stresses maps one can observe that the resistance of the bone and, especially, of the spongy tissue drops by 50% for a degree of osteoporosis of 15%, therefore at 20% osteoporosis the fractures of the humeral head are imminent. One can observe also that the most dangerous zone is located at the neck of the humeral head where, in fact, the fractures occur frequently.

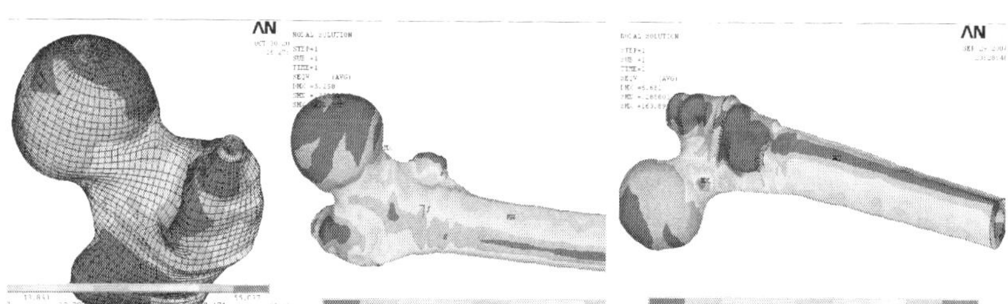

Fig. 29. Von Misses stresses for 0%, 15%, 20% osteoporotic bone

The proposed plate used for the fractures of the osteoporotic bones has two lateral legs with divergent longitudinal directions one to the other, having sharp heads and fixing devices and also a transversal arm which connects the two legs with a configuration which presents a spatial curvature, with a convex profile. The plate is designed in such a way that the lateral legs are different in shape in relation to the way the metaphisis is penetrated or to the implantation in the cortical bone. The lateral legs are united through a transversal arm by connection zones internally and externally, conveniently curved to obtain a better elasticity of the lateral legs and, more specifically, of the structure of the plate as a unit. The lateral legs have on their inner surface a series of teeth directed to the interior of the transversal arm and at the end of the inner surface of each one of the lateral legs one can observe the conical surfaces directed outwardly. This fact constrains the surgeon to augment the distance between the lateral legs during the implantation of the osteoporotic plate. The inner surface of the transversal arm presents an augmented rugosity in order to allow micro-vascularisation and, therefore, cortical callus formation. Moreover, in the case of lower limb bone osteotomy, the implant must be inserted on the longitudinal axis of the bone. In conceiving this implant we established a convex profile of the transversal arm of the plate with the same curvature as the bone. The advantage of added elasticity to the lateral legs is important because, when the human body temperature is attained, they exert compression force on the bone fragments and amplify the automatic effect of retaining the bone fragments on all fracture sides. The proposed implant for the osteoporotic bone can be perfectly implanted into the bone, offering a strong holding effect of the bone fragments on each side of the fracture line.

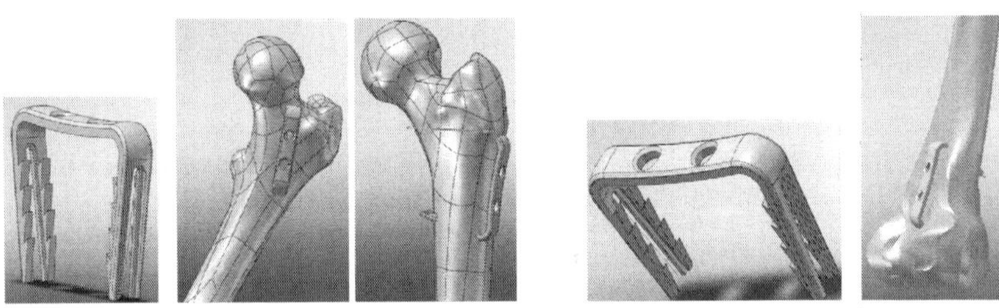

Fig. 30. The plate is implanted in the proximal epiphysis of the femur (first variant), the plate is implanted in the distal epiphysis of the femur (second variant)

4.5 Modular adaptive orthopaedic network based on shape memory alloys

The problem which this modular-adaptive implant proposal solves is that the implant ensures a modular adaptive network to the fracture due to the properties of the material from which the network is made (Nitinol), an elastic coupling and the stimulation of the rehabilitation of the bone continuity. As a function of the severity and particularity of the case, in the central area of all modules that form the network or just in the case of a small number of modules the simulative corresponding drugs can be stored. The central area can be perforated by the surgeon so the drugs can be administrated locally, in the traumatised area, the flow depending on the dimension of the penetrating needle. The smart material (for example Nitinol) that makes the modular network is characterised by superelasticty similar to the bone structures, a good image revealed by radiological investigations and a good physical and chemical compatibility which can be assimilated by an augmented resistance to the electrolytic effect of the biological environment. Due to the pseudoelastic property of shape memory alloys, even when resorption occurs between the two fragments, the implant maintains its compressive effect, which has a positive influence on fracture healing.

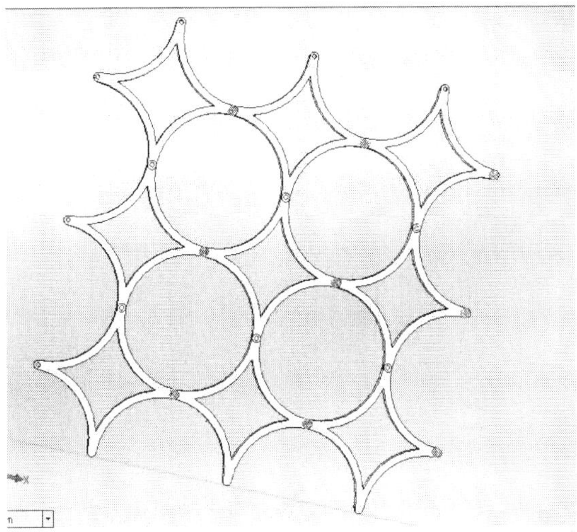

Fig. 31. The schema of the modular adaptive orthopaedic network

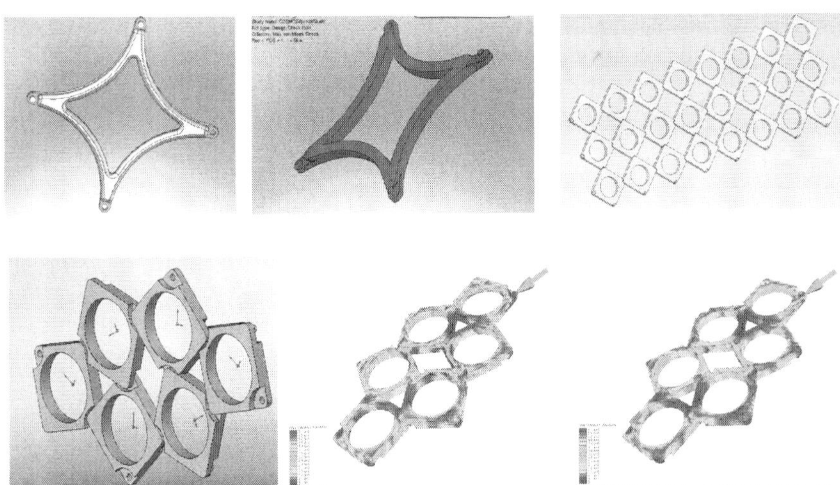

Fig. 32. For a force given by equation F=-800*sin(6.282*time) on the OX axis we present the stress maps corresponding to the network in two different moments of the dinamic load

A comparison between classical implants and proposed modular implants based on shape memory alloys is presented:

Traditional implants	Proposed implants
Big dimensions, configuration which results in the redundant bone callus	Small dimensions, completely adaptable to the fracture
Invasive surgical interventions in order to couple the implants	Minimal invasive surgical techniques are used for this types of implants - micro-incisions
Medium risk of postsurgical infections due to the surgical intervention	Minimal risk due to reduced area of surgical intervention
Neutral from the point of view of the bio-stimulation bone restoration	Bio-stimulation properties for bone growth, reduced time for healing the fracture zone
Require an important number of physical connections (holes) for implant fixation	Small number and reduced dimensions for the fixation holes (in some cases the number of holes can be zero)
The fixation problems related to classical implants can cause pseudo arthritis	Due to the constant pressure that the implants make the fracture fragments are well compacted, no micro-movements are allowed, avoiding in this way the pseudo arthritis

5. Theoretical and experimental studies for NiTi staples

5.1 Decomposition of the elasticity matrix for Nitinol structure phases

The form of the elasticity matrix contains the restrictions done by the symmetry theory of classical crystallography and it permits a simple geometrical interpretation of the relationship between stress and strain regardless of the degree on anisotropy. These restrictions are reflected in the invariant structures of the spectral decompositions. The spectral forms are determined by the symmetry groups, and are independent of the values of the elastic constants. In (Cowin & Mehrabadi, 1987, 1990) the eigenvalues and eigenvectors for anisotropic elasticity were determined. (Ting, 1987) has discussed the eigenvalue problem in connection with his study of the invariants of the elasticity tensor. The first spectral decomposition of the elasticity tensor was made in (Rychlewski & Zhang, 1989), using tensorial products. Then, (Sutcliffe, 1992) developed this method and they used it for different types of symmetries. A more simple method, using matrix 6x6 was used in (Theocaris & Philippidis, 1989) for the decomposition of the rigidity matrix of the transversal isotropic materials.
In the case of the linear-elastic materials, the dependence between the deformation matrix components and the stress matrix components can be written as a linear dependence:

$$\sigma_{ij} = \sum_{k=1}^{3}\sum_{l=1}^{3} S_{ijkl}\,\varepsilon_{kl} \tag{1}$$

This dependence can be written on the following form:

$$(\sigma) = [S](\varepsilon) \tag{2}$$

where:

$$(\varepsilon)=\begin{Bmatrix} \varepsilon_{11} \\ \varepsilon_{22} \\ \varepsilon_{33} \\ \sqrt{2}\,\varepsilon_{23} \\ \sqrt{2}\,\varepsilon_{13} \\ \sqrt{2}\,\varepsilon_{12} \end{Bmatrix};\quad (\sigma)=\begin{Bmatrix} \sigma_{11} \\ \sigma_{22} \\ \sigma_{33} \\ \sqrt{2}\,\sigma_{23} \\ \sqrt{2}\,\sigma_{13} \\ \sqrt{2}\,\sigma_{12} \end{Bmatrix} \tag{3}$$

$$[S]=\begin{bmatrix} S_{1111} & S_{1122} & S_{1133} & \sqrt{2}S_{1123} & \sqrt{2}S_{1113} & \sqrt{2}S_{1112} \\ S_{2211} & S_{2222} & S_{2233} & \sqrt{2}S_{2223} & \sqrt{2}S_{2213} & \sqrt{2}S_{2212} \\ S_{3311} & S_{3322} & S_{3333} & \sqrt{2}S_{3323} & \sqrt{2}S_{3313} & \sqrt{2}S_{3312} \\ \sqrt{2}S_{2311} & \sqrt{2}S_{2322} & \sqrt{2}S_{2333} & 2S_{2323} & 2S_{2313} & 2S_{2312} \\ \sqrt{2}S_{1311} & \sqrt{2}S_{1322} & \sqrt{2}S_{1333} & 2S_{1323} & 2S_{1313} & 2S_{1312} \\ \sqrt{2}S_{1211} & \sqrt{2}S_{1222} & \sqrt{2}S_{1233} & 2S_{1223} & 2S_{1213} & 2S_{1212} \end{bmatrix} \tag{4}$$

with:

$$S_{ijkl} = S_{jikl} = S_{ijlk} = S_{klij} \tag{5}$$

Basically, SMA presents two well-defined crystallographic phases, i.e., austenite and martensite. Martensite is a phase that is easily deformed, reaching large strains (~8%), and in the absence of stress, is stable only at low temperatures; in addition, it can be induced by either stress or temperature. The kinematics associated with the martensitic phase transformation in a single crystal is described for a cubic to tetragonal and cubic to monoclinic transformation, and the lattice invariant strain by plastic slip is discussed (Patoor et al.,2006). When the martensitic transformation takes place, numerous physical properties are modified. During the transformation, a latent heat associated with the transformation is absorbed or released based on the transformation direction. The forward, austenite-to-martensite transformation is accompanied by the release of heat corresponding to a change in the transformation enthalpy (exothermic phase transformation). The reverse, martensite-to-austenite transformation is an endothermic phase transformation accompanied by absorption of thermal energy. For a given temperature, the amount of heat is proportional to the volume fraction of the transformed material.

5.2 Symmetry cases of Nitinol crystallographic phases

We present the elasticity matrix for the crystallographic phases of Nitinol. For the trigonal crystallographic structure, the matrix [S] has the expression:

$$[S]=\begin{bmatrix} C_{11} & C_{12} & C_{13} & 0 & -\sqrt{2}C_{15} & 0 \\ C_{12} & C_{11} & C_{13} & 0 & \sqrt{2}C_{15} & 0 \\ C_{13} & C_{13} & C_{33} & 0 & 0 & 0 \\ 0 & 0 & 0 & C_{44} & 0 & 2C_{15} \\ -\sqrt{2}C_{15} & \sqrt{2}C_{15} & 0 & 0 & C_{44} & 0 \\ 0 & 0 & 0 & 2C_{15} & 0 & C_{11}-C_{12} \end{bmatrix} \tag{6}$$

In this case, the eigenvalues are:

$$\begin{aligned}
\lambda_1 &= \frac{1}{2}\left[C_{11}+C_{12}+C_{33}+\sqrt{(C_{11}+C_{12}-C_{33})^2+8C_{13}^2}\right]\\
\lambda_2 &= \frac{1}{2}\left[C_{11}+C_{12}+C_{33}-\sqrt{(C_{11}+C_{12}-C_{33})^2+8C_{13}^2}\right]\\
\lambda_3=\lambda_6 &= \frac{1}{2}\left[C_{11}-C_{12}+C_{44}+\sqrt{(C_{11}-C_{12}-C_{44})^2+16C_{15}^2}\right]\\
\lambda_4=\lambda_5 &= \frac{1}{2}\left[C_{11}-C_{12}+C_{44}-\sqrt{(C_{11}-C_{12}-C_{44})^2+16C_{15}^2}\right]
\end{aligned} \tag{7}$$

and the matrix of eigenvectors is:

$$[X]=\begin{bmatrix}
\frac{1}{\sqrt{2}}\sin\alpha & -\frac{1}{\sqrt{2}}\cos\alpha & \frac{1}{\sqrt{2}}\cos\beta & 0 & \frac{1}{\sqrt{2}}\sin\beta & 0\\
\frac{1}{\sqrt{2}}\sin\alpha & -\frac{1}{\sqrt{2}}\cos\alpha & -\frac{1}{\sqrt{2}}\cos\beta & 0 & -\frac{1}{\sqrt{2}}\sin\beta & 0\\
\cos\alpha & \sin\alpha & 0 & 0 & 0 & 0\\
0 & 0 & 0 & \cos\beta & 0 & \sin\beta\\
0 & 0 & -\sin\beta & 0 & \cos\beta & 0\\
0 & 0 & 0 & -\sin\beta & 0 & \cos\beta
\end{bmatrix} \tag{8}$$

where:

$$\sin\alpha=\frac{|\lambda_2-C_{11}-C_{12}|}{\sqrt{2C_{13}^2+(\lambda_2-C_{11}-C_{12})^2}};\ \cos\alpha=\frac{|\lambda_1-C_{11}-C_{12}|}{\sqrt{2C_{13}^2+(\lambda_1-C_{11}-C_{12})^2}};$$

$$\sin\beta=\frac{|C_{11}-C_{12}-\lambda_3|}{\sqrt{(C_{11}-C_{12}-\lambda_3)^2+4C_{15}^2}};\ \cos\beta=\frac{|C_{11}-C_{12}-\lambda_4|}{\sqrt{(C_{11}-C_{12}-\lambda_4)^2+4C_{15}^2}} \tag{9}$$

Particular cases:

a. In the case of the cubic crystallographic structure:

$$C_{12}=C_{13};\ C_{33}=C_{11};\ C_{44}=C_{11}-C_{12};\ C_{15}=0 \tag{10}$$

$$[S]=\begin{bmatrix}
C_{11} & C_{12} & C_{12} & 0 & 0 & 0\\
C_{12} & C_{11} & C_{12} & 0 & 0 & 0\\
C_{12} & C_{12} & C_{11} & 0 & 0 & 0\\
0 & 0 & 0 & C_{44} & 0 & 0\\
0 & 0 & 0 & 0 & C_{44} & 0\\
0 & 0 & 0 & 0 & 0 & C_{44}
\end{bmatrix} \tag{11}$$

The eigenvalues are:

$$\lambda_1=C_{11}+2C_{12};\ \lambda_2=\lambda_3=C_{11}-C_{12};\ \lambda_4=\lambda_5=\lambda_6=C_{44} \tag{12}$$

The matrix of eigenvectors is:

$$[X]=\begin{bmatrix} 1/\sqrt{3} & -1/\sqrt{6} & 1/\sqrt{2} & 0 & 0 & 0 \\ 1/\sqrt{3} & -1/\sqrt{6} & -1/\sqrt{2} & 0 & 0 & 0 \\ 1/\sqrt{3} & 2/\sqrt{6} & 0 & 0 & 0 & 0 \\ 0 & 0 & 0 & 1 & 0 & 0 \\ 0 & 0 & 0 & 0 & 1 & 0 \\ 0 & 0 & 0 & 0 & 0 & 1 \end{bmatrix} \qquad (13)$$

b. In the case of monoclinic crystallographic structure:

$$[S]=\begin{bmatrix} C_{11} & C_{12} & C_{13} & 0 & 0 & C_{16} \\ C_{12} & C_{22} & C_{23} & 0 & 0 & C_{26} \\ C_{13} & C_{23} & C_{33} & 0 & 0 & C_{36} \\ 0 & 0 & 0 & C_{44} & C_{45} & 0 \\ 0 & 0 & 0 & C_{45} & C_{55} & 0 \\ C_{16} & C_{26} & C_{36} & 0 & 0 & C_{66} \end{bmatrix} \qquad (14)$$

The eigenvalues are:

$$\lambda_4=\frac{1}{2}\left[C_{44}+C_{55}+\sqrt{(C_{44}+C_{55})^2+4C_{45}^2}\right];\ \lambda_5=\frac{1}{2}\left[C_{44}+C_{55}-\sqrt{(C_{44}+C_{55})^2+4C_{45}^2}\right] \qquad (15)$$

and $\lambda_1,\lambda_2,\lambda_3,\lambda_4$ are the roots of the equation:

$$\lambda^4-I_1\lambda^3+I_2\lambda^2-I_3\lambda+I_4=0 \qquad (16)$$

where I_k is the sum of the diagonal minors of k degree obtained by cutting the fourth and the fifth columns and rows in matrix [S].

c. In the case of orthorhombic crystallographic structure:

$$[S]=\begin{bmatrix} C_{11} & C_{12} & C_{13} & 0 & 0 & 0 \\ C_{12} & C_{22} & C_{23} & 0 & 0 & 0 \\ C_{13} & C_{23} & C_{33} & 0 & 0 & 0 \\ 0 & 0 & 0 & C_{44} & 0 & 0 \\ 0 & 0 & 0 & 0 & C_{55} & 0 \\ 0 & 0 & 0 & 0 & 0 & C_{66} \end{bmatrix} \qquad (17)$$

The eigenvalues are:

$$\lambda_4=C_{44};\ \lambda_5=C_{55};\ \lambda_6=C_{66} \qquad (18)$$

and $\lambda_1,\lambda_2,\lambda_3$ are the roots of the equation:

$$\lambda^3-I_1^{'}\lambda^2+I_2^{'}\lambda-I_3^{'}=0 \qquad (19)$$

where $I_k^{'}$ is the sum of the diagonal minors of k degree obtained by cutting the last three columns and rows in matrix [S].
We can conclude that the eigenvalues depend on the values of the elastic constants, but the eigenvectors are, in part, independent of the values of the elastic constants

5.3 The analytical expression for the staple compression force

The stress vector can be written:

$$(\sigma)=\sum_i(\sigma_i)=\sum[E_i]\cdot(\sigma) \tag{20}$$

Therefore, the specific deformation energy is:

$$U=\frac{1}{2}\cdot\sum_{(i)}\frac{1}{\lambda_i}\cdot(\sigma_i)^t\cdot(\sigma_i) \tag{21}$$

The orthopedic staple can be modeled as a bar which has an initial shape. When temperature increases the staple suffers deformations, changing its shape. Taking into account mechanical considerations, the deformation can be accepted as being caused by an exterior force which is applied to the free extremity. Thus, an increase of temperature, ΔT produces a displacement of the free extremity, Δw. The same displacement can be produced by a force (ΔP) which is applied in the free extremity. In fact, the force (ΔP) is a force to be applied in the free extremity. The total deformation energy is:

$$U=\frac{1}{2}\cdot\sum_{(i)}\frac{1}{\lambda_i}\cdot\iiint_{(D)}(\sigma_i)^t\cdot(\sigma_i)\cdot dv \tag{22}$$

According to the Castigliano theorem energy, the derived strains of an elastic body compared with force value ΔP are similar to the displacement projection of the application point of the direction force (fig.1).

$$\Delta w=\frac{\partial U}{\partial(\Delta P)} \tag{23}$$

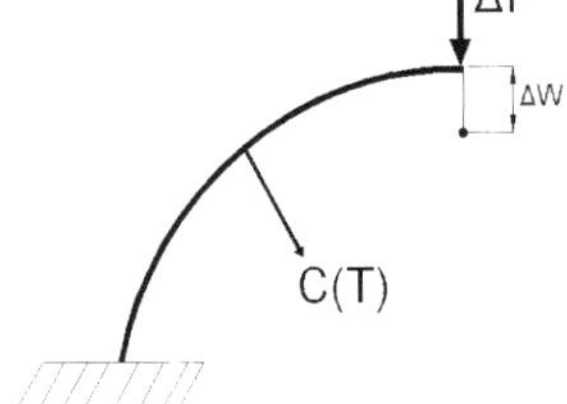

Fig. 35. The loading schema for the Nitinol staple

In the case of small deformations we can accept that the stresses developed in the staple are proportional to the variation force ΔP. In these conditions, we can write:

$$\Delta w = \Delta P \cdot \sum_{(i)} \frac{1}{\lambda_i} \cdot \iiint_{(D)} (e_i)^t \cdot (e_i) \cdot dv \tag{24}$$

where:

$$(e_i) = \frac{\partial(\sigma_i)}{\partial(\Delta P)} \tag{25}$$

The vectors (e_i) depend only on the staple shape. We call J_i the triple integrals which occur in the relation (24) depend on the temperature, but in a measure much smaller than the eigenvalues. Therefore the intégrals can be considered constants. In this case, by passing to the limit, the relation becomes:

$$\dot{w} = \dot{P} \cdot \sum_{(i)} \frac{1}{\lambda_i} \cdot J_i \tag{26}$$

The temperature variation on time is:

$$T = T_e - (T_e - T_i) \cdot e^{-c \cdot (t - t_i)} \tag{27}$$

T_i = initially temperature of staple; t_i = initially value of time; c = a coefficient which depends on the material thermal conductivity of the staple.
The eigenvalues λ_i of the elasticity matrix depend on the temperature and on the value $e^{-c(t-t_i)}$. Experimentally, it is demonstrated that the staple deformation is produced with constant speed. In (Kul'kova et al., 1995) were tested three Nitinol wire specimens: a commercially available superelastic (W_1) wire and two shape memory. It is demonstrated that the dependence of recovery force function on temperature is linear.

Developing in factors series as a function of term $e^{-c(t-t_i)}$ the functions of the proper values and keeping only the first order term, the variation in time of the compression force exerted by the staple is done by:

$$P = P_i + \frac{1}{c} \cdot f(T_e; T_i) \cdot \left(1 - e^{-c(t-t_i)}\right) \tag{28}$$

where: P_i is the exerted force at the initial moment t_i.

5.4 Experimental studies for the Nitinol staple

In order to determine the law of variation for the compression force which can be developed by the Nitinol staple as a function of variable environmental temperature and also to validate the compression potential of the staple through constant pressure at the temperature of the human body, we developed an experimental stand (Fig.36).
The experimental stand is made from: -experimental device used to mount the modular adaptive implant; -Spider 8 – a numerical acquisition system, 12 bits resolution, used to measure mechanical parameters, such as: forces, mechanical stresses, pressures, accelerations, velocities, displacements, temperatures.; -S2-100N force transducer, 0.1% linearity, Hottinger type; -FLIR B200 termographic camera; -IBM ThinkPad R5 notebook.

The Nitinol staple was stored for 15 minutes in NaCl liquid solution, 30% concentration, at -20^{0}C in a freezer. At this temperature the material of the staple enters in martensitic phase and the lateral pins of the staple are parallel.

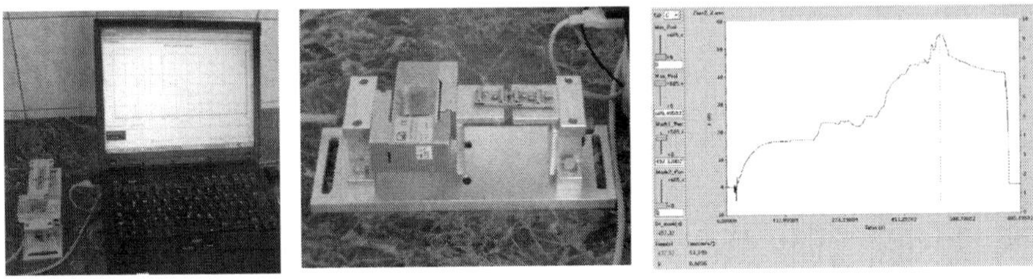

Fig. 36. The experimental stand and the diagram obtained for the staple compression force function on time

Having this shape, the staple was extracted from the NaCl solution and was easily inserted in special channels of the two implant modules fixed in the device. The staple was then left to attain room temperature (29^{0}C), thereby compressing the two modules. Afterwards, a jet of hot air was blown onto the staple increasing his temperature in different stages: first, to 31^{0}C, in a time period of 120 sec, then, to 35^{0}C in a time period of 120 sec and, finally, to 37^{0}C, the temperature of the human body. The hot air jet was then stopped and after the staple returned to room temperature it was extracted from the modular implant. Finally, we obtained the force-time diagram (Fig.36). One can observe a maxim value of 54 N which corresponds to 37^{0}C temperature for which the material of the staple entered in the cubic austenite phase. In order to correlate the staple deformation with the developed compression force, the temperature increase has been controlled with the aid of a termographical camera ThermaCam Flir B200. Afterwards, these pictures have been processed and analysed (Fig.37).

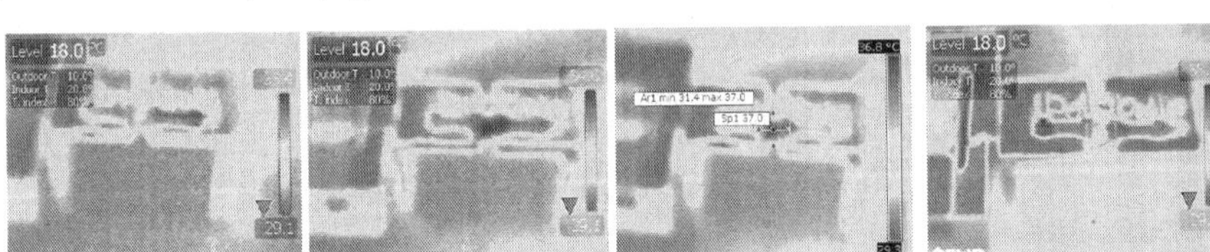

Fig. 37. A few successive images taken with Thermacam

Using the SIMI Motion software, the kinematical parameters of the both extremities of the staple were obtained. In order to link the action mode of the staple and the displacements of the extremity points of the pins during the shape transformation process from the martensitic stage to the austenitic stage, a SIMI Motion acquisition data system was used to obtain the kinematical parameters of the staple. The acquisition data system is composed of: -specialized software; -a Lenovo laptop; -two Sony video cameras (60 frames/sec); -markers.

The main stages of video capture analysis using SimiMotion software are:Camera calibration. 2. Definition of the studied points. 3. Settlement of the points connections. 4. Tracking the points. 5. Extraction of the results.

By attaching markers, the software automatically generates the equivalent model of the studied system and tracks the displacement of the markers in real time from each frame captured by the video camera, recording and analyzing the positions of the markers which allow us to obtain the motion law. The analysis procedure is based on the attachment of two markers which have been applied on the extremities of the two pins of the staple. A plane was chosen to calibrate the camera, plane given by two axes (OX and OY).
Two successive positions of staple deformation process are presented in Fig.38. In the same figure, the displacement diagram [mm], as functions of time, for the left point is presented. One can be observed that the dependence displacement-time is linear. This observation was used for the determination of the compression force theoretical expression.

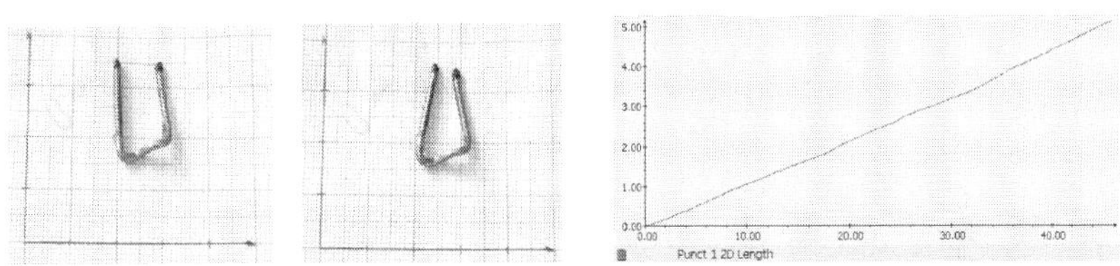

Fig. 38. Two successive positions of staple deformation process and the displacement diagram for the left extremity of the staple

We consider that the staple finishes its deformation when the difference between its temperature and room temperature is $\leq 1^{0}C$. In this hypothesis, the coefficient c can be determined with the relation:

$$c = \frac{\ln(T_e - T_i)}{\Delta t} \tag{29}$$

where Δt is the staple deformation time.
Experimentally, we can see that Δt =45sec, corresponding to the interval [-20; 29] ^{0}C of temperature variation (Fig.11). In this case, the resulted value for c is 0,086sec^{-1}. This value corresponds to the studied staple, so, taking into account the concrete experimental conditions, it is a constant for this product. Any other product made from Nitinol will have other value for c. The experimental diagram presented in fig.4 shows the stages of the compression force variation corresponding to the stages of the temperature variation (Table 1).

Temperature variation (^{o}C)	Compression force variation (N)	Values for $f(T_e-T_i)$ (N)
-20.....29	0.....17	f(29;-20)=17
29......31	17....24	f(31;29) = 7
31......35	24....44	f(35;31)=20
35......37	44....54	f(37;35)=10

Table 1. Experimental compression force values

Using the values for $f(T_e-T_i)$ as input data in the relation (50), we made a numerical simulation in Maple12 and we obtained the graphic presented in Fig.12. For the numerical simulation, we respected the same temperature increasing stages as in the experimental case. This explains the allure of the numerical graphic. For first temperature increase, from -20^{0}C to 29^{0}C, the force variation is nonlinear, and for the other three stages we observe that the force increasing is less than 10 N for a temperature increasing with 2^{0}C, the force variation is linear. For constant temperatures, the force remains constant. The diagram force-displacement proves the maximum of the compression force (54 N) is obtained in the Nitinol staple at the body temperature, 37^{0}C. This properties of the Nitinol staple allows its using in orthopedic applications, like simple orthopedic implants, or adaptive modular implants.

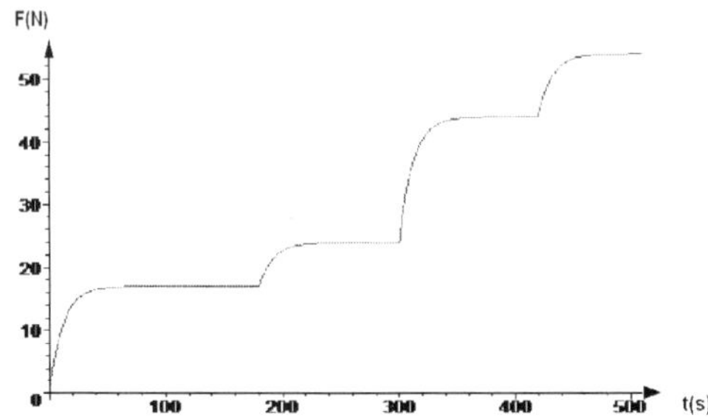

Fig. 39. The compression force-time numerical graphic

5.5 Electrochemical study on corrosion resistance of Nitinol in physiological media

The metal materials used as implants must be biocompatible. Biocompatibility means absence of corrosion or allergic reactions. Corrosion is one of the most important processes that affect the functionality and the duration of medical devices made of metals and their alloys used as implants. The failures of the implants were due to significant phenomena of localised corrosion. Corrosion as a test of biocompatibility is a very important factor, which produces metal ions in the biological medium and leads to the degradation of implants. There have been made electrochemical studies "in vitro" in order to determine the corrosion reactions, which are necessary for foreseeing the behaviour of the materials used in implantology. The degradation of metals and alloys in the human body is a combination of effects due to corrosion and mechanical activities. The surface roughness, texture and localized corrosion resistance are the most important characteristics for stabilizing tissue-implant interface. Although several studies have demonstrated the good corrosion resistance and biocompatibility of NiTi, the high nickel content of the alloy (55 weight % Ni) and its possible dissolution by corrosion still remains a concern (Ryhänen et al., 1997; Shabalovskaya, 1996; Venugopalan & Trepanier, 2000; Wever et al., 1998). Tissues in the human body contain water, dissolved oxygen, proteins and various ions, such as chloride and hydroxide, and they present an aggressive environment to metals or alloys used for implantation (Shrier et al., 1995). Corrosion resistance of a metallic implant is thus an important aspect of its biocompatibility (Black, 1992). In addition to the release of ions in the physiological environment, the corrosion process will also result in the deterioration of dimensional parameters of the corroding body (Fontana, 1986). NiTi corrosion behaviour can be significantly improved after specific surface treatments such as electropolishing (Trepanier et al., 1998). In this study the behaviour of Nitinol in physiological serum (PS) and glucose is discussed according to electrochemical measurements and microscopic images (Samide et al., 2008), which were obtained for the material before and after corrosion tests.

5.6 Experimental stand

The Nitinol used had the following composition (weight %): Ni 49,6% and Ti 50,4%.The samples were degreased with acetone and dried. Physiological serum (PS - 0.9 % NaCl) and 5 % glucose were used as the corrosion tests solutions. For the polarization study, a standard corrosion cell with a working electrode made of Nitinol wire with an active surface of 0.314 cm^2 was used. The Ag/AgCl electrode was used as a reference electrode. The auxiliary electrode was a platinum electrode (surface area-1 cm^2). The potentiodinamic polarization was conducted with a scan rate of 20 mVs^{-1}, in an electrochemical system, VoltaLab 40, with a personal computer and VoltaMaster 4 software (Figurel). The immersion time of the plates in the respective media was 4 minutes in open circuit, at room temperature. The morphology of the Nitinol surface before and after treatment in the above mentioned solutions was examined using a metallographic microscope Euromex, with Canon camera and included software (Figure 40).

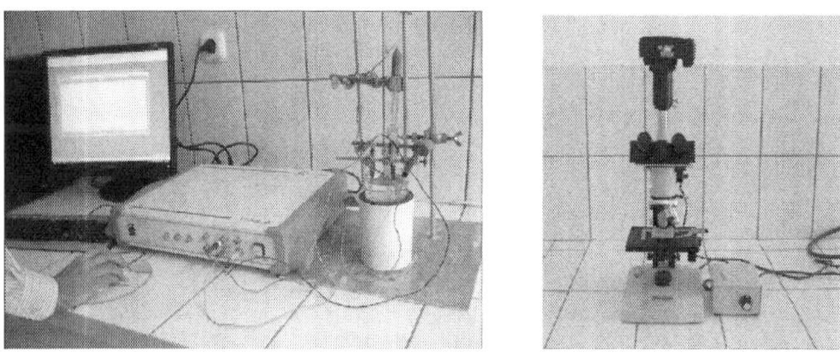

Fig. 40. Electrochemical assembly used for corrosion tests and the metallographic microscope type EUROMEX

5.7 Electrochemical measurements

Potentiodinamic curves

The polarization curves of nitinol wire obtained in physiological serum (PS) and glucose are presented in Fig41.

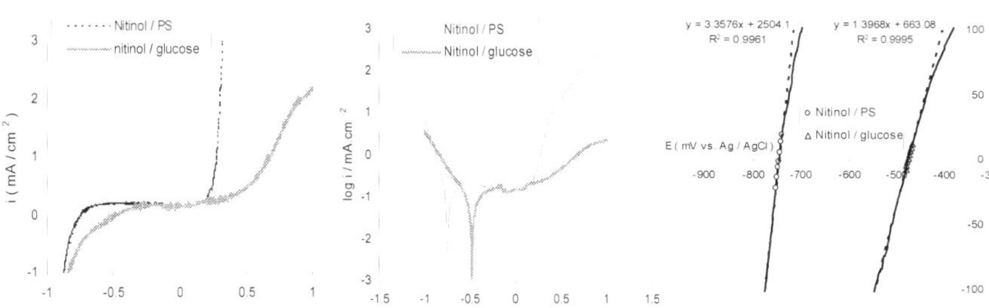

Fig. 41. Polarization curves of Nitinol wire obtained in physiological serum and glucose, after immersion time in open circuit of 2 minutes, at room temperature; Tafel diagram for Nitinol staple corroded in physiological serum and glucose; Polarization resistance (R_p) of Nitinol wire corroded in physiological serum and glucose

The study of the response Nitinol given by polarizing in physiological serum (PS) and glucose solutions, simulating the tissue fluid conditions indicate that the critical potential in pitting (E_{cp}) are shifted to a higher value, when corrosion study of Nitinol in glucose carried out. It has also been observed that the critical potential in pitting decrease from 504 mV in glucose to 246 mV in physiological serum (Table 2).

Medium	E_{cp} *(mV/Ag/AgCl)*	E_{corr} *(mV/Ag/AgCl)*	i_{corr} *(μA cm^{-2})*	R_p *(Ω. cm^{-2})*
Physiological serum	246	-746	2.3	297
Glucose	504	-474	0.94	716

Table 2. Electrochemical parameters obtained for NiTi corroded in physiological serum and glucose, at room temperature

This suggests that glucose acts by adsorption at site on the metal surface and it was formed, more adherent and more uniform passive layer than in physiological serum.

Tafel polarization. In Tafel domain, the polarization curves were performed in the potential range -1000mV to 1000 mV, with a scan rate of 20 mV/sec. The polarization curves obtained after 2 minutes of immersion are presented in Figure 4. The performed tests showed that:

- glucose leads to a corrosion *(E_{corr})* potential shifted to more positive values;
- the corrosion potential shifted to more positive values is correlate with a significant corrosion current *(i_{corr})* decrease;
- glucose solution disturbs significantly cathodic reaction and reduces the anodic reaction in a considerable manner;
- the electrochemical parameters presented in table 1 were calculated using VoltaMaster4 software at smoothing 9, calculi zone 1800 and segment 600 mV.

Polarization resistance method-Stern Method. The polarization curves obtained in the potential ranges near to corrosion potentials were recorded with a scan rate of 10 mV s^{-1}. The linearization was accomplished in the domain of over-voltages values ± 10 mV (Figure 5). The slopes $(di/dE)_{E\to Ecorr}$ of the lines from Figure 5 represent the polarization conductance. Polarization resistance (R_p -k Ω cm^2) was calculated using relation 1.

$$\left(\frac{di}{dE}\right)_{E\to E_{corr}} = \frac{1}{R_p} \tag{30}$$

The values of polarization resistance *(R_p)* increase in glucose, reaching a value of 716 Ω cm^2. The numerical values of the electrochemical parameters on behavior of Nitinol in PS and in glucose were calculated using VoltaMaster 4 software with an error of ±1.5 %, and are presented in Table 1.

Surface morfology. The electrochemically-corroded Nitinol samples in PS, glucose and aminosteril were also tested using the microscopic images, which indicate the formation of a superficial film providing a passivation on the corroded electrode in these solutions. The microscopic images of Nitinol surface before corrosion (Figure 42a) and after taking place the corrosive processes in PS (Figure 42b) and in glucose (Figure 42c) are presented.

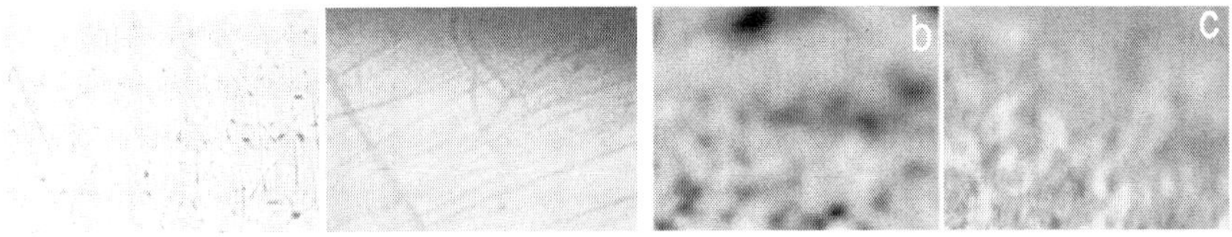

a) b) c)

Fig. 42. Microscopic images of the Nitinol surface: a) - before corrosion; b - after corrosion in physiological serum; c - after corrosion in glucose;

Un-corroded sample did not show any particular feature in microscopic imaging than small defects (Figure 6a). The results of microscopy for corroded sample in physiological serum, showed evidence of corrosion pits, and the formation of an un-continuous film on the Nitinol surface was observed. (Figure 42b). In the presence of glucose the micrograph showed no evidence of corrosion pits, but the formation of a more uniform film on the Niti surface was observed (Figure 42c). We can conclude that while correlating the data obtained by the used electrochemical methods it has been observed that the used physiological serum has a quite high corrosive action. It has also been observed that the potential of corrosion in pitting decrease from 504 mV in glucose to 246 mV in physiological serum. All the experimental data obtained show that the physiological serum has a more pronounced corrosive character as compared to a simple solution of 5% glucose. The results of microscopy for corroded sample in physiological serum, showed evidence of corrosion pits, and the formation of an un-continuous film on the Niti surface was observed. In the presence of glucose the micrograph showed no evidence of corrosion pits, but the formation of a more uniform film on the Nitinol surface was observed.

5.8 Experiment with NiTi springs used to actuate an external fixator device

The experiment aims to simulate "in vitro" bone fracture osteosynthesis, which is based on the Nitinol spring actuators and the laws of variation of heating temperature of the Nitinol actuators commuting a mobile bone fragment of a larger fixed bone fragment. This was done by mounting the two Nitinol actuators (like springs) in two cylindrical enclosures equipped with two channels that can slide alonga length determined by the two bolts used to fasten the bone fragments. One of the enclosures is provided with a rectangular cut that serves to mount the temperature sensor.
Materials used:

1. Two Nitinol springs (www.memory-metalle.de)
2. Temperature Sensor TMP 02 (www.sparfun.com)
3. Sharp IR proximity sensor GP2D120XJ00F (www.sparkfun.com)
4. FSR type force sensor (www.interlinkelec.com)
5. PCI data acquisition and control Mega Arduino 2560 (www.arduino.cc)
6. PCI data acquisition and control with Arduino Duemilanove (www.arduino.cc)
7. DFRobot Relay Shield (ww.dfrobot.com)
8. Power supply AC/DC 220/5V, 30 A.

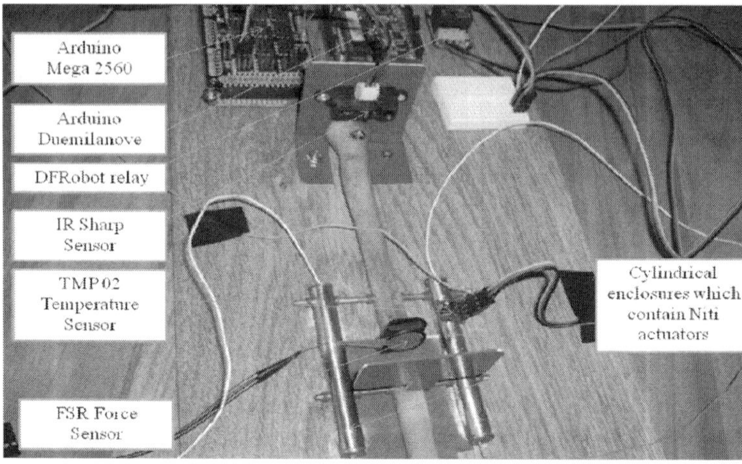

Fig. 43. The experimental layout used to measure the temperature and compression force generated by the Nitinol actuators which can be used in an external fixator device

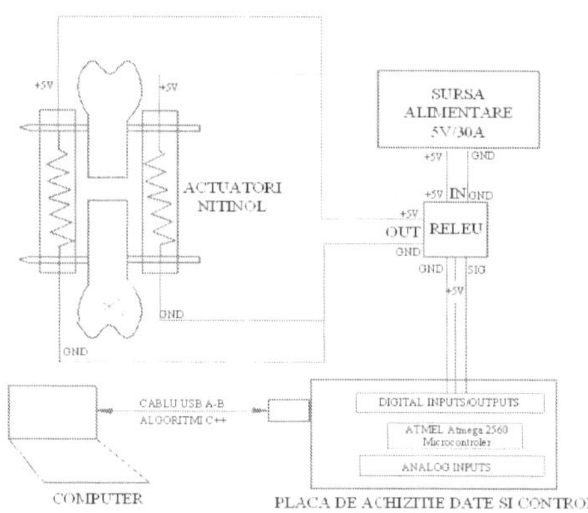

Fig. 44. The actuation scheme used in the experiment

The board data acquisition and control Arduino Mega2560 is designed to collect information from temperature, displacement and force sensors and to return the information on a computer screen, where it can be stored and later processed to obtain graphs and charts characterizing the physical process. The Arduino board is programmed with code written in C/C++ and communicate with the computer via serial interface. The Arduino Duemilanove board also is loaded with a program, written in C/C++, which establishes the time interval for opening (actuator of Nitinol are supplied from the power source) or closing (power supply interruption, springs of Nitinol are allowed to cool) the DFRobot relay. The results are shown in Fig.45

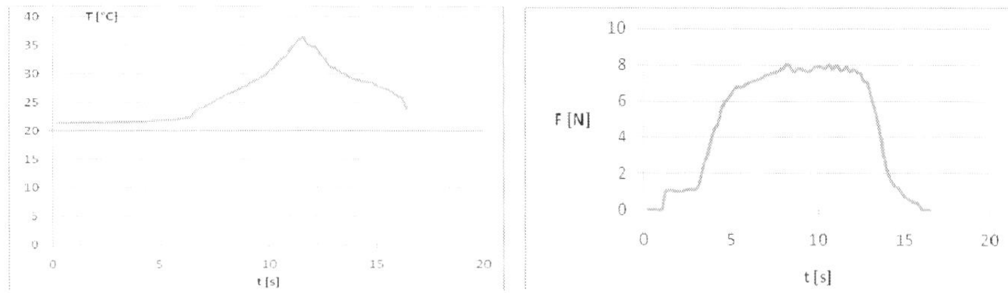

Fig. 45. The evolution of the temperature and bone compression force in time

5.9 In vitro experiment on the cadaver

We carried out experiments on the humerus bone of a cadaver.

The surgical technique is the following: One of the module was positioned on the proximal fragment. Using the drilling machine and the spiral, two channels in the cortical were made. Afterwards, two screws were mounted into the channels, making an assembly through which the implant was fixed to the bone. A similar approach involved the distal fragment of the bone. The second implant was positioned on the bone so it could be coupled with the first implant and, at the same time, to allow the longitudinal sliding of the two implants and of the two sectioned bones by 2 mm.

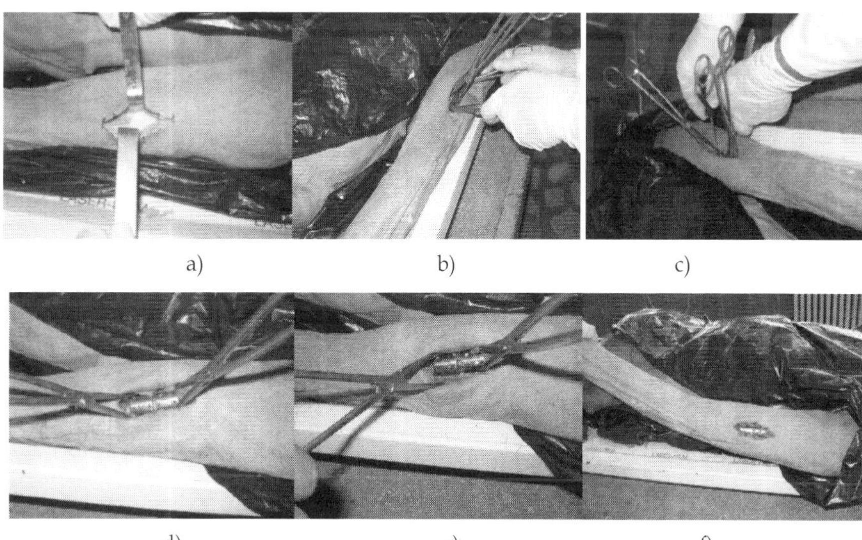

Fig. 46. Main stages of the surgical experiment on the humerus bone of a cadaver: a) establishing the fracture zone on the cadaver humerus; b) the skin is cut; c) the mounting of the modules; d) the initial coupling of the modules; d) the modules are coupled by two staples; f) the final assembly, before the skin closing.

After the second implant was mounted by means of the two screws, the implants were coupled by means of the Nitinol staple, which was previously cooled to -20^{0}C in a NaCl liquid solution kept in a refrigerator. By cooling, the staple is opened and driven into each of the two mounted modules. As the staple warms (possibly just upon heating to body temperature) the pins return to their original shape, pulling the fracture together, determining the translation of the modules and the separated parts of bone are compressed, reducing the risks of wrong orientation or additional bones callus. Main stages of the surgical experiment on the humerus bone of a cadaver are presented in Fig.46.

6. Acknowledgment

This work was supported by the funds of Ideas_92 Research Grant

7. References

Black, J. (1992). Biological performance of materials:fundamentals of biocompatibility. 2nd edn. New York: Marcel Decker, 1992: 38–60

Cowin, S.C. & Mehrabadi, M.M.(1987), "On the Identification of Material Symmetry for Anisotropic Elastic Materials", Quarterly Journal of Mechanics and Applied Mathematics, Vol.40, Part 4, pp. 451-476.

Cowin, S.C. & Mehrabadi, M.M. (1990), 'Eigentensors of Linear Anisotropic Elastic Materials", Quarterly Journal of Mechanics and Applied Mathematics, Vol.43, pp. 15-41.

Duerig, T.W.; Pelton, A.R. & Stockel, D. (1999). An overview of Nitinol medical applications, Materials Science and Engineering A, pp. 273-275,149

Farouk, O.; Krettek, C., Miclau, T. et al. (1999). Minimally Invasive Plate Osteosynthesis: Does Percutaneous Plating Disrupt Femoral Blood Supply Less Than the Traditional Technique?, Journal of Orthopaedic Trauma: 1999;13:401-06

Fontana, M.G. (1986). Corrosion engineering: modern theory and applications. 3rd edn. New York: McGraw-Hill, 1986: 445–502

Friend, C.M. & Morgan, N.B. (1999). Medical applications for Shape-Memory Alloys (SMA), Professional Engineering Publishing Ltd., UK, 1999

Gray's anatomy of the human body, twentieth edition, revised and re-edited by Warren h.Lewis, Newyork: bartleby.com, 2000

Gupta, S. & Manohar, C.S. (2005) Probability distribution of extremes of von mises stress in randomly vibrating structures, *Journal of Vibration and Acoustics Copyright*, 2005,Vol.127,547

Heim, U. & Pfeiffer, K.M. (1988) Internal fixation of small fractures, 3rd Ed. Berlin, Springer-Verlag, 1988:151-160

Hu, K.Z.; Zhang, X.L., Wang, C.T. et al. (2009). The contour of cementless femoral stem has minor effect on initial periprosthetic von Mises stress distribution. *A 3-dimensional finite element Saudi Medical Journal*, 2009;30:947-951

Jubel, A.; Andermahr, J., Bergmann, H. et al. (2003). Elastic stable intramedullary nailing of midclavicular fractures in athletes, Br J Sports Med 2003;37:480–484

Kregor, P.J.; Stannard, J., Zlowodzki, M. et al. (2001). Distal femoral fracture ixation utilizing the Less Invasive Stabilization System: The technique and early results, 2001,32, Supplement 3, Pages 32-47

Kapanen, A.; Ilvesaro, J., Danilov, A. et al. (2002). Behaviour of Nitinol in osteoblast-like ROS-17 cell cultures, Biomaterials, 2002;23:645-650

Karahan, O. & Bingul, Z., Robotics, Automation and Mechatronics, 2008 IEEE Conference, 2008;21-24:78-83

Kul'kova, S.E.; Beketov, K.A., Egorushkin,V.E. & Muryzhnikova, O.N. (1995), J. Phys. IV 5

Mantovani, D. (2000). Shape memory alloys: Properties and biomedical applications. Journal of the Minerals, Metals and Materials Society, 2000; 52:36-44

Mei, F.; Ren, X. & Wang, W.T. (1997). The biomechanical effect and clinical application of a Ni-Ti shape memory expansion clamp, Spine 1997, 22, 2083

Muller, M.E.; Nazarian, S., Koch, J. & Schatzker, J. Fractures classification. AO classification of the long bones fractures, Edition in Rom. language from Tomoaia, Gh., Edit. Risoprint, Cluj Napoca, 2006

Musialek, J.; Filip, P. & Nieslanik, J. (1998). Titanium-nickel shape memory clamps in small bone surgery, Arch Orthop Trauma Surg 117:341–344.

Patoor, E.; Lagoudas, D., Entchev, P., Brinson, L. & Gao, X., Shape memory alloys, Part I: General properties and modeling of single crystals, Mechanics of Materials, 38 (2006) 391–429

Pelton, A.R.; Stochel, D. & Duerig, T.W. (2000). Medical uses of Nitinol, Mater Sci Forum, 2000:327–328:63-70.

Psalman, V. (2008). Facta Universitatis, Series: Physical Education Sport, Dynamic balance and its diagnostics by using 3D biomechanical analysis. 2008;6:105-109

Raghubir, S. & Dahotre, B., Corrosion degradation and prevention by surface modification of biometallic materials , Journal of Materials Science: Materials in Medicine, Volume 18(5):725-751, DOI: 10.1007/s10856-006-0016-y

Rychlewski, J. & Zhang, J.(*1989*), Anisotropy degree of elastic materials. Arch. Mech. 47 (5), 697–715.

Ryhänen, J.; Niemi, E., Serlo, W. et al. (1997). Biocompatibility of nickel–titanium shape memory metal and its corrosion behaviour in human cell cultures. J BIOMED MATERRES 1997; 35: 451–7.

Ryhanen, M.; Kallionen, J. & Tuukkanen J. (1999). Medical applications for Shape-Memory Alloys (SMA), Professional Engineering Publishing Ltd., 1999:53

Samide, A.; Bibicu, I., Oprea, B. & Tutunaru, B. (2009) J.Optoelectronics Advanced Materials, 10 2156 (2008)

Sanders, J.O.; Sanders, A.E., More, R. et al. Electrochemical and surface characterization of a nickel–titanium alloy, Spine, 1993,18,1640.

Shabalovskaya, S.A. Biological aspects of TiNi alloy surfaces, Journal de Physique IV, C8, 5, 1995, 5/2(8):C8.1199–C8.12041199

Shabalovskaya, S.A. On the nature of the biocompatibility and on medical applications of NiTi shape memory and superelastic alloys. J BioMed Mater Res 1996;6: 267–89

Shrier, L.L.; Jarman, R.A. & Burstein, O.T. Corrosion–metal/environment reactions. 3rd edn. Jordan Hill, Oxford: Butterworth-Heinemann, 1995: 2: 3–2: 164

Smith, G.F. & Rivlin, R.S., "The Strain Energy Function for Anisotropic Elastic Materials", Transactions of the American Mathematical Society, Vol.88, pp.175-193, 1958.

Sutcliffe, S. (1992), "Spectral Decomposition of the Elasticity Tensor ", Journal of Applied Mechanics, Vol. 59, pp 761-773.

Tarnita, D.; Tarnita, D.N., Tarnita, R., Berceanu, C. & Cismaru, F. (2010). Modular adaptive bone plate connected by Nitinol staple, Materialwissenschaft und Werkstofftechnik, Materials Science and Engineering Technology, Special Edition Biomaterials, Willey-Vch., Matwer 40 (1-2) 1-120 (2009) ISSN 0933-5137

Tarnita, D.; Bolcu, D., Berceanu, C. & Cismaru, F. (2010).Theoretical and experimental studies for an orthopedic staple made up Nitinol, Journal of Optoelectronics and Advanced Materials, Vol. 12, No. 11, November 2010, p. 2323 - 2332 (0,33626)

Theocaris P.S. & Philippidis, E.(1989), "Elastic Eigenstates of a medium with transverse Thoma, T.Y., Proc Nat. Acad. Sci. U S A. 1955 November 15; 41(11), 908

Ting, T.C.T. (1987), "Invariants of Anisotropic Elastic Constants", Quarterly Journal of Mechanics and Applied Mathematics, Vol.40, Part 3, pp. 431-448.

Trepanier, C.; Tabrizian, M., Yahia, L.H. et al. Effect of the modification of the oxide layer on NiTi stent corrosion resistance, JBMR (Appl Biomater) 1998; 43: 433–40

Tsung-Jung, H., Wei-Hsiang, L., Journal of the Chinese Institute of Engineers, 2010, 33, No.1,121

von Mises, R., *Mechanik der Festen Korper im plastisch deformablen Zustand.* Göttin. Nachr. Math. Phys., 1913;1:582–592

Venugopalan, R. & Trépanier, C. Assessing the corrosion behaviour of Nitinol for minimally-invasive device design, Min Invas Ther & Allied Technol 2000: 9(2) 67–74

Wever, D.J.; Veldhuizen, A.G., de Vries, J. et al. Electrochemical and surface characterization of a nickel–titanium alloy. Biomaterials 1998; 19: 761–9

Yang, P.J.; Zhang, Y.F., Ge, M.Z. et al. Internal fixation with Ni-Ti shape memory alloy compressive staples in orthopaedic surgery: a review of 51 cases. Chin Med J (Engl) 1987,100,712

Yeung, K.W.; Poon, R.W., Chu, P.K. et al. Cheung Journal of Biomedical Materials Research Part A. Aug 2007, Vol. 82A, No. 2: 403-414

19

A Mechanical Cell Model and Its Application to Cellular Biomechanics

Yoshihiro Ujihara, Masanori Nakamura and Shigeo Wada
Osaka University, Japan

1. Introduction

1.1 Importance of understanding the mechanical behavior of cells

Cells are the structural and functional units of all living organisms. Cells are continually subjected to mechanical loads from a wide variety of sources. It is known that normal cellular functions, including motility (Haga et al. 2000), differentiation (Titushkin et al. 2007), and gene expression (Shieh and Athanasiou 2007) involve mechanical properties. To date, studies have provided a biochemical framework for understanding the mechanotransduction processes and responses of cells to mechanical stimuli (Cohen et al., 1997). Nevertheless, it remains controversial as to how cells sense mechanical stimuli and trigger subsequent biochemical reactions. Understanding these cellular behaviours and their underlying mechanisms could be advanced by exploring the mechanical properties of cells and the intracellular components that confer such mechanical properties.

1.2 Previous studies on cellular mechanics

To date, numerous studies have investigated the relationships between the mechanics of subcellular components and either the local (Wang, 1998; Titushkin et al. 2007) or the entire mechanical properties of the cell (Miyazaki et al., 2000; Nagayama et al., 2006). Although these studies have provided valuable information for understanding cellular mechanics, the highly complex and heterogeneous structures of the subcellular components, such as cytoskeletal filaments, result in difficulties in understanding their behaviour. For example, the diameter of actin filaments is of the order of submicrometers, actin filaments are connected to the cell membrane and other cytoskeletal filaments, and the subcellular components frequently interact. Despite recent advances in imaging techniques, visualizing structural changes in actin filaments during cell deformation remains a challenging task. In this regard, no reported study has successfully measured the mechanical properties of cells while simultaneously observing the behaviour of subcellular components through quantification of their mechanical properties as a cell deforms. Thus, it is not yet feasible to understand the mechanical properties of cells from the level of subcellular components, solely on the basis of these experiments.

Computational approaches can complement the experimental studies of cell mechanics. The currently developed computational approaches are classified into continuum and discrete approaches. Continuum approaches assume that the smallest length scale of interest is larger than the dimensions of the microstructure. Continuum approaches have been widely used to describe how strains and stresses are distributed within a cell (Karcher et al., 2003; Vaziri et al., 2007). The disadvantage of a continuum model lies in its ability to deal with discrete components, such as cytoskeletons, making it difficult to interpret the mechanical behaviours and interactions with discrete components, and their contribution to the mechanical properties of a cell. In contrast to the continuum approaches, discrete approaches treat the cytoskeleton as the main structural component and have been developed, in particular, to investigate the cytoskeletal mechanics in adherent cells (Satcher and Dewey, 1996; Stamenović et al., 1996). The microscopic spectrin-network model was developed for suspended cells, such as erythrocytes, to investigate the contribution of the cell membrane and spectrin network to the large deformation of red blood cells (Boey et al., 1998; Li et al., 2005). The tensegrity model consists of stress-supported struts, which play the role of microtubules, and cable-like structures, which play the role of actin filaments (Ingber, 2003). The tensegrity model depicts the cytoskeleton as a prestressed network of interconnected filaments, investigating the effects on cellular shape and stiffness (Stamenović et al., 1996). Because the tensegrity model is quite conceptual and does not consider other cellular components, such as the cell membrane and cytoplasm, difficulties arise when relating its findings to the physical relationships between the mechanical properties of a whole cell and its subcellular components.

1.3 Basic concept of the mechano-cell model

The mechanical properties of a cell are the result of the structural combination of subcellular components, such as the cell membrane, nuclear envelope, and cytoskeleton. To understand the underlying process of how these subcellular components contribute to the cell as a whole, it is essential to develop a cell model that displays continuum behaviour as a whole. Although one way to express the continuum nature of a cell is to use the continuum model, this has difficulties considering discrete elements, such as the cytoskeleton, which may reorient passively concomitant with cell deformation. Thus, we depict a cell as an assembly of discrete elements, including a cellular membrane, in an attempt to express the continuum behaviour of the cell as a whole. Using computational biomechanics in conjunction with experimental measurements, it should be possible to establish a new platform that helps to provide a more complete picture of cellular remodelling rather than the collection of information being solely dependent on the measurement technology.

2. Development of the mechano-cell model

2.1 Overview

We have developed a cell model, termed the "mechano-cell," that is capable of simulating the mechanical behaviour of a cell (Ujihara et al. 2010a). As shown in Fig. 1, the model

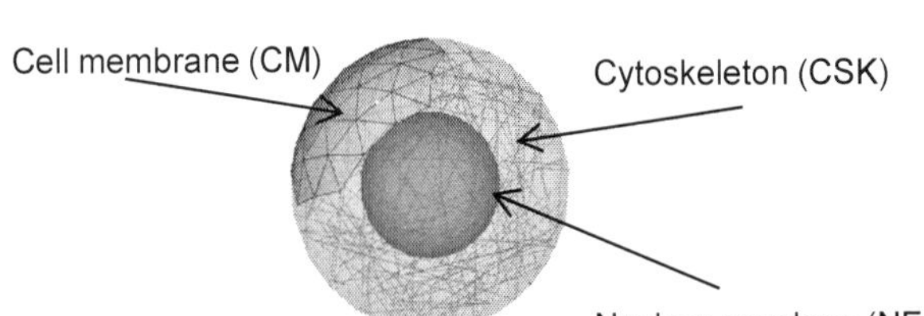

Fig. 1. Overview of the mechano-cell model.

consists of the cell membrane (CM), nuclear envelope (NE), and cytoskeletons (CSKs). The model changes shape such that the sum of the various elastic energies generated during cell deformation converges towards a minimum.

2.2 Modelling of a cell membrane and a nuclear envelope

The CM and NE are lipid layers, reinforced with cytoskeletal networks (Fig. 2). The cytoskeletal networks are firmly anchored to the CM and NE via various transmembrane proteins and/or membrane-associated proteins. It was thus assumed that the cytoskeletal network would not tear from the CM and NE.

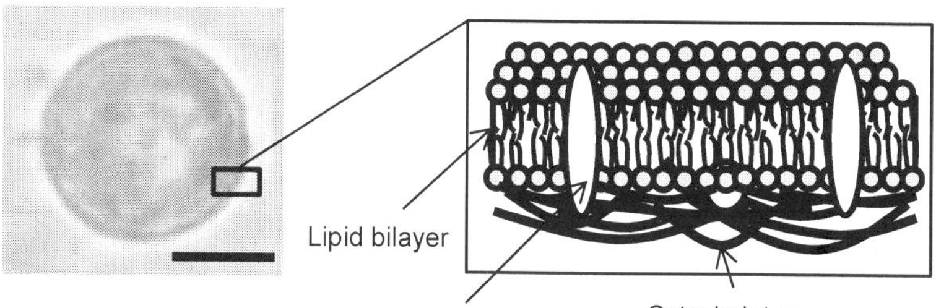

Fig. 2. Phase-contrast micrograph of a floating cell and schematic of the cell membrane structure. Scale bar = 10 μm.

In this study, the mechanical nature of the cytoskeletal network was included in the model of the CM and NE. The cytoskeletal networks beneath the CM and NE are known to resist in-plane deformation (stretch and area change), whereas the lipid bilayer is relatively permissive to in-plane deformation (Mohandas and Evans, 1994). Moreover, the CM and NE within cytoskeletal networks resist bending because of their thickness.

Spring network modelling was adopted to express the mechanical nature of the CM and NE (Wada and Kobayashi, 2003). Figure 3(a) shows the networks of the CM and NE and Figure 3(b) illustrates a magnified view of the triangular meshes. The black dots on the vertexes of the mesh are nodes, and are linked by a spring of spring constant k_s. Neighbouring elements are connected with a bending spring of spring constant k_b to prevent membrane folding. $\mathbf{r}_i$ is the positional vector of the node i, $\mathbf{n}_{l1}$ and $\mathbf{n}_{l2}$ are normal vectors to individual neighbouring meshes, and θ_l is the angle between $\mathbf{n}_{l1}$ and $\mathbf{n}_{l2}$. The stretching energy W_s and bending energy W_b generated are modelled as

$$W_s = \frac{1}{2} k_s \sum_{i=1}^{N_s} (L_j - L_{0j})^2 \tag{1}$$

$$W_b = \frac{1}{2} k_b \sum_{l=1}^{N_b} L_l \tan^2\left(\frac{\theta_l}{2}\right) \tag{2}$$

where N_s and N_b are the number of springs for stretching and bending, and L_{0j} and L_j are the lengths of the spring in the natural state after deformation. The tangent function is adopted in eq. (2) to infinitize the energy when the membrane is completely folded ($\theta_l = \pi$). By vector analysis, we rewrote eq. (2) as

$$W_b = \frac{1}{2}k_b \sum_{l=1}^{N_b} L_l \frac{1 - \mathbf{n}_{l1} \cdot \mathbf{n}_{l2}}{1 + \mathbf{n}_{l1} \cdot \mathbf{n}_{l2}} \tag{3}$$

The resistances to changes in the surface area of the whole membrane and to an area change of a local element are both modelled. The former corresponds to the situation whereby lipid molecules can move freely over the cytoskeletal network, while the latter corresponds to the situation where movement of the lipid molecules is confined to a local element. The area expansion energy W_A is thus formulated as a summation of the energy due to a change in the whole membrane area and due to a change in the local area:

$$W_A = \frac{1}{2}k_A \left(\frac{A - A_0}{A_0}\right)^2 A_0 + \frac{1}{2}k_a \sum_{e=1}^{N_e} \left(\frac{A_e - A_{0e}}{A_{0e}}\right)^2 A_{0e} \tag{4}$$

where A is the area of the whole membrane, subscript 0 denotes the natural state, and k_A is a coefficient for the whole area constraint, A_e is the area of the element, k_a is a coefficient for the local area constraint, and N_e is the number of elements. The total elastic energy stored is thus expressed as:

$$W^j = W_s^j + W_b^j + W_A^j \tag{5}$$

where j denotes CM ($j = c$) and NE ($j = n$).

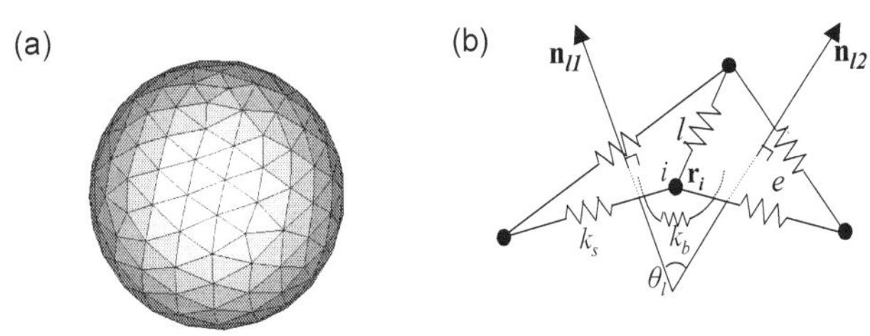

Fig. 3. (a) Mesh of the cellular membrane and nuclear envelope and (b) mechanical model of the cell membrane.

2.3 Modelling of CSK

As demonstrated in various studies (Wang, 1998; Nagayama et al., 2006), CSKs play a pivotal role in cellular mechanics. The CSK consists primarily of actin filaments, microtubules, and intermediate filaments (see Fig. 4). Here, these were modelled as CSK regardless of the type of cytoskeletal filament. For simplicity, a CSK is expressed as a straight spring that generates a force as a function of its extension. The energy W_{CSK} generated is thus modelled as

$$W_{CSK} = \frac{1}{2}k_{CSK} \sum_{i=1}^{N_{CSK}} (l_i - l_{0i})^2 \tag{6}$$

where k_{CSK} is the spring constant of the CSK, l_{0i} and l_i are the length of CSK$_i$ at the natural state and after deformation, and N_{CSK} is the total number of CSKs.

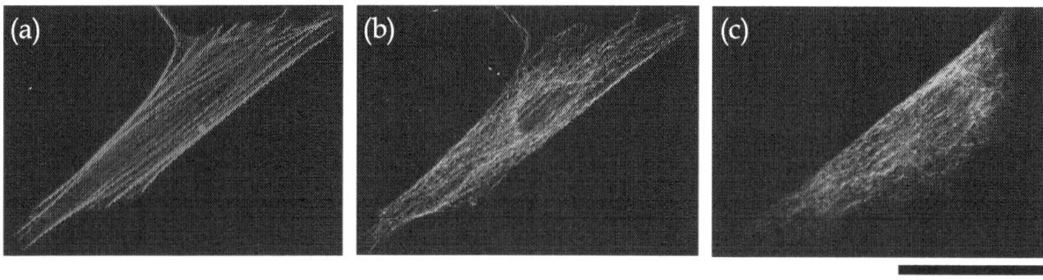

Fig. 4. Confocal laser scanning micrographs of (a) actin filaments, (b) microtubules and (c) intermediate filaments in adherent fibroblasts. Scale bar = 50 μm.

2.4 Interaction between the cell membrane and nuclear envelope

The organelles and cytosol are present between the CM and NE. The interaction between the CM and NE is expressed by a potential function with respect their distance apart. Figure 5 shows a conceptual diagram and potential function of the interaction between the CM and NE. We define the potential energy Ψ_{ij} between node i on the CM and node j on the NE as

$$\Psi_{\mathrm{ij}} = \begin{cases} k_n \left(\dfrac{\pi y_{ij}}{2} - \tan\left(\dfrac{\pi y_{ij}}{2} \right) \right) & (-1 \le y_{ij} \le 0) \\ 0 & (0 \le y_{ij}) \end{cases} \tag{7}$$

where k_n is a parameter to express the interaction between the CM and NE, and $y_{ij} = (d_{ij} - d_0)/d_0$, d_{ij} is the distance between node i on the CM and node j on the NE, and d_0 is the difference in the radius between the CM and NE at their natural state. The total potential energy Ψ is calculated by taking a summation of Ψ_{ij} as

$$\Psi = \sum_{i=1}^{N_n^c} \sum_{j=1}^{N_n^n} \Psi_{ij} \tag{8}$$

where N_n^c and N_n^n are the number of nodes on the CM and NE, respectively.

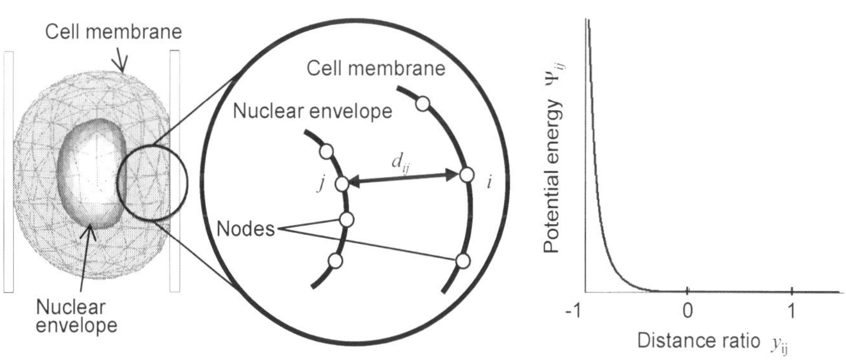

Fig. 5. Interaction between the cell membrane and nuclear envelope.

2.5 Minimum energy problem

The shape of the CM and NE can be determined from the elastic energies of the CM, NE, and CSKs, and from the interaction between the CM and NE if we provide constraints on the volumes encapsulated by CM V^c and NE V^n. By vector analyses, energies (5), (6), and (8) are rewritten as functions of the positional vector of nodal points $\mathbf{r}_i$. Thus, the shape of the CM and NE were determined as a minimum energy problem under a volume constraint. Mathematically, this is phrased as calculating the positional vectors that satisfy a condition such that the total elastic energy W_t is minimum, under the constraint that the volume V^c and V^n are equal to V_0^c and V_0^n

$$\begin{gathered}\text{Minimize } W_t \text{ with respect to } \mathbf{r}_i \\ W_t = W^c + W^n + W_{CSK} + \Psi \\ \text{subject to } V^c = V_0^c \text{ and } V^n = V_0^n\end{gathered} \tag{9}$$

where superscript c and n denote the CM and NE, and subscript 0 denotes the natural state. A volume elastic energy W_V is introduced as

$$W_V^j = \frac{1}{2} k_V^j \left(\frac{V^j - V_0^j}{V_0^j} \right)^2 V_0^j \tag{10}$$

where j denotes the CM (j = c) and NE (j = n), and k_V is the volume elasticity. Including eq. (10) in the minimum energy problem, eq. (9) is rewritten as

$$\begin{gathered}\text{Minimize } W \text{ with respect to } \mathbf{r}_i \\ W = W^c + W^n + W_{CSK} + \Psi + W_V^c + W_V^n\end{gathered} \tag{11}$$

2.6 Solving method

A cell shape is determined by moving the nodal points on CM and NE such that the total elastic energy W is minimized. Based on the virtual work theory, an elastic force $\mathbf{F}_i$ applied to node i is calculated from

$$\mathbf{F}_i = -\frac{\partial W}{\partial \mathbf{r}_i} \tag{12}$$

where $\mathbf{r}_i$ is the position vector of i. The motion equation of a mass point with mass m on node i is described as

$$m\ddot{\mathbf{r}}_i + \gamma \dot{\mathbf{r}}_i = \mathbf{F}_i \tag{13}$$

where a dot indicates the time derivative, and γ is the artificial viscosity. Discretization of eq. (13) and some mathematical rearrangements yield

$$\mathbf{v}_i^{N+1} = \frac{m\mathbf{v}_i^N + \mathbf{F}_i^N \delta}{m + \gamma\delta} \tag{14}$$

where $\mathbf{v}$ is the velocity vector, N is the computational step number, and δ is an increment of time. The position of node i $\mathbf{r}_i^{N+1}$ is thus calculated from

$$\mathbf{r}_i^{N+1} = \mathbf{r}_i^{N} + \mathbf{v}_i^{N+1}\delta \tag{15}$$

2.6 Procedure for computation

A flowchart for the simulation is illustrated in Fig. 6. The flowchart has two iterative processes. The external loop is a real-time process, while the internal loop is instituted to minimize the elastic energy by a quasi-static approach. Based on the virtual work theory, an elastic force $\mathbf{F}_i$ applied to node i is obtained from eq. (12). It is followed by updating the positional vector $\mathbf{r}$ of the nodal points by eq. (15) and calculating the total elastic energy W. If a changing ratio of the total elastic energy W is smaller than a tolerance ε, the boundary conditions are renewed to proceed to the next real-time step. If not satisfied, force $\mathbf{F}$ and positional vector $\mathbf{r}^N$ of the nodal points are repeatedly calculated under the same boundary conditions.

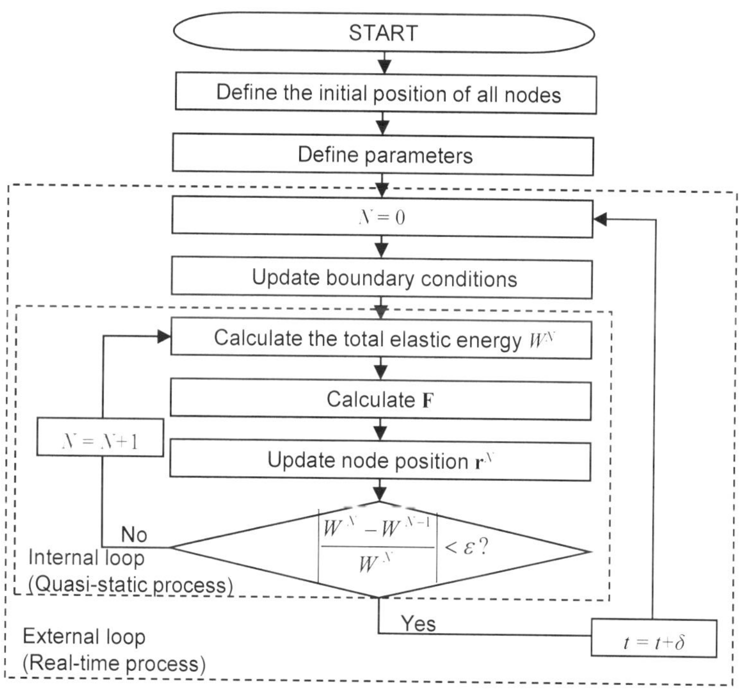

Fig. 6. Flowchart for the mechanical test simulation.

2.7 Parameter settings

The CM and NE were assumed as spheres at their natural state, with a diameter of 20 μm and 10 μm, respectively. In the model, N_s and N_b = 519, N_n^c and N_n^n = 175, N_e = 346, N_{CSK} = 200 and γ = 1.0×10^6 μg/s. For the CM, m = 1.0×10^{-9} μg, k_s = 5.6×10^5 μg/s^2, k_b = 9.0×10^3 μg·μm/s^2, k_A = 2.7×10^7 μg/s^2, k_a = 3.0×10^6 μg/s^2, k_V = 5.0×10^6 μg/(μm·s^2). For the NE, the mass was set to half of the CM, while the other parameters were set to double the CM.

The spring constants k_s, k_A, and k_a were estimated by the tensile test simulations such that the elastic energy generated in the mechano-cell equaled the strain energy W_D obtained when the CM was modelled as a continuum. According to the theory of continuum mechanics, the strain energy W_D is defined as

$$W_D = \frac{1}{2}\sum_{e=1}^{N_e} A_e h \boldsymbol{\varepsilon}_\mathbf{e}^\mathbf{T} \mathbf{D} \boldsymbol{\varepsilon}_\mathbf{e} \tag{16}$$

where N_e is the number of elements, A_e is the area of each element, and h is the thickness of the CM, $\boldsymbol{\varepsilon}_\mathbf{e}^\mathrm{T} = (\varepsilon_{Xe}, \varepsilon_{Ye}, \gamma_{XYe})$ is the strain vector of each element. $\mathbf{D}$ is the elastic modulus matrix under a plane strain condition. The parameters in eq. (16) were set to h = 0.5 μm, elastic modulus of the CM E_{CM} = 1000 Pa, and Poisson's ratio v = 0.3 by reference to Feneberg et al. (2004) McGarry et al. (2004), and Mahaffy et al. (2004). Note that the elastic modulus and Poisson's ratio appear in the elastic modulus matrix $\mathbf{D}$.

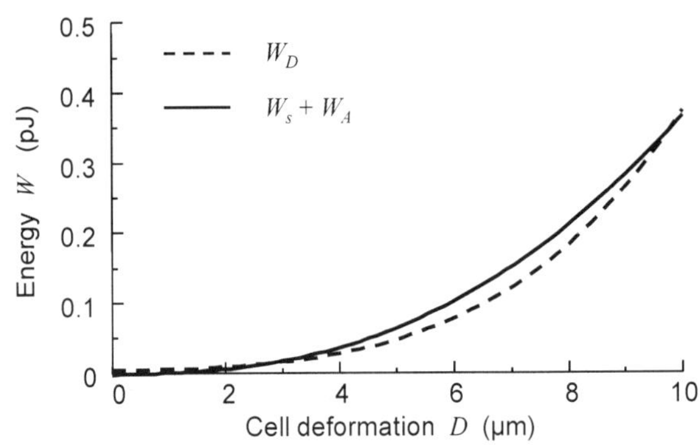

Fig. 7. Elastic energy of the in-plane deformations ($W_s + W_A$) stored in the mechano-cell (solid line) and the strain energy W_D obtained when the CM was modelled as a continuum (dashed line).

The spring constant of the bending spring k_b was determined such that the bending energy W_b calculated from eq. (2) at the initial state of the cell equaled the bending energy W_B analytically calculated (Wada and Kobayashi, 2003). Analytically, the bending energy W_B of a sphere is given by

$$W_B = \frac{1}{2} B \int_\Omega (C_1 + C_2)^2 dA \tag{17}$$

where B is the bending stiffness and C_1 and C_2 are the principal curvatures. Applying eq. (17) to the cell, allowing Ω to be CM and given that $B = 2.0\times10^{-18}$ J (Zhelev et al., 1994) and $C_1 = C_2 = 1/R_0$ (R_0 = 10 μm, initial radius of a cell), it follows that $k_b = 9.0\times10^3$ μg·μm/s^2.
The spring constant of the CSK k_{CSK} was set to 1.5×10^6 μg/s^2, based on the elastic modulus of an actin bundle (Deguchi et al., 2005). The CSKs were assumed to have a natural length when the cell was in its natural state. The CSKs were chosen randomly from all possible candidates of CSKs that were made by connecting two nodes on the CM. The spring

constants of the volume elasticity (k_V) were determined to assure cell incompressibility. Because no data is presently available for k_n, it was determined that the load-deformation curves obtained by the simulation, fit the range of the experimental data.

3. Tensile tests

3.1 Tensile tests

The mechanical behavior of a cell during a tensile test was simulated. The tensile test was simulated by fixing the nodes of CM at one side, while moving those at the opposite side in the direction of cell stretching.

3.2 Simulation results

Figure 8 shows the deformation behaviour of a cell in the tensile test where a fibroblast is stretched, obtained by simulation of the model (left) and experimentally (right). Similar to the experimental data, the simulation showed that the cell and nucleus were elongated in the stretched direction. CSKs were randomly oriented prior to loading and were passively aligned in the stretched direction as the cell was stretched.

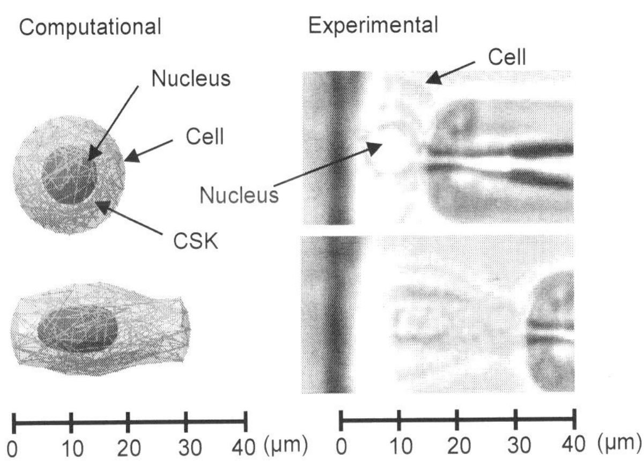

Fig. 8. Snapshots of a cell during the tensile test simulation (left) and experimental system (right). The scale is indicated at the bottom of the figure.

Load-deformation curves obtained from the simulation and experimental systems are presented in Fig. 9. Note that, in addition to the model with randomly oriented CSKs (Fig. 8), the data obtained from the models with parallel-oriented, oriented, and perpendicularly oriented CSKs, in addition to with no CSK are presented for comparison. The curve obtained from the simulation of the model with randomly oriented CSKs appeared to increase non-linearly. The curve of the model with randomly oriented CSKs lay within the variation of the experimentally obtained curves (simulation = 0.48 μN, experimental = 0.43-1.24 μN at 20 μm cell deformation). Moreover, the curves obtained from the experiments were between the curve of the parallel-oriented model and that of perpendicularly oriented model.

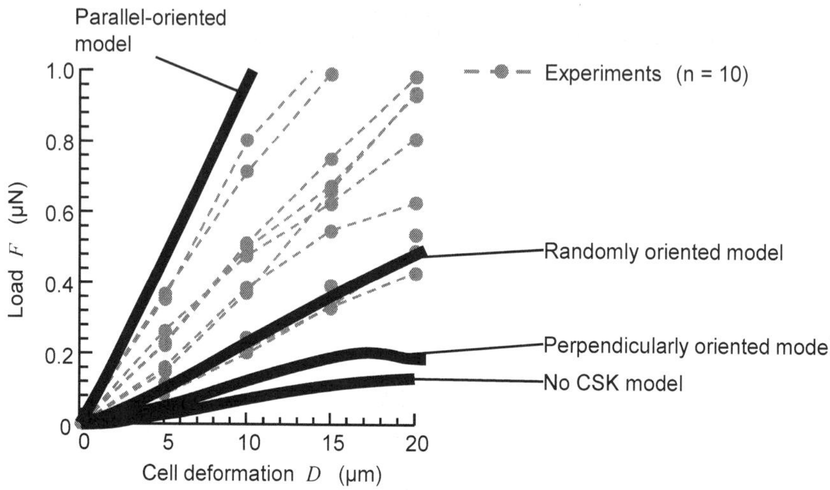

Fig. 9. Load-deformation curves obtained from the simulation and experimental system (n = 10).

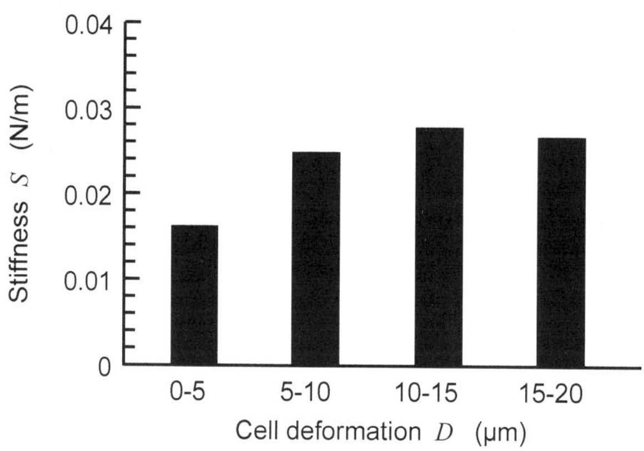

Fig. 10. Changes in cell stiffness of a model with randomly oriented CSKs with cell deformation.

An increase in the cell stiffness with cell elongation is manifested from Fig. 10 that illustrates the cell stiffness (*S*) of a model with randomly oriented CSKs between 0–5, 5–10, 10–15, and 15–20 μm deformation (*D*). The cell stiffness (*S*) increased by ~1.5-fold as the cell deformation (*D*) increased from 0 to 15 μm, while decreases were evident if the cell was stretched further.

The increase in cell stiffness with cell elongation is explained by the realignment of CSKs. Figure 11 provides a histogram of the existence probability of the orientation angles (P_θ)

of the CSKs of a randomly oriented model at a cell deformation (D) of 0, 10, and 20 μm. The CSKs at D = 0 μm were distributed uniformly over all angles. With elongation of the cell, the distribution of the orientation angle of the CSK became skewed towards 0° (Fig. 11), demonstrating that the CSKs tend to become passively aligned in the stretched direction. This passive re-alignment gradually increased the elastic resistance of the whole cell against the stretched direction, causing the load-deformation curve to be non-linear (Fig. 9).

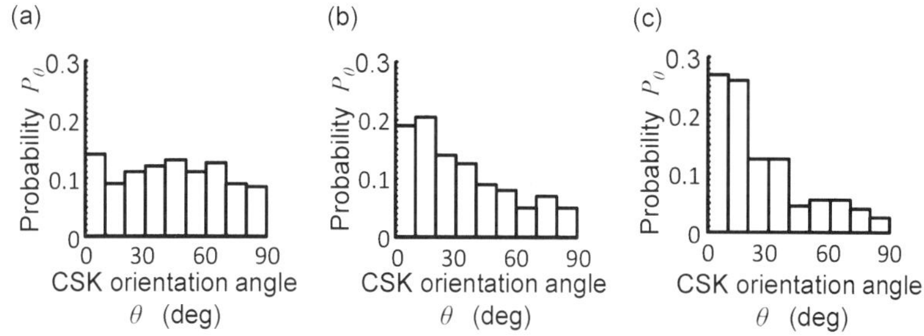

Fig. 11. Histogram of the existence probability of the orientation angles P_θ of the CSK the randomly oriented model during a cell deformation (D) value of (a) 0, (b) 10, and (c) 20 μm.

Not all the CSKs were stretched as the cell elongated. Figure 12 shows a histogram of stretch ratios P_λ of the CSK of the randomly oriented model at a deformation D of 0, 10, and

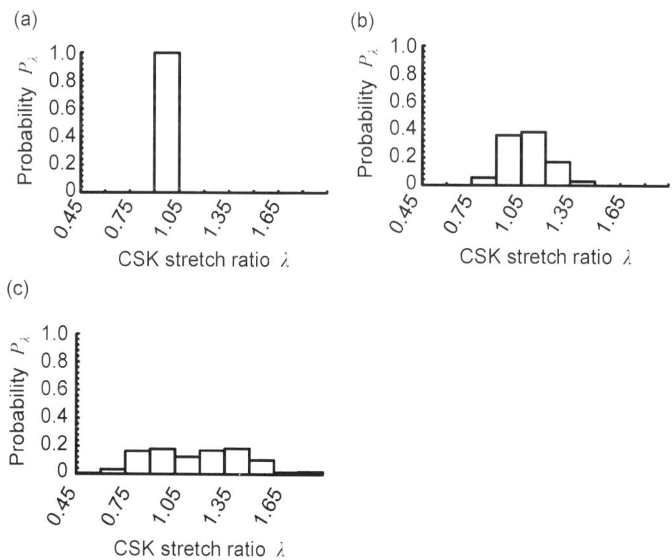

Fig. 12. Histogram of the stretch ratio P_λ of the CSK of the randomly oriented model at a cell deformation (D) value of (a) 0, (b) 10, and (c) 20 μm.

20 μm. As evident in Fig. 12 (a), the stretch ratio of all CSKs was 1 at a deformation D of 0 μm. Elongation of the cell resulted in the broadening of the distribution towards both positive and negative values of the stretch ratio, indicating that compressed, as well as stretched CSKs were present while the cell was stretched. A combination of these stretched and compressed CSKs, in addition to the shapes of the CM and NE, determine the mechanical properties of the whole cell. Thus, although all subcellular components, including CSKs, are expressed by a linear elastic element, the cell as a whole appears to display clear non-linear deformation properties.

3.3 Summary

In this section, a cellular tensile test was simulated, using the cellular model, to investigate the effects of mechanical behaviours of the subcellular components on the mechanical properties of the cell. Analysis of the mechanical behaviours of the CSKs showed that they were randomly oriented prior to loading, and tended to become passively aligned in the stretched direction. These results attribute the non-linearity of the load-deformation curve to a passive reorientation of the CSKs in the stretched direction.

4. Compressive tests

4.1 Compressive tests

A compressive test was simulated on the basis of the compressive experiment (Ujihara et al., 2010b). Contact between the plate and cell was assumed when a node on the CM came to within 0.01 μm of the plate. Once contacted, the node was assumed to move together with the plate. Spring constants to express the interaction between the CM and NE and the volume elasticity were set to 8.0×10^5 μg·μm/s^2 and 5.0×10^5 μg/(μm·s^2), respectively. Other parameters were identical to those defined in Section 2.7.

4.2 Simulation results

Figure 13 presents snapshots of a cell during cell deformation, with values of D = 0, 4, and 8 μm. While the cell was initially spherical, as it compressed, it elongated vertically due to the Poisson's effect by which a cell retains its volume. The CSKs that were oriented randomly prior to loading appeared to be passively aligned in a direction perpendicular to the compression.

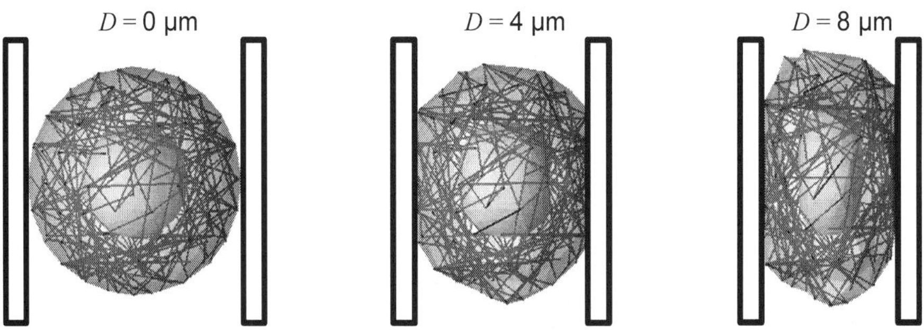

Fig. 13. Snapshots of the mechano-cell model with CSKs during the compressive test.

Similar to the tensile test, the load-deformation curves of the model obtained by the simulation and experimental systems were assessed in Fig. 14. Here, the results from a cell model in the presence or absence of CSKs are presented. The load required to compress the model with CSKs was larger than that for the model without CSKs. However, regardless of the presence of CSKs, the load increased non-linearly as the cells were compressed, similar to that observed in the experimental system. The curve of the model with CSKs was within the variation of the experimental results.

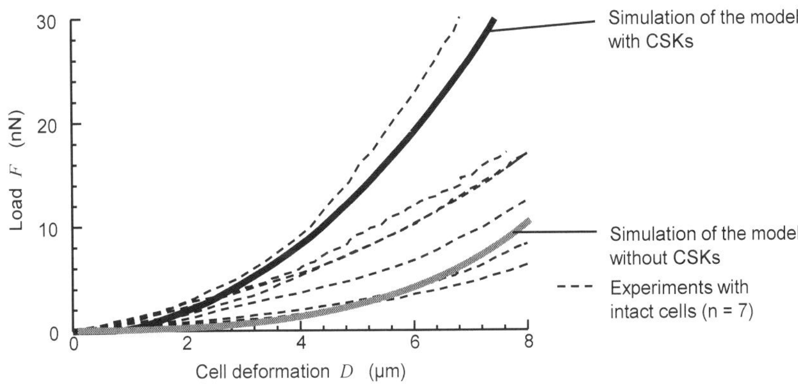

Fig. 14. Load-deformation curves of the model with and without CSKs and the experimental system (n = 7).

Compression induced an increase in the cell stiffness, as is evident in Fig. 15 that plots the stiffness S of the models with and without CSKs between 0–2, 2–4, 4–6, and 6–8 μm deformation (D). Here, the stiffness (S) is defined as the slope of the load-deformation curve for every 2-μm deformation (D) from 0 to 8 μm, on the basis of the assumption that

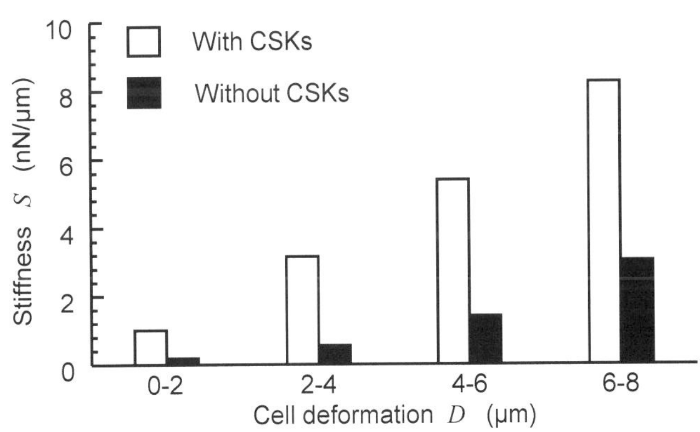

Fig. 15. Stiffness of the models ± CSKs.

the curve is piecewise linear. Regardless of the presence of the CSKs, the stiffness was markedly elevated during cell compression. The stiffness of the model with the CSKs at an interval of 2 μm was larger than that of the model without CSKs. Such an increase in cell stiffness correlated with the elevation of the mean orientation angle θ of all CSKs. Figure 16(a) shows that the mean θ elevated with cell deformation, indicating that the CSKs were passively oriented perpendicularly to the compressed direction. Concomitantly, the CSKs that were vertical were stretched as a result of the vertical elongation of the cell. Consequently, the CSKs exerted a contractile force and gave rise to an increase in the resistance against the vertical elongation of the cell. This increase in resistance is reflected in the elevation of the stiffness of the whole cell. With the progress of compression, a larger number of CSKs were inclined in the vertical direction, causing a gradual increase in the cell stiffness. In support of this, a positive relationship between the mean orientation angle of the CSKs and the cell stiffness during cell compression is illustrated in Fig. 16(b).

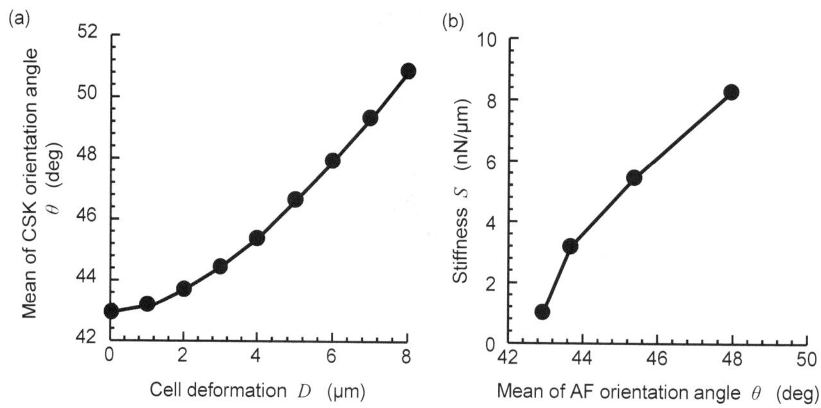

Fig. 16. Plot of (a) the mean orientation angle θ of CSKs against the cell deformation D, and (b) the stiffness against the mean CSK orientation angle θ.

4.3 Discussion and summary

In this section, the mechano-cell model was used in a compression test. The results addressed the significant contribution of the CSKs to the global compressive properties of a cell. The passive reorientation of CSKs in a direction perpendicular to the compression gave rise to an increase in the elastic resistance against the vertical elongation of the cell, thereby increasing the stiffness of the entire cell against the compression.

5. Other applications of the mechano-cell model

In addition to the tensile and compressive tests, the mechano-cell model is capable of expressing the cell behaviour in mechanical tests to examine the local mechanical properties of a cell, including micropipette aspiration and atomic force microscopy, as exemplified in Figs. 17(a) and (b). Moreover, the model can simulate the behaviour of an adherent cell on a substrate (Fig. 17(c)). Such a simulation may be useful in grasping the mechanical status of a cell during culture under mechanical loads, such as cyclic stretch of the substrate. Further applications of the mechano-cell model are illustrated in Fig. 17(d) where the mechano-cell model was embedded in a tissue. Here, tissue behavior was described with continuum mechanics under the assumption of an isotropic linear elastic material, and the behaviours of the CSKs within a cell upon the stretch of a tissue were examined. The combined use of the mechano-cell model with the continuum model will help achieve structural integration across the physical scales of biomechanical organization from CSKs to tissue.

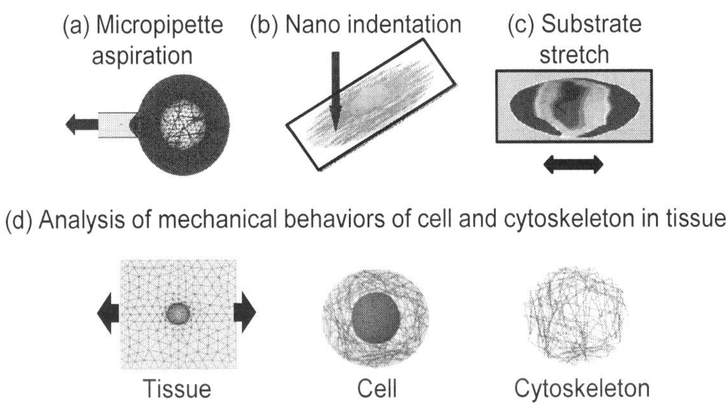

Fig. 17. Applications of the mechano-cell model.

6. Summary

In this study, we aimed to develop a cell model that mechanically describes cellular behaviour as an assembly of subcellular components, and its applications in exploring the relationship between the mechanics of the subcellular components and the global mechanical properties of a cell. The model revealed how subcellular components alter their structure during cell deformation and demonstrated how such changes reflect the mechanical properties of the cell. The model provided a physical interpretation of the relationships between cellular deformation, the mechanical properties of a cell, and the mechanical behaviour of the subcellular components.

A deep understanding of the mechanical characteristics of the subcellular components will offer valuable insight into the structure-function paradigm. However, it is hindered by the complex and heterogeneous structures of the subcellular components. Despite the recent advances in imaging techniques, the visualization methods of the structural changes in the CSKs of living cells during mechanical tests have not been well established. Furthermore, it is challenging to quantify the contribution of individual subcellular components to the overall mechanical response of a cell, solely from experimental data. The mechano-cell model is expected to help overcome these experimental drawbacks.

The results described here address the use of the mechano-cell model in aiding our understanding of the behaviour of heterogeneous intracellular structures and the cell as a whole.

7. Acknowledgment

This work was supported in part by a Grant-in-Aid for JSPS Fellows (21•1007) from the Japan Society for the Promotion of Science (JSPS) and "The Next-Generation Integrated Simulation of Living Matter", part of the Development and Use of the Next-Generation Supercomputer Project of the Ministry of Education, Culture, Sports, Science and Technology (MEXT). We thank Dr. Hiroshi Miyazaki, Dr. Kenichiro Koshiyama and Mr. Ray Noguchi for their useful comments on this work.

8. References

Boey, S.K.; Boal, D.H. & Discher, D.E. (1998). Simulations of the Erythrocyte Cytoskeleton at Large Deformation. I. Microscopic Models. *Biophysical Journal,* Vol.75, No.3, (September, 1998), pp. 1573-1583, ISSN 0006-3495

Cohen, C. R.; Mills, I. Du, W. Kamal, K. & Sumpio B. E. (1997). Activation of the Adenylyl Cyclase/Cyclic AMP/Protein Kinase A Pathway in Endothelial Cells Exposed to Cyclic Strain. *Experimental Cell Research,* Vol.231, No.1, (February, 1997), pp. 184-189, ISSN 0013-4827

Deguchi, S.; Ohashi, T. & Sato, M. (2005). Evaluation of Tension in Actin Bundle of Endothelial Cells Based on Preexisting Strain and Tensile Properties Measurements. *Molecular and Cellular Biomechanics,* Vol.2, No.3, (September, 2005), pp. 125-133, ISSN 1556-5297

Feneberg, W.; Aepfelbacher, M. & Sackmann, E. (2004). Microviscoelasticity of the Apical Cell Surface of Human Umbilical Vein Endothelial Cells (HUVEC) within Confluent Monolayers. *Biophysical Journal,* Vol.87, No.2, (August, 2004), pp. 1338-1350, ISSN 0006-3495

Haga, H.; Nagayama, M. Kawabata, K. Ito, E. Ushiki, T. & Sambongi, T. (2000). Time-lapse Viscoelastic Imaging of Living Fibroblasts Using Force Modulation Mode in AFM. *Journal of Electron Microscopy,* Vol.49, No.3, pp. 473-481, ISSN 0022-0744

Ingber, D.E. (2003). Tensegrity II. How Structural Networks Influence Cellular Information Processing Networks. *Journal of Cell Science,* Vol.116, No.8, (April, 2003), pp. 1397-1408, ISSN 0021-9533

Karcher, H.; Lammerding, J. Huang, H. Lee, R.T. Kamm, R.D. & Kaazempur-Mofrad MR. (2003). A Three-dimensional Viscoelastic Model for Cell Deformation with Experimental Verification. *Biophysical Journal,* Vol.85, No.5, (November, 2003), pp. 3336-3349, ISSN 0006-3495.

Li, J.; Dao, M. Lim, C.T. & Suresh, S. (2005). Spectrin-level Modeling of the Cytoskeleton and Optical Tweezers Stretching of the Erythrocyte. *Biophysical Journal,* Vol.88, No.5, (May, 2005), pp. 3707-3719, ISSN 0006-3495

Mahaffy, R.E.; Park, S. Gerde, E. Kas, J. & Shih, C.K. (2004). Quantitative Analysis of the Viscoelastic Properties of Thin Regions of Fibroblasts Using Atomic Force Microscopy. *Biophysical Journal,* Vol.86, No.3, (March, 2004), pp. 1777-1793, ISSN 0006-3495

McGarry, J.G. & Prendergast, P.J. (2004). A Three-dimensional Finite Element Model of an Adherent Eukaryotic Cell. *European Cells and Materials,* Vol.7, (April, 2004), pp. 27-33, ISSN 1473-2262

Miyazaki, H.; Hasegawa, Y. & Hayashi, K. (2000). A Newly Designed Tensile Tester for Cells and Its Application to Fibroblasts. *Journal of Biomechanics,* Vol.33, No.1, (January, 1999), pp. 97-104, ISSN 0021-9290

Mohandas, N. & Evans, E. (1994). Mechanical Properties of the Red Cell Membrane in Relation to Molecular Structure and Genetic Defects. *Annual Review of Biophysics and Biomolecular Structure,* Vol.23, pp. 787-818, ISSN 1056-8700

Nagayama, K.; Nagano, Y. Sato, M. & Matsumoto, T. (2006). Effect of Actin Filament Distribution on Tensile Properties of Smooth Muscle Cells Obtained From Rat Thoracic Aortas. *Journal of Biomechanics,* Vol.39, No.2, pp. 293-301, ISSN 0021-9290

Satcher, R.L. Jr. & Dewey, C.F. Jr. (1996). Theoretical Estimates of Mechanical Properties of the Endothelial Cell Cytoskeleton. *Biophysical Journal,* Vol.71, No.1, (July, 1996), pp. 109-118, ISSN 0006-3495

Shieh, A.C. & Athanasiou, K.A. (2007). Dynamic Compression of Single Cells. *Osteoarthritis Cartilage,* Vol.15, No.3, (March, 2007), pp. 328-334, ISSN 1063-4584

Stamenović, D.; Fredberg, J.J. Wang, N. Butler, J.P. & Ingber, D.E. (1996) A Microstructural Approach to Cytoskeletal Mechanics Based on Tensegrity. *Journal of Theoretical Biology,* Vol.181, No.2, (July, 1996), pp. 125-136, ISSN 0022-5193

Titushkin, I. & Cho, M. (2007). Modulation of Cellular Mechanics during Osteogenic Differentiation of Human Mesenchymal Stem Cells. *Biophysical Journal,* Vol.93, No.10, (November, 2007), pp. 3693-3702, ISSN 0006-3495

Ujihara, Y.; Nakamura, M. Miyazaki, H. & Wada, S. (2010a). Proposed Spring Network Cell Model Based on a Minimum Energy Concept, *Annals of Biomedical Engineering,* Vol.38, No.4, (April, 2010), pp. 1530-1538, ISSN 0090-6964

Ujihara, Y.; Nakamura, M. Miyazaki, H. & Wada, S. (2010b).Effects of Actin Filaments on the Compressive Properties of a whole cell, *6th World Congress of Biomechanics Abstract,* pp. 478, Singapore, August 1-6, 2010

Vaziri, A. & Mofrad, M.R. (2007). Mechanics and Deformation of the Nucleus in Micropipette Aspiration Experiment. *Journal of Biomechanics,* Vol.40, No.9, pp. 2053-2062, ISSN 0021-9290

Wada, S. & Kobayashi, R. (2003) Numerical simulation of various shape changes of a swollen red blood cell by decrease of its volume. *Transactions of the Japan Society of Mechanical Engineers A,* Vol.69, No.677, (January, 2003), pp. 14-21, ISSN 0387-5008, (in Japanese)

Wang, N. (1998) Mechanical Interactions among Cytoskeletal Filaments. *Hypertension,* Vol.32, No.1, (July, 1998), pp. 162-165, ISSN 0194-911X

Zhelev, D.V.; Needham, D. & Hochmuth, R.M. (1994). Role of the Membrane Cortex in Neutrophil Deformation in Small Pipets. *Biophysical Journal,* Vol.67, No.2, (August, 1994), pp. 696-705, ISSN 0006-3495